READINGS IN SPEECH FOLLOWING TOTAL LARYNGECTOMY

READINGS IN SPEECH FOLLOWING TOTAL LARYNGECTOMY

edited by
Bernd Weinberg, Ph.D.
Professor and Head
Department of Audiology and Speech Sciences
Purdue University

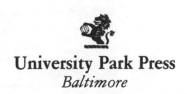

University Park Press
Baltimore

UNIVERSITY PARK PRESS
International Publishers in Science, Medicine, and Education
233 East Redwood Street
Baltimore, Maryland 21202

Composed by University Park Press, Typesetting Division
Manufactured in the United States of America by
The Maple Press Company

Sincere appreciation is extended to the authors and publishers of the articles in this volume for granting permission to reprint their work.

Library of Congress Cataloging in Publication Data

Main entry under title:
Readings in speech following total laryngectomy.
Includes index.
1. Esophageal speech—Addresses, essays, lectures.
2. Artificial larynx—Addresses, essays, lectures.
3. Laryngoplasty—Addresses, essays, lectures.
4. Laryngectomy—Addresses, essays, lectures.
I. Weinberg, Bernd. [DNLM: 1. Voice production,
Alaryngeal. 2. Laryngectomy. WV540 R287
RF540.R4   617'.53301   79-28540
ISBN 0-8391-1570-9

CONTENTS

PREFACE

Comprehensive understanding of the methods of speech used by patients who have undergone total laryngectomy surgery represents an important field of study within professional training programs developed for speech pathologists and head and neck surgeons. The eclectic nature of this field of inquiry creates special problems for those engaged in both teaching and learning about this subject. For example, papers dealing with fundamental aspects of this field have appeared in a wide variety of journals and books. Hence, the instructor and the student often find it difficult to obtain an accessible set of readings that provide an adequate and representative sampling of important facets of this field. *Readings in Speech Following Total Laryngectomy* was developed to meet this need.

The development of this reading text rests on the premise that students must become familiar with primary sources and seminal articles within this specialized field of clinical and academic study. Current texts in the area of alaryngeal speech tend to emphasize clinical techniques more than the basic or applied research upon which such techniques should be based. A primary feature of this offering is its orientation to research articles, an orientation used to provide speech and medical specialists with sufficient information upon which clinical techniques might be evaluated and developed. This offering of readings serves either as a core text or as collateral reading for courses of study in speech after laryngectomy.

Several criteria were used to select readings for this volume. First, an effort was made to secure representation of a reasonably wide variety of disciplines and topics. An attempt was made to include what many would regard as primary sources. Examples of experimental research, descriptive work, and review papers are included. Some contributions were selected to illustrate a program of clinical endeavor or research. Finally, other offerings were selected because they were relatively inaccessible.

The stylistic variations of various authors and sources have been maintained in many of the reproductions that make up this volume. This procedure is used to familiarize the student with a variety of journal and author styles.

A difficult problem encountered in the preparation of a book of readings is organization. The determination of categories for major sections and the ordering of contributions within each section may, to some, appear somewhat arbitrary. The rationale for category determination and ordering of contributions within each section is given in the narrative discussion which precedes each major section of this text. Although one arrangement may suit one instructor, others may find the sequence awkward or completely unworkable. It is the editor's sincere hope that his colleagues engaged in the teaching and study of speech following laryngectomy will find the present organization useful.

In the preparation of this offering, I have been impressed again by the kindness, generosity, and willingness that characterizes the clinicians and scientists who wrote the original articles. I remain grateful to them.

PART I

HISTORICAL PAPERS

The two articles reprinted in Part I are classics in the field and both are relatively inaccessible. "A Case of Total Extirpation of the Larynx," written by Roswell Park, M.D., provides an informative and somewhat entertaining account of one of the earliest total laryngectomy procedures performed in America. Readers will be particularly interested in reading about the early postsurgical use of a pneumatic artificial larynx developed by Gussenbauer. The world famous Roswell Park Memorial Institute of Buffalo, New York bears the name of the eminent head and neck surgeon who authored this work. The Park work was originally published in the *Annals of Surgery* (1886).

The second paper, "Speech Without Using the Larynx," was written by the famous speech scientist, E. W. Scripture. This offering provides an informative account of speech production using a phonautograph. Interesting insights about methods used to study speech in patients with laryngeal disability are offered in this article, which appeared in the *Journal of Physiology* (1916).

A CASE OF TOTAL EXTIRPATION OF THE LARYNX

Roswell Park, A.M., M.D.

*Professor of Surgery, Medical Department, University of Buffalo;
Attending Surgeon to the Buffalo General Hospital*

American cases of total extirpation of the larynx have been so few in number that I do not hesitate to report the following in this place, although a clinical lecture based upon it has already appeared.[1] The case was in the person of a medical gentleman, 64 years of age, whom I first saw in consultation with Dr. F. W. Hinkel, of this city. The doctor has kindly furnished me with some notes on the case from which I extract the following:

"Dr. P., first seen October 9, 1884. His voice was shrill, discordant, and very stridulous. He gave his age as 63 years. He had the appearance of rugged health, but stated that while a youth he had been "sent away to die of phthisis." After his graduation in medicine he developed perfect general health, which he had since retained, in spite of much abuse in civil and military life, and by excessive smoking. Said he had used as many as twenty cigars a day. He dated his throat trouble from an attack of acute laryngitis after great exposure in the early years of our civil war. Since then, has been annoyed by occasional attacks of hoarseness and sore throat, which gradually became more frequent, continuous and severe until, in the last few months, his voice had fallen into its present condition. Lately there were occasional darting pains through the region of the larynx. He had a hacking cough—especially at night—with little expectoration and no pain. Occasionally he had attacks of dyspnoea, which he termed "asthmatic attacks." Otherwise his personal and family history were good. He had never had a laryngoscopic examination.

"The oro-pharynx was found unusually small in proportion to size of patient, much inflamed and extremely irritable. The arches of the palate were swollen and red. The uvula was of a purplish-red color, much thickened and covered with corrugated mucous membrane, but not oedematous nor elongated. The laryngoscopic examination was made with difficulty, owing to excessive faucial irritability. It revealed deep congestion and puffiness of the mucous membrane in the supraglottic portion of the larynx. The ventricular bands were swollen, deep red in color, and not clearly defined. The location of the vocal bands was filled with two reddish-grey, irregular, sessile growths, apparently filling the ventricles on either side and covering both vocal bands. By careful examination they could be seen to extend on each side over the lateral walls of the sub-glottic portion of the larynx, so that the bulk of the growth was sub-glottic. The glottis was much and irregularly encroached upon. A tooth-like process from the posterior third of the right growth, and a similar process from the anterior portion of the left growth, transformed

Reprinted by permission from *Annals of Surgery*, 1886, *3*, 28–38.

[1]*Med. Press* of Western New York, December, 1885.

the chink into an irregular Z-shaped opening. The sub-glottic larynx was irregularly contracted in its lateral dimensions, rendering it impossible to see beyond the growths. The further encroachment upon this small breathing space by the swelling incident to acute congestion readily explains the 'asthma' from which he suffered at times. There was no ulceration present. The cushion of the epiglottis was swollen, but probing did not show marked tenderness over it or the growths. These latter I regarded as papillomata, but feared there was beginning epitheliomatous degeneration. Believing their complete removal *per os* to be impossible, I made use of soothing alterative applications, and warned the patient of the great possibility of malignant degeneration at his age, and of the possible future advisability of thyrotomy or even extirpation of the larynx.

"After a few days he disappeared suddenly from my observation. He came under my care again for a few days on January 8, 1885. He had been under Dr. Elsberg's care, in New York, in the interim. The condition and appearance of his throat were much the same as when first examined. On April 20 I saw him again. He stated there had been some operative procedures by Dr. Elsberg. Owing to the unfortunate death of that eminent laryngologist it has been impossible to obtain, with any exactness, his prognosis or treatment of the case. An examination showed but little change in the growths, and that for the worse, the glottis being smaller and the growths more redundant. The patient was suffering at the time from a severe pharyngitis. The uvula was much inflamed, and dyspnoea was quite marked. Under treatment this disappeared, and the patient with it.

"I again saw him on June 10. In the interval he had visited Philadelphia, and was there seen by Drs. Seiler, J. Solis Cohen, and others. His condition was now changed much for the worse. There were darting pains through larynx and into left ear. Voice was gone completely. His breathing was noisy, difficult and hurried. Pulse rapid and weak. Sleep was disturbed, and had often to be taken sitting up, on account of sudden attacks of dyspnoea. He was losing his strength and spirits. The left ventricular band presented, on its anterior third, a smooth, rounded tumor, of deep red color and considerable density, shading into the surrounding congested mucous membrane. The growths over the vocal bands had increased somewhat in size, but were not ulcerated. There was exquisite sensitiveness over the cushion of the epiglottis and over the new formation in the ventricular band, when probed. The case being now plainly one of epithelioma, I seriously broached to him thyrotomy, or extirpation of the larynx, as the only means of relief from the disease, and explained that tracheotomy might be rendered necessary by the slightest diminution of his air-space by inflammatory swelling. Some indiscretion on his part precipitated an acute congestion of his larynx, and on the morning of June 14 I found him in my office, laboring for breath, weak, excited and somewhat cyanosed, after a sleepless night spent in a struggle for life. Finding tracheotomy necessary at once, I hurried him home."

It was in the condition thus described that I found the patient. As he was in danger of immediate suffocation there was no difference of opinion as to the immediate necessity for tracheotomy. This was consented to, and at once performed. So little breathing space was there that we even feared to give an anaesthetic; we therefore urged that it be borne without. A syringe full of cocaine (four per cent) solution, was injected under the skin in the middle line of the neck, and the ether spray used as a local anaesthetic. With Dr. Hinkel's kind assistance operation was at once begun.

But pain was by no means abolished, and on this account the procedure was prolonged. Finally, after dissection was partly accomplished, and the deep parts so far exposed that, in case of necessity, the trachea could be roughly and quickly opened, the patient's demand for chloroform was acceded to, and it was carefully administered.

No small difficulty was experienced in properly exposing the trachea, and the operation was, hence, annoyingly prolonged. Even after its exposure the proper introduction of the tracheal tube was rendered very difficult; and the introduction of wire sutures through skin edges and the margins of the tracheal opening, as I had contemplated, was impossible. Full anatomical explanation of these difficulties was furnished by the subsequent operation, which showed that the trachea not only lay at an unusual depth, but had undergone a considerable calcification (senile) by which it had lost most of its elasticity. Desisting then from this effort a tracheal tube was finally introduced. Relief was immediate, and in two days he was up and about his room and had recovered from the physical exhaustion of his nearly complete apnoea.

During the latter part of the first week there was a mild amount of nocturnal delirium, which we were then inclined to ascribe to the influence of opiates, but which, in the light of subsequent developments, we had to consider traumatic in origin.

The tracheotomy wound granulated so rapidly that in the absence of sutures the tube could not be kept in place, but was crowded up and out by the healing process. But the more or less inflamed and tortured larynx, even though filled up with growth as it was, had had a week's rest, and after the removal of the tube he breathed with considerable ease.

The time had now come when the patient, who had a full realization of his predicament, must either decide on some still more radical measure or await death from extension of the disease. In favor of extirpation spoke the excellent physical condition and powers of endurance of the patient, and the facts that no cancerous cachexia was to be noted, and that there was no sign of any involvement of parts outside the laryngeal box. Against it, spoke only the known dangers of the operation. Our advice was in favor of operation, and this was also the advice of Dr. Carl Seiler, of Philadelphia, who saw him while on a trip to the West. The patient made his choice of radical operation, after a full presentation of its advantages and dangers.

Accordingly, he took a private room in the Buffalo General Hospital, where he was prepared for operation. On June 28, 1885, complete extirpation of the larynx was performed. During it I had the valuable assistance of Dr. Phelps, who kindly took charge of the anaesthetic (chloroform with 1% of amyl nitrite), of several other of my colleagues of the hospital staff, and of Drs. Seiler and Hinkel.

It was necessary to make a long incision, in the middle line, which ran from a little in front of the body of the hyoid to one inch below the upper end of the sternum; this, as the head was drawn backward over pillows, made it about six inches long. In it were included the remains of the previous tracheotomy incision. Careful dissection was then made down on either side of the larynx and trachea; the muscles attached to the sides of the larynx were peeled back with a sharp periosteum elevator. This separation of soft parts on either side was carried as high as the hyoid bone and as low as the second or third ring of the trachea. Vessels were caught in haemostatic forceps as fast as they bled, and tied later with catgut; a few larger veins were tied twice and cut between ligatures; about twenty-five haemostatic forceps were employed, once or twice all being in use at the same time. Up to this time patient had breathed his chloroformized air by the mouth. At this time, after the deep parts had been well exposed, and the lateral portions held aside with retractors, and after my fingers had pretty completely separated the trachea from the oesophagus, it was thought best to open the thyroid cartilage for exploratory purposes. This was no easy task, and sharp cutting bone forceps were necessary before it could be accomplished, so firmly was it calcified. By this exploration it was quickly noted that the growth was well confined within the laryngeal walls. So without further loss of time the trachea was divided, first longitudinally through its upper three rings, and then transversely between the first and second ring. A Trendelenberg tampon tracheal canula was then inserted, but its rubber balloon proved faulty; consequently, I packed sponge around its main tube and used it as an ordinary tracheal tube, save that the tube and funnel for the anaesthetic connected with it were utilized during a part of the remaining time.

The larynx and upper tracheal ring were now rapidly separated from the oesophagus, and, after this separation was complete from below, the thyro-hyoid membrane was divided and then the remainder of the lateral walls of the lower pharynx. The constrictors were dissected off from their insertions into the larynx, and the whole removed in one piece. Haemorrhage was checked, and then the parts explored for evidences of any extralaryngeal suspicious tissue. None was found here, but I decided to remove the uvula, which had been for some time very sensitive, and in which a little firm nodule was felt. The upper part of the epiglottis, with its glossal and lateral connections, was also left *in situ*.

Particular attention was then given to every bleeding point, and haemorrhage, which had at no time been alarming or uncontrollable, was perfectly checked. A little blood had run down the trachea and was coughed up at intervals. The tracheal tube was then removed and a strong silk suture introduced on either side, through the skin and the upper tracheal ring which, it will be remembered, had been split vertically. These were the only sutures used, and were for the purpose, not of trying to pull the trachea up in the neck, but simply of holding it well to the front. A large single trachea tube of aluminum, made for the purpose, was then introduced and held by tapes around the neck. Over its upper surface fell the anterior cut margin of the oesophagus. Iodoform was dusted sparingly throughout the wound, and the whole cavity carefully packed with iodoform gauze, so arranged that a pathway to the oesophagus was left, this latter being lightly plugged with the same material.

Further details of the case and of its after treatment are deemed unnecessary here. I will simply add that shock was comparatively slight and reaction satisfactory. Beginning five hours after completion of the operation food was regularly administered every four to six hours, the oesophageal tube being introduced through the wound.

Convalescence was only broken by one incident, but this came near being disastrous. On the fifth and sixth days it was noticed that he seemed a little dazed, and his written messages were somewhat incoherent; and I was reminded of his similar condition after his previous operation. Late in the evening of the sixth day, while apparently asleep, and being watched by one pupil of the training school for nurses, he suddenly jumped out of bed, threw up a window (second story) and made ready for a spring. The nurse seized him by his night-clothes and pulled him back. Then ensued a severe struggle, during which she was severely bruised, he endeavoring to escape and she to hold him back; in a moment her calls for assistance were answered and he was put back in bed. His acute mania was soon subdued. Next morning his temperature was only 99°, and he showed no evidences of his wild night, save that his thoughts were incoherent. In two days he had practically recovered, though his mind was not quite clear for two weeks afterward. This could not have been iodoform intoxication nor the effects of opium, because both had been used in minimum amounts; I therefore class it among those obscure cases of so-called "traumatic mania," about whose etiology we know practically nothing.

Nevertheless, after this his wound was dressed with cotton steeped in a saturated solution of salicylic acid and potassium chlorate, and to the stimulating effect of the latter I ascribe the remarkably rapid granulating process by which the wound closed. In three weeks the feeding tube was introduced through the mouth instead of by the wound, which was no longer sufficiently open. In five weeks he was wearing the tracheal portion of his artificial larynx; in six weeks the pharyngeal portion of it, was breathing through his nose once more, and was able to whisper so that he could be heard across the room. In seven weeks he was able to swallow soft solids, when the obturator of the upper tube was introduced. In eight weeks he was able, by means of the vibrating reed inserted in the tubes, to articulate with perfect distinctness.

As nearly as I can gather, never have the processes of repair occurred with greater rapidity than here; in fact, as I recall the formidable wound, it seems almost incredible that healing could have taken place as rapidly as it did.

The patient is now wearing an almost exact copy of Gussenbauer's *artificial larynx,* made from pure silver, from a model in the writer's possession. As this has never received adequate illustration in this country a description of it is subjoined.

It consists of a tracheal tube of large size *(A)* with rings at its lower end permitting a slight motion, corresponding to the natural flexibility of the trachea. Through its front plate and through an opening on its upper curvature passes a second or pharyngeal tube *(B),* made also flexible (or not, according to the case); with an opening on its lower curved surface, so placed that a stream of air may play freely through both tubes, even though the external outlet be closed. The upper end of the pharyngeal tube lodges behind and below the epiglottis, if this has been left *in situ,* or behind and below the base of the tongue, as the case may be. Around it the oesophagus granulates and closes, so that after the healing process is complete the only passage from the pharynx into the larynx is by way of the metal tube. In order that fluids and solids may not pass through this, an obturator *(C)* is provided, which is passed through the external opening and up through the tube, so that its rounded upper end plugs the upper end of the pharyngeal opening, thus preventing passage of anything into the trachea. But since this would also shut off the air, the obturator is attached below, not to a solid plug, but to a ring, as seen, which fits accurately into the external opening of the instrument, through which, then, the patient breathes so long as this plug is worn. Except at meal times a simple stopper *(E)* is worn, so

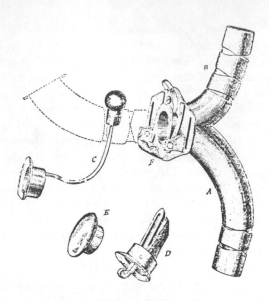

FIG. 1. Gussenbauer's Artificial Larynx.

that at all other times he breathes naturally through the nose and mouth. After a time, by an instinctive education of the pharyngeal and buccal muscles, the upper end of the tube is protected during the process of deglutition, and patients wearing these instruments learn to swallow readily without the assistance of the obturator.

Nothing now is lacking save a substitute for the vocal cords, something which, by vibrating in the air current, may produce a distinct *tone.*

Such a substitute is provided by a free metallic reed, like a melodeon reed, playing freely in a movable slotted bar *(D),* and fitted inside of a stopper like the other one. This movable bar carrying the reed has an external lever, by means of which the wearer is enabled, with a touch of the finger, to throw it into or out of the air current, and thus— as it were—to voluntarily open or close the glottis. With this part of the instrument *in situ,* and with the reed in the air current, the metal strip vibrates as it does in the jew's-harp, and the sound thus produced is converted, by the articulating parts above, into something more than a whisper—*into distinct speech.*

The voice, thus produced, though a monotone, is nevertheless a perfect voice in every respect save *pitch.*

This apparatus does not represent the first efforts that were made, even by Gussenbauer who was the first to succeed, to devise a substitute for the larynx, but it shows the instrument in form more perfect for the majority of cases than the mechanisms of Foulis or Bruns.

At date of writing, nearly six months after the operation, the details of which have been thus given, its subject is apparently in perfect health, has gained largely in flesh and strength, goes on extensive journeys and has even been out on a hunting trip.

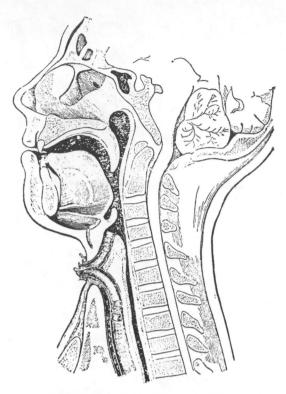

FIG. 2. Artificial Larynx in Position. [This figure, modified from one of Schüller's represents the instrument *in situ*. The artist's notions of topographical anatomy have led to some distortion of the anatomical relations, but without interference with the main purpose of the illustration.]

Microscopic examination of the intra-laryngeal mass revealed typical epitheliomatous structure.

In the table of cases of complete laryngectomies given by Cohen in the *International Encyclopaedia of Surgery* (vol. v., p. 764 *et seq.*), two only by American operators are given.

No. 28, by Dr. Lange, of New York. Recurrence of sarcomatous growth with death from asthenia seven months after operation.

No. 67, by Dr. Hodgen, of St. Louis. Death after four days.

Speech Without Using the Larynx

E. W. Scripture

Since the publication of an account of speech without a larynx by Czermak in 1859, cases of this kind have been observed repeatedly. It has been reported of several of them that they could speak with a fair degree of audibility and could produce sounds that seemed to have something of a laryngeal tone in them. Happening to meet such a case I thought it would be worth while to make a record of the speech with a view of investigating the source of this apparent laryngeal tone.

The girl, F. H., seventeen years old, had undergone tracheotomy at the age of three. Ever since that time she has breathed through a tracheotomy tube and has been unable to breathe when the tube is stopped or removed. Observation with the laryngoscope shows that the top of the pharynx is closed over the larynx and no air passes through. On retching the larynx is brought up and becomes visible. Under no circumstances can she make any air pass through the larynx. She can speak quite distinctly and correctly in a faint, almost toneless voice. Such a condition seems quite astonishing, because all speech sounds require breath. Without breath the person may go through all the movements of enunciation but he will produce no sound; his speech is visible but not audible.

The patient's method of producing audible speech was studied with the aid of the phonautograph. In this method the person speaks into the mouthpiece of a wide tube leading to a flexible membrane. The movements of the membrane are amplified by a light lever and registered on a blackened revolving surface. The arrangement is shown in Fig. 1.

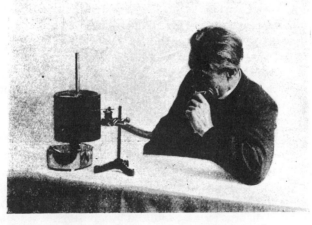

FIG. 1.   Recording speech by the Phonautograph.

Reprinted by permission from *Journal of Physiology*, 1916, *50*, 397–403.

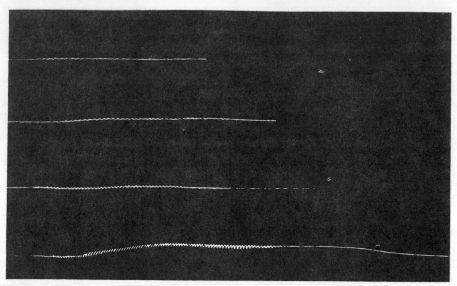

FIG. 2.   Record of 'ah-ah-ah-ah' sung on the notes, *c, e, g, c'* by a normal female voice. Each wave records one vibration of the larynx.

A record of 'ah-ah-ah-ah' sung on the notes *c, e, g, c'* by a normal female voice are produced in Fig. 2. The small waves record the voice tone, or the vibrations from the glottis. They become shorter in each successive record as the tone is raised; in the last note they are just half as long as in the first one. The waves run along evenly and smoothly as is usual in normal voices.

A record of 'ah-ah-ah-ah' sung on the notes *c, e, g, c'* by F. H. is reproduced in Fig. 3. It begins with a jerky line that records the efforts at intake of air. This is followed by quite regular waves. The succeeding records of 'ah' show faint and fairly regular waves. These waves become successively shorter as the pitch is raised.

Careful observation of F. H. reveals the mechanism by which she produces these tones. A movement of the muscles at the side and front of her neck, just under and behind the jaw, can be seen from the outside; the movement is of a kind that might contract the pharynx. With the mouth open the tongue can be seen to be raised tightly against the rear edge of the palate and the front part of the velum (Fig. 4). There is some slight movement on attempting to change the pitch. The mechanism is evident. The air in the pharynx is compressed; it is allowed to escape between the tongue and the velum in such a way as to produce a tone. The tone is produced by causing the surfaces of the tongue and the palate to vibrate somewhat as the vocal cords do. The change in pitch is produced by changes in the tension. In short, the lacking glottis is replaced by an imitation glottis formed by the tongue and the velum.

It might be asserted that the tone is produced by arousing the vibrations of the resonance cavity of the mouth just as by blowing across the opening of a bottle, and that the change of tone is produced by altering the size of the cavity. This cannot be true, because alteration of the size of the mouth cavity changes the character of the vowel. A normal person can raise the tongue against the palate and produce a rough tone by forcing the

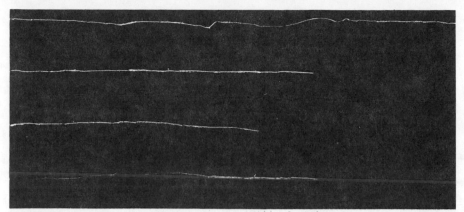

FIG. 3.   Record of 'ah-ah-ah-ah' sung on the notes *c, e, g, c'* by F. H. without the use of her larynx. The fall in the line at the start shows that air is being taken into the mouth. The following rises and falls show that air is sometimes emitted and sometimes taken in. Finally there is a rather explosive puff followed by fine waves. These waves are quite regular; they were heard as a tone. They record the tone of the voice. In any other record they would be attributed to the vibrations of the vocal cords; here they are due to vibrations of a kind of artificial glottis formed by the tongue against the velum. The shortening of these waves in the succeeding records shows that this tongue-velum glottis can be adjusted to produce notes of different pitch. The irregularities in the last line show that the vibration is not so smooth and regular as in the real glottis.

breath through; he can also raise the tone, but as he does so the vowel changes from 'ah' to 'ee.' He can also produce and raise the tone with an ordinary whisper and with the same result. This patient keeps the 'ah' quality throughout; therefore the tone she produces is not a cavity tone. There is additional proof that the tone she uses is not a cavity tone. Such tones are of much higher pitch; they never register with the phonautograph. The record in Fig. 3 shows definite waves; these must have been produced by some body equivalent to the larynx.

The different vowels are produced by F. H. by varying the mouth cavity. For 'ah' the mouth is open. The vowel 'oh' starts with a rather open mouth but the lips are soon rounded. A similar movement produces 'oo.' For 'awe' the lips are rounded and then opened. For 'eh' and 'ee' the appropriate lip positions are taken; the vowel 'ee' is spe-

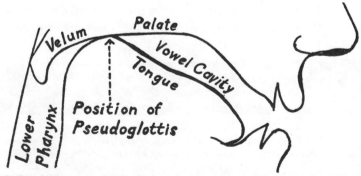

FIG. 4.   Method of producing a pseudo-glottis when the larynx is not used. Air is collected by enlarging the lower pharynx. The back of the tongue is raised against the velum. The contraction of the lower pharynx presses the air out between the tongue and the velum, producing a tone. The pitch of this tone is regulated by muscular contraction of the tongue and velum.

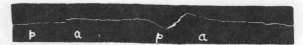

FIG. 5. (upper tracing). Record of 'papa' by a normal female voice. The straight line at the start registers the time during which the lips are closed and no breath is emitted. The sharp upward jerk is due to the sudden puff of air that escapes as the lips are opened. This is followed by the fine waves that register the vibrations of the larynx while the mouth is open for the vowel. The sudden fall registers the closure of the lips for the second 'p,' and so on.

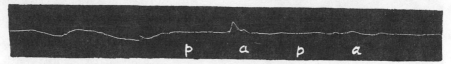

FIG. 6. (lower tracing). Record of 'papa' by F. H. The waving of the line at the start shows the variation in taking in air in order to supply air for the word. The straight line for the time during which the lips are closed (the occlusion) in the 'p' is followed by a sharp and rather forcible jerk upward that registers the explosion as the lips open. The fairly regular small waves thereafter register the vibrations of the vowel that were produced by the tongue-velum glottis and not the real one. As much of the air contained in the pharynx has been spent, the second 'p' does not have so forcible an explosion.

cially distinct. To produce the occlusives 'p, b, t, d' etc., the breath is cut off for a moment at some point in the air passage. A normal record of 'papa' with both syllables equally accented is shown in Fig. 5. During 'p' the lips are closed and the glottis open; during the vowel the mouth is open and the glottis is vibrating. A record of 'papa' by F. H. is given in Fig. 6. The air 'swallowed' into the pharynx is used to produce the explosions for 'p' and to vibrate the tongue-palate glottis that imitates the laryngeal vibrations of the vowels.

A record of 'tata' by F. H. is shown in Fig. 7. It reveals a marvel of skill in vocal mechanics. After making 't' by putting the tip against the palate to produce an occlusion and an explosion, the tongue rapidly readjusts itself to a new position in order to form the imitation glottis required for the following vowel.

The patient always made a distinction between 'p' and 'b,' 't' and 'd,' etc. In normal speech the greatest difference lies in the absence of laryngeal vibrations in 'p,' 't,' etc., and the presence of them in 'b,' 'd,' etc.; the patient could not make this difference. Another difference lies in the fact that in normal speech the explosions are stronger for 'p,' 't,' etc., than for 'b,' 'd,' etc. This latter difference was marked in the speech

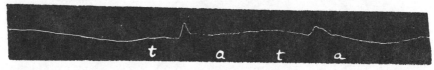

FIG. 7. Record of 'tata' by F. H. The downward movement of the line registers the intake of air into the pharynx. This is followed by a straight line for the time during which the point of the tongue is closed against the palate (the occlusion). The sharp jerk upward is produced as the tongue releases a puff of air (the explosion). Not long afterward the faint vowel waves appear. These are produced not by the larynx but by the vibration of the back of the tongue against the velum. To get the tongue in this position its tip must be released at the end of 't' and the back must be raised; this is what is happening during the time of the rather irregular line after the explosion of 't' and before the vowel waves.

FIG. 8.   Record of 'baba' by F. H. There is less violent intake of breath than in Fig. 6 because there is less needed for 'baba' than for 'papa.' The explosions are weaker.

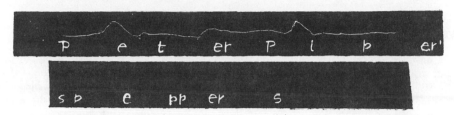

FIG. 9.   Record of 'Peter Piper's peppers' by F. H. The lower part of the figure follows on the upper part. Each 'p' has a sharply marked occlusion and a well-defined explosion. The explosion becomes steadily weaker; for the last 'p' it is hardly visible. There is practically no 's' for 'Piper's' but there is an exaggerated one at the end, when there was no need of economising air in the pharynx and all the rest might be safely used.

of F. H. as may be seen in comparing the record of 'baba' in Fig. 8 with that of 'papa' in Fig. 6.

A normal 'l' is made by passing air along one or both edges of the tongue while the larynx vibrates. F. H. produces the rubbing sound of the air along the passage but cannot use her pseudo-glottis at the same time. Her 'l' is therefore toneless or surd. It sounds exactly like the surd 'll' in Welsh.

The nasals are produced like the corresponding occlusives but there are no explosions. 'Mama,' 'nana' and 'sing' sound like 'papa,' 'tata' and 'sick.'

The patient has such skill in using the pharyngeal air supply that she can speak quite long sentences. Fig. 9 shows a record of 'Peter Piper's peppers.' The 'p's' are all very sharply and forcibly made but they gradually become weaker as the air is exhausted. Except in this respect and in the faintness of the vowel waves the record does not differ from a normal one.

Three years ago I reported a case of laryngectomy of a man of sixty-five. His speech was quite inaudible after the operation. To produce the explosive 'p' he was taught to close his lips and compress the air in his mouth and pharynx by tension on the cheeks and in the back of the throat. On opening the lips there was a puff of air that produced a quite audible 'p.' For 't' he placed the point of the tongue against the palate and compressed the air in his throat. By releasing the closure of the tongue he produced a distinct 't.' For 'k' the back of the tongue was raised and released with pressure in the same way.

In normal speech 'b,' 'd,' 'g' are distinguished from 'p,' 't,' 'k' mainly by the presence of a tone from the larynx. This patient could not produce a tone and the sounds could not be distinguished. He was taught to give the puffs of air through the cannula for 'b,' 'd,' 'g' and thereby to make a distinction between the two groups of sounds by adding a rushing noise to one group.

For the vowels there was no closure of the mouth that would enable this patient to compress any air; consequently the vowels were blanks and his speech consisted wholly of consonants. He was taught to give puffs from his cannula during the vowels, whereby they became distinguishable from pauses.

The patient died in a few months by extension of the carcinomatous growth. He did not have time to learn—and at his age would probably never have been able to learn—the really remarkable mechanism that F. H. has developed of her own accord.

REFERENCES

For a summary of cases of speech without a larynx: Kussmaul, Störungen der Sprache, 2. ed. (by Gutzmann), 267, 360, Leipzig, 1910; Gutzmann, Sprachheilkunde, 2. ed. 524, Berlin, 1912. For the case of laryngectomy referred to: Scripture, Speech without a Larynx, Jour. Amer. Med. Assoc. 1913, May 22, LX. p. 1601. For detailed accounts of the methods of recording speech: Scripture, Elements of Experimental Phonetics, Yale University Press, 1902; Stuttering and Lisping, Macmillan, New York and London, 1913.

PART II

INTRINSIC FORMS OF ALARYNGEAL VOICE AND SPEECH: BUCCAL AND PHARYNGEAL SPEECH

Intrinsic forms of alaryngeal voice and speech refer to nonsurgical-prosthetic methods of voice and speech production used by laryngectomized patients. The term *intrinsic* highlights the fact that the forms of speech and voice production described in this section rely upon the intrinsic human anatomical structures remaining following laryngeal extirpation. By contrast, forms of speech and voice production that depend upon extrinsic, man-made voicing prostheses or surgically created structures developed specifically for the purpose of voice production are covered in Parts IV and V of this text.

Esophageal speech is clearly the most widely employed form of oral communication used by laryngectomized individuals. Hence, the bulk of information covered in this section deals with important aspects of this intrinsic form of alaryngeal voice and speech.

The articles in this section describe two forms of alaryngeal speech: buccal speech and pharyngeal speech. The two articles, "A Study of Buccal Speech" (1971) and "A Study of Pharyngeal Speech" (1973), both by Weinberg and Westerhouse provide information about physiological mechanisms, acoustic properties, and perceptual characteristics of buccal speech and pharyngeal speech. The major clinical contribution of these works supports the belief that neither buccal speech nor pharyngeal speech should be regarded as desirable or practical primary methods of alaryngeal speech for laryngectomized patients.

A Study of Buccal Speech

Bernd Weinberg and Jan Westerhouse

Indiana University Medical Center, Indianapolis, Indiana

An intensive study of a normal-speaking subject, proficient in the use of buccal speech, was conducted. With respect to voice fundamental frequency variability, phonation time, and speaking rate his buccal speech characteristics compared favorably with those reported for excellent esophageal speakers. However, the reduced intelligibility of his buccal speech on rhyme-test words, the high average fundamental frequency of his buccal voice, and his conspicuous buccal gestures during speech represent distinct vocal liabilities.

Buccal speech represents one of several types of alaryngeal speech; however, its use as a primary method of communication is rare (Diedrich and Youngstrom, 1966). Damste (1958) and Lauder (1968) have offered the clinical hypothesis that buccal speech does not represent either a desirable or a practical primary method of alaryngeal speech. Experimental support for this hypothesis has not been reported. Moreover, descriptions of the acoustic characteristics, intelligibility, and the ultimate limits of performance for excellent buccal speech are also not available. The present investigation was undertaken to provide such information through an intensive study of a normal subject who is proficient in the use of buccal speech.

METHOD

The Subject

The subject was a normal-speaking adult male who taught himself buccal speech during childhood. Before his experiment he regarded buccal speech as a novelty. He has practiced buccal speech for more than 15 years, since, as a professional singer and entertainer, he uses buccal voice as an alternative method of singing. The authors judged him to be an excellent buccal speaker.

Procedures

Sound-synchronous motion-picture studies were used to describe the location of the vicarious air chamber and the mechanism of phonation for buccal speech. High-quality recordings of the subject's buccal speech were made as he (1) read the first paragraph of Fairbank's Rainbow Passage (1960), (2) gave a 60-sec sample of extemporaneous speech, (3) produced a series of maximally sustained vowels, and (4) sang the musical scale.

    To derive voice fundamental frequency (VFF), rate, and phonation time characteristics, the recording of the Rainbow Passage was duplicated and the second sentence was extracted. The experimental sentence was played at half-speed by a high-quality tape

Reprinted by permission from *Journal of Speech and Hearing Research*, 1971, *14*, 652–658.

recorder to one channel of a Honeywell Visicorder Model 1508. For calibration purposes, a counter-monitored 1000-Hz signal was played into the second channel of the Visicorder. Visicorder chart speed of 2000 mm/sec and mirror galvanometers M-5000 were used. The Visicorder record of the experimental sentence was segmented into categories of quasiperiodic phonation, aperiodicity, and silence. The individual periods of each wave form within each quasiperiodic segment and the aperiodic and silent interval segment lengths were measured. VFF means, standard deviations, ranges, and phonation times were derived from these measurements. The lengths of the Visicorder tracings for the series of maximally sustained vowels were measured to derive maximum phonation duration.

To permit evaluation of the intelligibility of buccal speech, the subject recorded the six 50-item word lists of the rhyme test described by House et al. (1965). The words were recorded without instrumental monitoring; however, the subject was instructed to maintain a constant level of vocal effort. Since the subject was experienced in recording materials, it was assumed that (1) the range of levels for the vocalic maxima of words was similar to that usually found for vowels produced by normal talkers and (2) the average level among the six lists did not vary significantly. Consequently, the recordings were not adjusted for level variations. The recorded word lists were presented to 15 normal-hearing, young adult listeners via high quality earphones and listening equipment. The average level of the speech presented to the listeners was 70 dB SPL measured under the headphones.

RESULTS

Mechanism of Buccal Phonation

Sound synchronous motion-picture studies indicated that the subject exhibited the classical mechanism of buccal phonation originally described by Van Gilse (1949). That is, he created a vicarious air chamber between the left upper jaw and the cheek and used this cavity as an accessory lung for speech. A neoglottis was created between the upper jaw, the teeth, and the cheek (Figure 1).

Voice Fundamental Frequency, Phonation Time, and Rate Characteristics of Buccal Speech

The subject had a range of more than three octaves (69 Hz to 571 Hz) for sung buccal voice. For buccal speech, his average VFF level was 323 Hz, the range was 20.3 semitones, and the standard deviation was 3.6 semitones.

The maximum duration of buccal phonation for a series of sustained vowels was 2 sec. During oral reading, 52% of total speaking time was spent producing quasiperiodic phonation, 15% was aperiodicity, and 33% was silence. His speaking rate for oral reading of the first paragraph of the Rainbow Passage was 131 wpm.

Buccal Speech Intelligibility

The intelligibility of the subject's buccal speech was evaluated using rhyme-test procedures and materials. His average intelligibility on rhyme-test words was 76% correct. The

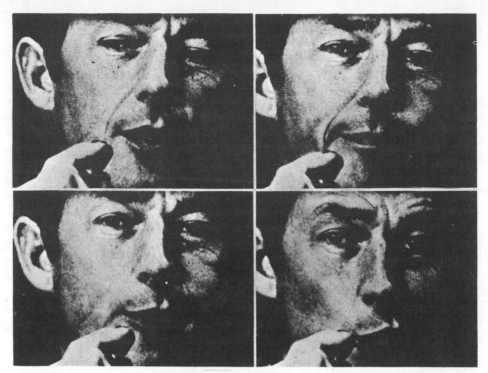

FIGURE 1. Photographic study of buccal phonation. Upper left: subject at rest. Upper right: subject fills his left buccal cavity. Lower left: subject begins to speak. Note that the vicarious air chamber is filled with air and that the buccinator and adjacent lip musculature contract to effect a unique neoglottis. Lower right: subject just prior to the end of utterance. Note that the buccal cavity is almost depleted with air and that the buccinator and lip musculature are vigorously contracted.

average intelligibility of each of the consonants under test is shown in Table 1. The recognition scores for individual consonants are of particular interest since they provide information about the articulatory patterns that characterize the buccal speech of the subject and provide a basis for understanding the listener's total impression of intelligibility. No significant differences in average intelligibility were found (1) between word-initial and word-final consonants (74 vs 77% correct) and (2) between voiced and voiceless consonants (75 vs 77% correct). With respect to consonant type, the order of correct identification, from most to least intelligible, was glides, fricatives, plosive, affricates, and nasals.

DISCUSSION

A review of the literature suggests that considerable confusion exists regarding the nature of and the differences among the behaviors termed buccal, pharyngeal, and esophageal speech. For example, Damste (1958) wrote:

> Another type of purely buccal speech was seen by us in a case of a 17-year-old boy. . . . Here the vibrations are generated by the lateral edge of the tongue against the lingual side of the upper alveolar process. Air from the pharynx is pressed through this pseudo-glottis by a backward movement of the root of the tongue. (p. 3)

Table 1. Average intelligibility (% correct) of consonants. Initial (I), final (F) and combined (IF) initial-final word position are tabulated.

Consonant	I	F	IF	Consonant	I	F	IF
p	59	77	68	f	92	42*	79
b	90	86	88	v	100**	65*	71
t	68	57	62	θ	80**	70*	72
d	77	82	80	ð	53**	47**	50
k	72	97	89	s	92	91	91
g	76	92*	83	z	†	85	85
				ʃ	100*	†	100
				tʃ	†	78*	78
				dʒ	77**	60**	71
m	77	71	74	h	66	†	66
n	57**	40	42				
ŋ	†	69*	69	w	52	†	52
				r	94	92	94
				l	90	100**	96

*Indicates that a sound in a given position is in at least two but less than six forms.
**Indicates that a sound occurs in only one test form.
†Consonant not tested in this word position.

Damste also used the term *parabuccal speech* to describe another method of alaryngeal phonation:

> Air is pressed from an air bubble high in the cheek through a "rima glottidis" that is formed between the upper alveolar process and the mucosa of the mouth tensed by the buccinator muscle. (p. 3)

Diedrich and Youngstrom (1966) have suggested that the behaviors termed buccal, pharyngeal, and esophageal phonation (or speech) be described and differentiated on the basis of the location of the vicarious air supply and the site of the neoglottis. We concur with their suggestion. Specifically, we suggest that the term *buccal phonation* (or speech) be used to describe a method of alaryngeal phonation in which both the vicarious air chamber and the neoglottis are formed between the cheek and upper jaw. The term *pharyngeal speech* should be used to describe a second method of alaryngeal speech, in which the air supply for phonation is in the pharynx and the neoglottis is formed between the tongue and the upper alveolus, the palate, or the pharyngeal wall. *Esophageal voice* should refer to the method of alaryngeal speech in which the air supply for phonation comes from the esophagus and the site of the neoglottis is the pharyngo-esophageal segment.

The need for standard use of terms to describe specific methods of alaryngeal speech represents more than a semantic issue. Buccal, pharyngeal, and esophageal speech represent three entirely different methods of alaryngeal speech production, and the terms used to describe the behaviors associated with these mechanisms should accurately reflect their differences. In light of these suggestions, we believe that the 17-year-old boy cited by Damste (1958) as an example of "purely buccal speech" used pharyngeal rather than buccal speech. Similarly, the subject described in the present investigation, the patient described by Van Gilse (1949), and the "para-buccal speaker" described by Damste (1958) all employ buccal speech.

With particular reference to the present experiment, a number of informative comparisons can be made between buccal, esophageal, and normal speech. Specifically, the 323-Hz average VFF level found for buccal speech is more than two octaves above that reported for male esophageal speakers (Curry and Snidecor, 1961) and almost an octave above that reported for any esophageal speaker (Shipp, 1967; Damste, 1958). Phonation time for buccal speech compared favorably with that reported for esophageal speakers (Shipp, 1967) yet was smaller than that reported for normal subjects (Hanley, 1951).

The maximum buccal phonation duration for sustained vowels of 2 sec corresponded closely to phonation durations reported for average esophageal speakers but was shorter than those reported for superior esophageal speakers (Berlin, 1963). The shorter maximum phonation duration for buccal speech is not unexpected when one compares the air reservoir capacity of the buccal cavity with that of the esophagus. The speaking rate for buccal speech of 131 wpm was (1) slightly faster than the median rate of 122.5 wpm reported for superior esophageal speakers (Curry and Snidecor, 1961), (2) slower than the 169 and 153 wpm rates reported for two esophageal speakers (Hoops and Noll, 1969; Snidecor and Isshiki, 1965), and (3) slower than the average rate reported for normal speakers (Darley, 1940).

With respect to intelligibility for rhyme-test words, the average intelligibility for buccal speech corresponded closely to that reported for two trained normal speakers' recordings of rhyme tests presented at a signal-to-noise ratio of -8 dB (House et al., 1965). Under the optimal S/N conditions used in the present experiment, normal and excellent esophageal speakers would be expected to demonstrate near-perfect intelligibility for rhyme-test words (House et al., 1965; Griffiths, 1967; Owens and Schubert, 1968; and unpublished work of the first author of this paper). For buccal speech, the average intelligibility of word-initial and word-final consonants was essentially the same. For normal and esophageal speech, consonants in the word-initial position are generally more intelligible than word-final consonants (House et al., 1965; Hyman, 1955). For buccal speech, the average intelligibility of voiced and voiceless consonants was also comparable. For esophageal speech, voiced consonants are more intelligible than voiceless consonants (Hyman, 1955; Sacco, Mann, and Schultz, 1967).

The intelligibility data were also analyzed to examine the types of errors made by listeners. The results showed that the buccal speaker had considerable difficulty producing the feature "nasality." Nasal consonants were the least intelligible (57% correct) of all consonants spoken in buccal speech. Moreover, listeners misidentified 35% of the nasal consonant items as nonnasal. The reasons underlying this difficulty merit future study. A careful analysis of voicing errors was also made, since it was hypothesized that a buccal speaker might also have difficulty producing voiced/voiceless oppositions. This hypothesis was rejected, since only 6% of the voiceless consonant items were misidentified as voiced. Although both buccal and esophageal forms of alaryngeal speech provide a vocalic carrier, the present data showed that our buccal speaker was considerably more proficient in achieving contrast between voiced and voiceless consonants than is the typical esophageal speaker (Hyman, 1955; Sacco, Mann, and Schultz, 1967).

It is our clinical opinion that the subject studied has excellent buccal speech. With respect to fundamental frequency variability, phonation time, and speaking rate his buccal speech characteristics compare favorably with those reported for excellent esophageal speakers (Curry and Snidecor, 1961). However, other findings provide experimental support for the clinical hypothesis that buccal speech does not represent either a desirable or a practical primary method of alaryngeal speech. Specifically, the speaker's reduced intelligibility on rhyme-test words in buccal speech, his high average buccal fundamental frequency, and his conspicuous buccal gestures during speech represent distinct vocal liabilities.

ACKNOWLEDGMENT

This research was supported in part by Grant No. 29-854-16 from the Delaware County Cancer Society, Muncie, Indiana. Computations of acoustic measures were supported in part by Public Health Service Grant No. RR162-06 given by General Medical Sciences and performed in the Research Computation Center, Indiana University Medical Center. WFBM TV-Radio, Indianapolis, Indiana, provided facilities, produced the motion-picture studies, and arranged for the recording of the subject. We gratefully acknowledge the assistance and cooperation of the experimental subject, Ross Barbour of the Four Freshmen. A recording of Ross Barbour's use of buccal voice may be heard on the LP album, Capitol ST 1860.

REFERENCES

Berlin, C. I., Clinical measurement of esophageal speech: I. Methodology and curves of skill acquisition. *J. Speech Hear. Dis.,* 28, 42–51 (1963).

Curry, E. T., and Snidecor, J. C., Physical measurement and pitch perception in esophageal speech. *Laryngoscope,* 71, 415–424 (1961).

Damste, P. H., *Oesophageal Speech After Laryngectomy.* Groningen: Gebr. Hoitsema (1958).

Darley, F. L., *A Normative Study of Oral Reading Rate.* Master's thesis, State Univ. of Iowa (1940).

Diedrich, W. M., and Youngstrom, K. A., *Alaryngeal Speech.* Springfield, Ill.: Thomas (1966).

Fairbanks, G., *Voice and Articulation Drillbook.* New York: Harper (1960).

Griffiths, J., Rhyming minimal contrasts. A simplified diagnostic articulation test. *J. acoust. Soc. Amer.,* 42, 236–241 (1967).

Hanley, T. D., An analysis of vocal frequency and duration characteristics of selected samples of speech from three American dialects. *Speech Monogr.,* 18, 78–93 (1951).

Hoops, H. R., and Noll, J. D., Relationship of selected acoustic variables to judgments of esophageal speech. *J. Communication Dis.,* 2, 1–13 (1969).

House, A. S., Williams, C. E., Hecker, M. H. L., and Kryter, K. D., Articulation-testing methods: Consonantal differentiation with a closed-response set. *J. acoust. Soc. Amer.,* 37, 158–166 (1965).

Hyman, M., An experimental study of artificial larynx and esophageal speech. *J. Speech Hearing Dis.,* 20, 291–299 (1955).

Lauder, E., *Self-Help for the Laryngectomee.* San Antonio, Texas (1968).

Owens, E., and Schubert, E., The development of constant items for speech discrimination testing. *J. Speech Hear. Res.,* 11, 656–667 (1968).

Sacco, P. R., Mann, M. B., and Schultz, M. C., Perceptual confusions among selected phonemes in esophageal speech. *J. Indiana Speech Hear. Assoc.,* 26, 19–33 (1967).

Shipp, T., Frequency, duration, and perceptual measures in relation to judgments of alaryngeal speech acceptability. *J. Speech Hear. Res.,* 10, 417–427 (1967).

Snidecor, J. C., *Speech Rehabilitation of the Laryngectomized.* Springfield, Ill.: Thomas (1962).
Snidecor, J. C., and Isshiki, N., Air volume and air flow relationships of six male esophageal speakers. *J. Speech Hearing Dis.*, 30, 205–216 (1965).
Van Gilse, P. H. G., Another method of speech without larynx. *Acta Otolaryng. Suppl.*, 78, 109–110 (1949).

Received September 14, 1970.

A Study of Pharyngeal Speech

Bernd Weinberg and Jan Westerhouse

Speech Research Laboratory, Indiana University Medical Center, Indianapolis, Indiana

Pharyngeal speech represents one of several types of alaryngeal speech; however, its use as a primary method of communication is rare. This report relates the principal findings of an intensive study of a 12-year-old girl with laryngeal papillomatosis who has used pharyngeal speech as an exclusive method of oral communication since age two. The unique physiologic mechanisms of pharyngeal speech are described and differentiated from other forms of alaryngeal speech. This girl's reduced pharyngeal speech intelligibility for consonant and vowel rhyme-test words, her unfavorable phonation time and maximum phonation duration characteristics, her low average fundamental frequency, and her markedly hoarse pharyngeal voice quality all are distinct vocal liabilities. These findings lend strong support to the hypothesis that pharyngeal speech should not be regarded as a desirable or practical primary method of alaryngeal speech.

There has been considerable confusion about the underlying mechanisms used to produce buccal, pharyngeal, and esophageal forms of alaryngeal speech (Diedrich and Youngstrom, 1966). Recent research has shown that these three forms of alaryngeal speech can be differentiated on the basis of their differing air supply locations and neoglottis sites. For example, during the production of esophageal speech the air supply for phonation comes from the esophagus, with the pharyngoesophageal segment functioning as a neoglottis (Diedrich and Youngstrom, 1966). For buccal speech, the air supply for phonation comes from a vicarious air chamber created in the buccal cavity, with the cheek and upper jaw forming a neoglottis (Van Gilse, 1949; Damste, 1958; Weinberg and Westerhouse, 1971). During pharyngeal speech, the air supply comes from the pharynx. A neoglottis is created between the tongue and the upper alveolus, the palate, or the pharyngeal wall (Diedrich and Youngstrom, 1966; Weinberg and Westerhouse, 1971).

Although buccal and pharyngeal speech are two available forms of alaryngeal speech, their use as primary methods of communication is rare. Various authors have suggested that both buccal and pharyngeal speech do not represent desirable primary methods of communication (Lauder, 1971; Damste, 1958). Weinberg and Westerhouse (1971) have recently provided evidence supporting this hypothesis for buccal speech. Unfortunately, detailed analyses of the acoustic features, intelligibility characteristics, and perceptual dimensions of pharyngeal speech are not available. The present investigation was undertaken to provide such information. We conducted an intensive study of a 12-year-old girl who has used pharyngeal speech as her exclusive method of oral communication since age two. Results are discussed in relation to the question of whether pharyngeal speech should be regarded as a practical or efficient primary method of alaryngeal speech.

Reprinted by permission from *Journal of Speech and Hearing Disorders*, 1973, *38*, 111–118.

METHOD

The Subject

The subject is a 12-year-old girl with laryngeal papillomatosis. At age two, she underwent a tracheotomy because of respiratory difficulty associated with her disease. Immediately after her tracheotomy, she taught herself pharyngeal speech and continues, to date, to use pharyngeal speech as an exclusive method of oral communication. This otherwise normal girl has never received remedial speech training.

Procedures

Sound-synchronous cinefluorographic studies were used to describe the location of the vicarious air chamber and the mechanism of pharyngeal phonation. High-quality recordings of the subject's pharyngeal speech were also made. To measure fundamental frequency (f_o), duration, and phonation time characteristics, her recording of the Rainbow Passage (Fairbanks, 1960) was duplicated, and the second sentence was extracted for acoustic analysis. The sentence recording was played by a high-quality tape recorder to one channel of a Honeywell Visicorder Model 1508. For calibration purposes, a counter-monitored 1000-Hz signal was played simultaneously into the second channel of the Visicorder. Visicorder chart speed of 1000 mm/sec and mirror galvanometers M-5000 were used. The Visicorder record of the patient's speech was segmented into categories of quasiperiodicity, aperiodicity, and silence. The individual periods of each quasiperiodic wave form were measured. The lengths of aperiodic and silent intervals were also measured. Fundamental frequency mean, standard deviation, range, and phonation time characteristics were derived from these measurements. The lengths of the Visicorder tracings for a series of maximally sustained vowels were measured to obtain an estimate of maximum phonation duration.

To permit evaluation of the intelligibility of her pharyngeal speech, the subject recorded the six 50-item word lists of a consonant rhyme-test described by House et al. (1965) and the six 240-item word lists of a vowel rhyme-test recently developed by Horii (1969). The words were recorded without instrumental monitoring; however, the subject was instructed to maintain a constant level of vocal effort. Since the talker was not experienced in recording speech materials for analysis or related uses, her success in following these instructions was investigated. Accordingly, the recorded words were played into a Bruel and Kjaer graphic-level recorder (Model 2305), and the level of the vocalic maxima of each word was measured relative to a 1000-Hz reference signal. Within each 50-word consonant list the SD of vowels levels was about 2 dB; for vowel lists the SD was about 3 dB. The average level of the six consonant test lists varied by only 1.5 dB; the variation for the six vowel test lists was 2.5 dB. Consequently, the recordings were not adjusted for level variations. The word lists were presented to 19 normal-hearing, young adult listeners through high-quality listening equipment. The average level of speech was 70 dB SPL measured under the headphones.

Quantitative measures of the intelligibility of the subject's pharyngeal speech were obtained by counting the number of correct responses to each rhyme-test word. These

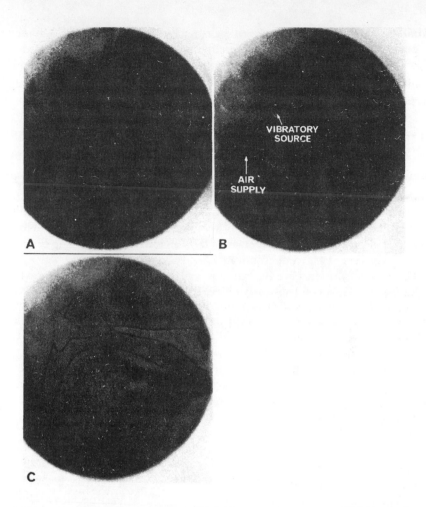

FIGURE 1. Radiographic study of pharyngeal speech. (A) Subject preparing to say /a/. (B) Subject saying /a/; neoglottis is formed between tongue and palate (see arrow). (C) /a/ completed; subject returning to postural rest.

numbers were used to calculate the percentages of correct identification (articulation scores) and the average intelligibility characteristics of pharyngeal speech for consonant and vowel rhyme-test materials.

RESULTS

Mechanism of Pharyngeal Phonation

Sound-synchronous cinefluorographic studies showed that this girl used her pharynx as a vicarious lung for speech. Air was directed from the pharynx through a neoglottis created between the tongue and the palate (Figure 1). Vibratory motions of the tongue dorsum against the palate interrupt the moving airstream to effect phonation. Of importance to the evaluation of pharyngeal speech intelligibility was the expected observation that this talker used her tongue simultaneously as both a phonatory and articulatory organ. This unique feature of pharyngeal speech might be expected to reduce her speech intelligibility, since the tongue is not free to function solely as an articulator.

Fundamental Frequency, Phonation Time, and Duration Characteristics of Pharyngeal Speech

The subject's average fundamental frequency during oral reading was 69 Hz, f_o standard deviation was 3.6 semitones, and full-range was 19 semitones. With respect to phonation time characteristics, 29% of her total speaking time was quasiperiodic, 24% was measured aperiodicity, and 47% was silence. Her speaking rate during oral reading of the first paragraph of the Rainbow Passage was 156 wpm. The maximum duration of pharyngeal phonation for a series of sustained vowels was one second.

Pharyngeal Speech Intelligibility

The average intelligibility of this girl's pharyngeal speech for consonant rhyme-test words was 76% correct. The average intelligibility of each of the consonants under test is shown in Table 1. The recognition scores for individual consonants are of particular interest since they provide information about the articulatory patterns that characterize the pharyngeal speech of the subject and provide a basis for understanding the listeners' total impression of intelligibility. Significant differences in average intelligibility were found between word-initial and word-final consonants (85 vs 67% correct) and between voiced and voiceless consonants (62 vs 90% correct). With respect to consonant type, the order of correct identification, from most to least intelligible, was affricates, fricatives-glides, plosives, and nasals.

Table 1. Average intelligibility (% correct) of consonants. Initial (I), final (F), and combined (IF) initial-final word position are tabulated. Superscript * indicates that the sound was in at least two but fewer than six word lists; † indicates that the sound was in only one word list; †† indicates that the consonant was not tested in this word position.

Consonant	I	F	IF	Consonant	I	F	IF
p	92	62	76	f	99	95*	98
b	83	40	66	v	95†	73*	76
t	97	98	97	θ	100†	82*	85
d	55	31	41	ð	74†	84†	79
k	90	83	85	s	100	93	97
g	94	49*	75	z	††	74	74
				ʃ	97	††	97
				tʃ	††	95*	95
				dʒ	100†	95†	97
m	49	68	59	h	87	††	87
n	20†	25	24				
ŋ	††	32*	32	w	97	††	97
				r	98	97	98
				l	55	100†	81

Table 2. Average intelligibility (percentage correct) of vowels.

Vowel	Percentage Correct	Vowel	Percentage Correct
ɝ	99	ʌ	59
o	86	ɔ	55
e	75	ɪ	50
ɛ	72	i	47
æ	65	a	32
ʊ	63	u	22

For vowel rhyme-test words, the average intelligibility of this girl's pharyngeal speech was 60% correct. The average intelligibility of each of the vowels under test is shown in Table 2. Of interest were the findings that mean intelligibility of diphthongized /o/ and /e/ were 86 and 75% correct, while for the semivowel /ɝ/ it was 99% correct. For the remaining nine pure vowels under test, the average intelligibility was only 52% correct.

DISCUSSION

There has been considerable confusion about the underlying mechanisms used to produce buccal, pharyngeal, and esophageal speech. Buccal, pharyngeal, and esophageal speech represent three entirely different methods of alaryngeal speech. The differences in their productive mechanisms have significant effects on the speech produced. One of the most profound differences between pharyngeal and buccal or esophageal forms of speech is the role of the tongue. The unique feature of pharyngeal speech is the simultaneous use of the tongue as both a vibratory and articulatory organ. As suggested earlier, this feature might be expected to reduce speech intelligibility, particularly for voiced sounds, since the tongue is not free to function solely as an articulator. For the pharyngeal talker studied here, a marked reduction in the intelligibility of both vowels and voiced consonants was observed.

With reference to our research, a number of informative comparisons can be made between pharyngeal, buccal, esophageal, and normal speech. Specifically, the 69-Hz average fundamental frequency of pharyngeal speech is comparable to that of male esophageal speakers (Curry and Snidecor, 1961; Weinberg and Bennett, 1972), but far below that of children her age. The inadequacy of this girl's pharyngeal voice is documented further in her phonation time characteristics. Specifically, she spent almost half (47%) of her total speaking time in silence. Moreover, she spent only 29% of her speaking time producing quasiperiodic sound and about the same proportion of time (24%) producing noise. By comparison, high-rated and excellent esophageal speakers spend about 50% of their speaking time in periodicity and less than 20% of their time producing noise (Shipp, 1967; Weinberg and Bennett, 1972). In short, this pharyngeal speaker spent about equal time producing periodicity and aperiodicity and almost half of her total speaking duration in silence. We would speculate that this talker's disproportionate amount of noise production may account for our perceptual impression of an unpleasant, markedly hoarse voice quality which was consistently evident in her pharyngeal speech (Yanagihara, 1967).

Her maximum pharyngeal phonation duration for sustained vowels (one second) is markedly shorter than that reported for even average esophageal speakers (Berlin, 1963), a factor that accounts for the marked increase in silent time exhibited by this talker. The speaking rate of 156 wpm was significantly faster than the median rate of 122 wpm reported for superior esophageal speakers (Curry and Snidecor, 1961) and slower than the average rate for normal speakers (Darley, 1940). Considering the patient's unfavorable phonation time characteristics, her speaking rate of 156 wpm is too rapid.

Her spontaneous speech is generally unintelligible to persons not acquainted with her or with the content of her discourse. With respect to consonant rhyme-test words, the average pharyngeal speech intelligibility (76% correct) was identical with that reported for a buccal speaker (Weinberg and Westerhouse, 1971) and comparable to that reported for two trained normal speakers' recordings of these rhyme-test materials presented at a signal-to-noise ratio of − 8 dB (House et al., 1965). For pharyngeal speech, consonants in the word-initial position were generally more intelligible than word-final consonants. For buccal speech, the average intelligibility of word-initial and word-final consonants are essentially the same (about 75% correct), while for esophageal and normal speech, consonants in the word-initial position are generally more intelligible (House et al., 1965; Hyman, 1955). For pharyngeal speech, voiceless consonants were significantly more intelligible than voiced consonants. For esophageal speech, voiced consonants are generally more intelligible (Hyman, 1955; Sacco, Mann, and Schultz, 1967), while for buccal speech the average intelligibility of voiced and voiceless consonants are comparable (Weinberg and Westerhouse, 1971).

With respect to vowel rhyme-test words, the average intelligibility (60% correct) to pharyngeal speech was comparable to that reported for trained normal speaker's recordings of these materials presented at a signal-to-noise ratio of − 10 to − 12 dB (Horii, 1969). Under the optimal S/N conditions used in our research, normal and excellent esophageal speakers demonstrate near-perfect intelligibility for consonant and vowel rhyme-test words (House et al., 1965; Owens and Schubert, 1968; Horii, 1969; and unpublished work of Bernd Weinberg and Y. Horii, 1972).

In summary, the poor intelligibility of this pharyngeal speaker's consonant and vowel rhyme-test words, her unfavorable phonation time and maximum phonation duration characteristics, her low-average fundamental frequency, and her poor voice quality all are distinct vocal liabilities. These results suggest that, like buccal speech (Weinberg and Westerhouse, 1971), pharyngeal speech should not be regarded as a desirable or practical primary method of alaryngeal speech.

We believe that these findings have direct clinical relevance to speech pathologists who provide alaryngeal speech instruction. For example, early attempts by the laryngectomized to produce esophageal voice are sometimes realized by the production of pharyngeal phonation. The clinician should differentiate between esophageal and pharyngeal phonation. Moreover, he should not praise or reinforce the patient's production of pharyngeal sound. Rather, he should make the patient aware of the differences between pharyngeal and esophageal phonation, and he should help the patient to replace his pharyngeal voice with consistent esophageal phonation. We believe that attempts by the laryngectomized to produce pharyngeal rather than esophageal speech represent an undesirable clinical behavior. The results of our research suggest that the basic mechanisms that underlie pharyngeal speech preclude the development of highly intelligible speech. Our clinical experience, coupled with direct measures of this girl's speech, suggest that pharyngeal speech has an unpleasant quality and is difficult to understand.

The patient studied in this research has provided and will continue to provide an informative "experiment in nature." To our knowledge, this girl is the first person with laryngeal papillomatosis to develop pharyngeal speech as an exclusive method of oral communication. Unfortunately, this type of speech does not provide her with a satisfactory method of communication. It should be emphasized that this girl's method of speaking was self-acquired and that she has never received any remedial speech training. These observations are particularly striking since she was seen regularly by a number of physicians and attended public schools where speech services were offered. She was initially referred to the Speech Research Laboratory at age 12 by an otolaryngologist. Our future goal is to help her develop other, more efficient, methods of speech. Our efforts to achieve this goal represent the substance of a newly initiated remedial speech program. The effectiveness of this clinical program will be evaluated in subsequent research using methods similar to those reported in this paper.

ACKNOWLEDGMENT

This project was supported in part by a grant from the Delaware County Cancer Society, Muncie, Indiana, and PHS Grant-NS-09262 from the National Institute of Neurological Diseases and Stroke. We gratefully acknowledge the assistance of Raleigh Lingeman in referring this patient for study. The Department of Audiology and Speech Sciences, Purdue University, provided listeners and made group listening facilities available. Requests for reprints should be directed to Bernd Weinberg, Speech Research Laboratory, Rotary Building, Indiana University Medical Center, Indianapolis, Indiana 46202.

REFERENCES

Berlin, C. I., Clinical measurement of esophageal speech: I. Methodology and curves of skill acquisition. *J. Speech Hearing Dis.*, 28, 42–51 (1963).

Curry, E. T., and Snidecor, J. C., Physical measurement and pitch perception in esophageal speech. *Laryngoscope*, 71, 415–424 (1961).

Damste, P. H., *Oesophageal Speech After Laryngectomy*. Groningen, the Netherlands: Hoitsema (1958).

Darley, F. L., A normative study of oral reading rate. Master's thesis, State Univ. of Iowa (1940).

Diedrich, W. M., and Youngstrom, K. A., *Alaryngeal Speech*. Springfield, Ill.: Thomas (1966).

Fairbanks, G., *Voice and Articulation Drillwork*. New York: Harper (1960).

Horii, Y., Specifying the speech-to-noise ratio: Development and evaluation of a noise with speech-envelope characteristics. Ph.D. dissertation, Purdue Univ. (1969).

House, A. S., Williams, C. E., Hecker, M. H. L., and Kryter, K. D., Articulation-testing methods: Consonantal differentiation with a closed-response set. *J. acoust. Soc. Amer.*, 37, 158–166 (1965).

Hyman, M., An experimental study of artificial larynx and esophageal speech. *J. Speech Hearing Dis.*, 20, 291–299 (1955).

Lauder, E., *Self-Help for the Laryngectomee*, San Antonio, Texas (1971).

Owens, E., and Schubert, E., The development of constant items for speech discrimination testing. *J. Speech Hearing Res.*, 11, 656–667 (1968).

Sacco, P. R., Mann, M. B., and Schultz, M. C., Perceptual confusions among selected phonemes in esophageal speech. *J. Ind. Speech Hearing Ass.*, 26, 19–33 (1967).

Shipp, T., Frequency, duration, and perceptual measures in relation to judgments of alaryngeal speech acceptability. *J. Speech Hearing Res.*, 10, 417–427 (1967).

Van Gilse, P. H. G., Another method of speech without larynx. *acta Otolaryng. Suppl.*, 78, 109–110 (1949).

Weinberg, B., and Bennett, S., Selected acoustic characteristics of esophageal speech produced by female laryngectomees. *J. Speech Hearing Res.*, 15, 211–216 (1972).

Weinberg, B., and Westerhouse, J., A study of buccal speech. *J. Speech Hearing Res.*, 14, 652–658 (1971).

Yanagihari, N., Significance of harmonic changes and noise components in hoarseness. *J. Speech Hearing Res.*, 10, 431–441 (1967).

PART III

INTRINSIC FORMS OF ALARYNGEAL VOICE AND SPEECH: ESOPHAGEAL SPEECH

The articles in this section deal with esophageal speech. ''The Mechanism of Esophageal Speech,'' written by William Diedrich (1968), is the finest review article on esophageal speech ever written and should prove to be one of the most widely read articles in this book. Diedrich provides an exceptionally thorough review of major issues related to esophageal speech production: air intake, theories and correlates of esophageal voice production, characteristics of esophageal speech, issues of controversy, and knowledge gaps. Readers seeking to obtain an accurate and comprehensive overview of important aspects of esophageal speech production are encouraged to read this article early in their studies. Readers with knowledge about the topic of esophageal speech production will often refer to this paper for rapid retrieval of critical information. Finally, persons using this volume as an initial introduction to the field of alaryngeal speech rehabilitation will find it useful to read this article early in their studies and to refer to it again as they complete their study of specific subtopics.

AIR INTAKE

The surgical removal of the larynx is a procedure commonly performed on patients with laryngeal cancer. Total laryngectomy necessitates the removal of the entire laryngeal framework. In this procedure, all structures located between the hyoid bone and the upper tracheal rings are sacrificed. The trachea is rotated forward and sutured to a surgically created opening. This leads to the creation of a permanent stoma, or opening, to the external neck wall for respiratory purposes and results in an anatomical, but not functional, separation between the pulmonary airway and the digestive tract.

Total laryngectomy surgery always results in a sacrifice of tissue essential to normal vocal function and in considerable alteration of the anatomy and physiology of the speech mechanism. As a result, the normal processes of speech are modified to such a great extent that there is always a complete loss of the ability to produce voice by conventional means. Laryngectomized patients compensate for this loss by using alternative methods of voicing to support speech production. Currently, the most common form of alaryngeal speech is esophageal speech.

Production of esophageal voicing necessitates use of the esophagus as an accessory lung and use of the pharyngoesophageal (P-E) segment as a voicing source. The pharyngoesophageal segment is the upper sphinter of the esophagus and serves to divide the pharynx from the esophagus. In normal humans, this segment consists of the cricopharyngeus muscle, fibers of the pharyngeal inferior constrictor, and upper fibers of esophageal muscle. The pharyngoesophageal segment does undergo major morphological and functional change as a result of laryngeal extirpation. Larynx removal results in a significant sacrifice of tissue critical to postsurgical esophageal voice acquisition. Moreover, the morphological and physiological characteristics of the P-E segment in laryngectomized patients are highly variable. Hence, the P-E segment in laryngectomized patients represents a surgical residue, i.e., an aggregate of structures remaining following tumor removal and reconstruction by the operating surgeon.

On an oversimplified basis, the production of esophageal voicing can be described as a two-part process: air intake and voicing. The esophageal speaker must effect a pressure drop across the pharyngoesophageal segment to effect either air intake or voicing.

Esophageal speakers insufflate air into the esophagus by means of the injection or the inhalation methods of air intake. The injection method of air intake is a positive pressure·respiratory maneuver. Basically, persons using this method complete tongue compression maneuvers and/or articulatory gestures to generate increased oral and pharyngeal pressure. The magnitude of these pressures must be large enough to override pressure in the P-E segment, causing the segment to open and permit air to enter the esophagus. Moolenaar-Bijl (1953), a Dutch speech therapist, provides the original description of what is now known as consonant injection and was the first person to advance the notion that esophageal insufflation can occur as a result of pressure build-up associated with the production of certain types of consonants. Weinberg and Bosma (1970) describe a second type of injection, now known as glossal or glossopharyngeal press. In this case, the compression maneuver is a separate act analogous to glossopharyngeal, or frog, breathing.

By contrast, the inhalation method of air intake is a pulmonary activated method of air insufflation. Although firm experimental verification of this method is not available, Isshiki and Snidecor (1965) provide some indirect descriptions of this approach and a very concise explanation is given by Diedrich (1968). Since inhalation is a pulmonary activated method, air is taken into the esophagus synchronously with pulmonary inhalation. In this method, air is directed into the esophagus by having patients inhale pulmonary air, a behavior that causes the magnitude of negative pressure in the esophagus to increase. Patients are instructed either to keep their mouths open or to sniff during pulmonary inhalation. Under these two conditions, air pressure in the mouth will be positive, i.e., roughly equivalent to atmospheric pressure. Hence, air will flow from the area of positive pressure (mouth and pharynx) to the area of increased negative pressure (esophagus), provided that the resistance of the P-E segment can be overcome.

Following insufflation of air into the esophagus, the speaker must develop a transpseudoglottal pressure differential to drive the P-E segment into oscillation. In this case, the differential pressure relationship is always characterized by esophageal pressures that exceed the resistance offered by the P-E segment. Stated differently, the speaker must develop positive esophageal pressure of sufficient magnitude to exceed the resistance offered by the closed P-E segment, causing the segment to vibrate for voicing.

ACOUSTIC, TEMPORAL, AND PERCEPTUAL
CHARACTERISTICS OF ESOPHAGEAL SPEECH

A large body of research has been conducted in order to describe some of the important characteristics of esophageal speech. Since total laryngectomy always results in a sacrifice of tissue essential to normal vocal function, clinicians and investigators have assumed that the principal factors affected by laryngectomy are those related to the voicing source. Hence, there have been a number of studies completed to specify the fundamental frequency (f_0) and phonation time characteristics of esophageal speech. A review of this information reveals that the fundamental frequency characteristics of esophageal speakers are now well understood. The three Snidecor and Curry (1959, 1960, 1961) papers are primary references for this topic. The results of their work indicate that the average f_0 for male esophageal speakers was about 65 Hz, a value approximately one octave below that expected for normal adult speakers. In addition, the magnitude of measured f_0 variability (approximately four semitones) indicates that the amount of f_0 variation present in connected discourse produced by esophageal speakers is equal to, and often greater than, that measured for normal speakers. Subsequent acoustic studies (Shipp, 1967; Hoops and Noll, 1969; Weinberg and Bennett, 1971, 1972) provide data that verify these early observations. Weinberg and Bennett (1971, 1972) reveal that average f_0 characteristics of esophageal speech may differ as a function of speaker sex and may highlight the extensive variation in average f_0 exhibited by esophageal speakers.

Although it is reasonable to conclude that the fundamental frequency characteristics of esophageal voice are reasonably well understood, information concerning fundamental aspects of esophageal phonation is lacking. For example, the nature of anatomical and physiological mechanisms underlying the regulation of f_0 and vocal intensity are not understood. Information concerning acoustic characteristics of esophageal voice other than f_0, for example, source spectral characteristics, is also not available. Such information is essential to future understanding of quality attributes of esophageal voice and to the development of models or theories of esophageal phonation. In this context, Smith, Weinberg, Feth, and Horii (1978) reveal that the depth of ambiguity surrounding our understanding of esphageal voice quality attributes and underscores the usefulness of examining clinically disordered speakers in order to provide insights into fundamental questions concerning the nature of speech production and perception, in general.

It is clear that until recently the majority of research and clinical work dealing with esophageal speech has been directed toward problems associated with voice reacquisition and toward description of selected attributes of esophageal voice. The results of recent work make it apparent that total laryngectomy surgery also causes substantial changes in the nonphonatory aspects of speech production. For example, Snidecor and Curry (1959, 1960) have clearly demonstrated that the speech rate of esophageal speakers is markedly reduced. The speaking rate of six superior esophageal speakers ranged from 85 to 129 words per minute, with the group average of 113 words per minute. The assumption has always been that the decrement in rate of esophageal speech is due to the increase in the amount of time these speakers spend in silence. This increase in silent time results from the esophageal speaker's limited ability to sustain voicing. For example, the esophageal speaker produces an average of five words per air charge compared to a mean of 12.5 words per breath group produced by normal speakers (Snidecor and Curry, 1961). Hence, the esophageal speaker must pause more often for air intake. In addition, Snidecor and Curry (1960) observe differential length in pauses occurring in esophageal speech. For example, phrase limiting pauses (i.e., junctural pauses) were approximately 1.41 times longer than air intake pauses. The mean duration of pauses signaling juncture in esophageal speech was also greater than the mean duration of junctural pauses measured for a normal speaker.

Although comprehensive knowledge about articulatory changes due to laryngeal extirpation is lacking, there is experimental evidence to support the notion that total laryngectomy surgery does alter articulatory behavior. For example, the hyoid bone is typically removed during total laryngectomy and its removal necessitates disruption of much of the musculature of the suprahyoid complex and supporting musculature of the tongue. Such disruptions, coupled with the deprivation of pulmonary support, are likely to affect the articulatory dynamics of laryngectomized patients. Diedrich (1968) notes a number of changes in articulatory dynamics of esophageal speakers. For example, esophageal speakers evidenced more continuous movement of the tongue and shorter duration of articulatory contact of the tongue or lips in comparison with durations sampled on a preoperative basis in this group of patients. Dealing with formant frequency characteristics of esophageal speech, Sisty and Weinberg (1972) show that removal of the larynx does alter vocal-cavity transmission characteristics. The observation that the average vowel formant frequency values associated with esophageal speech were elevated was interpreted to support the view that laryngectomized patients exhibit a reduced vocal tract length. Sacco, Mann, and Schultz (1967), Creech (1966), and Tikofsky (1965) provide strong support for the general beliefs that, on the average, esophageal speech is characterized by a reduction in intelligibility and that efficient contrast of the voicing (voiced versus voiceless) feature is difficult for esophageal speakers to achieve. These results lend credence to the view that extirpation of the larynx results in substantial changes in both phonatory and nonphonatory aspects of speech production.

Horii and Weinberg (1975) emphasize the effects that broadband masking noise has on the intelligibility of speech and suggests that esophageal speech is more vulnerable to deterioration by noise than normal speech supported by laryngeal voice sources. Taken together, the results of studies in this section of the text lend credence to the view that extirpation of larynx results in substantial changes in both phonatory and nonphonatory aspects of speech production.

It is apparent that the bulk of research and clinical studies have been descriptive in nature. Only recently have investigators been interested in examining, in a serious fashion, linguistic aspects of esophageal speech. For example, studies of the degree to which larynx removal affects the realization of rule-governed features or linguistic contrasts have only recently been undertaken. In this context, Christensen and Weinberg (1976) reveal that esophageal speakers do exhibit changes in articulatory behavior as evidenced by altered durational characteristics of vowels. Although this observation is true, the inherent, rule-governed relationship between vowel duration and voicing features of consonant environment was not altered in esophageal speech. The latter finding was interpreted to support the belief that some inherent, rule-governed durational features of English are retained following laryngeal extirpation. Christensen, Weinberg, and Alfonso (1978) provide information about productive voice onset time (VOT) characteristics of esophageal speech. In this regard, it is now well known that normal speakers of English systematically vary the timing of voice onset to distinguish prevocalic, voiceless stops, /p/, /t/, and /k/, from their so-called voiced counterparts, /b/, /d/, and /g/. Esophageal speakers were also found to be capable of systematically varying VOT to distinguish prevocalic stops /p/, /t/, and /k/ from /b/, /d/, and /g/. This observation is intriguing in light of the striking differences between the voice and speech producing systems of normal and esophageal speakers. The data of this project were interpreted, in part, to support the notion that esophageal speakers are capable of effecting systematic and linguistically appropriate variation in the timing of voicing onset. Although this general conclusion was made, these data also revealed that esophageal speakers were far less consistent than normal speakers in effecting phonological contrasts.

By way of summary, it should be noted that a large number of forms of linguistic contrast have not been examined in esophageal speech. For example, information concerning the efficacy with which esophageal speakers are able to effect intonation, stress, and junctural contrasts is nonexistent, but of some considerable theoretical and clinical interest.

ANATOMICAL AND PHYSIOLOGICAL ASPECTS OF ESOPHAGEAL VOICING AND SPEECH

The current state of knowledge about physiological aspects of esophageal phonation and speech is limited. For example, reference was made earlier to the fact that information about the anatomical and physiological mechanisms underlying control of fundamental aspects of esophageal phonation is lacking. In addition, studies of anatomical and physiological mechanisms underlying the control of articulatory and suprasegmental behaviors of esophageal speech production are also lacking.

Early classic investigations in this area attempted to delineate the nature of change in the structure and the function of the pharynx and the esophagus resulting from laryngectomy. For example, Kirchner, Scatliff, Dey, and Shedd (1963) sought answers to these questions in data obtained from cinefluorographic examinations and intraluminal pressure measurements of the pharynx and the esophagus. Kirchner et al. (1963), coupled with the review provided by Diedrich (1968), make it apparent that the points of attachment of a large number of extrinsic laryngeal muscles along with the cricopharyngeus muscle are sacrificed during total laryngectomy surgery. The data reviewed in these articles provide ample support for the notion that the voicing source used to support esophageal speech can properly be regarded as a surgical residuum characterized by extensive intersubject variability. Moreover, the information presented in this section of the text reveals that the relationships between speech or vocal proficiency and morphological or physiological characteristics of the P-E segment or esophagus remain unspecified.

The evidence provided by Kirshner et al. (1963), by Diedrich (1968) and by Winans, Reichbach, and Waldrop (1974) suggest that total laryngectomy effects slight alterations in the anatomy and physiology of the esophagus. As stated earlier, laryngeal attachments of the cricopharyngeus muscle are, of necessity, cut when removing the larynx. This may account for the observations of weakened contractions of the cricopharyngeus muscle postsurgery (Kirchner et al., 1963; Winans et al., 1974) and for altered patterns of contraction in the upper esophagus in some laryngectomized patients. Namely, the observations of Kirchner et al. (1963) revealed that the amplitude of esophageal peristalsis was depressed in the area of the upper esophagus in some laryngectomized patients. Peristaltic activity of the lower esophagus and function of the lower esophageal sphincter were not observed to be altered by disturbances of the function of the upper esophagus or of the cricopharyngeus muscle. The body of the esophagus in laryngectomized patients, like that of normal speakers, is bound at both ends by a zone of elevated pressure, while intraesophageal pressure was negative relative to atmospheric pressure.

The pharyngoesophageal segment does undergo major morphological and functional change as a result of laryngeal extirpation. The observations of Diedrich (1968) and of Kirshner et al. (1963) reveal that some laryngectomized patients exhibit well-defined single P-E segments, typically located between cervical vertebrae 4 and 6. In other patients, more than one segment was observed. For example, some patients exhibited double and triple segments. Finally, Diedrich and Youngstrom (1966) fail to observe a well defined P-E segment during voice production in a small number of esophageal speakers. The high degree of variability in the morphological characteristics of the segment represents a consistent, reasonable, and clinically relevant observation. The observation that the morphology of the P-E segment in laryngectomized patients is highly variable is not surprising, since the postsurgical characteristics of the segment might properly be regarded as surgical residue. Stated differently, the P-E segment in laryngectomized patients represents an aggregate of structures remaining following tumor removal and reconstruction by the operating surgeon.

Winans, Reichbach, and Waldrop (1974) describe how intraluminal manometry techniques might be applied to the study of P-E segment and esophageal function in laryngectomized patients. The strengths of this article lie in the description of intraluminal manometry and in the description of function of the esophagus and segment of laryngectomized patients during swallow and rest. The degree to which observations of function during nonspeech tasks relate to function during speech production is not clear. In view of the known differences between speech and nonspeech motor behavior, conclusions concerning the nature of physiological differences between "good" and "poor" esophageal speech seem highly tenable, if not unwarranted.

Shipp (1970), using excellent experimental procedures and design, provides useful insights into the nature of pharyngoesophageal muscle function in esophageal speakers. Electromyographic measurements were obtained from 18 laryngectomized subjects during speech and nonspeech tasks. The article by Shipp is particularly intriguing for persons seeking to use biofeedback techniques as part of a diagnostic/therapeutic speech rehabilitation program for laryngectomized patients.

"Air Volume and Air Flow Relationships of Six Male Esophageal Speakers" (Snidecor and Isshiki, 1965) continues to serve as a primary reference about the aerodynamics of esophageal voice and speech. Using time-honored experimental techniques, Snidecor and Isshiki provide the most comprehensive information about air flow and volume characteristics of esophageal speech. One of the more salient findings stemming from this work is the observation of diminished air flow and volume characteristics associated with the production of esophageal voice. For example, the mean flow rate associated with sustained vowels produced by esophageal speakers ranged from about 30–70 cc/sec. These values are markedly lower than those associated with normal vowel production, where flow rates range from about 100–200 cc/sec. These data, coupled with information about esophageal pressures during vowel production provided by Diedrich (1968), shed light upon the efficacy of the P-E segment as a voicing generator. Specifically, esophageal pressure ranges between about 20–60 cm H_2O during sustained vowel production by esophageal speakers. In this case, the pressure values are markedly higher than those associated with normal vowel production where subglottic pressure typically ranges between about 3–10 cm H_2O.

Taken together, current data suggest that the resistance (pseudoglottal resistance) offered by the voicing source associated with esophageal phonation is an order of magnitude larger than that offered by the larynx. Thus, in addition to being a surgical residuum devoid of abductor-adductor properties, the voicing source of esophageal speech appears to be a heavily mass-loaded, high impedance source.

EVALUATION AND ASSESSMENT

The first total laryngectomy was performed just over a century ago. Hence, the history of implementing esophageal speech and voice retraining into speech rehabilitation programs for laryngectomized patients is both long and rich. In view of its rich history and the fact that esophageal speech continues to represent the primary method of speech for laryngectomized patients, methods of evaluation and assessment merit critical study. Evaluation and assessment should be considered in terms of assessing the ultimate proficiency of esophageal speech, measuring speech changes occurring as a consequence of therapeutic intervention and evaluating factors known to either facilitate or interfere with the development of proficient esophageal speech.

For example, Wepman, MacGahan, Rickard, and Shelton (1953) provide an early attempt to develop a rating scale used in the evaluation of esophageal speech proficiency.

The Wepman et al. scale has been widely used, and serious students of alaryngeal speech must become familiar with this rating scale. The Wepman et al. scale is a general scale that incorporates arbitrary or empirically derived proficiency levels. The scale uses broad categories or classifications that, although useful, do not provide a system of proficiency classification that is universally accepted.

Berlin (1963), Berlin and Zo Bell (1963), and Berlin (1965) deal primarily with the problem of measuring patient progress during treatment. The major thrust of Berlin's work centers on the measurement of four skill-building behaviors essential to the supporting alaryngeal speech with esophageal voicing. The four skills, which appear to have a certain degree of face validity relationship with the production of esophageal speech adequacy, are the ability 1) to phonate reliably on demand, 2) to maintain short latency between esophageal insufflation and voicing, 3) to maintain adequate duration of phonation, and 4) to sustain phonation during articulation. Clinicians will find that the Berlin measures can be effectively used to chart patient progress, particularly during the early stages of esophageal speech development.

Berlin and Zo Bell (1963) suggest that specific changes in the ability of esophageal speakers to maintain adequate duration of phonation may provide an early sign of recurrence of cancer in the hypopharyngeal area.

Creech (1966) and Tikofsky (1965) deal with evaluating esophageal speech in terms of intelligibility criterion. Speech intelligibility clearly represents an important measure related to the perceived proficiency or acceptability of esophageal speech. Creech (1966) and Tikofsky (1965) have also revealed how speech pathologists can obtain ratings of the relative intelligibility of esophageal speech. The statement by Creech that "...as an esophageal speaker approaches 60 percent intelligibility, serious consideration should be given to dismissing him from therapy..." (1966, p. 18) is both unwarranted and misleading. The goal is to develop near-perfect intelligibility is esophageal speakers. Hence, the recommendation made by Creech seriously undercuts therapeutic efficacy and may fail to lead many laryngectomized speakers to their ultimate speech potential.

The problem of speech assessment of esophageal speech is attacked from slightly different perspectives by Shipp (1967) and by Hoops and Noll (1969). The purpose of their work was to identify acoustic and temporal characteristics of esophageal speech that influence listeners' ratings of speech acceptability or proficiency. To accomplish this objective, they subjected recordings of esophageal speech to several forms of acoustic and temporal analysis and perceptual evaluation. Basically, the results of their work revealed that a number of variables (speech rate, phonation time characteristics, and severity of respiratory, or stomal, noise ratings) were significantly related to judgments of speech acceptability. Although these works may appear somewhat technical and experimental to clinically oriented readers, the results of these two pieces are highly clinically relevant. Namely, speech pathologists seeking to increase the proficiency of esophageal speech should endeavor to decrease the level of stomal noise, to increase speech rate, to decrease the amount of time speakers spend in silence, and to increase the amount of time speakers spend voicing.

Finally, there is the issue of identifying factors that may limit or preclude either the acquisition of esophageal voicing or the development of functionally serviceable esophageal speech. This is not a trivial issue for clinical speech pathologists or surgeons, and it has been addressed by Shames, Font, and Matthews (1963) who sought to identify biographical, medical, personality-social, communication, and speech training variables that correlated with speech proficiency. Comparative information about the relationship between these factors is also provided for users of artificial larynges. Although significant relationships were found between a sizable number of variables and speech proficiency, such data should not be interpreted to support the view that predictors for esophageal voice and speech acquisition have been established.

GENERAL AND PSYCHOSOCIAL FACTORS

Comprehensive review of the literature on total laryngectomy and esophageal speech rehabilitation reflects a predominant interest in such areas as the diagnosis of laryngeal malignancy, surgical and nonsurgical treatment regimes, anatomical and physiological determinants of alaryngeal voice and speech production, and characteristics of speech after laryngectomy. Fundamental to any discussion of laryngeal malignancy, total laryngectomy, and speech rehabilitation is the fact that we are dealing with people. Hence, serious study of the topic of speech after laryngectomy must include an examination of such issues as patient's reactions to the diagnosis of laryngeal cancer and the subsequent surgery, presurgical and postoperative anxieties, fears and trauma, and reactions to altered physical appearance, body state, and related medical and social problems. In addition, readers must examine the extent to which psychosocial factors may be related to the successful acquisition of speech after laryngectomy. For example, Du Guay (1966) provides useful information about the presurgical views of laryngectomized patients concerning the nature of their postsurgical speech. Du Duay highlights some dramatic and, in some cases, pathetic, misconceptions harbored by patients and provides rehabilitation specialists with practical suggestions on alleviating those misconceptions. Gardner (1966) emphasizes the special problems encountered by women undergoing total laryngectomy and alaryngeal speech rehabilitation. Readers not familiar with the historical aspects of this field should recognize that Dr. Gardner, a speech pathologist thoroughly experienced in all facets of alaryngeal speech rehabilitation, is the founder of the International Association of Laryngectomees, an organization solely devoted to the care and treatment of individuals undergoing total laryngectomy.

Amster, Love, Menzel, Sandler, Sculthorpe, and Gross (1972) provide a comprehensive examination of psychosocial factors and speech after laryngectomy. Their study, coupled with their extensive literature and bibliographic review, is essential reading for persons seriously interested in the problems of alaryngeal speech. More recently, Gilmore (1974) explores the social and vocational acceptability of esophageal speakers and normal speakers. The results of this work, which revealed that esophageal speakers experience reductions in social and vocational status, are of considerable significance to all professionals involved in the treatment of laryngectomized patients.

THE MECHANISM OF ESOPHAGEAL SPEECH

William M. Diedrich

Hearing and Speech Department
University of Kansas Medical Center
Kansas City, Kan.

INTRODUCTION

Extirpation of the larynx because of cancer results in radical changes, not only in man's basic physiology, but also in his social process of communication. The broader term "communication" is used here because the removal of the larynx affects not only the vocal function in speech but also the articulation of speech. In addition, there is a disturbance of the extralinguistic vocal behaviors (coughs, "uh-huhs," and "hmms"), the inflection and intensity, and the emotional expressions of laughing and crying. Vicarious and artificially devised methods have provided compensatory mechanisms for speaking, but not for these more subtle vocal expressions. Four general types of alaryngeal speech are used: buccal, pharyngeal, esophageal, and artificial larynx. In this paper, the specific mechanisms of esophageal speech will be discussed in detail.

Following removal of the larynx, the trachea is sutured to the base of the neck to provide a permanent stoma for respiratory purposes. The patient no longer breathes through his nose, and consequently there is no longer a need for the complex valvular action provided by the larynx for closing off the airway during deglutition. Furthermore, to acquire esophageal speech, a patient must learn to insufflate air into his esophagus and expel the air for phonatory purposes. The detailed description that follows will attempt to describe the processes of air intake, air expulsion, phonation, and articulation during esophageal speech.

AIR INTAKE

The basic problem in air intake is to get the air through the closed pharyngo-esophageal (P-E) vestibule and into the esophagus. The normal physiological contraction of the pharyngo-esophageal fibers prevents air from entering the esophagus. This becomes a special problem in cases with functional spasm of the cricopharyngeal sphincter (van den Berg & Moolenaar-Bijl, 1959). However, Dey and Kirchner (1961) have shown that the normal tonic contraction (10 mm Hg) of the esophageal sphincter is usually diminished (5 mm Hg) and may be absent in the laryngectomized patient. Furthermore, they state that the sphincter alone does not prevent esophageal respiration.

Methods of Air Intake

Some cinefluorographic studies (Schlosshauer & Möckel, 1958; Motta *et al.*, 1959) have observed three methods of air intake: deglutition, aspiration, and injection. Other cinefluorographic studies (Damsté, 1958; Diedrich & Youngstrom, 1966) have stressed just two methods—inhalation and injection. Deglutition was differentiated from air injection on the basis of the dynamic movement patterns observed in the tongue, palate, and pharynx (Diedrich & Youngstrom, 1966).

Reprinted by permission from *Annals of the New York Academy of Sciences*, 1968, *155*, 303–317.

During *inhalation* the patient maintains a patent airway either between the lips and the esophagus or between the nose and the esophagus. As the patient inhales pulmonary air, there is a subsequent decrease in the negative pressure that normally exists in the esophagus. In other words, the negative pressure in the esophagus at rest, which is several mm Hg below atmospheric pressure (Atkinson *et al.,* 1957), increases to about −10 to −15 mm Hg during pulmonary inhalation. Thus a partial vacuum is created in the esophagus. Atmospheric air pressure in the mouth and hypopharynx will push air into the esophagus if the tonic closure of the pharyngo-esophageal fibers is relaxed.

During the *injection* procedure, air in the oropharyngeal cavities is compressed by movements of the tongue into the esophagus. Usually a tongue-tip-alveolar-ridge contact prevents the air from going out of the mouth, and velopharyngeal closure prevents the air from going into the nasal passages. As the tongue injects the air from the oropharyngeal cavities into the esophagus, one or both of two things must happen: Either the compressed air in the oropharyngeal cavities must override the tonic contraction of the P-E segment fibers and/or the P-E segment fibers must relax, allowing the compressed air to be pushed into the esophagus.

Speed of Air Intake

Several studies have shown that the air intake speed is quite rapid. Damsté (1958) found in 23 patients that they averaged 0.21 sec for air intake. He had a range of 0.12–0.27 seconds. He found that one patient in his series who used inhalation required an average of 0.6 sec for air intake. The remaining patients were injectors. Snidecor and Curry (1959) found by electropneumographic and electrical-photographic techniques that the air charge took approximately one-half second for superior speakers (mean values of 0.42 to 0.80 sec). Isshiki and Snidecor (1965), using air pressure variation in a pneumograph sensitized by a strain gauge pressure transducer, recorded mean durations of air intake of 0.11 to 0.32 sec, with a median of 0.18 seconds. Diedrich and Youngstrom (1966) found that, from a position of rest, air intake speed averaged about 0.5 seconds. They also found that there was a *prephonation* time between the end of air intake and actual phonation that was approximately one-fifth of a second. This is approximately the same time that Berlin (1963) obtained with mean values of 0.24 sec for a period of latency that occurred between an audible inflation and phonation. In a later study using the Brujl and Kjaer graphic recorder, Berlin (1965) found mean latency times between air intake and phonation to be about 0.4 seconds.

Temporal Occurrence

Air intake may occur during esophageal speech at two different times in a given speech utterance (Diedrich & Youngstrom, 1966). This is different from air intake in normal speakers, which usually occurs only at rest or during an interphrase pause. However, during esophageal speech, air intake may occur not only from a position of rest or during an interphrase pause but also during the intraphrase interval (speech pulse or speech utterance). Air may be inhaled or injected from a position of rest or during the interphrase interval; however, air can only be injected (not inhaled into the esophagus) during an intraphrase interval. As a result of the intraoral ballistic movements that are necessary during the articulation of the voiceless consonant sounds, it is hypothesized that air may be injected into the esophagus, usually in the releasing (initial) but not in the arresting (final) position. The plosive and sibilant sounds and the sibilant-plosive blends seem especially useful for this type of air injection, although articulation of other voiceless fricatives may achieve the same result. Further discussion of the interrelationship between air intake and articulation during esophageal speech will be discussed under the section on articulation.

Recent airflow studies (Snidecor & Isshiki, 1965a and 1965b; Isshiki & Snidecor, 1965) have shown that during the intraphase interval air may flow into the esophagus with voicing. Although not a frequent phenomenon, it occurs more often than imagined from clinical observation.

Air Intake Phase Relationships with Pulmonary Function

Probably no one aspect of esophageal speech has been subject to more controversy over the years than that of whether the esophageal speaker uses insufflation of air into the esophagus in synchrony with pulmonary inhalation or not. Robe and colleagues (1956) summarized the historic clash, and their work indicated that asynchrony did not exist. However, airflow studies of Snidecor and Isshiki (1965a) and Isshiki and Snidecor (1965), using more recent techniques, have provided evidence that asynchrony and synchrony do occur, not only for different speakers but for the same speaker. The phenomenon is complicated by the temporal occurrence of the air intake and the method of air intake.

They have categorized eight different periods of airflow:

1. Oronasal airflow *in,* with no phonation; tracheal airflow *in.*
2. Oronasal airflow *in,* with phonation; tracheal air *in.*
3. Oronasal air *in,* with no phonation; tracheal air *out.*
4. Oronasal air *in,* with phonation; tracheal air *out.*
5. Oronasal airflow *out,* with no phonation; tracheal airflow *in.*
6. Oronasal air *out,* with phonation; tracheal air *in.*
7. Oronasal air *out,* with no phonation; tracheal air *out.*
8. Oronasal air *out,* with phonation; tracheal air *out.*

In general, synchrony predominates for both methods of air intake, especially with those who use inhalation. Inhalation of esophageal air cannot be done during pulmonary exhalation. Those who use the injection method of air intake were found more often to be asynchronous. The reason for this is that air injection can occur on plosive or sibilant sounds during the intraphrase interval, i.e., during pulmonary exhalation. It also should be remembered that good speakers used both methods of air intake.

Isshiki and Snidecor (1965) also have shown that esophageal speakers reading the Rainbow Passage have a range of respirations from 3 to 36, with a median of 24, as compared to six respirations for one normal speaker. They found that four out of six good esophageal speakers insufflated a larger percentage of *air volume* in synchrony with inhalation of pulmonary air than they did with exhalation. They also found that four out of the six speakers spent *more time* taking air into the esophagus with exhalation than they did with exhalation of pulmonary air. One surprising finding was the percentage of air volume that was voiced during insufflation. There was a range of 14 to 67%, with a median of 28%; in other words, over one-fourth of the insufflation was voiced during the reading of the passage. One good speaker phonated over two-thirds of the time during esophageal air intake and was classified as an injector. Since voice on air intake is usually associated with the inhalation method—and not during injection, at least in my experience—this finding is even more unique.

Airflow Rates on Air Intake

Again the Snidecor and Isshiki (1965a) studies provide information regarding rates of airflow during esophageal intake. The median mean rate for dominate air intake method was 94 cc/sec as compared to 976 cc/sec for one normal subject. When total volume and total speech time were computed, the median rate of air intake for the six esophageal subjects was found to be 29 cc/sec (Isshiki & Snidecor, 1965).

Extraneous Noises

A variety of noises may accompany air intake. The klunking sound is observed during injection, not inhalation, and may occur when air intake is done from the rest or interphrase interval, but it is not observed during the articulation of an intraphase interval (Diedrich & Youngstrom, 1966). It was observed that when the tongue retrudes to force air into the esophagus, the hypopharynx is frequently obliterated, and when the tongue moves forward, the klunking is heard when air fills this cavity (Diedrich & Youngstrom, 1966; Isshiki, 1966); however, klunking also was heard when the hypopharynx was not occluded, and it may be the result of air implosion into the esophagus.

Stoma noise (whistling, breathing, or blowing) frequently is associated with air intake (Diedrich & Youngstrom, 1966:103):

> Those who use the inhalation method of esophageal air intake tend to make stoma noises on both inhalation and exhalation of pulmonary air. Those who inject air usually do not make noise on inhalation of pulmonary air, but stoma noise may be heard on expulsion of the esophageal air in synchrony with pulmonary exhalation. Stoma noise may be heard during air intake from rest or during interphrase pauses, but it is not heard on air intake (which can only be injection) during intraphrase intervals.

THE AIR RESERVOIR

Esophagus

In the older literature (Kallen, 1934), it was often believed that the stomach participated as an air reservoir. From x-ray data, Ragaglini and associates (1956) concluded that the source of the air supply for phonation was in the hypopharynx. Most workers using radiographic techniques (Hodson & Oswald, 1958; Schlosshauer & Möckel, 1958; Kamieth, 1959; Motta, *et al.*, 1959; Vrtička & Svoboda, 1961, 1963) have concluded that the normal air reservoir in esophageal speech is the esophagus. Snidecor and Isshiki (1965b) reported an unusual case of a patient who had the rare ability to insufflate over 600 cc, but they quickly pointed out that he usually did not use these amounts of air during conversation. Since 80 cc of air is generally considered the capacity of the esophagus (van den Berg & Moolenaar-Bijl, 1959), this patient was obviously using the stomach, in addition to the esophagus, to contain this volume of air.

Volume of Air Use

Up to 50 cc of air may enter the esophagus at the beginning of a swallow; at the end of the swallow, the same amount generally leaves the esophagus (Isshiki & Snidecor, 1965). The median dominant airflow rates for air intake was 94 cc per sec, and since the median air intake time was 0.18, this means that only about one-fourth to one-half of the esophagus (based on a 40- to 80-cc capacity) is actually being refilled during a reading passage. The data of Snidecor and Isshiki (1965a) indicated that there was a range in volume of 372 to 1,115 cc for 51 words—a median of 935 cc, as compared to 3,020 cc for the normal. This means that the range of volume of air per syllable during continuous speech for 51 words was 5.0 to 15.9 cc, with a median of 13.4 cc per syllable for the six subjects. An average of 43.1 cc per syllable was obtained for one normal speaker for the same passage.

It can be concluded from this research that air volume per se was not related to the type of speaker; rather, the airflow rates on exsufflation were important. These rates are determined by volume of air trapped, amount of pressure developed in the esophagus, and amount of resistance supplied by the vibrator. These last two factors will be discussed in more detail in the next two sections.

AIR EXPULSION

Intraluminal Pressures

The intraesophageal air pressure at rest is -4 to -7 mm Hg below atmospheric pressure (Kramer et al., 1957; Ingelfinger, 1958), this may decrease to -15 mm Hg (Dey & Kirchner, 1961) on pulmonary inspiration. No oronasal airflow is detected in the laryngectomee (Isshiki & Snidecor, 1965).

During esophageal speech, the negative pressures may reach -15 to -20 mm Hg in the esophagus, and after insufflation of air, the pressure is immediately reversed and positive pressures of 25 mm Hg (Dey & Kirchner, 1961) and 50 cm H_2O (Salmon, 1965) have been recorded during phonation. Average positive pressures of 10 to 30 cm H_2O are sufficient to produce audible sound, and 50 to 75 cm H_2O are sufficient for high pitch and high intensity. In patients who have cricopharyngeal spasms, up to 100 or more cm H_2O pressure have been recorded (van den Berg & Moolenaar-Bijl, 1959) before phonation is heard. Damsté (1958) observed 30 to 40 cm H_2O pressure in good esophageal speakers. Vrtička and colleagues (1965), using a manometer device similar to van den Berg's, found an average of 35 mm Hg pressure in 43 laryngectomees. In good esophageal speakers, pressure as low as 20 mm Hg was recorded, while slow rehabilitation was noted for those who had 40 to 80 mm Hg. For pressures of 90 mm Hg, the phonatory effort was described as a "rattled voice." Frint and Pauka (1965) used another variation of the van den Berg technique and examined 22 laryngectomized patients. The good speakers averaged 17 cm H_2O and the poor speakers 35 cm H_2O after they had emptied the esophagus. With good speakers, spontaneous eructation occurred with pressures of 7 to 29 cm H_2O, and poor speakers registered 30 to 56 cm H_2O. Frint and Pauka also found that spontaneous eructation pressures were lower than those of voluntary eructation. Low esophageal pressures in good speakers rose to above 30 cm H_2O when functional spasm of the cricopharyngeal sphincter occurred. Because of the tremendous amount of pressure variability found in her study, Salmon (1965) questioned whether good and poor speakers can be predicted on the basis of intraesophageal pressure measurements.

Air Flow

In esophageal speakers, Snidecor and Isshiki (1965a) found mean flow rate values during continuous speech for voiced air expulsion that ranged from 25 to

97 cc/sec, with a median of 61 cc/sec. This compares with normal voiced air-flow during continuous speech of 219 cc/sec.

They reported (1965b) flow rates for sustained /a/ in a superior esophageal speaker of 20 to 75 cc/sec for soft or medium voice and 85 to 100 cc/sec for a loud voice, with a mean flow of 72 cc/sec for "easy" phonation. These values are much greater than those for most esophageal speakers. The flow rate in normals for comfortable sustained /a/ was 70 to 180 cc/sec. These authors point out that the mean flow rates are comparable to those estimated by van den Berg and coworkers (1958).

Mechanisms for Air Expulsion

As pulmonary air is expelled, there is a subsequent increase in the positive pressure within the esophagus and the air is forced upward through the P-E segment, which results in phonation. If the understanding of the mechanisms of air intake is not clear and seems complex, the dynamics of air expulsion are still more enigmatic. There are several problems to be resolved, including the morphology and physiology of the esophagus, its cephalad and caudad sphincters, the position of the esophagus within the chest cavity, and the effect on the esophagus of intrapulmonary pressure changes, diaphragmatic tension, stomach pressures, and abdominal muscle contractions.

Van den Berg and associates (1958) attempted to answer the question of what keeps the pressure in the esophagus constant during escape of air:

(1) A voluntary active contraction of the striated muscles of the upper part of the oesophagus . . . the primary consequence would be an obstruction for the escape of air from the oesophagus.

(2) A direct compression of the region of the cardia by the diaphragm. . . . The oesophageal pressure would be scarcely affected, as the air might escape to other regions of the oesophagus, passively distending the walls.

(3) The passive behavior of the non-muscular component of the wall of the oesophagus, giving rise to a volume-pressure relationship like that of many vessels of our body, which behave as elastomeres, having a certain region in which the volume can vary much at a nearly constant pressure.

(4) The passive increase of the oesophageal pressure by expiratory movements of the thorax. In the average normal subject this increase amounts to 0.17 cm of water/100 ml/sec of expired air during normal breathing . . . this effect becomes extremely important with a filled oesophagus during loud speech or with a strong effort to speak, a new glottis being formed in the trachea by local distention of the oesophagus into the trachea. . . . Eventually, air may be trapped in the bronchi, with very high oesophageal pressures at a negligible flow.

(5) The passive increase of the oesophageal pressure by the decrease of the volume of the lungs during expiration. In the normal average subject this increase amounts to 0.3 to 0.5 cm. of water/100 ml. lung volume. At the end of a maximal expiration, however, this increase can attain very high values, as the tissue itself is compressed then. Normally, this effect is unimportant. . . . Mechanisms 3 and 4, the latter here without an increased air resistance of the lungs, are sufficient to explain the constancy of oesophageal pressure during the pronunciation of the vowel a. . . . During a cough the velocity of the air in the trachea may approach the velocity of the sound, by the decrease of the diameters of the air-passages.

... Normally, a large increase of the oesophageal pressure of the subject was preceded by a quick traction of the abdominal muscles, pushing the diaphragm in the upper direction, and by a contraction of the muscles of the neck, limiting and eventually diminishing the area available for trachea and oesophagus, which are separated by a flexible wall. The increase of the resistance of the air-passages is here, with a filled oesophagus, even much more prominent than during a cough with an empty oesophagus, as a new glottis is formed in the trachea, the oesophagus protruding into the trachea. This increase accounts for the steep increase of the oesophageal pressure without a corresponding increase of the flow from the lungs.

Salmon (1965) pointed out that the pressure in the esophagus is not constant, but in fact is increased, as phonation is prolonged.

THE VIBRATOR

Morphology

Most workers agree that the cervical level of the P-E segment is between C_4 and C_6 in the vast majority of patients. Many have attempted to define the morphology of the pharyngo-esophageal junction. Some examples are: *hemisphere* and *half-egg-shaped* (Vandor, 1955); *thin* and *coarse* pseudoglottis (Schwab, 1957); *bulky* pseudoglottis as well as *ventral* and *dorsal* pseudoglottis (Schlosshauer & Möckel, 1958); *thickening* of the anterior, posterior and lateral walls of the P-E tract (Motta *et al.*, 1959); *transverse* torus, a *vertical flat* torus, and a *half sphere* (Böhme & Schneider, 1960); and *round flat*, and *irregular* (Vrtička & Svoboda, 1961).

Diedrich and Youngstrom (1966) described the neoglottis as being composed chiefly of tissue on the dorsal, the ventral, or the dorsal-ventral side of the pharyngeal-esophageal lumen. In 78 vowel phonations (26 patients, each saying three isolated vowels), they found a distribution of 20 ventral, 29 dorsal, and 17 ventral-dorsal, and 12 had no obvious bulge or constriction at the P-E junction. In the rest position, no bulge or constriction was observed in 25 out of 26 patients. Kirchner and colleagues (1963) described how the bulge may occur on the dorsal wall because of contracted inferior pharyngeal constrictors, but no satisfactory explanation has been made for the ventral (anterior) wall constriction.

Most workers (Damsté, 1958; van den Berg & Moolenaar-Bijl, 1959; Levin, 1962) have stated that the neoglottis in laryngectomized subjects is composed primarily from the cricopharyngeal muscle. Anatomical studies (Batson, 1955; Decroix *et al.*, 1958) have shown that the cricopharyngeal muscle is from 12 to 15 mm in length. Intraluminal pressure studies in normals (Ingelfinger, 1958) and in normals and laryngectomized subjects (Dey & Kirchner, 1961) have indicated that there is an area of constriction at the pharyngo-esophageal junction of about 30 to 40 mm in length. These studies suggested that fibers from the upper esophagus and the lower pharynx, in addition to those from the cricopharyngeus, contribute to the sphincter mechanism.

A mean P-E segment length during phonation of 21 mm as measured from cinefluorograms and 29 mm as measured from spot films was found by Diedrich and Youngstrom (1966). During phonation, some contraction of the P-E segment occurs, which accounts for the smaller range of 21 to 29 mm of actual distance as compared to the 30 to 40 mm of distance during the resting stage found by the intraluminal studies. The constricted P-E segment during phonation was at least 5 mm, and as much as 15 mm, longer than that presumably covered by the cricopharyngeus muscle. Therefore they concluded that the P-E segment in laryngectomized subjects was not comprised solely of the cricopharyngeus.

Although different workers (Robe *et al.*, 1956; Schwab, 1957; Damsté, 1958; Schlosshauer & Möckel, 1958) had postulated that the narrower the P-E segment, the better the phonation ability, Diedrich and Youngstrom were unable to find any significant correlations between speech skill and axial length of the P-E segment. Other workers (Hodson & Oswald, 1958; Černoch & Zbořil, 1961; Kirchner *et al.*, 1963) also had confirmed that the length of the neoglottis is not related to speech skill.

Some interesting variance in the morphology of the P-E segment observed on cinefluorograms has been reported (Diedrich & Youngstrom, 1966). Out of 24 subjects observed during phonation, four were found with a double segment, one with a triple segment, and two with no obvious bulge. Other workers (Vandor, 1955; Böhme & Schneider, 1960) noted no obvious bulging of the P-E segment in some of their subjects. Using intraluminal pressure techniques, Dey and Kirchner (1961) reported the lack of any obvious constriction at the P-E junction in subjects with good esophageal speech.

Innervation

There are two reasons for the interest in the structure and innervation of the P-E segment: (1) regulation of the flow of air into the esophagus during pre-phonation, and (2) regulation of the control of closure for phonation.

One of the better descriptions of the innervation of the upper esophageal sphincter is by Ingelfinger (1958):

> On anatomic grounds, the sphincter appears innervated by an overlapping supply of elements derived from the nucleus ambiguus and dorsal vagal nucleus, and carried by the X and to a lesser degree, from the IX and XI nerves. The resting tonicity of the sphincter and its opening are under influences carried by these nerves. . . . Because of its high resting tone, the obvious response of the sphincter is to the inhibitory component of the peristaltic impulse. Although the sphincter also opens under conditions other than swallowing, the responsible mechanisms are unknown.

> It is likely, however, that voluntary, like involuntary, relaxation of the upper esophageal sphincter is not easily elicitable by itself, but is one step in an arrangement of multiple performances.

Decroix and coworkers (1958), in their extensive study of the anatomical and physiological bases of esophageal speech, provided some tentative evidence that there may be proprioceptive fibers present in the muscle tracts of the pharyngo-esophageal sphincter. Proprioceptive innervation demonstrated by the presence of neuromuscular spindles in the esophageal wall can explain the contraction in the lower part of the sphincter and permits the control and the precise degree of voluntary contraction needed in esophageal voice. In the dissections of 50 pharyngo-larynges, the Decroix group demonstrated the constancy of the branches of the recurrent nerve intended for the "mouth of esophagus." They stressed the importance of preserving as much of the innervation of this area as possible.

Storchi and Micheli-Pellegrini (1959) carried out 32 dissections of the recurrent laryngeal nerve (in 16 cadavers) with the intent of finding some practical confirmation of the pipe organ concepts of phonation expressed by Micheli-Pellegrini. They reiterated the difficulties of precise definition concerning the fine innervation of the cricopharyngeal muscle and confirmed the existence of a system of branchlets that originate from the recurrent nerve and distribute themselves towards the pharyngeal-esophageal sphincter. Decroix and colleagues believe these branchlets must originate in almost all cases directly from a branch of the recurrent nerve. From their preparations, Storchi and Micheli-Pellegrini believe the branches proceed towards the pharyngeal-esophageal sphincter, both as single, isolated, trunks and as multiple fillets which are derived from the extralaryngeal branch of the recurrent nerve and which contain motor fibers as well as sensory fibers. They do not ascribe to the Decroix group's neurochronaxic theory of esophageal phonation.

In an electromyographic (EMG) procedure for studying muscle activity of the inferior constrictors and the cricopharyngeus, Shipp (1966) found during inflation of the esophagus, just prior to phonation, simultaneous bursts of EMG activity from both the inferior constrictor and the cricopharyngeus muscles. These were interpreted as being a passive stretch reaction to the bolus of air being injected. He found a latency period between esophageal insufflation and phonation accompanied by low-level activity from both muscle sites, which would support the notion of a prephonation period (Diedrich & Youngstrom, 1966). During the onset of phonation, there was increased activity from the cricopharyngeus and often some parallel activity in the inferior constrictor muscle that diminished rapidly upon completion of phonation.

In several subjects who were classified as good esophageal speakers, the EMG pattern showed inhibition of both the cricopharyngeus and the inferior constrictors during phonation. This finding may mean that the resting tonicity of the P-E segment is so high that in order for phonation to occur, relaxation (inhibition) of the tonus must occur. Shipp (1966) found that poor speakers displayed either extremely weak or uncoordinated and inconsistent EMG patterns of the cricopharyngeus muscle during phonation. In either case, the latter finding would support the view that good phonatory ability is based on a neurally intact P-E segment function. Despite the fact that the morphology and tonicity measured by intraluminal studies are not equivocal in their relationship to speech skills, EMG studies may point the way to innervation deficits of the mechanism.

Pitch

Spectrographic studies (van den Berg & Moolenaar-Bijl, 1959) have shown mean fundamental frequency ranges of 50 to 100 Hz, and Damsté (1958) had the same ranges with a median of 68 Hz, reporting that one individual approximated 185 Hz. Kytta (1964) found a mean of 50.4 Hz in 18 subjects. On the other hand, Perry and Tikofsky (1965), using narrow-band spectrography in conjunction with oscillographic wave tracings, reported mean fundamental frequencies for esophageal vowels to be in the 29 to 37 Hz range, with about 56% of the fundamentals below 30 Hz.

In their study of six superior esophageal speakers, using phonelloscopic tracings, Curry and Snidecor (1961) found a fundamental frequency range of 17 to 135 Hz with a median of 63 Hz. Shipp (1967) utilized an optical oscillograph write-out system to determine fundamental frequency. The better speakers had a mean of 84.4 Hz and the poorer speakers a mean of 64.7 Hz.

Isshiki's findings in normals (1964) are also relevant to the development of a higher pitch in esophageal speakers. To obtain increased intensity at a high pitch, the flow rate must be increased. Since esophageal speakers have only one-third the flow rate of normals, it is not surprising that they cannot obtain good intensity levels at higher pitches.

Curry (1962) noted the special perceptual difficulties associated with esophageal speech. He cites Damsté's (1958) observation in this regard, which points out that measured frequencies and perceived pitch at low frequencies are not readily detected. In their data, Curry and Snidecor (1961) found a mean total frequency range of 13.21 tones for the superior esophageal speakers and only 10.5 tones for the superior adult speakers with normal laryngeal function. Since the esophageal mean is on that part of the tonal scale where range in fundamental frequency within a tonal interval is small and the normal tonal interval is large, then ". . . variation in fundamental frequency around the esophageal mean would be less than the variation around the normal mean" (Perry, 1963b).

Intensity and Quality

Loudness (intensity) is related to the amount of pressure exerted on the esophageal tube that increases the rate of expelled airflow out of the tube and to the resistance at the mouth of the esophagus.

Isshiki's (1964) findings regarding airflow rates and pitch in normals are particularly relevant here. He stated that at very low pitch the intensity of voice is increased by increasing the glottal resistance rather than increasing the flow rate; furthermore, with low resistance of the glottis, increase in flow rate would cause the glottis to remain open and the voice to become weak.

Clinical experience has shown that digital compression of the neoglottis in the esophageal speaker results in increased intensity of the voice. In fact some laryngectomees must wear a special collar or band around their neck in order to obtain the necessary tension of the neoglottis for good phonation (van den Berg & Moolenaar-Bijl, 1959; Diedrich & Youngstrom, 1966). Nichols (1962) also has pointed out that when the esophageal speaker attempts to get increased intensity he must exert some kind of pressure in the P-E segment. Frequently this pressure becomes too great — which may result in a complete lack of voice. Drummond (1965) reported using masking noise through headphones to increase the intensity of the esophageal voice.

Hyman (1955) studied sound pressure levels in three groups of speakers and found that at a reference level of 50 db re 0.0002 dynes/cm² the artificial larynx users were 33 db, normal speakers 29 db, and esophageal speakers 23 db. McKinley (1960) also found that the average intensity of esophageal speech is about 6 to 7 db below normals.

Snidecor and Isshiki (1965b) showed that a superior male esophageal speaker was capable of intensity levels of 85 db, with a range of 20 db for both the upward and the downward intensity sweeps. When the voice is high in pitch, the noise component is relatively great and the pitch is more unstable, as shown by irregular vertical striations on wide-band sonograms. They noted that pitch and intensity vary ". . . almost entirely by air flow with secondary participation through action of the pseudoglottis." Later they state:

> Since there is much less control of the pseudoglottis in esophageal speakers than for the glottis in normal subjects, it is assumed that the mean flow rate of of greater importance in controlling the intensity, than in normal speakers.

Although the quality of esophageal speech is observed to be visually different on spectographic analyses (Nichols, 1962), the description of esophageal speech quality has not been adequately done. Various terms—"hoarseness," "huskiness," and "harshness," as well as "breathy" and "watery"—are used to describe the voice. In addition, the nasal resonance qualities can be discussed but not very well described. It has been shown previously (Diedrich & Youngstrom, 1966) that esophageal speakers usually maintain velopharyngeal closure on nasal sounds.

Waldrop and Toht (cited in Nichols, 1962) plotted frequency-amplitude displays of vowels emitted by normal, pharyngeal, esophageal, and buccal speech. The pharyngeal speech was closer in pattern than the others were to normal speech. However, they did not have x-ray data to indicate where either the air chamber or the neoglottis was located.

Both Damsté (1958) and Diedrich and Youngstrom (1966) showed that it is possible to have a "pharyngeal" voice with a small air column at C_4 and C_5. The air was located deep in the hypopharynx but above the lip of the esophagus, and the neoglottis was formed by tissue at the base of the tongue, which vibrated against the posterior wall of the pharynx. The quality of this pharyngeal speech is hard to describe; it has less intensity, is higher in pitch, and contains poorer resonance (oral-pharyngeal) characteristics than a true esophageal voice has.

Theories of Phonation

Decroix and colleagues (1958) made a valiant attempt to defend a neuro-chronaxic theory of esophageal voice production. They did not believe that the subglottal pressure produced by air trapped in the esophagus is great enough to support phonation. They noted that the neoglottis adapts itself to a neuromuscular function that is identical to that of the old laryngeal function and thereby ". . . becomes the seat of a new and imposed vibratory movement."

Another theory (Micheli-Pellegrini, 1957) of phonation has been to compare the neoglottis to a fixed tube (pipe organ) with sound produced by the generation of eddies in a narrow part of the tract, with subsequent cavity resonance. Van den Berg and Moolenaar-Bijl (1959) admit that this theory of phonation may be true for certain types of esophageal speech where no definitive neoglottis is present. They point out that the vibrating structure may be damped to such a degree that the cavity is less damped and determines the fundamental frequency of the vibration.

Most workers (van den Berg & Moolenaar-Bijl, 1959) believe that the neoglottis functions in an aerodynamic manner similar to the normal larynx. The stroboscopic observations reported by Damsté (1958) and high-speed cinematography of the neoglottis by Rubin (1959) clearly show an undulating mucosal wave starting from the inferior surface of the neoglottis and moving upward to the superior surface, just as it is observed in the vibratory movement of the normal vocal fold.

ARTICULATION

Investigation of esophageal speech generally has concerned the site of the neoglottis, the air reservoir, and the manner of air intake. The process of articulation and the dynamic relationships between air intake and esophageal phonation have largely been ignored. There have been several excellent intelligibility studies (Anderson, 1950; Hyman, 1955; Di Carlo et al., 1955; Shames et al., 1963), but these have not carefully considered why differences exist in articulation of esophageal speech and normal speech.

Consonants

Air pressure tracings in the mouth (Di Carlo *et al.*, 1955; Damsté, 1958) showed higher peaks of pressure in normals for the production of the /p/ than they did for the /b/. For the esophageal speaker, the tracing showed equal pressure for the /p/ and the /b/ sounds, and both are greater than the /p/ sound in normals. Cinefluorograms made of one patient prior to his operation and 12 months post-laryngectomy (Diedrich & Youngstrom, 1966) indicated that the tongue had more continuous movement during the articulation of esophageal speech than it had in preoperative speech, the contact positions of the tongue or lips in normal phonation had a longer duration than they had in esophageal speech, and the /s/ morphology (position of the tongue) showed the greatest difference in posture of all sounds studied.

Tikofsky and associates (1964) found that substitution of a voiced consonant in the initial position when none was intended represented 55% of all the misidentification of esophageal words. It was also found that listeners will tend to make more misidentifications of initial consonants than they do of final consonants. As they pointed out:

> The reduction in control appears not to occur because of the esophageal speaker's inability to produce voicing. . . . [but] there is a tendency for the esophageal speaker to anticipate the voicing requirements of the vowel which will follow the initial consonant, and to begin to produce a vibratory pattern too soon.

Vowels

Normal speakers have been compared with esophageal speakers in producing the /i/, /ɔ/ and /u/. The results indicated (Perry, 1963a) that the esophageal speakers were less able to imitate vowels than normal speakers were, and the reason given is that the "laryngectomy appear[s] to result often in a significant restriction in the range of the tongue's mobility." The pre- and postoperative cinefluorographic studies by Diedrich and Youngstrom (1966) indicated that tongue mobility was not restricted after a laryngectomy, but that the supralaryngeal and hypopharyngeal resonators were altered. As a matter of fact, the tongue makes compensatory movements that the normals do not need.

Interrelationship between Articulation and Air Intake

The temporal relationships in esophageal speech air intake and articulation have been emphasized (Diedrich & Youngstrom, 1966). Air intake may occur from a rest or interphrase interval. The same individual may accomplish air intake by utilizing inhalation in one interval and injection in the other. Air intake may also occur within an intraphrase interval. Air may be injected, not inhaled, during the articulation of voiceless consonant sounds.

Airflow data (Isshiki & Snidecor, 1965) have indicated that voicing may occur on air intake more frequently than is generally recognized. Furthermore, these airflow studies have shown that some speakers possess the ability to release esophageal air without phonation, and this means that it may be possible to use esophageal air as driving pressure for the voiceless stop plosives. However, the intelligibility studies of Tikofsky and coworkers (1964) seem to provide evidence that the majority of articulation errors are in the other direction, i.e., the esophageal speaker has difficulty in preventing esophageal tone when he wants a voiceless sound.

SUMMARY

This review indicates the tremendous complexity of the mechanisms of esophageal speech. Although a great deal is known about the process, some of the following areas need further clarification:

1. Air intake, especially in regard to those mechanisms that relax the P-E segment.

2. Air expulsion: What are the critical variables, e.g., contraction of the esophageal walls, increased intrathoraxic pressure, and/or abdominal pressure?

3. The vibrator and the nature of its physiological function: Does it become more tonic, or, in some cases, must it relax for phonation?

4. Can control over the P-E segment be such as to allow release of esophageal air, without phonation, in order to build up those pressures necessary for the production of voiceless consonant sounds that are made in the oral-pharyngeal cavities?

REFERENCES

ANDERSON, J. O. 1950. A descriptive study of elements of esophageal speech. Unpublished Ph.D. Dissertation. Ohio State University. Columbus, Ohio.
ATKINSON, M., P. KRAMER, S. M. WYMAN & F. J. INGELFINGER. 1957. The dynamics of swallowing. I. Normal pharyngeal mechanisms. J. Clin. Invest. 36: 581–588.
BATSON, O. V. 1955. The cricopharyngeus muscle. Ann. Otol. 64: 47–54.
BERLIN, C. I. 1963. Clinical measurement of esophageal speech. I. Methodology and curves of skill acquisition. J. Speech Hearing Dis. 28: 42–51.
BERLIN, C. I. 1965. Clinical measurement of esophageal speech. III. Performance of non-biased groups. J. Speech Hearing Dis. 30: 174–183.
BÖHME, G. & H. G. SCHNEIDER. 1960. Die Pathophysiologie des Laryngektomierten im Zusammenhang mit der Güte der Sprechfunktion. Z. Laryng. Rhinol. Otol. 39: 512–520.
ČERNOCH, Z. & M. ZBOŘIL. 1961. Rentgenkinematograficke zaznamy Jicnovereci. Cesk. Rentgenol. 15: 85–92.
CURRY, E. T. 1962. Frequency measurement and pitch perception in esophageal speech. In Speech Rehabilitation of the Laryngectomized, by J. C. Snidecor. Charles C. Thomas, Publisher. Springfield, Ill.
CURRY, E. T. & J. C. SNIDECOR. 1961. Physical measurement and pitch perception in esophageal speech. Laryngoscope 71: 415–424.
DAMSTÉ, P. H. 1958. Oesophageal Speech. Gebr. Hoitsema. Groningen, The Netherlands.
DECROIX, G., C. LIBERSA & R. LATTARD. 1958. Bases anatomiques et physiologiques de la reéducation vocale des laryngectomisés. J. Franc. Otorhinolaryng. 7: 549–573.
DEY, F. L. & J. A. KIRCHNER. 1961. The upper esophageal sphincter after laryngectomy. Laryngoscope 71: 99–115.
DI CARLO, L. A., W. W. AMSTER & G. R. HERER. 1955. Speech after Laryngectomy. Syracuse University Press. Syracuse, N. Y.
DIEDRICH, W. M. & K. A. YOUNGSTROM. 1966. Alaryngeal Speech. Charles C. Thomas, Publisher. Springfield, Ill.
DRUMMOND, SHEILA. 1965. The effects of environmental noise on pseudovoice after laryngectomy. J. Laryng. 79: 193–202.
FRINT, VON T. & K. PAUKA. 1965. Erfahrungen mit der intra-ösophagealen Druckmessung bei Laryngektomierten. Monatsschr. Ohrenheil. Laryngo-Rhinol. 99: 284–288.
HODSON, C. J. & M. V. OSWALD. 1958. Speech Recovery after Total Laryngectomy. E. and S. Livingston, Ltd. Edinburgh, Scotland, and London, England.
HYMAN, M. 1955. An experimental study of artificial larynx and esophageal speech. J. Speech Hearing Dis. 20: 291–299.
INGELFINGER, F. J. 1958. Esophageal motility. Physiol. Rev. 38: 533–584.
ISSHIKI, N. 1964. Regulatory mechanisms of voice intensity variation. J. Speech Hearing Res. 7: 17–30.
ISSHIKI, N. 1966. Personal communication.
ISSHIKI, N. & J. C. SNIDECOR. 1965. Air intake and usage in esophageal speech. Acta Otolaryng. 59: 559–574.

KALLEN, L. A. 1934. Vicarious vocal mechanisms. Arch. Otolaryng. (Chicago) 20: 360–503.

KAMIETH, VON H. 1959. Vergleichende röntgenologische Untersuchungen bei der Ösophagus-sprache Kehlkopfloser. Radiol. Clin. (Basel) 28: 88–101.

KIRCHNER, J. A., J. H. SCATLIFF, F. L. DEY & D. P. SHEDD. 1963. The pharynx after laryngectomy. Laryngoscope 73: 18–33.

KRAMER, P., M. ATKINSON, S. M. SYMAN & J. J. INGELFINGER. 1957. The dynamics of swallowing. II. Neuromuscular dysphagia of pharynx. J. Clin. Invest. 36: 589–595.

KYTTA, J. 1964. Finnish oesophageal speech after laryngectomy. Sound spectrographic and cineradiographic studies. Acta Otolaryng. Suppl. to 195: 94.

LEVIN, N. M. 1962. Voice and Speech Disorders: Medical Aspects. Charles C. Thomas, Publisher. Springfield, Ill.

McKINLEY, S. 1960. Correlates of stress patterns in esophageal speech. Unpublished Master's Thesis. Vanderbilt University. Nashville, Tenn.

MICHELI-PELLEGRINI, V. 1957. On the so-called pseudo-glottis in laryngectomized persons. J. Laryng. 71: 405–410.

MOTTA, G., A. PROFAZIO & T. ACCIARRI. 1959. Osservazioni roentgencinematografiche sulla fonazione nei laringectomizzati. Otorinolaring. Ital. 28: 261–286.

NICHOLS, A..C. 1962. Loudness and quality in esophageal speech and the artificial larynx. In Speech Rehabilitation in the Laryngectomized, by J. C. Snidecor. Charles C. Thomas, Publisher. Springfield, Ill.

PERRY, P. S. 1963a. A selective disability in esophageal vowel articulation. ASHA Convention Report. (Appendix VII and VIII in Phonetic Characteristics of Esophageal Speech. 1965. R. S. Tikofsky, Ed. ORA Project 05539. Office of Research Administration. University of Michigan, Ann Arbor, Mich.)

PERRY, P. S. 1963b. An investigation of the lowest frequency in normal and esophageal vowel phonation. Unpublished Ph.D. Dissertation. University of Michigan. Ann Arbor, Mich. (Appendix V in Phonetic Characteristics of Esophageal Speech. 1965. R. S. Tikofsky, Ed. ORA Project 05539. Office of Research Administration. University of Michigan. Ann Arbor, Mich.)

PERRY, P. S. & R. S. TIKOFSKY. 1965. The occurrence of low valued, weak intensity frequencies in normal and esophageal phonation. (Appendix VI in Phonetic Characteristics of Esophageal Speech. 1965. R. S. Tikofsky, Ed. ORA Project 05539. Office of Research Administration. University of Michigan. Ann Arbor, Mich.)

RAGAGLINI, G., M. TERAMO & V. MICHELI-PELLEGRINI. 1956. Ulteriori richerche roentgencinematografiche nello studio della fonazione dei laringectomizzati. Nunt. Radiol. 22: 156–163.

ROBE, EVELYN Y., P. MOORE, A. H. ANDREWS, JR. & P. H. HOLINGER. 1956. A study of the role of certain factors in the development of speech after laryngectomy: 1. Type of operation, 2. Site of pseudoglottis, 3. Coordination of speech with respiration. Laryngoscope 66: 173–186 (Part 1), 382–401 (Part 2), and 418–499 (Part 3).

RUBIN, H. 1959. High-speed cinematography of the pathologic larynx. (Film.) Cedars of Lebanon Hospital. Los Angeles, Calif.

SALMON, SHIRLEY J. 1965. Pressure variations in the esophagus, pharyngeal-esophageal constriction and pharynx associated with esophageal speech production. Unpublished Ph.D. Dissertation. State University of Iowa. Iowa City, Iowa.

SCHLOSSHAUER, B. & G. MÖCKEL. 1958. Answertung der Röntgentonfilm aufnahmen von Speiseröhrensprechern. Folia Phoniat. 20: 154–166.

SCHWAB, W. 1957. X-ray cinematographic investigations in substitute speech after a laryngectomy. Acta Otorinolaryng. Iber. Amer. 8: 270–273.

SHAMES, G. H., J. FONT & J. MATTHEWS. 1963. Factors related to speech proficiency of the laryngectomized. J. Speech Hearing Dis. 28: 273–287.

SHIPP, F. T. 1966. Personal communication.

SHIPP, F. T. 1967. Frequency, duration, and perceptual measures in relation to judgments of alaryngeal speech and acceptability. J. Speech Hearing Res. 10: 417–427.

SNIDECOR, J. C. & E. T. CURRY. 1959. Temporal and pitch aspects of superior esophageal speech. Ann. Otol. 68: 623–636.

SNIDECOR, J. C. & N. ISSHIKI. 1965a. Air volume and air flow relationships of six male esophageal speakers. J. Speech Hearing Dis. 30: 205–216.

SNIDECOR, J. C. & N. ISSHIKI. 1965b. Vocal and air use characteristics of a superior male esophageal speaker. Folia Phoniat. 17: 217–232.

STORCHI, O. F. & V. MICHELI-PELLEGRINI. 1959. A proposito dell'innervazione ricorrenziale del muscolo cricofaringeo e della sua importanza nella fonazione dei laringectomizzati. Boll. Mal. Orecch. 77: 3–14.

TIKOFSKY, RITA, T. GLOTTKE & P. S. PERRY. 1964. Listener identification of esophageal production of voiced and voiceless consonants. ASHA Convention Report. (Appendix XII in Phonetic Characteristics of Esophageal Speech. 1965. R. S. Tikofsky, Ed. ORA Project 05539, Office of Research Administration. University of Michigan. Ann Arbor, Mich.)

VAN DEN BERG, J. & A. J. MOOLENAAR-BIJL. 1959. Cricopharyngeal sphincter, pitch, intensity, and fluency in oesophageal speech. Pract. Otorhinolaryng. (Basel) 21: 298–315.

VAN DEN BERG, J., A. J. MOOLENAAR-BIJL & P. H. DAMSTÉ. 1958. Oesophageal speech. Folia Phoniat. 10: 65–84.

VANDOR, F. 1955. Röentgenuntersuchung der Pseudoglottis von Laryngektomierten. Fortschr. Roentgenstr. 82: 618–625.

VRTIČKA, K. & M. SVOBODA. 1961. A clinical and x-ray study of 100 laryngectomized speakers. Folia Phoniat. 13: 174–186.

VRTIČKA, K. & M. SVOBODA. 1963. Time changes in the x-ray picture of the hypopharynx, pseudoglottis, and esophagus in the course of vocal rehabilitation in 70 laryngectomized speakers. Folia Phoniat. 15: 1–12.

VRTIČKA, K., H. GUNDERMANN & M. PETRIK. 1965. Enfaches Metsgerät zur Feststellung der Spannung des oberen Oesophagusmundes bei Laryngektomierten. HNO 13: 175–177.

Connection between Consonant Articulation and the Intake of Air in Oesophageal Speech *

By A. MOOLENAAR-BIJL, Groningen

The mechanism for bringing air into the oesophagus, used by those patients who, after laryngectomy, have to adapt themselves to a new way of producing voice, was formerly thought to consist in "swallowing". As early as 1924, however, *Gutzmann* [1] suggested "aspiring" as a possibility. Since then, many authors have agreed that "aspiring" is the method used by patients who have achieved fluent oesophageal speech (e. g. *Luchsinger* [2] to whom we owe a recent extensive study). The impression is, however, that in Europe speech treatment has

Reprinted by permission from *Folia Phoniatrica*, 1953, 5, 212–216.

gained little benefit from this recognition. Only *Marland* [3] indicates that learning to aspire air should be started by means of pumping movements with the throat.

Besides swallowing there are two other ways of bringing air into the oesophagus, two modifications of aspiration: "direct inhalation" and "injection". Our experience with 36 laryngectomised patients has taught us that neither swallowing nor inhaling is the mechanism to be preferred. I need hardly say that swallowing interrupts speech audibly after every 6–10 syllables and is a tiring process which should be avoided as far as possible. "Direct inhalation", though not tiring or conspicuous in itself, keeps pace with tracheal respiration and therefore makes breathing frequent and superficial: speech tends to be jolting, syllabic and lacking in dynamic variation.

The "injection method", which we now use by preference in Groningen, consists of insufflating air into the oesophagus by means of a small, nearly imperceptible movement with the lips or the tongue. This movement resembles a very slightly articulated p, t or k. Air is thus brought in quickly and unobtrusively. This mechanism requires much less energy than swallowing and it enables the patient to speak more smoothly and continuously than is possible with inhalation.

In my lecture at the 8th Convention of this same Association I mentioned this method and supposed (as others have done before, e. g. *Stetson* [4] some 16 years ago) that air might be brought into the oesophagus by means of the articulation of certain consonants. My supposition was the result of observing several laryngectomised patients, especially one who was (and still is) our best oesophageal speaker. He could easily repeat syllables with p, t and k 20–40 times without any further intake of air; but syllables with m, l, b, d, and so on, he could pronounce only 7 or 8 times in succession.

We have tried to benefit from this observation, viz. that voiceless explosives could be used as a starting point in speech therapy and would probably be more effective than air swallowing or special exercises for aspiration. We now always start speech treatment very simply with the syllable "pah" or "tah", and as soon as there is some oesophageal voice, we pass on to monosyllabic words with voiceless explosives (such as put, cap, tick). It proved to be much easier for nearly every patient to produce oesophageal voice with these words than with isolated vowels or initial vowels, which used to be the classic way in the swallowing method. After these monosyllabic words we very soon pass on to words of two syllables, especially those with the accent on the second syllable. These words should always have an initial voiceless explosive in both syllables. In English: e. g. catarrh, tattoo, complete, contract, percuss, perplex, cartoon, perturb, propose, protect, concoct, compact; in Dutch there are plenty of these, in German and French even more.

In accordance with these findings and as a consequence of this method, our more advanced pupils are able to repeat several times over a short sentence containing many voiceless explosives (e. g. "Kapitein Pieters kocht twee prachtige kakatoes", or "Captain Peters took a cup of tea sitting in the cockpit"), – whereas they are hardly able to repeat, even once, a short sentence with many liquids (e. g. "Hij wil zeeën bevaren en landen bereizen", or "We have never been in England nor in Holland").

These empiric facts indicate that the articulation of the voiceless explosives, especially p and t, plays a part in the act of aspiring air into the oesophagus. We tried to substantiate this supposition by an X-ray examination; and for this we are greatly indebted to Professor *Keyser*, Director of the Groningen Radiological Institute. Although the results seem to corroborate the theory, I am fully aware that they are obtained from one patient only. We intend testing them on other patients in due course.

We see the following on the X-ray screen: In repose the oesophagus is entirely closed. The moment the patient prepares to pronounce a series of syllables "mah", the oesophagus fills with air and then empties gradually while the syllable "mah" is pronounced six times.

When the patient utters a series of syllables "pah", the oesophagus fills up with the first "p", and we can then see the walls giving way a little with each "ah" and expanding again maximally with each "p". Thus after the patient has repeated "pah" 15 or more times, the air volume is exactly as large as it was at the beginning.

As a final proof a roentgenogram was taken at the moment when an isolated voiceless "p" was being formed. Here too we can see the oesophagus, closed in repose, filling with air when the "p" is artiulated.

Coming back to speech treatment and the use of this phenomenon: as soon as the patient has gained some skill in pronouncing syllables with p and t, he has no difficulty at all with initial vowels. It is possible that the tiny aspiring movement preceding the initial vowel may sometimes give the impression of a real p or t; this movement should therefore be made very lightly and not quite joining the word.

Those patients who can without difficulty produce a belch at the beginning of speech treatment, may as easily pronounce a syllable with p or t. The first phase of the ructus, as described by *Van Gilse* [5], is thus substituted by a real element of speech. Those who cannot produce a belch at will should, voicelessly, practise syllables with p and t, until after a very short time they are accompanied by oesophageal voice.

It is needless to say that speech therapy of laryngectomised patients should begin as soon as possible after the operation. Of our 36 patients, operated upon by Professor *Eelco Huizinga*, 30 obtained reasonable to very good (pharyngeal-)oesophageal speech.

Summary

The preferable method of insufflating air into the oesophagus in speech after laryngectomy is by "injection". The movements of the mouth achieving this are identical with the articulation of certain consonants, especially p, t and k. These consonants should therefore be taken as a starting point in speech therapy; they facilitate the intake of air into the oesophagus in a natural way and make soda-water and muscle-training superfluous auxiliaries in most cases. Roentgenograms show how the oesophagus fills with air on pronunciation of an isolated "p", the air volume in the oesophagus remaining constant during repetition of the syllable "pah", but diminishing on repeated pronunciation of the syllable "mah".

Zusammenfassung

Die bevorzugte Methode der Lufteinschlürfung während der Ösophagussprache ist die «Injektion». Die Bewegungen des Mundes, die dabei ausgeführt werden, sind identisch mit denjenigen bei der Artikulation von gewissen Konsonanten, speziell bei stimmlosen explosiven. Deshalb sollten diese Konsonanten als Ausgangspunkte für die Therapie benützt werden, um das Einschlürfen in den Ösophagus auf natürliche Weise zu erleichtern. Röntgenaufnahmen zeigen das Füllen des Ösophagus bei der Aussprache verschiedener Silben.

Résumé

La méthode de choix d'insufflation d'air dans l'œsophage chez le laryngectomisé est «l'injection». Le mouvement de la bouche achevant cet acte est identique à l'articulation de quelques consonnes, spécialement des explosives sans voix. C'est pourquoi ces consonnes devraient être utilisées comme des points de repère en thérapie, car elles facilitent l'insufflation de l'air dans l'œsophage d'une manière naturelle. Des radiographies montrent le remplissage de l'œsophage lors de la prononciation de différentes syllabes.

Bibliography

[1] *Gutzmann, H. Jr.:* Deutsch. med. Wschr. *13*, 520, 1924. – [2] *Luchsinger, R.:* Pract. oto-rhino-laryng. *14*, 304, 1952. – [3] *Marland, P.:* Speech *13*, 4, 1949. – [4] *Stetson, R. H.:* Arch. néerl. Phon. exp. *13*, 95, 1937. – [5] *Van Gilse, P. H. G.:* Arch. néerl. Phon. exp. *5*, 37, 1930.

SIMILARITIES BETWEEN GLOSSOPHARYNGEAL BREATHING AND INJECTION METHODS OF AIR INTAKE FOR ESOPHAGEAL SPEECH

Bernd Weinberg

Indiana University Medical Center
Indianapolis

James F. Bosma

National Institute of Dental Research
Bethesda, Maryland

This article describes similarities between the respiratory maneuvers of glossopharyngeal breathing and injection methods of air intake for esophageal speech. The observations in this report were derived from two primary sources: (1) The first was cineradiographic studies of oral, pharyngeal, and upper esophageal function in postlaryngectomy and poliomyelitic persons. For the postlaryngectomy patients we obtained cineradiographic studies of speech and deglutition of 27 esophageal speakers from W. M. Diedrich and K. A. Youngstrom, of the University of Kansas Medical Center. (See Diedrich and Youngstrom, 1966, for a detailed description of the radiographic procedures and sample.) For the poliomyelitic persons, we obtained cineradiographic studies of glossopharyngeal breathing from the 16 mm film, *Glossopharyngeal Breathing*, by C. W. Dail and J. E. Affeldt. Additional radiologic studies of glossopharyngeal breathing were available from the work of one of us (J. B.) in other investigations of polio patients. (2) The second source was a review of pertinent clinical and experimental studies of glossopharyngeal breathing and esophageal speech.

Reprinted by permission from *Journal of Speech and Hearing Disorders*, 1970, *35*, 25–32.

Glossopharyngeal breathing (GPB), originally described by Dail, Affeldt, and Collier in 1955, is a method of breathing used by persons with respiratory paralysis. GPB is a form of intermittent, positive-pressure respiration in which the tongue functions as an important organ of respiration. Figure 1 illustrates the essential steps of GPB.

Briefly, GPB consists of pumping air into the lungs through coordinated stroking actions of the tongue, jaw, and pharynx. Initially, air is trapped in the oral and pharyngeal cavities. The mouth is closed by the lips or tongue, the palate is elevated to effect velopharyngeal closure, the upper esophageal orifice is shut, and the larynx is closed. The tongue moves upward and backward, as a rotary piston, forcing air

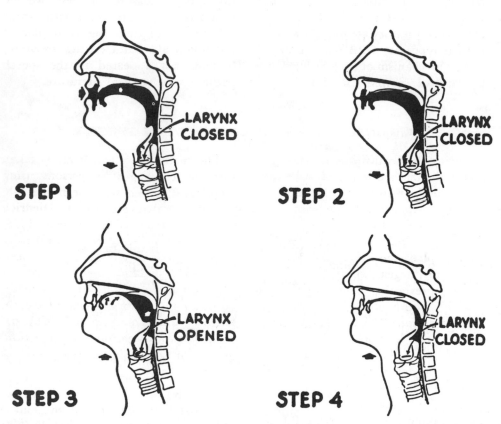

Figure 1. Steps taken during one stroke of glossopharyngeal breathing. Step 1, a mouthful and throatful of air is taken, depressing the tongue, jaw, and larynx to get maximum volume. Step 2, the lips are closed and the soft palate raised to trap the air. Step 3, the jaw, floor of mouth, and larynx are raised. This, with progressive motion of tongue, forces air through the opened larynx. Step 4, after as much air as possible is forced through the larynx, it is closed and the air is retained in the lungs until the cycle is reinstated.

(From Dail, Affeldt, and Collier, 1955, p. 446.)

into the pharynx. At the same time, the vocal cords open and air is forced into the trachea, where it is trapped by subsequent vocal cord closure.

These steps define the essential features of the glossopharyngeal "stroke." Ten or more rapidly repeated strokes constitute a cycle of inspiration and result in an accumulation of air in the lungs. After a sufficient volume of air has been pumped into the respiratory system, expiration occurs actively or passively, depending on the availability of expiratory musculature and the current respiratory pattern. The cycle is then repeated. GPB may be an exclusive mechanism of lung filling in the presence of complete disability of in-

spiratory motor function, or it may be a mechanism of supplementary inflation employed to improve vital capacity and to accomplish an adequate cough (Collier, Dail, and Affeldt, 1956).

The basic mechanism of GPB has been understood for over a decade. Yet its similarities to injection methods of air intake for esophageal speech remain essentially unknown. Although Damste (1958, 1959) first mentioned some of the common features of these two respiratory maneuvers, systematic study and review of their highly similar, if not identical, characteristics apparently have not appeared in the speech pathology or medical literature.

AIR INJECTION FOR ESOPHAGEAL SPEECH

During the acquisition of esophageal speech the laryngectomee must learn to overcome the resistance imposed by the pharyngoesophageal (P-E) segment.

In persons with a larynx, the P-E sphincter is reflexively controlled by the cricopharyngeal muscle. At rest, the upper esophageal sphincter is contracted, preventing penetration of air into the mouth of the esophagus during respiration (Negus, 1949; Ingelfinger, 1958). The importance of the reflex closure of the P-E segment is clearly evident during activities in which pharyngeal air pressure is high, as in sneezing, playing wind instruments, and speaking. Opening of the P-E segment during such activities would be unnatural and detrimental. Yet segment opening is precisely what the laryngectomee must learn if he is to produce esophageal speech (Damste, 1958).

The methods by which air is taken into the esophagus by persons using esophageal speech have been the subject of several investigations (Diedrich and Youngstrom, 1966; Damste, 1958; Isshiki and Snidecor, 1965). Two principal methods of air intake have been described: inhalation and injection.

Injection is the most frequent method of air intake for esophageal speech. Diedrich and Youngstrom (1966) described two variations of injection, glossal or glossopharyngeal press, as follows:

Glossal Press: The tip of the tongue [is] in contact with the alveolar ridge and frequently the middle of the tongue [contacts] the hard and soft palate. The posterior portion of the tongue [makes] a dorsal . . . movement but [does] not touch the posterior pharyngeal wall. Velopharyngeal closure [is] always present. The lips may or may not be open.

Glosso-Pharyngeal Press: Both the tip and middle portions of the tongue [are] in contact with the alveolus, hard palate, and soft palate. The posterior portion of the tongue [makes] a dorsal movement contacting the posterior pharyngeal wall which [makes] a ventral movement during this phase. The hypopharyngeal cavity [is] frequently obliterated by the backward movement of the tongue. The velopharyngeal port [is] always closed. The lips may or may not be open. (p. 37)

Figure 2 illustrates cinefluorographic tracings of glossal and glossopharyngeal press.

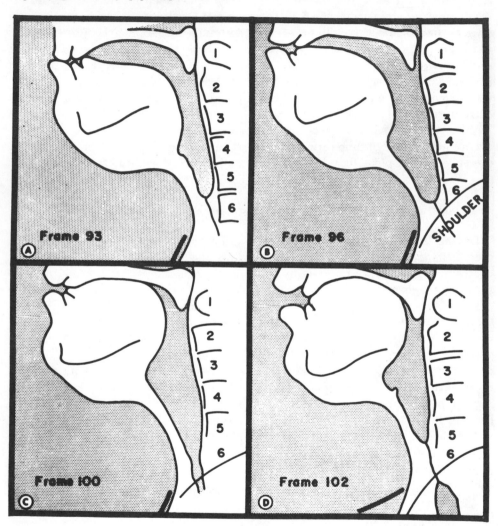

Figure 2a. Cinefluorogram tracings of subject using the glossal press method of air injection. The sequence started on Frame 93 and ended on Frame 103, prior to phonation of the /ʊ/ sound on Frame 106. (A) Frame 93, lips were closed, tongue against alveolus, palate closed from previous phonation of /a/. (B) Frame 96, palate now partially relaxed and hypopharynx becoming bigger. (C) Frame 100, tongue compressed against hard palate, P-E segment open. (D) Frame 102, maximum dorsal (backward) movement of the tongue, esophagus filled with air, P-E segment contracted.

General Physiological Properties

It is of prime importance to recognize the common pumping mechanism of these two different rehabilitation techniques (Damste, 1958). Physiologically, both GPB and injection represent intermittent, positive-pressure respiratory maneuvers. During GPB, air is pumped into the trachea and lungs,

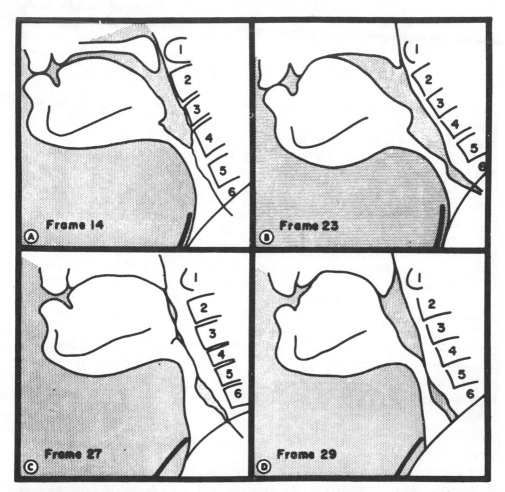

Figure 2b. Cinefluorogram tracings of subject using the glossopharyngeal press method of air injection. The sequence started on Frame 14 and ended on Frame 29, prior to phonation of the /i/ sound on Frame 32. (A) Frame 14, lips closed, palate elevated. (B) Frame 23, lips closed, anterior tongue against alveolus and posterior portion flattened, palate closed, P-E junction open. (C) Frame 27, lips parted, tongue compressed against the hard and soft palate, posterior pharyngeal wall has moved ventrad, hypopharynx has been obliterated. (D) Frame 29, tongue has moved ventrad and superior P-E segment has formed. (From Diedrich and Youngstrom, 1966, pp. 39-40.)

the tongue functions as a primary respiratory organ, and the larynx acts as an intermittent valve (Figure 1). During air injection for esophageal speech, air is pumped into the esophagus by identical rotary lingual motions; however, the P-E segment functions as the intermittent value (Figure 2). In this respect, the esophagus may be viewed as an accessory pneumatic chamber having a newly acquired and uniquely defined motor function.

During stroking for both GPB and air injection, the patient must maintain a hermetically sealed vocal tract. High pharyngeal air pressures, for example, greater than 20-30 cm H_2O have been recorded during both GPB (Harries and Lawes, 1957) and air injection (Salmon, 1965; Damste, 1958). Radiographic studies of the velopharyngeal area have demonstrated higher palatal elevation during the compression phase of both the GPB (Dail, Affeldt, and Collier, 1955) and the injection stroke (Diedrich and Youngstrom, 1966) than that found in normal speech. The consistent observation of excessive palatal elevation during GPB and air injection for esophageal speech is undoubtedly related to the generation of high pharyngeal pressures and to the necessity for effecting a hermetically sealed upper respiratory chamber.

Data obtained from respiratory studies of GPB and esophageal speech illustrate similarities in stroke duration and air volume. Harries and Lawes (1957), using spirographic techniques, found mean GPB stroke durations between 0.40 and 0.55 sec. These durations agree closely with latency measures for air injection for esophageal speech, which average approximately 0.50 sec

(Diedrich and Youngstrom, 1966; Berlin, 1963; Snidecor, 1962).

Furthermore, Harries and Lawes (1957) and Kelleher and Parida (1957) found a mean GPB stroke volume of 60 ml, with stroke volume ranges of 25 to 125 ml. More recently, Isshiki and Snidecor (1965) reported flow rates of 118 and 33 cc per sec during air intake for two "injector" type esophageal speakers. Since stroke volume may be calculated by dividing flow rate by duration of air intake, it becomes apparent that stroke volumes for GPB and injection of air for esophageal speech are comparable.

Clinical Similarities

Review of the literature on glossopharyngeal breathing highlights common clinical characteristics of GPB and air injection for esophageal speech.

Dail and his associates (1955) noted that some polio patients complained of pharyngeal drying and irritation during early GPB instruction. They found that pharyngeal irritation and drying were usually overcome following weeks of practice or after patients learned to take air in through the nose. Analogously, pharyngeal irritation or drying has been reported by several laryngectomized patients treated by one of us (B.W.). This complaint was most frequent during early phases of esophageal speech instruction and diminished with the passage of time or by altering the air intake route through the nose.

During GPB, polio patients have also complained of full sensations in the head and a feeling of faintness:

Theoretically, positive pressure breathing may interfere with venous return to the right side of the heart, which under normal circumstances, is compensated for by an intact circulatory system. (Dail et al., 1955)

This observation suggests an alternative explanation for the feelings of faintness or full-headedness reported by some laryngectomees learning to talk.

The time required to learn GPB varies from patient to patient. Dail et al. (1955) and Zumwalt et al. (1956) noted that some of their patients learned the basic GPB stroke in only one lesson. After learning the basic cycle most of their patients spent several weeks or months practicing to increase strength and endurance for appreciable breathing time. Similarly, many laryngectomees have learned to inject air into the esophagus and to phonate during the first lesson, but weeks and months of practice are required to establish consistent phonation and to increase speaking duration.

Zumwalt et al. (1956) wrote that a strong incentive is essential to the successful learning of GPB. Diedrich and Youngstrom (1966) and Shames, Font, and Mathews (1963) have emphasized the critical role of patient motivation and aspiration level in the learning of esophageal speech. In short, proficiency of GPB and esophageal speech may not be directly related to given morphologic or physiologic factors, but rather to variables such as personality, motivation, and aspiration levels of the patient.

Homologic Considerations

GPB has been called "gulping" and "frog breathing" because its basic mechanism is physiologically analogous to the respiratory motions of the frog and other amphibians. In human research, Bosma, Lind, and Gentz (1959) observed that:

> The oral and pharyngeal area motions of initial respiration in the newborns essentially resemble the distinctive glossopharyngeal inflation of the lung, similar to that described in poliomyelitic patients having severe motor respiratory deficiency and who have learned "frog breathing."

In view of the physiologic similarities between GPB, the initiation of respiration in newborns, and the injection method of air intake for esophageal speech, we consider injection a homologically primitive respiratory mechanism used by mature adults during esophageal speech. During esophageal speech, the esophagus assumes the role of an accessory lung, and, during injection, the upper respiratory system motions resemble the more primitive respiratory maneuvers of amphibia and newborns.

SUMMARY

This article describes the similarities between glossopharyngeal breathing and injection methods of air intake for esophageal speech. The observations were derived from cineradiographic studies of oral, pharyngeal, and upper esophageal function in laryngectomized persons employing esophageal speech and in poliomyelitic subjects using glossopharyngeal breathing. Pertinent clinical and experimental studies of glossopharyngeal breathing and esophageal speech illustrate the common physiologic, homologic, and clinical features of these two respiratory maneuvers.

ACKNOWLEDGMENT

We are grateful to W. M. Diedrich, Ph.D., and K. A. Youngstrom, M.D., of the University of Kansas Medical Center, for the cineradiographic materials they made available to us for this study; and to the National Foundation for Infantile Paralysis, New York, for their loan of the Dail-Affeldt film *Glossopharyngeal Breathing*. Figure 1 has been reprinted through the courtesy of the *Journal of the American Medical Association,* and Figures 2a-b, courtesy of Charles C Thomas, Publisher.

REFERENCES

Bosma, J. F., Lind, J., and Gentz, N., Motions of the pharynx associated with initial aeration of the lungs of the newborn infant. *Acta Paediat.,* 48, Suppl. 117, 117-122 (1959).

Berlin, C., Clinical measurement of esophageal speech. I. Methodology and curves of skill acquisition. *J. Speech Hearing Dis.,* 28, 42-51 (1963).

Collier, C. R., Dail, C. W., and Affeldt, J. E., Mechanics of glossopharyngeal breathing. *J. appl. Physiol.,* 8, 580-584 (1956).

Dail, C. W., Affeldt, J. E., and Collier, C. R., Clinical aspects of glossopharyngeal breathing. *J. amer. med. Asso.,* 158, 445-449 (1955).

Damste, P. H., *Oesophageal Speech After Laryngectomy.* Groningen: Boekdrukkerij Norheen Gebroeders Hortsema (1958).

Damste, P., The glossopharyngeal press. *Speech Path. Ther.,* 2, 70-76 (1959).

Diedrich, W. M., and Youngstrom, K. A., *Alaryngeal Speech.* Springfield, Ill.: Charles C Thomas (1966).

Harries, J. R., and Lawes, W. E., Spirographic studies in glossopharyngeal breathing. *Brit. med. J.,* 2, 1205-1206 (1957).

Ingelfinger, F. J., Esophageal motility. *Physiol. Rev.,* 38, 533-584 (1958).

Isshiki, N., and Snidecor, J. D., Air intake and usage in esophageal speech. *Acta oto-laryng.,* 59, 599-574 (1965).

Kelleher, W. H., and Parida, R. K., Glossopharyngeal breathing. *Brit. med. J.,* 2, 740-743 (1957).

Negus, V., *The Comparative Anatomy and Physiology of the Larynx.* London: N. Heinemann (1949).

Salmon, S., Pressure variations in the esophagus, pharyngo-esophageal constriction, and pharynx associated with esophageal speech production. *Ph.D. dissertation,* State Univer. Iowa (1965).

Shames, G. H., Font, J., and Mathews, J. Factors related to speech proficiency of the laryngectomized. *J. Speech Hearing Dis.,* 28, 273-287 (1963).

Zumwalt, M., Adkins, H. W., Dail, C. W., and Affeldt, J. E., Glossopharyngeal breathing. *Phys. Ther. Rev.,* 36, 455-460 (1956).

AIR INTAKE AND USAGE IN ESOPHAGEAL SPEECH

Nobuhiko Isshiki and John C. Snidecor
Los Angeles and Santa Barbara, California, U.S.A.

From the Department of Surgery, Medical Center, University of California, Los Angeles, and from the Department of Speech, University of California, Santa Barbara

Simultaneous recording of the rate and volume of oronasal air flow, respiratory movement and voice signal were made on six esophageal speakers during speech, swallowing and breathing. Analysis of the data indicated the following:

1. The method of air intake varied greatly with the individual. A plosive-injector charged most (91%) of his air during exhalation, while four speakers who utilized the inhalation and injection methods, insufflated more air without voice during inhalation than during exhalation.

2. In all subjects, except the plosive-injector, voice was produced predominantly with outward flow of air during exhalation.

3. The mean flow rates for comfortably sustaining vowel /a/ ranged from 27 to 72 cc/sec.

4. The inhalatory phonation was negligible for all speakers. Swallowing was not effective for air intake.

5. Some clinical implications of the experimental results and pneumotachographic method were discussed.

INTRODUCTION

The first and most important step in learning esophageal speech is the act of taking air into the esophagus. Because of its importance, various methods of air insufflation have been investigated and discussed by many writers. Historically, the methods postulated are inhalation (suction), injection (tongue pumping), plosive-injection and swallowing.

The inhalation method is supported by Seeman (1958), Burger & Kaiser (1925), Brighton & Boone (1937), Froeschels (1951) and Hodson & Oswald (1958). According to the inhalation method, air is sucked into the esophagus by (1) negative pressure in the esophagus created by the inhalatory movement and (2) simultaneous relaxation or opening of the pseudoglottis.

The injection method, on the other hand, emphasizes the movement of the articulatory organs such as the tongue, soft palate and mouth. The air

This research was supported by USPHS Research Grant NB-04430-03 from the National Institute of Neurological Diseases and Blindness. Research travel was supported by the Wood Glen Hall Research Fund.

Reprinted by permission from *Acta Oto-Laryngologica*, 1965, 59, 559–574.

in the closed glossopharyngeal cavity is pressed down (injected) into the esophagus chiefly by the downward and/or backward movement of the tongue. This phenomenon is variously described as "tongue pumping", "Pumpwerk", or "the initial stage of swallowing". Those who give general support to the injection method are Schilling (1927), Stetson (1937), van Gilse (1949) and Schlosshauer & Möckel (1958). This method has recently been recommended by van den Berg, Moolenaar-Bijl & Damsté (1958). They also emphasize the importance of plosive consonants in esophageal speech. Gutzmann (1909) pointed out that the plosive consonants are most easily learned by the esophageal speaker. Furthermore, the significance of the plosive consonant was reevaluated by Moolenaar-Bijl (1953) not only for the ease with which the plosive consonants can be produced, but also for their role in taking air into the esophagus. Most of the recent investigators appear to refute swallowing per se as a method of air intake in esophageal speech.

Methods of air intake and their respective proponents were classified as above for the sake of simplification. It should be mentioned, however, that definitions and opinions as to the method are different in detail depending on the investigators. For instance, Schlosshauer & Möckel (1958), expressing their doubt about the conventional classification of method of air intake, stated that the combination of various methods would be consonant with the physiological mechanism available for esophageal speech. Based on the cineradiographic findings, Diedrich & Youngstrom (1962) reported that "seven subjects used the inhalation method for trapping air and 20 subjects were classified as using the injection method".

Compared with the wealth of information regarding the method of air intake, very little work has been done in the actual measurement of air flow rate and volume for esophageal speech. Kaiser (1926), using a Gad's air volume recorder, studied the aerodynamic aspect of esophageal voice for the first time. She reported that an excellent esophageal speaker insufflated air, generally a little less than 100 cc, before speech. Based on the spirometric or radiographic findings, the volume of air per syllable or per word was reported by Stetson (1937), Howie (1947) and Snidecor (1962). Sugano (1962) stated that the air volume expired out of the esophagus ranged from 45 cc to 140 cc. So far as the available literature is concerned, no systematic and analytic measurement of air flow rate or its volume during esophageal speech appears to have been previously reported.

The present paper is one part of a series of three studies. The detailed description of an excellent esophageal speaker (W) and the interrelationship between speech fluency and air flow characteristics are reported elsewhere. The topics discussed in this paper include: (1) individual variation in the method of esophageal speech; (2) advantage and disadvantage of each different method of air intake; (3) synchrony or asynchrony between the air intake and respiration; (4) synchrony or asynchrony between vocalization and respiration.

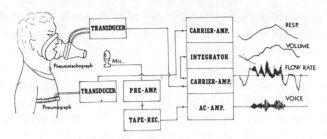

Fig. 1. Diagram of the experimental arrangement.

PROCEDURE

Subject. Six male esophageal speakers were studied in the present investigation. All of the speakers were intelligible, and even the poorer speakers were judged as belonging in the automatic category described by Wepman *et al.* (1953).

Tasks. The tasks the subjects performed included reading a part of the Rainbow Passage, sustaining phonations of the vowel /a/, counting as high as possible with one breath, articulating CVC syllables, swallowing, and breathing. The Rainbow Passage that the subjects read follows:

> When the sunlight strikes raindrops in the air, they act like a prism and form a rainbow. The rainbow is a division of white light into many beautiful colors. These take the shape of a long round arch, with its path high above, and its two ends apparently beyond the horizon.

Equipment. An outline of the experimental arrangement is illustrated in Fig. 1. Four measurements were made simultaneously during esophageal speech: (1) the voice; (2) respiratory (thoracic) movement; (3) rate and (4) volume of air flow through the oronasal passage. The subjects wore an air-tight mask during speech so that no air could leak between the face and mask. Voice signals were recorded on a tape recorder through a condenser microphone. The output of the tape recorder was, in turn, connected via an AC amplifier to a four channel poly beam recorder to obtain an oscillographic recording of voice. The movement of the thorax was recorded by means of a pneumograph. A pressure variation in the pneumograph was sensitized by a strain gauge pressure transducer and recorded on another channel of the recorder.

A pneumotachograph was utilized to measure the rate of air flow in and out of the mouth and nose during speech. Electrical signals from the differential pressure transducer were amplified by a carrier amplifier and fed into one of the four channels of the poly beam recorder so that a tracing of the flow rate was secured. An integrating amplifier converted the flow rate signal into the volume automatically. The pneumotachograph was calibrated by frequent checks with a rotameter.

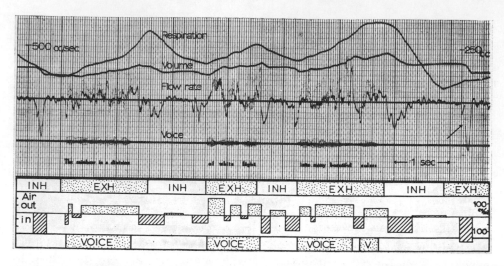

Fig. 2. From top to bottom the traces represent: (1) Respiration. Inhalation is represented by the downward slope, exhalation by the upward curve. (2) Volume of air intake and exsufflation (each heavy graduation, consisting of 5 fine graduations, corresponds to 25 cc). Inward air flow is represented by the downward slope, outward flow by the upward slope. (3) Air flow rate traces above the baseline represent outward flow, below the line inward flow. Each heavy graduation corresponds to 50 cc/sec. (4) Voice. These recordings are schematically shown below by block diagrams. In the second row of the diagram, flow rate is represented by the height of the block, volume by the area. The arrow indicates an asynchronous air intake.

An example of the recordings is shown in Fig. 2. A detailed description (Types and Number) of this instrument was given in a previous paper by Isshiki (1964).

Analyses of recordings

In analyzing the complicated sequence of events during esophageal speech, three parameters were taken into consideration, as schematically indicated in Fig. 2. These were respiratory movement, direction of air flow and voicing. According to all possible combinations of these three factors, the events during esophageal speech were classified into 8 different categories, as shown in Table 1. For each type of different event, analyses were made as to the volume and rate of air flow and the duration of the event. The data were summarized for each type of event in order to estimate which type was predominantly utilized for the intake of air and voice production. In interpreting the data for the air flow, special care was taken so that the flow measured by the pneumotachograph did not directly indicate the air flow into the esophagus. Some movement of air sensitized by the pneumotachograph simply resulted from the slight change in the oropharyngeal cavity because of the tongue movement. In general, it was noted that if the incoming and outgoing flow of air were limited within the cavity above the pseudoglottis, the inward flow of air was immediately followed by the same

TABLE 1.

Type	Direction of oronasal air flow	Phase relation between tracheal and oronasal air flow	Voicing or not	Remarks
1	In	Out-phase	No	Indicative of injection of air
2	In	Out-phase	Voice	Indicative of injection of air
3	In	In-phase	No	Indicative of inhalatory intake
4	In	In-phase	Voice	Inhalatory phonation
5	Out	Out-phase	No	Loss of air or voiceless consonant
6	Out	Out-phase	Voice	Asynchronous phonation
7	Out	In-phase	No	Loss of air or voiceless consonant
8	Out	In-phase	Voice	Synchronous phonation similar to normal

amount of outward flow of air. On the other hand, all the outgoing air flow accompanied by voice was judged as emanating from the esophagus or from below the pseudoglottis.

RESULTS

Total amount and rate of air intake

The total amount of air intake while reading the Rainbow Passage was about 1000 cc for each of the present subjects except for speaker P, as indicated by Table 2. The substantially smaller amount of air (325 cc) that

TABLE 2. *Air Intake[a]*.

Ranking ... Subject ...	1 W	2 A	2 V	3 C	3 M	4 P
Total volume of air intake in cc	948	1118	888	987	1189	325
Total speech time in sec	28	23	29	36	45	29
Rate of air intake in cc/sec	33.9	48.6	30.6	27.4	26.4	11.2
Synchronous intake of air (during inhalation) in volume percentage	76	9	62	64	71	44
Asynchronous intake of air (during exhalation)	24	91	38	36	29	56
Synchronous intake of air (during inhalation) in time percentage	66	16	48	49	64	43
Asynchronous intake of air (during exhalation)	34	84	52	51	36	57
Voiced air intake in volume percentage	14	67	35	21	21	45
Unvoiced air intake in volume percentage	86	33	65	79	79	55
Number of respirations	14	3	24	26	36	25

[a] The data were obtained from recording the air flow during the reading of the Rainbow Passage.

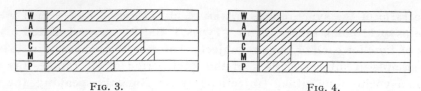

FIG. 3.   FIG. 4.

FIG. 3. Phase relationship between air intake and respiration, expressed in volume percentage. The slashed area represents the air intake during inhalation (synchronous intake), the blank area the air intake during exhalation (asynchronous intake).

FIG. 4. Relationship between air intake and voice production. The slashed area represents the voiced air intake, the blank area the voiceless air intake.

P insufflated may be responsible for his poor speech. The efficiency of air intake, however, should be judged not by the total amount of air intake but by the rate of air intake per unit of time (total air intake/total speech time including the pause between speech). *The rate of air intake*[1] per unit of time for the subjects ranged from 11.2 cc/sec to 48.6 cc/sec. It was noted that the better the speakers the more efficient the air intake. Speakers C and M, who were ranked 3rd in ability, could insufflate as much air, if not more, than the higher ranked subjects could, but speakers C and M required longer periods of time for this task.

Phase relationship between intake of air and respiration

The inhalation method implies, by definition, that the intake of air is synchronous with the inhalatory movement of the thorax, while in the injection method the intake of air takes place during exhalation as well as inhalation. If the air is insufflated during exhalation or asynchronously with the breathing, it appears that the air was taken in by a variation of the injection method, not the inhalation method. Therefore, an analysis of the phase relationship between the intake of air and respiration is helpful in judging the method of air intake which the esophageal speaker is utilizing.

For each of the six subjects, the percentages of air volume insufflated synchronously with the respiration (Types 3 and 4 in Table 1) during the reading of the Rainbow Passage were calculated and are shown in Table 2 and Fig. 3. It is clear from the table and figure that the means of air intake varies greatly with the individual. Speaker A obtained most (91%) of his air during the exhalatory phase. This asynchrony between air intake and respiration indicates that he is principally an injector. Four subjects, W, V, C, and M insufflated a greater amount of air during inhalation rather than during exhalation. However, all subjects secured some air (above 23% in this investigation) during the exhalatory phase (asynchronous intake of air).

[1] The rate of air intake should be distinguished from the mean flow rate of air which is calculated by dividing the total amount of air intake by the sum of the period of air intake (excluding the rest or expulsion period).

The ratio of the synchronous intake of air (Types 3 and 4 in Table 1) to the asynchronous intake of air (Types 1 and 2) was calculated also in terms of *time* for each of the six subjects. The results are shown in Table 2. For example in subject A, 84% of the total period of air intake was used for the asynchronous intake (injection) of air. Roughly speaking, the time ratio of the synchronous intake of air to the asynchronous intake for each speaker is similar to the ratio in terms of the *volume* which was mentioned in the preceding paragraph.

Air intake with or without voicing

If the air is suctioned into the esophagus through the pseudoglottis which is actively opened, the incoming stream of air is usually not accompanied by voice, although if the glottis is closed air intake may accompany the voicing. If the air is actively injected under a positive pressure through the closed glottis, the air flow is more likely to cause vocalization. From these concepts, the air intake was analyzed in relation to vocalization.

The volume ratio of air insufflation with voice (Types 2 and 4 in Table 1) to that without voice (Types 1 and 3) is shown in Table 2 and Fig. 4. A great individual variation in the ratio is noted. Subject A was unique in that a greater volume of air was taken with voicing than without voicing. This finding further indicates that he is an injector. The other subjects insufflated more air without vocalization than with vocalization. It is of great interest to note that this ratio between the voiced insufflation and unvoiced insufflation is quite similar to the ratio between synchronous insufflation and asynchronous insufflation. In other words, it appears that the voiced air intake occurs mostly during the exhalatory phase (voiced injection method) and very seldom during the inhalatory phase (inhalatory phonation).

Comparison of 4 types of air intake

When the two factors of vocalization and the phase relationship with breathing are taken into consideration, the intake of air can be classified into 4 types as shown in Table 1. In order to find the characteristics of each method, these four types of air intake were compared with one another in respect to the amount of air intake per trial, the flow rate, the efficiency and the duration of each trial. As shown in Table 3, for all subjects the volume of air insufflated by method 3 (in-phase, unvoiced) is greater than that obtained by the other methods. The intake of air by type 4 (synchronous with respiration, voiced), which represents the inhalatory phonation, is almost negligible because the number of occurrences and the total volume of air taken in this method are extremely small for all subjects. A greater resistance to the incoming air flow is expected when the air-intake is accompanied by voice, since during phonation the pseudoglottis is assumed to be closed. This greater resistance of the pseudoglottis to the air flow during phonation may explain why more air can be insufflated without vocaliza-

TABLE 3. *Mean volume cc of air intake during one performance using four different methods.*

Method	W	A	V	C	M	P	Mean
			Subject				
Type 1	14.4	11.0	10.0	11.8	9.1	7.0	10.55
Type 2	5.9	13.4	8.1	7.8	6.9	5.4	7.92
Type 3	29.9	17.0	17.0	18.5	21.7	9.9	19.0
Type 4	10.0	—	10.8	—	5.7	4.0	7.62

TABLE 4. *Mean duration sec of air intake during one performance using four different methods.*

Method	W	A	V	C	M	P	Mean
			Subject				
Type 1	.23	.12	.12	.18	.20	.12	.16
Type 2	.12	.11	.11	.17	.13	.16	.13
Type 3	.32	.30	.13	.20	.30	.25	.25
Type 4	.25	—	.09	—	.07	.13	.14

tion than with vocalization. So far as the amount of air intake is concerned, method 3 (indicative of the inhalatory method) appears most effective, but in respect to the amount of information, method 2 (indicative of the injection method) appears to be more efficient if the voice produced during the air intake is well articulated and intelligible.

As indicated in Table 4, one performance of method 3 consumed a longer period of time than did the other methods. If we regard method 1 and 2 as the injection methods and method 3 as the inhalation method, then the difference in duration of one action between the injection method (1 and

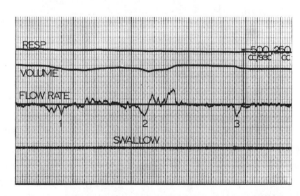

FIG. 5. Air flow during swallowing movement. The inward flow of air is generally followed by the outward flow.

TABLE 5. *Mean flow rate cc/sec of air intake for four different methods.*

Method	Subjekt						Mean
	W	A	V	C	M	P	
Type 1	62	96	83	64	46	57	68
Type 2	50	118	71	45	56	33	62
Type 3	94	58	135	95	73	39	82
Type 4	40	—	123	—	77	30	70

2) and the inhalation method (3) is quite conceivable, because in general the duration of the tongue movement appears shorter than that of the breathing movement.

The flow rate for the different types of air intake are shown in Table 5. It is seen that in subject W, V, C, and M who appeared to utilize primarily the inhalation method, the flow rate for method 3 (indicative of inhalation method) is higher than the flow rate for method 1 or 2 (indicative of the injection method). In contrast, the flow rate for method 1 or 2 (injection) was higher than the flow rate for method 3 (inhalation) for speaker A and P, who were regarded as principally using an injection method.

Generally, during one inhalatory movement, one or two substantial intakes of air occurred. The better speakers such as W and V were inclined to perform a greater number of air intakes—sometimes three—during one inhalatory phase, as indicated in Fig. 2.

The air flow through the oronasal passages during *swallowing* was recorded for all subjects. An inward flow of air (usually less than 50 cc) during the initial stage of swallowing was followed by an outward flow of air during the latter stage of swallowing (Fig. 5). This phenomenon appears to occur because most of the air movement is limited within the cavity above the pseudoglottis and a very small amount of air may be drawn inefficiently into the esophagus by swallowing.

The oronasal air flow during *breathing* indicated that the normal inhalation itself did not introduce any inward movement of air through the nose or mouth in any subjects.

Outward flow of air

As indicated in Table 6, most of the outward flow of air from the esophagus or oropharyngeal cavity occurred during the exhalatory phase of respiration (synchrony), regardless of the method of air intake. Table 6 also indicates the percentage of the outflow which is accompanied by vocalization. Again, speaker A, a plosive-injector, exhibits a different characteristic in this respect from the other speakers. He expels a greater amount of air without voice (unmodulated air flow) than with voice (modulated air flow). In the other speakers, most of the outflow of air expelled during the exhalatory phase was used for voice production. Unmodulated air flow

TABLE 6. *Outward flow of air: relationship with respiration and vocalization, expressed in volume percentage.*

	W	A	V	C	M	P
Synchronous outflow (during exhalation)	91	97	85	69	92	77
Asynchronous outflow (during inhalation)	9	3	15	31	8	23
Voiced outflow	83	44	74	50	81	59
Unvoiced outflow	17	56	26	50	19	41

TABLE 7. *Phonation: relationship with the direction of air flow and respiratory phase, expressed in volume percentage.*

Method	Subject					
	W	A	V	C	M	P
Type 8	84	40	61	65	73	58
Type 2	13	60	24	32	21	36
Type 4 & 6	3	0	15	3	6	6

does not necessarily mean the loss of air, because it may be contributing to the pronunciation of the voiceless consonants. It should be remembered that not all of the outflow without voice (unmodulated air flow) is expelled from the esophagus; some air flow may come from the pharyngeal cavity.

Phonation

When the direction of air flow and the phase relation with respiration are taken into consideration, voice production can be classified into four different types: (1) using the inward flow during exhalation (asynchronic); (2) using the inward flow during inhalation (synchronic); (3) using the outward flow during inhalation (asynchronic); (4) using the outward flow during exhalation (synchronic). These four different kinds of phonations correspond to the types 2, 4, 6, and 8 respectively in the classification in Table 1.

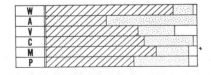

FIG. 6. Three different types of phonation. The slashed area: a phonation with outward air flow during exhalation (Type 8), the dotted area: a phonation with inward flow of air during exhalation (Type 2), the blank area: A phonation during inhalation (Type 4 and 6).

TABLE 8. *The mean flow rates cc/sec for two main types of phonation during speech.*

Method	Subject						Normal
	W	A	V	C	M	P	
Type 8	69	97	56	45	66	25	219
Type 2	50	118	71	45	56	33	

Table 7 and Fig. 6 show which of these four different methods of voice production is predominantly (in volume and time) employed by each speaker. In all of the subjects, except A (the plosive-injector), the voice was produced predominantly with the outward flow of air during exhalation (Type 8) and, to a lesser degree, produced with the inward flow of air during the exhalatory phase (Type 2). Speaker A produced voice more by utilizing the inward flow during exhalation than by utilizing the outward flow during exhalation. Regardless of the method of air intake used by the subjects, the vocal utterances during the inhalatory phase (Types 4 and 6) using either inward or outward air flow, were almost negligible. The mean flow rates while reading the Rainbow Passage for two main types of vocalization are shown in Table 8 (Types 2 and 8). The mean flow rate during phonation through the use of outward flow of air during exhalation (Type 8) ranged from 25 to 97 cc/sec. The mean flow rate for the poorest speaker (P) is substantially lower as compared with those for the other and better speakers. The plosive-injector A uses a very high rate of air flow for phonation. All of the foregoing data were obtained from recording the air flow during the reading of the Rainbow Passage.

The mean flow rates for comfortably sustained phonation of the vowel /a/ ranged from 27 to 72 cc/sec. Speaker W continued phonation for a maximum of 4.25 sec. The injectors, A and P, could not prolong the vowel /a/ as long as the other speaker could. The difference in the flow rates between voiceless consonants and voiced consonants was not as distinct in esophageal speech as in normal speech.

DISCUSSION

An analysis of the data revealed that the types of air intake and usage in connection with respiration and vocalization vary greatly with the speakers. Furthermore, it was suggested that most of the esophageal speakers, here studied, used a combination of methods of air intake. In order to contrast the differences among those methods, a comparison was made between speakers W and A, both of whom were superior in esophageal speech and were considered as representing the two different types of esophageal speech.

Speaker W took most of the air (76%) during inhalatory phase of respira-

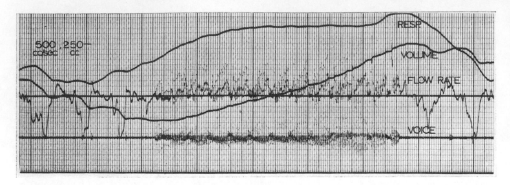

Fig. 7. Maximum repetition (14 times) of the syllable /ba/ with one breath by speaker W. Note that no air intake occurred in connection with the syllable /ba/.

tion (synchronous intake), while speaker A pumped in almost all the air (91%) during the exhalatory phase (asynchronous intake). A similar tendency was found in time-percentage of air intake: in W, 66% of total time of air intake was used for the synchronous intake (air intake during inhalation), while A used 84% of the total time of air intake for the asynchronous intake. In speaker W, only 14% of the total volume of air intake was accompanied by voice. In speaker A, 67% of the total air intake was voiced. The type and frequency of breathing are also quite different between the two speakers. Speaker W breathed 14 times while reading the 51 words passage, but A breathed only 3 times during the same passage; a normal subject took 6 breaths for the same passage.

In speaker A, the expiration occurred very gradually and slowly. The noise level produced by both speakers at the tracheostoma were too low to attract any attention. Both W and A were excellent in speech performances. For instance, the word per minute indicated 153 word/min. for W and 128 for A. The speeches by the two subjects were equally intelligible. A's speech, however, was characterized by his overaccentuation of consonant sounds. In the performance of prolonged phonation of the vowel /a/, speaker W was much superior to speaker A in that W sustained the vowel /a/ much longer than did A. Speaker W repeated syllable /ma/ as many times (14) as he did /ba/. This fact suggests that he did not inject air in connection with the plosive consonant (Fig. 7).

Since A charged most of the air during the exhalatory phase, it would be safe to conclude that he is an injector. From further analysis of the record of CVC syllable and perceptive judgment of his speech, speaker A appears to be a plosive injector. On the other hand, a synchronous intake of air (air intake during inhalation) alone, although highly indicative of the inhaler, is not sufficient to conclude that one is purely an inhaler, because the injection of air can occur theoretically during the inhalatory phase too. The question is whether or not he is using the tongue to pump air. The recording of air flow showed that the normal deep (not so quick as during speech) breathing movement itself, without any movement of the tongue, did not induce any substantial inflow of air through the oronasal passage.

Some portion of air was taken in also during exhalation (asynchronous intake) as indicated by the arrow in Fig. 2. The two separate intakes of air during one inhalatory phase, as shown in the same figure, appeared to correspond to two movements of the tongue. Furthermore, to an inquiry about his method of air intake, speaker W answered that he could not charge air without the movement of the tongue. From these findings, it was assumed that W was also using the tongue pumping method (injection). From reasoning similar to the above, the other subjects were also considered as using both inhalation and injection method, although the degree of dominance of one method over the other appeared to vary with the speakers.

Earlier work in this area appears to support one particular method and to refute the other methods. Moreover, some of the articles, although they support the various methods, give the impression that the speaker has to choose and use only one method: the methods appeared incompatible with each other. Within the limitation of the present data, we feel that many esophageal speakers are unconsciously employing a combination of methods of air intake, which, we think, is recommendable.

Naturally, insufflation of air into the esophagus by the tongue movement would be greatly facilitated by negative pressure in the esophagus. Actually one of the advantages of the inhalation method is a large amount of air intake per trial, which can be demonstrated by a sustained phonation of the vowel /a/. As previously mentioned, the mean volume of synchronous intake of air (during inhalation) is greater than the volume insufflated during the exhalatory phase (Table 3).

However, it should be mentioned that overexertion of the respiratory movement may result in various disadvantages which have been pointed out by many writers. These include parasitic noise at the tracheostoma, unfavorable effect on the lungs and vascular system, fatigue, and so on. The speakers who repeat deep breathing too frequently during speech with a great tracheal noise, should be taught more about the use of the tongue and lips in charging air in and the relaxation of the pseudoglottis as a means of compensation for respiratory overexertion. Too much dependence on the inhalation method may sometimes lead to these difficulties mentioned above. However, these difficulties or disadvantages do not lead to a refutation of the inhalation method at all. The important aspect is the balance of the respiratory effort.

Some of the earlier authors insisted on the necessity of dissociation among air intake, speech and respiration. Recent investigators, on the other hand, presented data favoring synchrony among these factors. Robe, Moore, Andrews & Holinger (1956), supporting the synchrony between oral and pulmonary air movement, still mention the need of dissociation among them in some speakers who produce much noise at the tracheostoma. The suppression of only the respiratory movement does not seem to solve the problem, because this will result in the reduction of the volume of air intake and in the decreased force of air expulsion during phonation. If those noise producing speakers learned to relax the pseudoglottis or the other method of air intake—tongue pumping, the respiratory exertion would naturally be reduced. No further need exists for respiratory overexertion.

The inhalatory phonation (using inflow, during the inhalatory phase) was very rare for all the speakers: the volume percentage of the inhalatory phonation to the total phonation ranged from 0 to 8. The swallowing method was not efficient in air charging. The volume of air swallowed was very small and the swallowing movement could not be repeated rapidly. For the air charge into the esophagus, a laryngectomized patient has to learn correct movements of the tongue and the lips which have not been used prior to laryngectomy.

Some movement of the tongue and the other articulatory organs which are used in normal speech before laryngectomy are similar to the movements necessary for air insufflation, and therefore can be utilized as cues to the new movements to be learned. These are, for instance, pronunciation of the plosive consonants and swallowing. Many investigators (van Gilse 1949; van den Berg, Moolenaar-Bijl & Damsté 1958; Schlosshauer & Möckel, 1958) have already described the initial phase of swallowing as resembling the action of the tongue required for air insufflation. It should be emphasized to the patient that the total action of swallowing is not appropriate for air intake but only the initial stage need be used.

A general discussion on the coordination of air intake with respiration would not be realistic, without a consideration of the method of air intake that the speaker is utilizing. In an inhaler, more synchrony between air intake and respiration is noted than in an injector. Actually, there would be no simple answer to this problem: synchrony or asynchrony. Most speakers employ both synchronic and asynchronic intake of air in various degrees depending on the method of air intake. In this study, the majority of speakers (inhalation and injection) charged more air synchronously than asynchronously.

The phase relationship between speech and respiration also depends on the method of air intake used. Most (85–100% in volume) of the phonations were made during the exhalatory phase using either inflow or outflow (Type 2 and 8 in Table 1). Excluding the plosive injector A, the present speakers produced voice mainly by utilizing the outward flow (Type 8).

As exemplified by the two superior esophageal speakers who were utilizing different methods, no one single method appeared best suited for any speaker. It was shown that a pneumotachographic technique for measuring flow rate presents a useful means of analyzing the sequence of events during esophageal speech. Further research through this technique alone or in combination with other methods is needed in this field, not only for superior speakers such as those studied here but also for less able speakers.

ACKNOWLEDGMENT

The authors express their appreciation to Hans von Leden, M.D., and Elvira Werner Kukuk, M.D. for their cooperation in this study. The subjects were nominated by Morton Cooper, Ph.D., and Robert Harrington, Ph.D., both of whom are experienced teachers of esophageal speech.

ZUSAMMENFASSUNG

Der Grad und Umfang des oronasalen Luftflusses, also respiratorische Bewegungen und Stimmsignale, wurden gleichzeitig an sechs Oesophagus-Sprechern, während diejenigen sprachen, schluckten und atmeten, registriert. Eine Analyse der Befunde hat Folgendes ergeben:

1) Die Methode der Luftaufnahme zeigte grosse individuelle Unterschiede. Ein Plosive-Injektor belastete sich mit der meisten (91%) ihm zur Verfügung stehenden Luft während der Ausatmung, dagegen sogen vier Sprecher, welche die Inhalations- und Injektionsmethode benutzten, stimmlos mehr Luft ein während der Inhalation als bei der Ausatmung.

2) Alle Testpersonen, mit der Ausnahme des Plosive-Injektors, erzeugten ihre Stimme vorwiegend mit Fluss der Luft nach aussen während der Ausatmung.

3) Der Luftfluss-Mittelwert für bequem aufrechterhaltenem Vokal /a/ lag zwischen 27 and 72 cc/sec.

4) Die Inhalationsphonation war für alle Sprecher nicht beachtenswert. Der Akt des Schluckens ist nicht empfehlenswert für Lufteinnahme.

5) Einige klinische Zusammenhänge der experimentellen Resultate und der pneumotachographischen Methoden wurden diskutiert.

REFERENCES

BERG, J. VAN DEN, MOOLENAAR-BIJL, A. J., and DAMSTÉ, P. H., 1958: Oesophageal speech. *Folia Phoniat.* (Basel), *10*, 65.

BERG, J. VAN DEN, and MOOLENAAR-BIJL, A. J., 1959: Crico-pharyngeal sphincter, pitch, intensity and fluency in oesophageal speech. *Pract. Otorhinolaryng.* (Basel), *21*, 298.

BRIGHTON, G. R., and BOONE, W. H., 1937: Roentgenographic demonstration of method of speech in case of complete laryngectomy. *Amer. J. Roentgenol.*, 38, 571.

BURGER, H., and KAISER, L., 1925: Speech without a larynx. *Acta Otolaryng.* (Stockh.), *8*, 90.

CURRY, E. T., and SNIDECOR, J. C., 1961: Physical measurement and pitch perception in esophageal speech. *Laryngoscope*, *71*, 3.

DAMSTÉ, P. H., 1958: *Oesophageal speech after laryngectomy.* Groningen.

DIEDRICH, W. M., and YOUNGSTROM, K., 1962: *An investigation of speech after laryngectomy.* Office of Vocational Rehabilitation Summary Report, Project No. 337.

FROESCHELS, E., 1951: Therapy of the alaryngeal voice following laryngectomy; a contribution. *Arch. Otolaryng.* (Chic.), *53*, 77.

GILSE, P. H. G. VAN, 1949: Another method of speech without larynx. *Acta Otolaryng.* (Stockh.), Suppl. *78*, 109.

GUTZMANN, H., 1909: Stimme und Sprache ohne Kehlkopf. *Z. Laryng. Rhinol. Otol.*, *1*, 221.

HODSON, C. J., and OSWALD, M. V. O., 1958: *Speech Recovery after Total Laryngectomy.* E. and S. Livingstones, Ltd., Edinburgh and London.

Howie, T. O., 1947: Rehabilitation of the patient after laryngectomy. *Occup. Ther., 26,* 372.

Isshiki, N., 1964: Regulatory mechanism of voice intensity variation. *J. Speech Hearing Res., 7,* 17.

Isshiki, N., and von Leden, H.: Hoarseness-Aerodynamic studies. *Arch. Otolaryng.* (Chic.), (in press).

Kaiser, L., 1926: Examen phonétique d'un sujet privé de larynx. *Arch. Néerl Physiol., 10,* 468.

Moolenaar-Bijl, A. J., 1953: Connection between consonant articulation and the intake of air in oesophageal speech. *Folia Phoniat.* (Basel), *5,* 212.

Robe, E. Y., Moore, P., Andrews, A. H., Jr., and Holinger, P. H., 1956: A study of the role of certain factors in the development of speech after laryngectomy. 3. Coordination of speech with respiration. *Laryngoscope, 66,* 481.

Schilling, R., 1927: Über die Pharynx- und Oesophagusstimme. *Z. Hals. Nas. Ohrenheilk., 9,* 893.

Schlosshauer, B., and Möckel, G., 1958: Auswertung der Röntgenfilmnahmen von Speiseröhrensprechern. *Folia Phoniat.* (Basel), *10,* 154.

Seeman, M., 1958: Zur Pathologie der Ösophagusstimme. *Folia Phoniat.* (Basel), *10,* 44.

Snidecor, J. C., 1951: Pitch and duration characteristics of superior female speakers during oral reading. *J. Speech Hearing Dis., 16,* 44.

— 1962: *Speech Rehabilitation of the Laryngectomized.* C. C. Thomas, Springfield, Illinois, 1962.

Stetson, R. H., 1937: Esophageal speech for any laryngectomized patient. *Arch. Otolaryng.* (Chic.), *26,* 132.

Sugano, M., 1962: Study on oesophageal speech. *J. Jap. Bronchooesophag. Soc., 13,* 135.

Wepman, J. M., MacGahan, J. A., Rickard, J. C., and Shelton, N. W., 1953: Progressive nature of esophageal speech development and its objective measurement. *J. Speech Hearing Dis., 18,* 247.

Nobuhiko Isshiki, M.D., Dept. of Otolaryngology, School of Medicine, University of Kyoto, Kyoto, Japan,
John C. Snidecor, Ph.D., Dept. of Speech, University of California, Santa Barbara, Calif., U.S.A.

Received July 28, 1964

TEMPORAL AND PITCH ASPECTS OF
SUPERIOR ESOPHAGEAL SPEECH

JOHN C. SNIDECOR, PH.D.

GOLETA, CALIF.

E. THAYER CURRY, PH.D.

URBANA, ILL.

John O. Anderson[1] in 1954 listed a bibliography of 88 items relative to esophageal speech. Since that time Robe, Moore, Andrews and Holinger[18] have contributed a major study to the field as have Bateman, Dornhurst, and Leathheart.[3] No doubt other studies are in the hands of the publishers or in progress.

The study of available source material dating from 1859 indicates a great deal of material on the incidence of cancer of the larynx and survival rate subsequent to laryngectomy,[16] the nature of the operation,[9,18] pedagogy,[2] and approximately 20 studies that agree in placing the usual locus of vibration at the level of the cricopharyngeus sphincter,[18] but which do not preclude other vibrators.[9,10] Among the more important considerations is the rather general agreement that the air-charge is usually small[22] and that for successful speakers it is taken into and expelled from the upper esophagus rather than from the stomach or lower esophagus[18] as assumed by early writers.

Generally speaking, available source materials have little to offer in the way of normative statistical information that gives direct answers to such important questions as: a) How many words and syllables can be spoken per charge of swallowed air? b) How long does it take to swallow a charge of air? c) What rate in words per minute can be achieved relative to normal speech? d) What characteristics of pitch level and variability can be anticipated in esophageal speech?

It is the purpose of this study to describe the time and pitch performances of six superior esophageal speakers utilizing speech sam-

John C. Snidecor is Professor of Speech, University of California, Santa Barbara. E. Thayer Curry is Professor of Speech, University of Illinois, Urbana, Illinois. The basic data for this study were obtained by the senior author while on Sabbatical leave at the Navy Electronics Laboratory, San Diego, California.

ples of adequate length for which norms for rate,[5] breathing,[21] and pitch[6] are already available for normal or superior speakers.

SELECTION OF SUBJECTS

Superior speakers were selected so that any generalizations arrived at might serve as suitable goals for those learning to speak without a larynx.

An initial group of 52 satisfactory performers from Southern California was obtained through contact with otolaryngologists, speech therapists, the Veterans' Administration, the American Cancer Society, the Lost Chord Club of Los Angeles, and the New Voice Club of San Diego. The senior author screened this group successively to 23 and finally to ten performers. At this stage the following passage from Fairbanks[7] was recorded for each of the ten performers:

"When the sunlight strikes raindrops in the air, they act like a prism and form a rainbow. The rainbow is a division of white light into many beautiful colors. These take the shape of a long round arch, with its path high above, and its two ends apparently beyond the horizon."

These ten recordings were presented, when necessary, by mail, to eight skilled and experienced judges, and included the following directions:

"Please number your papers from one to ten.

"You will presently hear ten brief readings of esophageal speech. These recordings have already been screened for general effectiveness from 23 performances which in turn were screened from 52 performances. This indicates that all of the final samples are reasonably effective for the type of speech under consideration.

"Please rate each speaker for general effectiveness on a one to five rating scale. One equals poor, two equals fair, three equals average, four equals good, and five equals excellent. Judge on these samples only, not on other samples of speech that you have heard.

"A brief word about general effectiveness. Its first attribute is intelligibility, but consideration is also given to those attributes of rate, loudness, pitch, quality, and articulation that make the content easy to assimilate without stress or discomfort on the part of the speaker.

"Do *not* penalize for misreading or mispronunciation.

"You will hear all performances through once before being asked to judge. Record your judgments only on the second playing of the record."

On the basis of these judgments six speakers were selected and utilized for the pitch study. Because of the serious illness of one speaker the next ranking speaker was chosen for the six speakers used for the duration measurements.

All of the speakers were males with at least four years of experience with esophageal speech. Three of the speakers were experienced teachers of esophageal speech. There were excellent female speakers in the original group, but none appeared to match the performance of the male subjects who were finally selected. Six judges were requested to select female voices from the male voices on the basis of recordings alone. Their complete lack of success tends to indicate marked similarity in the voices of male and female esophageal speakers.

Each of the six speakers performed at the highest level of esophageal speech as defined by Wepman, MacGahan, Richard, and Shelton.[23] In other words they spoke with continuity and without consciousness of the act of swallowing and eructation. The speech was easily and naturally produced without apparent thought or effort.

EXPERIMENTAL PROCEDURE

The air-charges were recorded by means of a sensitive light weight electropneumograph placed high on the chest and similar in design and construction to that previously described by Snidecor[21] for the recording of the breathing cycle for superior speakers. In this present study an intensity modulated 1,000 cycle tone served as an air-charge signal and was recorded on one channel of a dual channel magnetic tape recorder while speech was being recorded on the other channel. At a later time the information on each channel was transferred to the moving photographic tape of a Miller Light Writer traveling at 45 mm per second which supplied a visual record of "breathing" and speech that was amenable to measurements. The electrical and photographic means of achieving this final record can best be described by schematic drawings which are available from the senior author. The rise in esophageal air pressure which actuated the pneumograph is described by Bateman, Dornhurst, and Leathheart[3] as "... always accompanied by a sharp expiratory effort and loss of air from the lungs." This puff of air was audible and served to check the electrical recording. The writers believe that the recording of this puff might serve as an economical and reasonably accurate index of air-charge where it appeared desirable to make time estimates based on larger samples of speech.

As described under "Selection of Subjects," each subject recorded a portion of the Rainbow Passage.[7] This passage was used in selecting the subjects, and also for phonelloscopic analysis. All pitch data herein discussed are from this selection.

While recording both his voice and air-charges each speaker performed "as if speaking to an audience of 25 people." First, the subjects were requested to count to ten as many times as possible on one air-charge. The best of three trials was selected for study. Counting is commonly practiced and demonstrated by esophageal speakers. It will be noted that the count to ten requires the speaking of eleven syllables. Second, each subject read and was recorded for the Rainbow Passage[7] attempting to "breathe" at points he had marked as representing his best spots to pause for air. This performance can be dismissed briefly, but not thoughtlessly, by noting that these skilled speakers did not predict with any degree of success when they were going to take an air-charge. Those learning esophageal speech frequently mark passages and take air accordingly. Their skilled counterparts are no more conscious of air intake than normal conversational speakers. Third, each subject read the "Rate Passage"[7] with a break for rest at the end of the first paragraph. From 43 to 48 air charges from this passage were studied for each subject. All temporal data except counting are based on the results from this passage, a sample of which is presented later in this paper.

All temporal measurements were made directly from the photographic record with a simple analogue computer that read directly in seconds and decimals thereof. These results were checked against a one-tenth of a second time line recorded on the photographic tape.

Using the phonophotographic technique originated by Metfessel,[14] modified by Simon[19] and Lewis and Tiffin[12] and electrified by Cowan,[4] pitch curves were plotted from frequency measurements, and measures of pitch were computed.

On the apparatus used for this study, the recording drum circumference was 191.2 cm; the temporal extent of each measurement interval was 0.051 sec.

One of the best general measures of efficiency in speech is rate. Darley[5] established norms for the passage in question for normal speakers and found that the zero percentile was represented by 129 words per minute, the fiftieth percentile by 166 words per minute, and the one hundredth percentile by 222 words per minute. Franke[8] in an investigation of the judgment of rate found that critical listeners found rate too rapid if it exceeded 185 words per minute or too slow if it was less than 140 words per minute.

Perusal of Table I, Item 1 indicates that these superior esophageal speakers ranged from 85 words per minute to 129 words per minute for an extended performance. For the brief, 56 word "Rainbow Passage" speaking rate was somewhat more rapid than for the long passage. The range was from 108 to 137 words per minute with a median rate of 122.5. No speaker exceeded Darley's fifth percentile, nor did any speaker achieve a rate that would have been judged adequately rapid in terms of Franke's data. One hundred and twenty words per minute, or two words per second, is the rate at which efficient secretaries take shorthand. This rate is not slow enough to disturb the average listener. Too much should not be made of rate, for speaker Number three, Table I, was consistently judged as superior to speakers four, five, and six, yet his rate of 85 words per minute was considerably lower than the rates 109 words per minute, 120 words per minute, and 129 words per minute for these speakers.

The question obviously arises: can the esophageal speaker speed up his rate? The answer is that he can do so only within narrow limits without sacrifice of loudness or suitable phrasing. This fact was borne out by trial runs for more rapid rate which were largely unsuccessful. This lack of modifiability is readily explained by the need for frequent air-charges on the part of even highly efficient esophageal speakers.

Item 2 in Table I, that of counting, gives some idea of this problem as will further information in Table I. None of the six speakers exceeded the count of ten (11 syllables) in the three trials allowed each speaker. Speaker number five insisted that he could count to at least thirty without an air-charge. The electropneumograph proved that small air-charges were taken after the count of ten. This speaker was completely unconscious of this fact until he saw evidence of the air-charges on the instrument following the experimental run. It will be noted, however, that speaker five did read as high as 22 syllables on one air-charge, a figure exactly equal to the count of ten repeated

TABLE I

TEMPORAL RELATIONSHIPS

SPEAKER NUMBER	1	2	3	4	5	6	SUPERIOR "NORMAL" SPEAKER
1. Words per minute	120	114	85	109	120	129	140 to 185
2. Count, best of three trials	10	8	10	4	10	7	40 (estimate)
3. Mean words per air-charge	4.2	5.2	2.8	2.9	6.3	3.5	12.5
4. Range in words per air-charge	1-10	1-10	1-5	1-5	3-15	1-8	2-36
5. Sigma, words per air-charge	1.8	1.9	1.0	1.0	3.0	1.4	4.9
6. Mean syllables per air-charge	5.8	7.6	3.9	3.8	8.7	5.2	17.5 (estimate)
7. Range in syllables per air-charge	3-12	2-13	2-6	1-7	4-22	2-11	2-50 (estimate)
8. Sigma, syllables per air-charge	2.11	2.57	1.13	1.21	4.05	1.95	No data
9. Mean pause time for air-charge	.54	.76	.63	.42	.80	.64	.75 to .94
10. Mean duration of air-charge	1.54	1.75	1.04	1.00	2.25	1.25	4.19
11. Mean pause time for phrases	.72	1.13	1.05	.62	1.06	.76	.63

twice which contains 22 syllables due to the two syllables in the digit seven.

These and following data must be interpreted in relationship to the experimental situation lest the results be challenged by those[11] who insist that advanced esophageal speakers produce 200 syllables with one mouthful of air, and that they can count to 70 on one "breath." The esophageal speakers in this study were held to a loudness level suitable for an audience of 25 people. A check of sound level pressures indicated that they maintained these levels. Lowered intensity might well increase somewhat the number of syllables spoken. As has been stated, these superior speakers, without exception, took small charges of air efficiently and unconsciously. The superior speaker using normal breath while reading the same passage did not begin to produce the syllables per breath claimed for some esophageal speakers.

Table I, Item 3, indicates that mean words per air-charge range from 2.8 to 6.3 for esophageal speakers with 12.5 mean words per breath for normal breathing superior speakers. The extreme range for one esophageal speaker was 15 words (22 syllables) whereas one exceptional superior speaker under identical conditions spoke 36 words (50 syllables). These differences can be shown graphically by comparing the two passages[8] below. The oblique lines in the first passage represent the air-charges taken by an efficient esophageal speaker who "charges" as frequently as most of his selected colleagues. The lines in the second passage represent the breaths taken by a superior, normal breathing speaker, who breathes as frequently as his selected colleagues.

Your rate of speech will be adequate | if it is slow enough to provide | for clearness and comprehension, | and rapid enough to sustain interest. | Your rate is faulty if it is too rapid | to accomplish these ends. | The easiest way to begin work | on the adjustment of your speech | to an ideal rate | is to measure your present rate | in words per minute | in a fixed situation | which you can keep constant over a number of trials. | The best method | is to pick a page | of simple, factual prose | to be read. | Read this page in your natural manner, | timing yourself in seconds. | Count the number of words on the page, | divide by the number of seconds, | and multiply this result by sixty | to calculate the number of words per minute. | As you attempt to increase | or retard your rate, | repeat this procedure | from time to time, | using the same reading material, | to enable | you to check your success. |

Your rate of speech will be adequate if it is slow enough to provide for clearness and comprehension, | and rapid enough to sustain interest. | Your rate is faulty if it is too rapid to accomplish these ends. | The easiest way to begin work on the adjustment of your speech to an ideal rate | is to measure your present rate in words per minute in a fixed situation which you can keep constant over a number of trials. | The best method is to pick a page of simple, factual prose to be read. | Read this page in your natural manner, timing yourself in seconds. | Count the number of words on the page, divide by the number of seconds, and multiply this result by sixty to calculate the number of words per minute. | As you attempt to increase or retard your rate, | repeat this procedure from time to time, | using the same reading material, to enable you to check your success. | [7]

Performance one for the esophageal speaker demanded 30 charges of air, whereas performance two for the normal speaker demanded only 11 breaths, yielding word/breath scores of 4 and 12 for the 159-word passage.

Figure 1 illustrates the performance of each group of speakers in regard to the range and mean values of words per air-charge. The

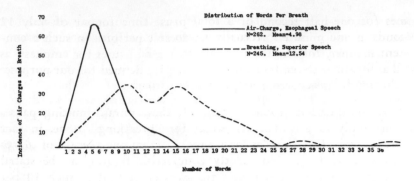

Figure 1

normal speaker reads aloud with an average of 12.54 words per breath, but has a wide range of performance, and tends to utilize breathing phrases of seven and fourteen words. The esophageal speaker averages 4.98 words per air-charge and has a much narrower range of performance.

Further information in Table I on syllabic performance is presented as description in addition to the grosser but more commonly used measure of words.

Our syllabic values, Item 6, are somewhat higher than those found by Stetson[22] who stated a limitation of from 3 to 4 syllables, whereas our lowest average value is 3.8 syllables, and our highest 8.7 syllables per air-charge. The number of speakers is greater in this study and also the speech sample is much larger. The Bateman, Dornhurst, and Leathheart data[3] based on three subjects and short speech samples agree with our data insofar as these are comparable. Our information, even when extreme values are considered, is far more conservative than some information given recent wide publicity.[11]

Esophageal speech despite frequent air-charges is relatively efficient and pleasant to hear. How can this be true? Table I, Item 9, answers this question in part. The skilled esophageal speakers gulped air in from .42 to .80 seconds, mean values considered. This is unbelievably rapid "breathing," fully as rapid in fact as most normal speakers breathe for speech, although it must be added that superior speakers usually breathe at phrasal limits.

If an esophageal speaker speaks at the rate of 120 words per minute, and stops for air after each five words, he would stop 24 times for one-half second or a total pause time for air of only 12 seconds in one minute. Actually he doesn't perform in such a consistent manner, for like the normal speaker he pauses for emphasis as well as breath at the ends of phrases which are defined for our purposes in this study as occurring at punctuation marks.

As indicated in Table I, Item 11, these phrase limiting pauses are markedly longer than his pauses for "breathing" alone, in fact approximately 1.41 times as long, ranging from one average of .62 to an average of 1.13. No exactly comparable figures can be stated for normal speakers, but pauses for phrases, judged as such 50 per cent or more of the time, average .63 seconds, whereas pauses infrequently judged as limiting phrases averaged only one-tenth of this value.[8] In brief, both classes of speakers pause appropriately for phrases, but it appears that the superior esophageal speaker pauses longer than the normal speaker in order that such pauses can contrast with pauses that are for air-charges only.

The value of .63 seconds for phrasal pauses for the normal speakers is shorter than the average time utilized for breathing which is probably explained by the fact that the normal speaker pauses for a number of phrases without taking a breath at these pauses.

As indicated in Item 10, the superior esophageal speaker can utilize his air-charge for approximately $1\frac{1}{2}$ seconds (1.00 to 2.25) during which time he averages from 2.8 to 6.3 words. This contrasts with the normal speakers who utilize their breath for 4.19 seconds and speak 12.5 words. If relative time or words per air-charge is taken as a measure of efficiency the normal speaker is from $2\frac{1}{2}$ to 3 times more efficient than the esophageal speaker.

It is probably much more reasonable to use total words per minute as a measure of efficiency and compare the average for esophageal speech of 113 words per minute with the rate of 166 words per minute for the average normal speaker. When this is done the normal speaker speaks at only 1.47 times the rate of the esophageal speaker, or conversely the esophageal speaker is 80 per cent as fast as the average normal speaker. The fact that the esophageal speaker will always be judged as too slow[8] is of little consequence if his efficiency is relatively satisfactory, and it appears to be quite satisfactory for speech samples of 300 words.

EXPERIMENTAL RESULTS, PITCH

Table II indicates selected measures of central tendency and variability for the frequencies recorded in the speaking performances of

TABLE II

GENERAL MEASUREMENTS OF VOCAL FREQUENCY

	SUPERIOR ESOPHAGEAL SPEAKERS	SUPERIOR ADULT SPEAKERS
Median Frequency Level (c.p.s.)	63.27	132.1
Nearest Musical Tone	C_2	C_3
Median Frequency Level (tones above 16.35 cycles per second)	11.70	18.24
Mean S. D. (tones)	2.30	1.88
Mean Frequency Level (c.p.s.)	62.8	128.1
Nearest Musical Tone	C_2	C_3
Mean Frequency Level (tones above 16.35 cycles per second)	11.65	17.87
Mean Extent of All Inflections (tones)	2.4	2.3
Mean Extent of All Shifts (tones)	2.8	2.6
Mean Rate of Pitch Change (tone per sec.) During Inflections During Shifts	7.9 4.3	17.7 7.0
Mean Total Frequency Range: Tones Octaves	13.21 2.2	10.50 1.75
Mean Effective Frequency Range: Tones Octaves	6.5 1.0	6.3 1.0

these superior esophageal speakers; results for the study group are contrasted with a standard set of measures on a group of selected superior normal speakers previously reported by Pronovost.[17]

The most striking feature of Table II is the difference of almost exactly one octave between the frequency levels of the superior esophageal speakers and the superior normal adult speakers, the respective median values being 63.27 and 132.1 c.p.s. These levels are very close to the musical notes of C_2 and C_3. For these carefully selected speakers, this table shows that for the superior esophageal group both the mean and median frequency used was essentially one whole octave lower than for the comparative group of superior normal speakers. This finding is graphically represented by Figure 2 which gives a distribution of the frequencies measured for the two groups of selected

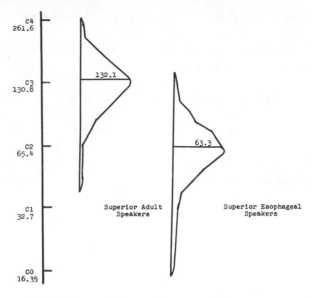

Fig. 2.—Distributions of frequencies measured for two groups of superior speakers.

superior speakers. The form of the two distributions is quite similar; the most obvious difference is, of course, the octave difference in the median frequency levels for the contrasted groups.

In addition to the difference in frequency level, the distributions of Figure 2 show a greater variability of frequency usage for the esophageal speakers than for the normal speakers. A comparison of the standard deviations presented in Table II statistically illustrates the differences. A study of the median frequency levels reported by Pronovost[17] indicates these values for the individual superior speakers of his experiment: 129.9, 116.5, 146.2, 128.8, 130.8 and 157.9 c.p.s. In contrast with these median values used by the normal speakers the highest values used by the selected superior esophageal speakers were: 115.9, 123.4, 118.7, 95.2, 112.3 and 106.6 c.p.s. Four of the esophageal speakers thus used a highest frequency which was lower than the median frequency used by the lowest of the superior normal group.

Both Table II and Figure 2 indicate the total range of frequencies used in the recorded performances; 13.2 tones for the superior esophageal speakers compared with 10.5 tones for the superior normal group. These measures exceed those reported in most previous studies for normal speakers. Lewis and Tiffin,[12] for example, found ranges between 3.8 and 9.9 tones. According to Murray and Tiffin,[15] the frequency ranges of poor, good and trained voices are 2.9, 4.5 and 6.3 tones, respectively. For actual reading, Lynch[13] reports total frequency ranges of 5.8 tones for untrained and 8.2 tones for trained readers. The Median 90 per cent Range is somewhat more meaningful than total range and is oftimes referred to as the "Effective Range." These values are essentially the same for both groups and indicate about one octave for both superior esophageal and superior normal speakers. Again, when values for individual speakers were considered, three of the esophageal speakers exceeded the effective range for the most variable normal speaker; two values were at the same value, and only one esophageal speaker was markedly less in effective range. Table II also indicates measures for frequency and pitch movements. Group values for the mean extent of inflections and shifts are quite similar. However, the group of superior normal speakers is indicated to have considerably larger values for mean rates of pitch change. During inflections the normal group value is 17.7 tones per second while the voices of the superior esophageal group moved only 7.9 tones per second. During shifts the comparable values are 7.0 and 4.3 tones per second. These measures for rates of pitch change during inflections and shifts are, in addition to the basic difference in median frequency level, the only striking contrasts between the vocal frequency usage of the superior esophageal and superior adult speaker groups. The difference in rate of pitch change may well be a simple function operating because of marked differences in rate of speech.

SUMMARY AND CONCLUSIONS

Utilizing a sensitive electropneumograph and phonophotographic techniques, the temporal and pitch factors in six superior esophageal speakers were studied. Major findings slightly generalized were:

1. The subjects spoke relatively easily and were no more conscious of the "breathing" function than normal speakers.

2. Three speakers counted to 4, 7, 8 respectively, and three speakers counted to 10 on one air-charge.

3. The speakers averaged five words (4.98) per air-charge, and performances averaged about 120 words per minute. A top limit of 11 to 12 syllables is very satisfactory. However, one speaker achieved an extreme range of 22 syllables.

4. The air-charge was gulped in about one-half second, a more rapid performance than that of the normal speaker inhaling for an intraphrasal breath pause.

5. The mean pitch level is almost exactly one full octave below that of the normal male speaker.

6. Pitch inflections, shifts, and total and functional pitch range are within normal limits for normal male speakers.

7. The rate of pitch change, in tones per second, is only half that of the normal speaker.

PRACTICAL SIGNIFICANCE

This study, in exploring superior esophageal speech, with adequate samples of speech, establishes realistic norms for those who must learn to speak in this unique way. Highly efficient air-charges encompassing many syllables as reported in recent popular literature are not apparent and in our opinion are reported because the air-charge becomes unconscious for the experienced speaker. Contrary to some reports, pitch variability is comparable to that in normal speech. It is, however, very doubtful that average pitch level can be raised much, if any, above 66 to 77 cycles per second.

REFERENCES

1. Anderson, J. O.: Bibliography on Esophageal Speech. J.S.H.D. 19:1:70-72 (Mar.) 1954.

2. Bangs, J. L., Lierle, D. M., and Strother, C. R.: Speech after Laryngectomy. JSD 11:171-176, 1946.

3. Bateman, G. H., Dornhurst, A. C., and Leathheart, G. L.: Oesophageal Speech. Brit. Med. Jour. 2:1177-78 (Nov. 29) 1952.

4. Cowan, M.: Pitch and Intensity Characteristics of Stage Speech. Ar. Sp. Suppl. 1936.

5. Darley, F. L.: A Normative Study of Oral Reading Rate. M.A. thesis, State Univ. of Ia., 1940.

6. Fairbanks, G.: Recent Experimental Investigations of Vocal Pitch in Speech. Jour. of Acous. Soc. of Amer. 11:457-460, 1940.

7. Fairbanks, G.: Voice and Articulation Drillbook. Harpers, p. 168, rainbow passage; p. 144, rate passage; 1940.

8. Franke, P. E.: Study of the Rate of Speech in Words Per Minute and Relation to Judgments of Rate. M.A. thesis, State Univ. of Ia., 1939.

9. Jackson, C. L.: The Voice after Direct Laryngoscopic Operations, Laryngofissure, and Laryngectomy. Arch. Otolaryng. 31:23-37 (Jan.) 1940.

10. Jackson, C., and Jackson, C. L.: Diseases of the Nose, Throat, and Ear. Phil., W. B. Saunders Co., 581-582, 1946.

11. King, H.: I Lost My Voice to Cancer. Sat. Eve. Post (Sept: 1) 1956.

12. Lewis, D., and Tiffin, J.: A Psychophysical Study of Individual Differences in Speaking Ability. Ar. Sp. 1:43-60, 1934.

13. Lynch, G. E.: A Phonophotographic Study of Trained and Untrained Voices Reading Factual and Emotional Material. Ar. Sp. 1:9-25, 1934.

14. Metfessel, M.: Techniques for the Objective Study of Vocal Art. Psychol. Monog. 36:1-40, 1927.

15. Murray, E., and Tiffin, J.: An Analysis of Some Basic Aspects of Effective Speech. Ar. Sp. 1:41-83, 1934.

16. Palmer, J. M.: Hoarseness in Laryngeal Pathology—A Review of Literature. Laryngoscope 66:500-15 (May) 1956.

17. Pronovost, W.: An Experimental Study of Methods for Determining Natural and Habitual Pitch. Sp. Monog. 9:111-123, 1942.

18. Robe, E. Y., Moore, P., Andrews, A. H., and Hollinger, P. H.: A Study of the Role of Certain Factors in the Development of Speech after Laryngectomy. Laryngoscope 66:3:173-186 (Part I); 66:4:382-401 (Part II); 66:5:481-499 (Part III); 1956.

19. Simon, C. T.: The Variability of Consecutive Wave Lengths in Vocal and Instrumental Sounds. Psychol. Monog. 36:41-83, 1927.

20. Snidecor, J. C.: An Objective Study of Phrasing in Impromptu Speaking and Oral Reading. Speech Mono. 11:97-104, 1944.

21. Snidecor, J. C.: Temporal Aspects of Breathing in Superior Reading and Speaking Performances. Speech Mono. 22:5:284-289, 1955.

22. Stetson, R. H.: Esophageal Speech for Any Laryngectomized Patient. Arch. Otolaryng., Chicago, 26:132-142, 1937.

23. Wepman, Joseph M., MacGahan, John A., Rickard, Joseph C., and Shelton, Niel W.: The Objective Measurement of Progressive Esophageal Speech Development. J.S.H.D. 18:249-50 (Sept.) 1953.

HOW EFFECTIVELY CAN THE LARYNGECTOMEE EXPECT TO SPEAK?

Norms for Effective Esophageal Speech.

JOHN C. SNIDECOR, Ph.D.,*

Santa Barbara, Calif.

and

E. THAYER CURRY, Ph.D.,†

Urbana, Ill.

The present sources of materials related to esophageal speech have little to offer in the way of direct information on how effectively the laryngectomee may reasonably expect to speak. The typical laryngectomee is concerned with such vital questions regarding his speech performance as the following:

1. How many words and syllables can be spoken per charge of swallowed air?

2. How long does it take to swallow a charge of air?

3. What rate in words per minute can be achieved relative to normal speakers?

4. What possibilities of pitch level and pitch variety can be anticipated for esophageal speakers?

The word *frequency* will hereafter be used in place of *pitch* because we measure frequency, which in turn is perceived as pitch. By way of example, we hear middle C and the octave below it as perceived pitches, but these are represented physically as 256 cycles per second and 128 cycles per second.

The laryngectomee would be benefited by some practical normative statistical information about the possibilities he could reasonably expect to achieve in successful esophageal speaking.

*Professor of Speech, University of California, Santa Barbara, Calif.

†Professor of Speech, University of Illinois, Urbana, Ill.

Reprinted by permission from *The Laryngoscope*, 1960, 70, 62–67.

105

It is the purpose of this report to describe generally the time and frequency performances of six superior esophageal speakers utilizing speech samples of adequate length for which norms for rate, breathing and frequency are already available for normal or superior speakers.

SUBJECTS.

Superior esophageal speakers were selected so that any generalizations might serve as suitable and attainable goals for those learning to speak without a larynx. An initial group of 52 satisfactory performers from Southern California was obtained through contact with otolaryngologists, speech therapists, the Veterans Administration, The American Cancer Society, The Lost Chord Club of Los Angeles, and the New Voice Club of San Diego. The senior author screened this group successively to 23 and ten. Eight skilled and experienced judges selected six of the ten performances as best on a rating scale of general effectiveness. The Fairbanks "Rainbow Passage"[2] was recorded for each performer, "as though speaking to an audience of 25 people."

All of the selected speakers were males with at least four years of experience with esophageal speaking. Three of the speakers were experienced teachers of esophageal speech. There were excellent female speakers in the original group, but none appeared to match the performance of the male subjects who were finally selected. Six judges were requested to select female voices from the male voices on the basis of recordings alone. The complete lack of success on the part of the judges tends to indicate marked similarity in the voices of male and female esophageal speakers.

Each of the six speakers performed at the highest level of esophageal speech, as defined by Wepman, MacGahan, Rickard and Shelton[5]; in other words, they spoke with continuity and without consciousness of the act of swallowing and eruction. The speech was easily and naturally produced without apparent thought or effort.

RESULTS.

The answers to our four basic questions can be presented

from the data obtained with the six selected speakers. Because of the brief nature of this report, the sensitive electropneumography, and phonophotographic techniques have not been described in detail.

1. How many words (or syllables) may the laryngectomee expect to speak on each charge of swallowed air? The answer to this question must be interpreted in the light of one feature of the particular experimental situation involved in this present study. The superior esophageal speakers in this study were held to a loudness level suitable for an audience of 25 people. A constant check of sound pressure levels indicated that the speakers did maintain this level. A lowered intensity might well have increased somewhat the number of syllables spoken. The experimental study indicated that without exception these superior speakers took small charges of air efficiently and unconsciously. It should be noted that the normal superior speakers while reading the same "Rainbow Passage," did not begin to produce the syllables per breath claimed by some esophageal speakers.

Our study indicates the mean words per air charge range from 2.8 to 6.3 for esophageal speakers; this should be compared with 12.5 mean words per breath for normal breathing superior speakers. The extreme range for one esophageal speaker was 15 words (22 syllables); contrast with this one exceptionally superior normal speaker who, under identical conditions, spoke 36 words (50 syllables). The normal speaker read aloud with an average of 12.54 words per breath. This speaker had a wide range of performance and tended to utilize breathing phrases of 7 and 14 words. On the other hand, the esophageal speaker averaged 4.98 words per air charge and had a much narrower range of performance.

The syllabic values found in this study are somewhat higher than those found by Stetson,[4] who stated a limitation of from three to four syllables. The lowest average value in the present study was 3.8 syllables and the highest 8.7 syllables per air charge. These values, even when highly efficient performances are considered, are much more conservative than some information given recent wide publicity.[3]

2. How long does it take to swallow a charge of air? Esophageal speech, despite frequent air charges, is relatively efficient and pleasant to hear. In order to understand how this can be true, we need to know that the skilled esophageal speakers gulped air in from .42 to .80 seconds, mean values considered. This is unbelievably rapid "breathing," as rapid in fact as most normal speakers breathe for speech. It should be pointed out that superior speakers usually breathe only at phrase limits. The esophageal speaker utilized his air charge for approximately one and one-half seconds, during which time he averaged 2.8 to 6.3 words, and so it is obvious that he needed air charges not only at phrase limits, but also many times in between. This is contrasted with the normal speakers who utilized their breath for 4.19 seconds and spoke 12.5 words. If relative time or words per air charge is taken as a measure of efficiency, the normal speaker was from $2\frac{1}{2}$ to 3 times more efficient than the esophageal speaker.

3. What rate in words per minute can be achieved relative to normal speakers? It is probably most reasonable to combine the factors of Questions *1* and *2*, and to use total words per minute as a measure of efficiency. When this was done, the average for the superior esophageal speakers was 113 words per minute, compared with a rate of 166 words per minute[1] for the average normal speaker for the same reading material. Considering this measure, the normal speaker spoke only 1.47 times the rate of the esophageal speaker. Stated another way, the esophageal speaker was 80 per cent as rapid as the average normal speaker. Although the esophageal speaker would be judged as "too slow" compared to normal speakers, this is of little consequence if his efficiency is relatively satisfactory. The superior esophageal speakers did perform efficiently with the 300-word speech samples in the present study.

Preliminary study indicated that the skilled esophageal speakers could not speed up their rate without sacrificing either loudness or suitable phrasing. Even with the superior speaker the ability to modify rate is severely limited by the need for frequent air charges.

4. What possibilities of frequency level and frequency variability can be anticipated for esophageal speakers? The results of the experimental frequency analysis indicated that the superior esophageal group (for both the mean and median frequency) was essentially one whole octave lower than the comparative group of superior normal speakers. This, in fact, represents a very low pitch and may be identified to the ear by striking the second C below middle C on the piano; however, despite the difference in frequency level the distribution of frequency usage showed greater variability for the esophageal speakers than for the normal speakers. The standard deviation values were 7.0 and 4.3 tones per second. Four of the esophageal speakers used the highest frequency which was lower than the median frequency used by the lowest of the superior normal group. The total range of frequencies was 13.2 tones for the superior esophageal speakers compared with 10.5 tones for the superior normal group.

This striking and unexpected finding clearly negates any assumption that the esophageal speaker must be monotonous in pitch. In fact, it supports the contention that esophageal speakers can learn to sing simple tunes at a slow pace. The wide range of the values in this study possibly could be attributed to a much longer reading selection and some improvement in the experimental equipment. It should also be pointed out that these frequency variations are taking place at a very low level in the frequency range.

CONCLUSIONS.

The authors feel that this study exploring the rate and frequency characteristics of superior esophageal speech may be useful in establishing realistic norms for those who must learn to speak in this unique way. This study has utilized much longer samples of speech than previous studies, and it is, therefore, believed that the results are highly reliable for these carefully selected superior speakers. All in all, the results are rather conservative, being much more optimistic for reasonably effective speech than earlier studies based on small samples, but far less optimistic than predictions for success in recent popular literature.

1. The esophageal speakers spoke relatively easily and were no more conscious of the "breathing" function than were normal speakers.

2. The speakers of this study averaged 5 words (4.98) per air charge and performances averaged about 120 words per minute. A top limit of 11 to 12 syllables was very satisfactory; however, one speaker did achieve an extreme range of 22 syllables.

3. The air charge was gulped in about one-half second, a more rapid performance than that of some normal speakers inhaling for an intra-phrasal breath pause.

4. The mean frequency (pitch) level is almost exactly one full octave below that of the normal male speaker.

5. Contrary to some reports, frequency (pitch) variability is quite comparable to that of normal speech.

6. It is, however, very doubtful that the average frequency level can be raised much, if any, above 66-70 cycles per second.

BIBLIOGRAPHY.

1. DARLEY, F. L.: "A Normative Study of Oral Reading Rate," M.A. Thesis, State University of Iowa, 1940.

2. FAIRBANKS, G.: "Voice and Articulation Drillbook." Harpers, 1940.

3. KING, H.: I Lost My Voice to Cancer. *Sat. Eve. Post*, Sept. 1, 1956.

4. STETSON, R. H.: Esophageal Speech for Any Laryngectomized Patient. *Arch. Otolaryngol.*, 26:132-142, 1937.

5. WEPMAN, JOSEPH M.; MACGAHAN, JOHN A.; RICKARD, JOSEPH C., and SHELTON, NIEL W.: The Objective Measurement of Progressive Esophageal Speech Development. *Jour. Speech, Hear. Dis.*, 18:249 250, 1953.

PHYSICAL MEASUREMENT AND PITCH PERCEPTION IN ESOPHAGEAL SPEECH.

E. Thayer Curry, Ph.D.,

Urbana, Ill.,

and

John C. Snidecor, Ph.D.,

Santa Barbara, Calif.

General Note.

The frequency (as well as the relative sound pressure) of an auditory stimulus can be measured in the complete absence and independently of any listener. The term "frequency" should be considered as a distinctly physical attribute of the auditory stimulus; the unit is the cycle per second (c.p.s.). On the other hand, "pitch" (as is loudness) is an auditory experience identified with the listener. Pitch should be thought of as the listener's personal reaction to the auditory (pure frequency) stimulus; the pitch unit is the mel. These distinctions between frequency and pitch will be carefully observed in the following discussion. For a more complete treatment of this psychophysical problem, the reader is referred to the pertinent discussion by Licklider entitled, "Basic Correlates of the Auditory Stimulus," Chapter 25, *Handbook of Experimental Psychology.*[1]

Section I.

LITERATURE MATERIALS ON FREQUENCY AND PITCH IN ESOPHAGEAL SPEECH.

Frequency.

When carefully analyzed, many of the literature references to "pitch" are obviously concerned with "frequency," if the terms pitch and frequency are used with the connotation

Reprinted by permission from *The Laryngoscope*, 1961, *71*, 415–424.

previously set forth. A good example of this predominant usage of the term pitch is illustrated by the following passage from van den Berg:[2]

"Generally, the pitch of oesophageal speech is rather low, between 50 and 100 c.p.s., on account of the rather large mass of the vibrating pseudo-larynx. Occasionally, however, this mass is smaller and a more agreeable pitch results. The relations between the original properties of the struc-

TABLE I.

Fundamental Frequency Measures in Esophageal Speech.

Frequency Identification				Median Frequency	
Interval (c.p.s.)	Upper Limit of Interval		Column I Damste's Patient Number	Column II Damste's 20 Subjects	Column III Snidecor/ Curry Subjects
	Tones Above 16.35 c.p.s.	Musical Equivalent			
164.81—185.00	21	F#$_3$	52	1	
146.81—164.80	20	E$_3$			
130.81—146.80	19	D$_3$			
116.51—130.80	18	C$_3$			
103.81—116.50	17	A#$_2$	45	1	
92.51—103.80	16	G#$_2$	43,55	2	
82.41— 92.50	15	F#$_2$			
73.44— 82.40	14	E$_2$	7,36,38,40	4	1
65.41— 73.43	13	D$_2$	8,17	2	2
58.27— 65.40	12	C$_2$	31,33	2	1
51.92— 58.26	11	A#$_1$	4,16,37,51	4	2
46.26— 51.91	10	G#$_1$	18,44	2	
41.21— 46.25	9	F#$_1$	22	1	
36.72— 41.20	8	E$_1$	26	1	
Median Frequency of Group (c.p.s)				67.5	63.3
Mean Frequency of Group (c.p.s)				78.5	62.8
Mean S. D. (Tones)				—	2.30

tures, the type of operation, the method of training and the resulting pseudolarynx are not yet clearly established. The best results are observed when the ultimate structure is rather thin and pointed . . ."

Detailed experimental studies of frequency usage among esophageal speakers are not numerous in the literature; however, one portion of Damste's excellent study of 1958[3] should be extensively considered in evaluating the frequency measures which describe the speech of laryngectomized individuals. In Table I, the frequency* data taken from Damste's Fig. 5 have been retabulated and contrasted with similar measures from the Snidecor and Curry[4] study. The "usual pitch" for

*Although Damste listed his measures as "pitch," the values were taken from the tape records and are indicated in c.p.s. units. The technique of converting the tape interval to c.p.s. is not stated in the published version of Damste's thesis.

each of Damste's 20 subjects has been indicated as the median frequency and shown in Column II. The median frequency for each of the six subjects of Snidecor and Curry has been listed in Column III. Damste's 20 subjects considered as a group have a median frequency of 67.5 c.p.s. This value is very close to the 63.3 c.p.s. measured as the median frequency for the Snidecor and Curry experimental group. Twelve of the Damste patients (60 per cent) have "usual pitch" in the four frequency intervals (tones) in which the median frequency values for all of the Snidecor and Curry subjects occur; however, the individual Damste patients show a much wider range of frequency production than do the Snidecor and Curry subjects. The highest "usual" frequency noted among any of the Damste speakers was 185 c.p.s.; this value is compared with 80.8 c.p.s. for the highest median frequency listed for any one of the Snidecor and Curry speakers. Actually, the highest frequency measured with any of the Snidecor and Curry subjects was 135.5 c.p.s.; this value is a full half octave lower than the "usual pitch" of Damste's patient No. 52. The lowest frequency measured in any of the Snidecor and Curry subjects was 17.2 c.p.s. The records of all six individuals in this group showed readily measurable periodicity in the octave between C_0 and C_1, that is between 16.35 and 32.70 c.p.s.

As a generalization, the combined data of Table I appear to substantiate the conclusion from Snidecor and Curry that the mean frequency level for most esophageal speakers is almost exactly one full octave below that of the normal adult male speaker. Other conclusions about the frequency abilities of superior esophageal speakers will be presented in the next section on frequency variability.

Pitch.

The rather obvious perceptual aspects of esophageal speech, *i.e.*, the "pitch" aspects, have been listed by many authors. A passage from van den Berg[2] is of particular pertinence:

"The variations in pitch which can be produced by the patient are much more limited than those which can be made in laryngeal speech. The reasons are obvious. In the larynx we have a very complicate (sic) and delicate complex of muscles which allow for compensatory mechanisms, while in the pseudolarynx only one muscle is present."

The literature is in practically complete agreement on at least two attributes of the voice of the laryngectomee: *1*. it is obviously very low in pitch; *2*. it is severely limited in the perceived range of pitch variability. This second problem of restricted variability has a very special and interesting psychophysical aspect which will be considered with the therapy recommendations.

SECTION II.

EXPERIMENTAL RESULTS OF SPEECH FREQUENCY USAGE AND VARIABILITY AS MEASURED WITH SUPERIOR ESOPHAGEAL SPEAKERS.

Snidecor and Curry have described their experimental results with a carefully selected group of esophageal subjects who were judged to be speaking in a highly superior manner using a standard reading passage, "The Rainbow Passage."[5] The measurements of fundamental speech frequency were obtained by utilizing the phonophotographic technique originated by Metfessel,[6] modified by Simon[7] and Lewis and Tiffin[8] and electrified by Cowan.[9] Frequency values were plotted on semi-logarithmic paper and measures of pitch were computed in the conventional manner.[9] The recording drum circumference was 191.2 cm. on the apparatus used for this particular study; the temporal extent of each measurement interval was 0.051 seconds.

The average reading time for each of the subjects was 28.3 seconds for the entire passage. This time was utilized as follows:

Silence 38.5%
Aperiodic sound 1.9%
Clearly periodic fundamental sound frequency...........59.6%

Table II presents a distribution of the fundamental frequency measures for the group of superior esophageal speakers. Variations among the individual speakers, as well as central tendencies for the group are readily observed. Some of these measures of frequency range and variability are further tabulated in Table III. The frequency value (in

TABLE II.

Measures of Fundamental Frequency in Experimental Group of
Superior Esophageal Speakers.

Measured Frequency Interval (in c.p.s.)	Speakers of Snidecor and Curry Study						Group Total
	1	3	5	7	8	6	
130.81—146.80	1						1
116.51—130.80	5	2	2				9
103.81—116.50	17		4	1	2		24
92.51—103.80	61	5	21	1	15	2	105
82.41— 92.50	67	6	30	1	30	8	142
73.44— 82.40	63M*	30	64	37	64	23	281
65.41— 73.43	33	54	62M*	64	78M*	34	325
58.27— 65.40	30	93M*	73	58	80	63	397M*
51.92— 58.26	10	73	46	63M*	37	56M	285
46.26— 51.91	11	42	19	49	15	54*	190
41.21— 46.25	14	9	15	27	6	44	115
36.72— 41.20	4	5	9	15	1	19	53
32.71— 36.71	3	1	5	6	2	13	30
29.12— 32.70	1	1	1	1		3	7
25.96— 29.11			1	1	3	5	10
23.12— 25.95				1	1	2	4
20.60— 23.11						3	3
18.35— 20.59					1		1
16.36— 18.34						1	1
Total Periodic Intervals	320	321	352	325	335	330	1983
Aperiodic Intervals	1	4	4	6	44	4	63
Silence	254	157	165	219	234	253	1282
Total Intervals	575	482	521	550	613	587	3328

M—Median frequency interval.
*—Mean frequency interval.

c.p.s.) for the highest and lowest measurable periodic interval is shown for each of the six subjects. The total range (in tones and octaves) between the highest and lowest frequency is indicated for each superior speaker. A somewhat more meaningful value, the median 90 per cent of frequencies produced (sometimes referred to as the "effective range"), shows this measure to be greater than one octave (six full tones) for five of the six superior subjects under study.

The two types of frequency movement during the speech of the superior esophageal subjects are indicated in Table IV; mean rates for both types are shown. Inflections are frequency movements during vocalization; shifts are frequency movements between vocalizations. Upward movements comprise 47 per cent of the inflectional change; the mean extent is 2.0 tones. Downward frequency movements comprise 53 per cent of inflectional changes with a mean extent of 2.8 tones. When frequency changes during shifts are considered, upward movements constitute 69 per cent of the total number; the mean extent is 3.1 tones. Downward frequency move-

TABLE III.

Measures of Frequency Range of Superior Esophageal Speaker Group.

	Speakers					
	1	3	5	7	8	6
Shortest Measurable Periodic Interval:						
Frequency (c.p.s.)	135.5	123.4	118.7	112.3	106.6	95.2
Tones above 16.35 c.p.s.	18.3	17.5	17.2	16.7	16.2	15.2
Longest Measurable Periodic Interval:						
Frequency (c.p.s.)	32.2	30.4	28.3	24.0	19.5	17.2
Tones above 16.35 c.p.s.	5.9	5.4	4.8	3.3	1.5	0.4
Total Range of Frequency Measured:						
Tones	12.4	12.1	12.4	14.8	13.4	14.7
Octaves	2.1	2.0	2.1	2.5	2.2	2.5
"Effective Range" Median 90 per cent:						
Tones	7.8	4.7	7.2	6.1	6.0	7.2
Octaves	1.3	0.8	1.2	1.1	1.0	1.2
Median Frequency:						
In c.p.s.	80.8	60.4	66.2	58.2	67.3	54.0
Tones above 16.35 c.p.s.	13.8	11.3	12.2	11.0	12.3	10.4
Mean Frequency:						
In c.p.s.	76.7	60.5	65.8	57.3	66.7	50.9
Tones above 16.35 c.p.s.	13.4	11.3	12.1	10.9	12.2	9.7

ments are smaller both in per cent of occurrence (31 per cent) and extent (2.0 tones). These frequency movements are similar to the speech of superior normal speakers. For both groups frequency moves upward primarily by means of shifts and primarily downward by means of inflections. Thus the general manner of frequency movement is similar for both normal and superior esophageal speakers. Table IV also indicates the relative rates of frequency movement; these values are 7.9 tones per second during inflections and 4.3 tones per second during shifts.

PITCH DISCRIMINATION ABILITY IN THE FREQUENCY RANGE OF ESOPHAGEAL SPEECH.

In Section I it was suggested that there are special perceptual problems associated with esophageal speech. Damste refers to this problem and discusses the acoustic properties of esophageal speaking as follows:

"The fundamental tone of an oesophageal voice is often difficult to determine. This is because the frequency is low and because the sound is very complex, in other words the fundamental tone is accompanied by a large number of relatively strong overtones. The ear is not very sensitive

TABLE IV.

Extents, Directions and Rates of Frequency Movement During Speech of Superior Esophageal Subjects.

Frequency Change During Inflections:	Up	Down	Total	
Number	275	309	584	
Per Cent of Total Number	47	53	100	
Mean Extent in Tones	2.0	2.8	2.4	
Mean Rate of Frequency Movement, tones per second:				7.9
Frequency Change During Shifts:	Up	Down	Total	
Number	121	54	175	
Per Cent of Total Number	69	31	100	
Mean Extent in Tones	3.1	2.0	2.8	
Mean Rate of Frequency Movement, tones per second:				4.3

in the frequency-range of the fundamental, much more sensitive in the range of the partials. And the latter contain a large part of the total sound-energy."

Damste's observation regarding the relative insensitiveness of the human ear at the frequency range of esophageal speech involves a psychophysical relationship peculiar to frequency and pitch in the low frequency region of most esophageal speech. Stevens and Volkmann[10] present experimental evidence which clearly indicates that in the frequency region below 100 c.p.s. the perceptual or pitch aspects of a stimulus are greatly reduced when compared with frequencies above 100 c.p.s.

The shape of the Stevens and Volkmann curve has important practical implications for the esophageal speaker who is attempting to improve his speaking performance by increasing the frequency variability of his pseudolaryngeal output. Snidecor and Curry in their study pointed out that the mean total frequency range was 13.21 tones for the superior esophageal speakers and 10.5 tones for superior adult normal speakers. In terms of measured frequency extent the superior esophageal speakers had significantly greater frequency variability than did the superior normal adult subjects. The mean effective frequency range values (median 90 per cent) for the two groups were 6.5 and 6.3 tones respectively. Despite this apparently favorable comparison between the frequency ranges for the two subject groups, the esophageal speakers were nonetheless considered to have a "restricted pitch range" when the tape recordings were evaluated. The frequency measures indicated a considerably greater movement than was apparent in pitch to the listener. This considerable lack of agreement between the measured (frequency) and perceptual (pitch) aspects of the low frequency speaking performances of these esophageal subjects can readily be understood from the Stevens and Volkmann experiment.

The esophageal speaker should continuously be encouraged to extend the range of frequencies used in his speaking performances; however, because of the particular frequency-pitch relationship in the frequency region of esophageal speech, the extensions of frequency range will not be as productive of perceptual variability as would be the case in the higher frequency regions characteristic of the normal speaking range.

SECTION IV.

SUGGESTIONS FOR INCREASING FREQUENCY VARIABILITY DURING ESOPHAGEAL SPEECH.

The work of van den Berg discusses certain aspects of increasing the frequency variability of esophageal speech:

"Therefore, pitch and intensity are correlated in oesophageal speech. A low pitch is produced with a low intensity of the voice, a high pitch with a high intensity. This increase of the pitch at increasing intensity, i.e., at increasing flow of air through the pseudo-glottis, is caused by the Bernoulli effect[11] of the air which escapes through the narrow opening. The walls are sucked towards each other by the negative pressure in the pseudo-glottis and this effect increases the effective stiffness of the muscular structures, which then vibrate at a higher frequency, as their mass remains the same."

"The speech of a clever patient sometimes gives the illusion of agreeable changes of pitch which objectively are not present. He uses his vocal cavities in such a way that the resonant frequencies, or formants, change during the pronunciation of the vowel in question. Occasionally, the range of tensions in the region of the pseudolarynx is very small. The range of pitches may then be improved by exerting an additional pressure, *e.g.*, by means of a finger, by compressing the neck against a collar or by bending the head downwards. A well designed collar may be very useful when the crico pharyngeal sphincter, or what is left of it, is so weak that the oesophageal air escapes at such a low pressure that the intensity of the voice is too low."

In another work[12] van den Berg shows spectra, vowel constant, with clear variation in frequency with pressure variations.

"Thus, the pitch is secondary compared with the intensity, and the subject had to make himself clear about how to produce the high pitch. Therefore, he always separated the section with a high pitch from that with a low pitch by a new breath and a new injection of air into the oesophagus."

Some general suggestions for increasing frequency variability would include:

1. Practice singing a familiar song as "Pop Goes the Weasel" or "Mary Had a Little Lamb." By choice of new melodies the laryngectomee can gradually extend the frequency needed to reproduce the song.

2. Produce frequencies in response to key stimuli from the piano. The frequency range may be gradually extended both up and down the keyboard.

3. Remember that higher pitch is related to greater intensity. By repeated trials, attempt to produce both greater intensity and higher pitch.

Special Note: The authors wish to emphasize clearly that all the speakers in the Curry and Snidecor experiment were esophageal speakers. None were pharyngeal speakers.

BIBLIOGRAPHY.

1. STEVENS, S. S.: *Handbook of Experimental Psychology*. New York. John Wiley & Sons, 1951.

2. VAN DEN BERG, J., and MOOLENAAR-BIJL, A. J.: Crico-Pharyngeal Sphincter, Pitch, Intensity and Fluency in Oesophageal Speech. *Prac. Oto-Rhino-Laryngol.*, 21:4. 1959.

3. DAMSTE, P. H.: *Oesophageal Speech After Laryngectomy*, Groningen, 1958.

4. SNIDECOR, JOHN C., and CURRY, E. THAYER: Temporal and Pitch Aspects of Superior Esophageal Speech. *Ann. Otol., Rhinol. and Laryngol.*, 68:3, 1959.

5. FAIRBANKS, G.: *Voice and Articulation Drillbook*. New York. Harpers, 1940.

6. METFESSEL, M.: Techniques for the Objective Study of Vocal Art. *Psychol. Monog.*, 36:1-40, 1927.

7. SIMON, C. T.: The Variability of Consecutive Wave Lengths in Vocal and Instrumental Sounds. *Psychol. Monog.*, 36:41-83, 1927.

8. LEWIS, D., and TIFFIN, J.: A Psychophysical Study of Individual Differences in Speaking Ability. *Arch. of Speech*, 1:43-60, 1934.

9. COWAN, M.: Pitch and Intensity Characteristics of Stage Speech. *Arch. of Speech*, Suppl., 1936.

10. STEVENS, S. S., and VOLKMANN, J.: The Relation of Pitch to Frequency. *Amer. Jour. Psychol.*, 53:329-353, 1940.

11. VAN DEN BERG, J., ZANTEMA, J. T., and DOORNENBAL, P., JR.: On the Air Resistance and the Bernoulli Effect of the Human Larynx. *Jour. Acoust. Soc. of Amer.*, 29:626-631, 1957.

12. VAN DEN BERG, J., MOOLENAAR-BIJL, A. J., and DAMSTE, P. H.: Oesophageal Speech. *Folia Phoniatrica*, Separatum, 10:2, 1958.

SELECTED ACOUSTIC CHARACTERISTICS OF ESOPHAGEAL SPEECH PRODUCED BY FEMALE LARYNGECTOMEES

BERND WEINBERG *and* SUZANNE BENNETT

Indiana University Medical Center, Indianapolis, Indiana

Voice fundamental frequency (VFF), phonation time, and duration characteristics were analyzed for 15 female and 18 male esophageal speakers to determine whether acoustic differences existed as a function of speaker sex. A significant difference was found between the mean fundamental frequency of esophageal speech produced by men and that produced by women. The average VFF of women was approximately seven semitones higher than that established for men. Without regard to speaker sex, the average voice fundamental frequency for the total sample of 33 talkers was 24.9 semitones (69 Hz). Mean fundamental frequencies for individual speakers ranged from 12.9–43.7 semitones (33–200 Hz). No significant sex differences were found for VFF variability, phonation time, and duration measures. The findings highlight the need for investigators to control for acoustic differences between male and female esophageal speakers.

The majority of previous acoustical research on esophageal voice has been directed toward specifying voice fundamental frequency, phonation time, and rate characteristics of male speakers (Kytta, 1964; Curry and Snidecor, 1961; Hoops and Noll, 1969; Shipp, 1967; and Damste, 1958). In some of these studies, the data suggest that isolated female laryngectomized speakers were used. However, in these experiments the sex of the experimental subjects was not always reported (Damste, 1958; Shipp, 1967). We failed to uncover a single published experiment specifically concerned with the voice characteristics of female esophageal speakers.

In view of the paucity of information concerning the physical characteristics of esophageal speech produced by laryngectomized women, an experiment was undertaken to specify selected acoustic characteristics of esophageal speech produced by females and to compare these characteristics with similar data for male esophageal voices.

METHOD

Subjects and Recordings

Thirty-three laryngectomees who had used esophageal speech as a primary method of speech communication for at least two years served as subjects.

Reprinted by permission from *Journal of Speech and Hearing Research*, 1972, *15*, 211–216.

The 15 female and 18 male speakers were rated for speech acceptability (Shipp, 1967) and for vocal effectiveness (Curry and Snidecor, 1961) by two speech pathologists experienced in esophageal voice rehabilitation. The 33 subjects were rated average to excellent speakers by each judge.

High-quality recordings were made of each subject reading the first paragraph of Fairbanks' Rainbow Passage (1960). The 33 recordings were duplicated, and the second sentence of the Rainbow Passage was extracted for acoustic analysis.

Acoustical Analysis

Each recording was played by a Nagra IV-D tape recorder to one channel of a Honeywell Visicorder Model 1508 to process voice fundamental frequency, phonation time, and duration data. Visicorder chart speed of 1000 mm/sec and mirror galvanometers type M-5000 were used. To control for variation in chart speed, a countermonitored 1000-Hz calibration signal was played simultaneously into the second channel of the Visicorder.

The fundamental frequency record of each subject was initially segmented into three basic categories: (1) periodic phonation, (2) aperiodicity, and (3) silence. Each wave form within the periodic segments as well as the segment lengths of aperiodicity and silence were measured to the nearest 0.5mm. From these measurements the following measures were computed for each subject: mean, standard deviation, full range, and 90% range of VFF; total speaking duration; percentage of total duration spent in periodic phonation, aperiodicity, and silence; and phonation time.

Statistical Analysis

To compare male and female esophageal speech, the data were subjected to a single classification analysis of variance. A preliminary Bartlett test of homogeneity of variance was performed. The Welch F' test was used in cases where heterogeneity of variance was found (Welch 1951). When F tests were significant ($p < 0.01$), comparisons between male and female group means for individual measures were evaluated by t-test procedures.

RESULTS AND DISCUSSION

Results of the acoustical analyses are presented for individual female esophageal speakers in Table 1 and for male esophageal speakers in Table 2. In these two tables, voice fundamental frequency and related measures are given in semitones ($\#ST = 39.86 \log VFF/16.35$) rather than in Hz, because statistical analysis of the data was in terms of semitones.

Without regard to speaker sex, the average VFF level for the entire sample of 33 esophageal talkers was 24.9 semitones (69 Hz). For females, the average fundamental frequency was 28.87 semitones (87 Hz), for males, 21.74 semitones (58 Hz). The difference of 7.1 semitones between the average VFF levels of male and female speakers was significant ($t = 2.84$, $df = 31$, $p < 0.01$).

TABLE 1. VFF, duration, and phonation time of 15 female esophageal talkers.

Talker	VFF-Mean*	VFF-SD (ST)	VFF-Range (ST)	VFF-90% Range (ST)
1	12.9	4.4	20.4	15.1
2	24.4	3.5	19.0	11.2
3	17.1	4.6	26.7	13.7
4	39.1	2.9	15.9	8.1
5	23.5	5.0	22.2	14.9
6	43.7	3.4	24.0	9.7
7	19.4	4.8	19.7	15.6
8	31.3	2.7	13.2	9.3
9	23.5	4.3	25.3	14.2
10	27.4	3.6	22.0	11.0
11	41.7	3.4	23.3	9.7
12	31.1	3.2	17.8	8.4
13	31.5	3.7	19.5	14.7
14	31.2	4.9	27.2	19.0
15	35.3	4.3	22.7	12.0
Mean	28.87	3.94	21.25	12.44

Talker	% Periodic	% Aperiodic	% Silence	% Phonation Time	Total Duration (Sec)
1	62	19	19	81	5.1
2	41	29	30	70	5.3
3	49	09	42	58	7.7
4	57	16	27	73	4.7
5	53	17	30	70	4.6
6	62	12	26	74	5.2
7	41	31	28	73	5.0
8	51	12	37	63	5.7
9	42	22	36	64	6.2
10	43	21	36	64	6.7
11	62	06	32	68	5.3
12	56	12	32	68	4.9
13	31	35	34	67	5.9
14	42	41	17	83	5.2
15	62	16	22	78	4.0
Mean	50.27	19.87	29.86	70.33	5.44

* ST above O FL = Semitones above 16.35 Hz

Even though female esophageal talkers had significantly higher mean VFFs than male esophageal talkers, there was no difference between female and male talkers on any of the other three measures of VFF shown in Tables 1 and 2. Neither was there any difference between female and male talkers with respect to measures of phonation time and total duration. In general, phonation time and duration data compared favorably with existing information about high-rated esophageal speakers (Table 3), suggesting that our subjects represented a sample of average-to-excellent speakers.

To compare these results with results from previous research, group data

TABLE 2. VFF, duration, and phonation time of 18 male esophageal talkers.

Talker	VFF-Mean*	VFF-SD (ST)	VFF-Range (ST)	VFF-90% Range (ST)
1	28.8	4.5	22.0	15.9
2	27.0	3.4	17.5	12.0
3	24.1	5.3	29.0	17.4
4	13.4	3.7	22.5	12.0
5	21.2	4.4	27.9	15.5
6	24.8	4.3	27.9	11.1
7	27.5	4.3	25.5	12.9
8	26.3	6.1	47.8	19.0
9	19.5	3.0	15.5	9.7
10	17.0	4.5	24.8	14.2
11	20.2	4.7	22.6	15.9
12	20.0	3.2	18.4	11.3
13	20.8	3.2	20.0	10.0
14	21.6	4.2	22.1	14.2
15	18.4	3.8	21.5	14.1
16	16.5	2.9	19.8	8.2
17	19.5	4.1	16.4	14.7
18	24.7	5.2	26.5	17.0
Mean	21.74	4.15	23.76	13.62

Talker	% Periodic	% Aperiodic	% Silence	% Phonation Time	Total Duration (Sec)
1	53	15	32	68	5.4
2	60	11	29	71	5.2
3	36	29	35	65	6.7
4	63	09	28	72	5.2
5	67	18	15	85	4.8
6	54	12	34	66	5.1
7	66	16	18	82	4.4
8	59	13	28	72	7.2
9	58	17	25	74	4.6
10	43	32	25	75	4.9
11	41	07	52	48	7.9
12	59	12	29	71	4.5
13	53	19	28	72	4.7
14	57	06	37	63	6.5
15	51	24	25	75	5.4
16	37	23	40	59	5.7
17	38	37	25	74	5.2
18	46	26	28	72	5.5
Mean	52.28	18.11	29.61	70.22	5.49

* ST above O FL = Semitones above 16.35 Hz

from the present experiment (Table 3) are shown together with information for 17 comparably rated speakers studied by Shipp (1967) and for six superior male speakers studied by Curry and Snidecor (1961). Although subjects in this study were given ratings of speech acceptability comparable to Shipp's (1967) high-rated speakers, their average fundamental frequency was consid-

TABLE 3. VFF, duration, and phonation time for speakers in the present study, for high-rated speakers studied by Shipp (1967), and for superior male speakers (Curry and Snidecor, 1961).

| Physical Measures | Present Study | | | Shipp (1967) Total (N = 17) | Curry & Snidecor (1961) Total (N = 6) |
	Total (N = 33)	Females (N = 15)	Males (N = 18)		
Fundamental Frequency					
Mean	69	87	58	84	63
SD	4.06 ST	3.94 ST	4.16 ST	2.27 Tones	2.30 Tones
Mid-90% Range	13.08 ST	12.44 ST	13.62 ST	7.60 Tones	6.5 Tones
Phonation Time					
Total Duration (sec)	5.47	5.44	5.49	5.54	6.01
% Periodic	51.36	50.27	52.28	48.3	–
% Aperiodic	18.91	19.87	18.11	13.3	–
% Silence	29.73	29.86	29.61	38.6	46.3
% Phonation Time (% Periodic + % Aperiodic)	70.27	70.14	70.39	61.4	53.7

erably lower than the 84-Hz value reported by Shipp (Table 3). Their average VFF was, however, markedly similar to the 63-Hz value found for six superior male esophageal speakers (Curry and Snidecor, 1961). Shipp (1967) attributed the discrepancies in mean VFFs between his subjects and those of Curry and Snidecor (1961) to differences in methods used to extract fundamental frequency. Specifically, Curry and Snidecor (1961) used averaging techniques to calculate fundamental frequency, while Shipp (1967) and the present investigators employed a wave-by-wave analysis. Further study is now in progress in our laboratory to determine whether the differences in average VFF reported by various investigators represent differences in sampling or method of analysis.

The present data for VFF are consistent with previous results which indicate that esophageal speakers exhibit a wide range of intersubject variation in mean VFF. The total range of average VFF for females (Table 1) was 12.9 to 43.7 semitones (33–200 Hz); for males (Table 2) the range was 13.4 to 28.8 semitones (34–83 Hz). Thus in the present samples, the lowest and highest average VFFs were for female speakers. It is important to note that eight of the 15 females had VFFs exceeding the upper limit of the range of VFFs seen for men.

The finding that average fundamental frequency of esophageal voice differed significantly as a function of speaker sex represents an original observation. This result, coupled with our recent observation that listeners could identify the sex of these esophageal talkers from recordings of their voices (Weinberg and Bennett, 1971), casts serious doubt upon the validity of the commonly accepted clinical assumption that the voices of male and female esophageal speakers are markedly similar (Snidecor, 1969). With respect to future research, these findings highlight the need to control for the acoustic differences which exist in the voices of male and female esophageal speakers.

ACKNOWLEDGMENT

This research was supported in part by U.S. Public Health Service Research Grant NS-09262-01, American Cancer Society Research Grant IN-46K, and the Delaware County Cancer Society, Muncie, Indiana. The assistance of James C. Shanks and Nancy Paras is gratefully acknowledged. James Norton served as statistical consultant. Research computation support was provided by USPHS Grant RR162-06 to the Research Computation Center, Indiana University Medical Center. Reprint requests should be addressed to Bernd Weinberg, Speech Research Laboratory, Indiana University Medical Center, Indianapolis, Indiana 46202.

REFERENCES

CURRY, E. T., and SNIDECOR, J. C., Physical measurement and pitch perception in esophageal speech. *Laryngoscope*, 71, 415-424 (1961).

DAMSTÉ, P. H., *Oesophageal Speech After Laryngectomy*. Netherlands: Univ. of Groningen (1958).

FAIRBANKS, G., *Voice and Articulation Drillbook*. New York: Harper (1960).

HOOPS, H. R., and NOLL, J. D., Relationship of selected acoustic variables to judgments of esophageal speech. *J. commun. Dis.*, 2, 1-13 (1969).

KYTTA, J., Spectrographic studies of the sound quality of esophageal speech. *Acta Otolaryng.*, Suppl. 188 (1964).

SHIPP, T., Frequency, duration, and perceptual measures in relation to judgments of alaryngeal speech acceptability. *J. Speech Hearing Res.*, 10, 417-427 (1967).

SNIDECOR, J. C., *Speech Rehabilitation of the Laryngectomized*. Springfield, Ill.: Charles C Thomas (1969).

WELCH, B. L., On the comparison of several mean values: An alternative approach. *Biometrika*, 38, 330-336 (1951).

WEINBERG, B., and BENNETT, S., A study of talker sex identification of esophageal voices. *J. Speech Hearing Res.*, 14, 391-395 (1971).

Received December 21, 1970.

A STUDY OF TALKER SEX RECOGNITION OF ESOPHAGEAL VOICES

BERND WEINBERG *and* SUZANNE BENNETT

Speech Research Laboratory, Indiana University Medical Center, Indianapolis, Indiana

This study investigated the ability of listeners to identify the sex of esophageal talkers on the basis of voice recordings. Recognition data are provided for 15 female and 18 male esophageal talkers. In general, the results support the hypothesis that naive listeners can reliably and accurately identify the sex of esophageal talkers from voice samples.

Snidecor and Curry (1959), Damste (1958), Kytta (1964), Shipp (1967), Rollin (1962), and others have investigated various acoustic characteristics of esophageal speech. In general, acoustic studies of esophageal speech have employed male talkers. In the few studies where a small number of female talkers have been used, the investigators have apparently assumed that no significant acoustic differences existed between the sexes.

At the perceptual level, Snidecor and Curry (1960) informally commented that "the complete lack of success on the part of the six judges to select female voices from the male voices on the basis of recordings . . . tends to indicate marked similarity in the voices of male and female esophageal speakers." More recently, Gardner (1966) reported that "the laryngectomized women were often mistaken for men over the telephone."

Currently, there is an absence of experimental data concerning (1) the accuracy and reliability of listeners to identify the sex of a talker on the basis of recordings of esophageal voices, (2) the acoustic features of esophageal voices produced by female laryngectomized talkers, and (3) the influence of selected acoustic measures on perception of talker sex.

Although the ratio of male to female laryngectomees favors men approximately 10:1 (Snidecor, 1968, pp. 62-63), a large number of female talkers now use esophageal speech as a primary method of communication. Moreover, masculinization of the female voice presumed in above reports represents a distressing and sometimes serious voice disorder that may create social, communication, and rehabilitative problems. Hence, the information gaps cited above merit systematic investigation. The present study—the first in a series—was designed to determine the accuracy and reliability of listeners to identify the sex of esophageal talkers on the basis of voice recordings.

Reprinted by permission from *Journal of Speech and Hearing Research*, 1971, *14*, 391–395.

METHOD

Talkers and Recordings

The talkers for this experiment were 15 adult female and 18 adult male laryngectomees who had employed esophageal voice as their primary means of speech communication for a minimum period of two years. Talkers were rated for speech acceptability (Shipp, 1967) by two speech pathologists experienced in esophageal voice rehabilitation. The 33 talkers were all judged as average-to-excellent esophageal talkers on independent rating trials performed by each judge.

High quality recordings were made of each subject reading the first paragraph of Fairbank's Rainbow Passage (1959). The 33 recordings were duplicated, and the second sentence of each recording of the Rainbow Passage was extracted. A 66-item experimental tape was produced so that each talker appeared twice in random order.

Listeners and Recognition Task

Eighty-eight young adults with little or no experience in judging speech or familiarity with esophageal voice served as listeners. The perceptual experiment was conducted in a low ambient-noise environment with judges seated facing a high-quality tape reproduce-speaker system. Listeners were told that they would hear each of 66 adult talkers read the experimental passage "The rainbow is a division of white light into many beautiful colors." They were also told that the talkers had lost their vocal folds and that they used a new method of talking called esophageal speech. Judges were instructed to listen to each experimental sentence and then indicate whether the talker was a man or woman. In short, a two-alternative forced choice experiment was conducted. Responses were recorded on an answer sheet provided to each listener.

RESULTS

Reliability

To provide an estimate of the reliability of listener recognition of talker sex, the percentage of agreement in sex identification of listeners in response to the first and second presentation of each talker was calculated. The 88 listeners demonstrated a 94% test-retest agreement in talker sex identification for all talkers, a 98% test-retest agreement for male talkers, and an 88% test-retest agreement for female talkers. These figures appeared sufficiently high to establish confidence that naive listeners were capable of making reliable judgments of talker sex from recordings of esophageal voices.

TABLE 1. Talker sex identifications of esophageal voices.

Stimulus	Response* Male	Female
Male	1547 (0.98)	37 (0.02)
Female	266 (0.20)	1054 (0.80)

*Responses are for 18 male talkers and 88 listeners and for 15 female talkers and 88 listeners.

Accuracy

The accuracy of listeners to identify the sex of esophageal talkers is summarized in Table 1. The entries in this matrix are those obtained from responses to the second presentation of the talkers. Although the first presentation of the 33 voices was initially intended as a practice and familiarity trial, analysis showed that no significant shift in the listeners' identifications occurred between trials. Judges identified the sex of the 33 esophageal talkers with 90% accuracy. Ninety-eight percent of the listener responses to male esophageal voices were correct. For the women talkers, 80% of the listener responses were correct. Thus, male esophageal talkers were rarely identified as female talkers, while 20% of the listener responses to female esophageal talkers were identified as male.

The results of this study based on group data are, however, somewhat misleading. A more realistic and detailed description of the findings is obtained by treating the listener responses to each talker as a separate experiment. Figure 1 plots the number of listeners responding "male" to each talker. The two horizontal lines in this figure represent the 99.9% confidence interval around the median number of possible identifications of a talker as being "male" (MacKinnon, 1964). As shown in Figure 1, each of the male talkers was correctly identified as a man at levels far exceeding chance. Moreover, 11 of 15 female esophageal talkers were correctly identified as women. Two female talkers (Subjects 1 and 21) were generally identified as men, while each of the remaining two women talkers (Subjects 5 and 26) were as likely to be identified as a man or woman.

DISCUSSION

In general, the results of this study support the hypothesis that naive listeners can reliably and accurately identify the sex of esophageal talkers from voice recordings. Assuming that the women sampled in this investigation represent a reasonable survey of the population of female esophageal talkers, it might be estimated that approximately one of every four to five female esophageal talkers may exhibit serious problems of vocal masculinization. Stated in more positive terms, naive listeners correctly identified approximately three of

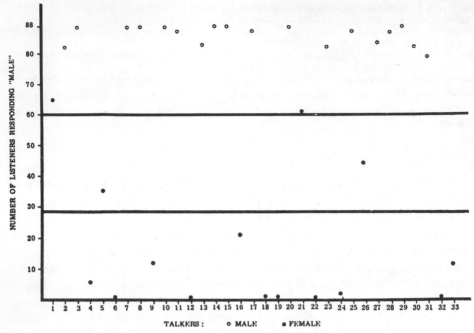

FIGURE 1. Number of listeners responding "male" to each talker.

every four women studied as female talkers. These perceptual findings suggest that there ought to be significant acoustic differences among some of the voices studied. Consequently, investigations are now being conducted to specify selected acoustic parameters of these 33 esophageal voices and to relate the influence of such parameters to perception of talker sex.

ACKNOWLEDGMENT

This investigation was supported by Public Health Service Research Grant NS-09262-01 from the National Institute of Neurological Diseases and Stroke; by Institutional Grant IN-46K from the American Cancer Society; and by a Reasearch Grant from the Delaware County Cancer Society, Muncie, Indiana. The suggestions and assistance of James C. Shanks, Nancy Paras, and James Norton are gratefully acknowledged.

REFERENCES

DAMSTE, P. H., *Oesophageal Speech after Laryngectomy*. Groningen, Neth.: Haitsema (1958).

FAIRBANKS, G., *Voice and Articulation Handbook*. New York: Harper (1959).

GARDNER, W. H., Adjustment problems of laryngectomized women. *Arch. Otolaryng.*, 83, 57-68 (1966).

KYTTA, J., Finnish oesophageal speech after laryngectomy: Sound spectographic and cineradiographic studies. *Acta. Otolaryng.*, suppl. 195 (1964).

MACKINNON, W. J., Table for both the sign test and distribution free confidence intervals of the median for sample sizes to 1,000. *J. Amer. statist. Ass.*, 59, 935-956 (1964).

ROLLIN, W. J., A comparative study of vowel formants of esophageal and normal speaking adults. Unpublished Ph.D. dissertation, Wayne State Univ. (1962).

SHIPP, T., Frequency, duration, and perceptual measures in relation to judgments of alaryngeal speech acceptability. *J. Speech Hearing Res.,* 10, 417-427 (1967).

SNIDECOR, J. C., and CURRY, E. T., Temporal and pitch aspects of superior esophageal speech. *Ann. Otol.,* 68, 623-636 (1959).

SNIDECOR, J. C., and CURRY, E. T., How effectively can the laryngectomee speak? *Laryngoscope,* 70, 62-67 (1960).

SNIDECOR, J. C., *Speech Rehabilitation of the Laryngectomized.* Springfield, Ill.: Charles C Thomas (1968).

Received May 29, 1970.

VOCAL ROUGHNESS AND JITTER CHARACTERISTICS OF VOWELS PRODUCED BY ESOPHAGEAL SPEAKERS

BONNIE E. SMITH, BERND WEINBERG, LAWRENCE L. FETH, and

YOSHIYUKI HORII

Purdue University, West Lafayette, Indiana

Audiotape recordings of sustained vowels produced by nine esophageal speakers were subjected to acoustic and perceptual analysis. Results indicated that (1) the magnitude of vocal jitter present in the vowels was substantially larger than that observed in normal speakers and speakers with laryngeal/vocal disturbance, (2) listeners could reliably rate the severity of vocal roughness in the vowels, (3) voices of esophageal speakers were characterized by varying degrees of vocal roughness, and (4) mean fundamental frequency, mean jitter, or jitter ratio measures did not serve as useful predictors of the perceived severity of vocal roughness. These findings are interpreted to suggest that the mechanism esophageal speakers employ to regulate fundamental frequency is substantially different from that employed by normal speakers and that the identity of physical variables underlying the perception of roughness severity in naturally produced human speech is not well understood.

During normal voice production, the vocal folds vibrate in a synchronous quasi-periodic manner, in which small, cycle-to-cycle variation in the frequency of vocal-fold vibration occurs. Within limits, such variations have no known adverse effects on voice quality and may contribute to the naturalness of human speech (Scripture, 1906; Moore and Von Leden, 1958; Lieberman, 1963; Lehiste, 1970).

It is widely known that the voices of esophageal speakers are characterized by the presence of varying degrees of vocal roughness. Systematic examination of physical properties of esophageal speech that might relate to the perception of rough vocal quality has not previously been conducted.

The work of Isshiki, Yanagihara, and Morimoto (1966), Yanagihara (1967a, b), Emanuel and Sansone (1969), Lively and Emanuel (1970), Sansone and Emanuel (1970), and Emanuel, Lively, and McCoy (1973) indicates that listener perception of the severity of vocal roughness is related to the magnitude of spectral noise. The investigations of Wendahl (1963, 1966), Coleman and Wendahl (1967), Lieberman (1963), and Moore and Thompson (1965) indicate that strong, positive relationships exist between the magnitude of cycle-to-cycle frequency variation (jitter) and the degree of perceived roughness.

The objectives of the present investigation were (1) to measure the mag-

Reprinted by permission from *Journal of Speech and Hearing Research*, 1978, *21*, 240–249.

nitude of cycle-to-cycle variation in fundamental frequency (jitter) in sustained vowels produced by esophageal speakers, (2) to assess the reliability of listener ratings of the perceived severity of vocal roughness present in the sustained vowel productions of esophageal speakers, and (3) to investigate the relationship between roughness ratings and vocal jitter measures. Vocal jitter measures were selected for initial inquiry because Wendahl (1966) and others have indicated that the correlations between stimulus jitter and listener ratings of the severity of auditory roughness were near unity.

METHOD

Speech Sample and Recording Procedure

Audiotape recordings were made of each subject producing a series of sustained /ɑ/-vowels. Recordings were made in a sound-treated room using a high-quality tape-recorder—microphone system. Subjects were seated and wore a custom-made headband that maintained the microphone 15 cm from the lips. The following instructions were given to each subject:

> For this experiment we would like you to sustain the vowel /ɑ/. As you produce each vowel, work hard to maintain a constant pitch and speech effort throughout each production. In other words, you are to produce /ɑ/ in *as steady a manner as possible* at a conversational level of loudness.

The /ɑ/-vowel samples were recorded on one channel of the recorder and a 100-Hz pulse-signal, produced by a unit pulse-generator and monitored by a countertimer, was recorded on a second channel. The 100-Hz signal served as a calibration signal and was used to assess the magnitude of jitter present in the measurement system.

Vocal Jitter Measurements

Two of the investigators listened to the recordings of each speaker and selected a sample vowel representing each speaker's most constant utterance (that is, the vowel with minimal variation in pitch and loudness). One-second segments were spliced from the midsections of each of the selected vowels. Oscillographic records of each of these segments were produced using a Honeywell Visicorder (Model 1508) operating at a transport speed of 2000 mm/sec, while the speed of the tape recorder was reduced by a factor of four. Period-by-period measurement of these records was used to obtain five acoustic measures: (1) mean fundamental frequency, (2) mean vocal jitter (expressed in milliseconds), (3) standard deviation of vocal jitter, (4) jitter ratio, and (5) percentage of total duration identified and measured as periodic. Mean fundamental frequency was calculated by measuring the length of each vocal period, converting these values to milliseconds, and calculating the average of these values in terms of mean period (msec) and fundamental frequency (Hz). Mean vocal jitter was calculated by measuring the difference in millimeters between each consecutive pair of vocal periods, converting this value to milliseconds, and computing the average of the differences. Jitter ratio (JR) was calculated using the formula offered by Jacob (1968)

$$JR = \frac{\overline{X}_j}{\overline{X}_p} \times 1000$$

where $\overline{X}_j$ is mean jitter in milliseconds and $\overline{X}_p$ is mean period in milliseconds. Jitter ratio measures were used to facilitate comparisons of variations in absolute jitter present with varying mean fundamental frequencies.

Roughness Ratings

The 1-sec vowel segments were used to develop stimulus tapes for the perceptual investigation. A paired-comparison approach was used to evaluate the severity of vocal roughness. Three master tapes were produced, each consisting of 36 randomly ordered vowel pairs. Intrastimulus duration was approximately 0.5 sec and interstimulus interval or listener response time was approximately 5 sec.

During the conduct of the roughness rating investigation, the randomly ordered vowel pairs were presented to listeners on three occasions. Initially, listeners were asked to select the vowel of each pair with the higher pitch. The objective of this task was to familiarize listeners with the nature of the stimuli and with the paired-comparison rating scheme. During the remaining two presentations, listeners rated the severity of vocal roughness of the vowel stimuli. Listeners were required to select the member of each vowel pair they perceived as "more rough." Repeated presentation was used to assess listener reliability.

Listeners were nine graduate students and eight professors in the Department of Audiology and Speech Sciences at Purdue University. All listeners were experienced in evaluating speech and participating in psychoacoustic research, were familiar with esophageal speech, and were trained in assessment of voice disorders.

The tape-recorded samples of vowel pairs were played to listeners on an Ampex Model AG 600-2 recorder and delivered binaurally through TDH-39 earphones mounted in MX-41/AR cushions. Stimulus levels were adjusted for comfortable listening. Listeners were run on an individual basis in a sound-treated room.

Analysis

Paired-comparison judgments of the severity of vocal roughness provided information concerning the number of more rough judgments each stimulus received in relation to other stimuli. Thurstone's (Torgerson, 1958) technique for analysis of paired-comparison data was used to transform the listener responses into scale scores. Scores for each vowel were obtained to provide a method of rank-ordering the degree of perceived vocal roughness on an interval scale. Interval-scale scores were used to facilitate comparisons of listener perceptions of vocal roughness with ratio-scaled acoustic (fundamental frequency and jitter) measures. Intercorrelation techniques were used to assess relationships between scale scores of perceived vocal roughness and acoustic measures of jitter ratio, mean vocal jitter, and mean fundamental frequency.

RESULTS

Measurement System Jitter

Period-by-period measurements were made of both the calibration signals and vowel samples. Mean jitter values for the nine calibration signals ranged from 0.07 to 0.13 msec. Jitter standard deviations ranged from 0.06 to 0.12 msec. These results revealed that the magnitude of jitter related to frequency variation in the analysis system was small. Jitter values for the calibration signals were substantially less than for the vowel samples (means ranged from 0.62 to 5.13 msec), indicating that jitter values obtained for the vowel stimuli largely reflect stimulus, rather than system-produced jitter.

Acoustic Characteristics of Vowel Stimuli

Periodicity and Fundamental Frequency. A determination was made of the percentage of periodicity/aperiodicity present in each of the vowel stimuli analyzed (see Table 1). Inspection of Table 1 reveals that the vowels were largely characterized by periodicity: Percentage range from 91 to 100.

Fundamental frequency means and standard deviations of the vowels are

TABLE 1. Periodicity and fundamental frequency characteristics of the nine vowel stimuli.

Vowel	% of Utterance Measured as Periodic	Mean Period (msec)	Standard Deviation of Period (msec)	Mean Fundamental Frequency (Hz)
1	100	33.1	4.3	30.2
2	95	14.2	3.3	70.4
3	96	15.6	3.2	63.9
4	91	18.2	1.7	54.9
5	91	15.7	2.6	63.6
6	100	13.8	0.8	72.4
7	100	18.7	2.8	53.4
8	97	11.4	0.9	87.8
9	100	35.2	6.0	28.4

also presented in Table 1. The mean period values ranged from 11.4 to 35.2 msec; hence, mean fundamental frequencies varied from 87.8 to 28.4 Hz. Standard deviations of the vocal periods extended from 0.8 to 6.0 msec.

Vocal Jitter Characteristics

Vocal jitter means, standard deviations, and jitter ratios for the vowel stimuli are summarized in Table 2. Average jitter values for this set of vowels

TABLE 2. Jitter characteristics of the nine vowel stimuli.

Vowel	Mean Jitter (msec)	Jitter Standard Deviation (msec)	Jitter Ratio
1	3.33	3.94	100.54
2	1.49	2.51	104.86
3	2.33	2.11	148.88
4	1.00	0.87	54.91
5	2.32	1.84	147.49
6	0.88	0.57	63.08
7	0.74	0.90	39.53
8	0.62	0.44	54.43
9	5.13	5.18	145.53

ranged from 0.62 to 5.13 msec. Jitter standard deviations ranged from 0.44 to 5.18 msec. Jitter ratios ranged from 39.53 to 148.88.

Listener Reliability

The reliability of vocal roughness judgments was assessed by two methods. The first involved calculating the percentage of agreement in listeners' more rough responses to repeated presentations of identical pairs of vowel stimuli. The overall test-retest agreement in listener responses was 80%. For individual listeners, the percentages of test-retest agreements ranged from 69 to 89. Ten of the listeners exhibited test-retest agreements exceeding 80%.

Reliability of listener judgments of vocal roughness was assessed secondly by comparing the frequency with which each of the nine vowel stimuli was judged more rough on Presentation 1 versus Presentation 2. The relationship between these two sets of data was assessed by correlation procedures and the resulting Pearson correlation coefficient was 0.997. Taken together, the results of the two approaches suggest that listeners were able to rate the severity of perceived vocal roughness in the vowels reliably.

Vowel Roughness Magnitude Characteristics

A determination of the magnitude of vocal roughness was made by computing the frequency of more rough judgments for each stimulus. Because the frequency of more rough judgments in response to each stimulus did not differ significantly as a function of presentation trial, perceptual data described hereafter are solely from ratings made during the first presentation.

Sign-test analyses were used to determine whether significant differences in the perceived severity of vocal roughness were present among the nine vowel stimuli. As discussed in the previous section, each vowel stimulus was paired with every other vowel. This resulted in the perceptual evaluation of 36 vowel pairs. Because 17 listeners participated, as many as 17 more rough ratings could have been assigned to one member of each vowel pair. On the basis of sign-test analysis, a member of a given vowel pair was perceived as being significantly ($p < 0.05$) more rough than its partner when 13 or more listeners assigned more rough ratings to that stimulus. Stated differently, the values 13 and four encompass the 95% confidence intervals around the median number of possible ratings of a vowel being more rough (MacKinnon, 1964).

The number of more rough ratings assigned to each vowel during the paired-comparison investigation are summarized in Table 3. Table 3 identifies stimulus pairs in which listeners perceived significantly ($p < 0.05$) more vocal roughness in one member of a vowel pair. The data indicate that listeners perceived significantly more vocal roughness in one member of 24 or 66.7% of the 36 vowel pairs rated.

As mentioned earlier, listener responses were transformed into scale scores

TABLE 3. Number of more rough ratings assigned to each vowel stimulus. A value in jth row, kth column represents the number of times kth stimulus was judged more rough than jth stimulus.

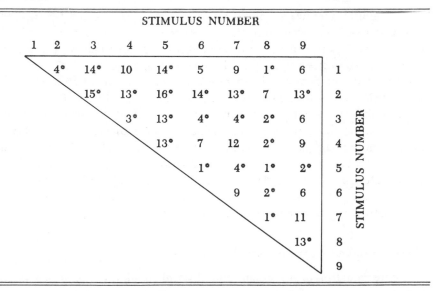

STIMULUS NUMBER

1	2	3	4	5	6	7	8	9	
	4*	14*	10	14*	5	9	1*	6	1
		15*	13*	16*	14*	13*	7	13*	2
			3*	13*	4*	4*	2*	6	3
				13*	7	12	2*	9	4
					1*	4*	1*	2*	5
						9	2*	6	6
							1*	11	7
								13*	8
									9

STIMULUS NUMBER

*$p < 0.05$

of vocal roughness. Scale values corresponding to each of the nine vowel stimuli are displayed in the list below. Stimuli are ordered in terms of their severity of perceived vocal roughness:

Vowel Stimulus	Scale Scores
5	2.02
3	1.61
7	1.15
1	1.14
4	1.03
9	0.97
6	0.95
2	0.31
8	0.00

Relationships Between Listener Ratings of Vocal Roughness and Acoustic Measures

Intercorrelation analyses were used to measure the relations between scale scores of vocal roughness and acoustic measures of mean fundamental frequency, mean jitter, and jitter ratio. Results of these analyses are summarized in Table 4, and indicate that mean fundamental frequency, mean vocal jitter,

TABLE 4. Intercorrelations between scale scores of vocal roughness, mean fundamental frequency, mean jitter, and jitter ratio.

Values	Mean f_0	Mean Jitter	Jitter Ratio
Scale Scores	−0.36	0.31	0.55
Mean f_0	−	−0.78*	−0.32
Mean Jitter		−	0.75

*$p < 0.05$

and jitter ratio measures were not significantly ($p < 0.05$) correlated with scale values of vocal roughness. The magnitudes of the correlations between roughness severity ratings and acoustic measures ranged from −0.36 (mean fundamental frequency) to 0.55 (jitter ratio), emphasizing that none of the acoustic measures served as useful predictors of perceived severity of vocal roughness. The intercorrelation data reveal that average voice fundamental frequency was significantly ($p < 0.05$) correlated with average vocal jitter, suggesting that approximately 60% of the variation in vocal jitter was predicted on the basis of average fundamental frequency. These observations indicate that the magnitude of vocal jitter increased as the fundamental frequency of the vowel decreased.

DISCUSSION

Jitter Characteristics of Vowels

Mean jitter values for vowels produced by the male esophageal speakers in this study ranged from 0.62 to 5.13 msec. Unfortunately, there is limited information concerning the magnitude of vocal jitter present in sustained vowel samples produced by normal male speakers. In one study, Hollien, Michel, and Doherty (1973) measured the magnitude of vocal jitter present in sustained vowels produced by normal male speakers. Mean jitter for four male speakers ranged from 0.01 to 0.06 msec. Jacob (1968) measured the magnitude of vocal jitter present in sustained vowels produced by 15 normal male and 15 normal female speakers. Mean jitter values for male speakers ranged from 0.02 to 3.06 msec. Jacob (1968) observed that jitter magnitudes exceeded 0.6 msec only 8% of the time, and that they exceeded 1.0 msec in only 6% of all utterances. The percentage of jitter values exceeding 1.0 msec was calculated for each of the vowel samples produced by the esophageal speakers in the present study. Percentage values ranged from 16 to 90 for the nine laryngectomized speakers.

Moore and Thompson (1965) reported jitter measures obtained from acoustic analyses of vowel samples produced by two subjects—one classified as having a severely hoarse voice and one judged to be hoarse to a moderate degree. The voice sample from the speaker with the voice judged as severely hoarse had a mean jitter value of 0.30 msec. The sample from the speaker with a moderately hoarse voice had a mean jitter value of 0.06 msec. Michel (1966) reported mean jitter values ranging from 0.07 to 0.57 msec in voices judged to be pathologic.

Jitter ratios for utterances produced by our esophageal speakers ranged from 39.53 to 48.88 Jacob (1968) observed that 70% of pitter ratio values for normal speakers were less than 6.42 and that 90% of these values were less than 8.74. Hollien, Michel, and Doherty (1973) found jitter ratios between 1.41 and 14.16 for four normal male speakers.

The findings of the present study indicate that the magnitude of vocal jitter (expressed in either absolute or relative terms) present in sustained vowels of esophageal speakers is generally substantially larger than that observed in comparable speech utterances produced by normal speakers and speakers with vocal/laryngeal pathologies. These observations are not altogether surprising in view of the relatively simple structural apparatus esophageal speakers use to effect voicing.

In the present work, the term vocal jitter was used to describe random cycle-to-cycle frequency variation associated with voicing. Specifically, jitter was used to define the variation in the period of successive vocal cycles, which occurs when an individual is attempting to sustain phonation at a constant frequency and effort level (Michel and Wendahl, 1971). In utterances of this type, variations in the duration of successive vocal cycles are presumed to be unintentional. The observation that the magnitude of random variation associated with esophageal voicing is large is interpreted to suggest that the mechanism esophageal speakers employ to regulate fundamental frequency is substantially different from that employed by normal speakers.

Roughness Ratings and their Relationship to Selected Acoustic Measures

Results of the perceptual part of this investigation indicated that listeners were able to provide reliable judgments of the severity of perceived vocal roughness of sustained vowel samples produced by esophageal speakers. The perceptual data also supported the notion that the voices of esophageal speakers are characterized by varing degrees of vocal roughness or hoarseness. Four degrees of roughness severity were identified in the voices of the nine esophageal speakers studied here.

The relationship between scale scores of perceived vocal roughness and acoustic measures of mean fundamental frequency, mean vocal jitter, and jitter ratio were assessed using correlation analyses. The perceived magnitude of vocal roughness present in sustained vowels produced by esophageal speakers was not significantly related to any of these acoustic measures. These findings were somewhat surprising in view of previous observations by Wendahl (1966) and Coleman (1969) suggesting that the perceived magnitude of vocal roughness was strongly related to the magnitudes of stimulus jitter, that is, correlations were near unity.

It is important to point out that there were significant differences in the types of stimuli used by Wendahl (1966) and Coleman (1969) and those used in the present study. For example, the stimuli used by Wendahl and Coleman were synthetically generated by an electrical analog of the larynx (LADIC). LADIC enabled the investigators to maintain control of such critical stimulus variables as fundamental frequency and amplitude. In the present study, stimuli were generated by human speakers. Hence, a number of important physical properties were not under investigator control.

Experiments with synthetic speech provide opportunities to evaluate the perceptual relevance of various physical properties of speech. However, the results of such studies should be interpreted cautiously, particularly in terms of developing assumptions about relations between elements of speech production that influence perception of naturally produced human speech attributes. Clearly, vowels produced by human speakers represent stimuli in which a number of properties vary. Hence, the observation that a single physical property, such as vocal jitter, did not strongly predict listener judgments of roughness severity should not be surprising.

ACKNOWLEDGMENTS

This article is based on a master's thesis completed by Bonnie E. Smith in the Department of Audiology and Speech Sciences, Purdue University. The authors wish to acknowledge the contributions of C. Binnie. Requests for reprints should be sent to Bonnie E. Smith or Bernd Weinberg, Department of Audiology and Speech Sciences, Purdue University, West Lafayette, Indiana 47907.

REFERENCES

COLEMAN, R., Effect of median frequency levels upon the roughness of jittered stimuli. *J. Speech Hearing Res.*, 12, 330-336 (1969).

COLEMAN, R., and WENDAHL, R., Vocal roughness and stimulus duration. *Speech Monogr.*, 34, 85-92 (1967).

EMANUEL, F., LIVELY, M., and McCOY, J., Spectral noise levels and roughness ratings for vowels produced by males and females. *Folia phoniat.*, 25, 110-120 (1973).

EMANUEL, F., and SANSONE, F., Some spectral features of "normal" and simulated "rough" vowels. *Folia phoniat.*, 21, 401-415 (1969).

HOLLIEN, H., MICHEL, J., and DOHERTY, E., A method for analyzing vocal jitter in sustained phonation. *J. Phonetics*, 1, 85-91 (1973).

ISSHIKI, N., YANAGIHARA, N., and MORIMOTO, M., Approach to the objective diagnosis of hoarseness. *Folia phoniat.*, 18, 393-400 (1966).

JACOB, L., A normative study of laryngeal jitter. Master's thesis, Univ. of Kansas (1968).

LEHISTE, I., *Suprasegmentals*. Cambridge, Mass.: MIT Press (1970).

LIEBERMAN, P., Perturbations in vocal pitch. *J. acoust. Soc. Am.*, 33, 597-603 (1963).

LIEBERMAN, P., Some acoustical measures of the fundamental periodicity of normal and pathological larynges. *J. acoust. Soc. Am.*, 35, 344-353 (1963).

LIVELY, M., and EMANUEL, F., Spectral noise levels and roughness severity ratings for normal and simulated rough vowels produced by adult females. *J. Speech Hearing Res.*, 13, 503-517 (1970).

MACKINNON, W., Table for both the sign test and distribution free confidence intervals of the median for sample sizes to 1,000. *J. Am. statist. Ass.*, 59, 935-936 (1964).

MICHEL, J., Acoustic correlates of perceived voice quality. Paper presented at the Annual Convention of the American Speech and Hearing Association, Washington, D.C. (1966).

MICHEL, J., and WENDAHL, R., Correlates of voice production. In E. Travis (Ed.), *Handbook of Speech Pathology*. (2nd ed.) New York: Appleton-Century-Crofts, 465-479 (1971).

MOORE, G., and THOMPSON, C., Comments on physiology of hoarseness. *Archs Otolar.*, 81, 97-102 (1965).

MOORE, G., and VON LEDEN, H., Dynamic variations of the vibratory pattern in the normal larynx. *Folia phoniat.*, 10, 205-238 (1958).

SANSONE, F., and EMANUEL, F., Spectral noise levels and roughness severity ratings for normal and simulated rough vowels produced by adult males. *J. Speech Hearing Res.*, 13, 489-502 (1970).

SCRIPTURE, E., *Researchers in Experimental Phonetics: The Study of Speech Curves*. Washington, D.C.: Carnegie Institution, Pub. 41 (1906).

SHIPP, T., and HUNTINGTON, D., Some acoustic and perceptual factors in acute-laryngitic hoarseness. *J. Speech Hearing Dis.*, 30, 350-359 (1965).

TORGERSON, W., *Theory and Methods of Scaling*. New York: John Wiley (1958).

VON LEDEN, H., MOORE, P., and TIMCKE, R., Laryngeal vibration: Measurement of the glottic wave. Part III: The pathologic larynx. *Archs Otolar.*, 71, 16-35 (1969).

WENDAHL, R., Laryngeal analog synthesis of harsh voice quality. *Folia phoniat.*, 15, 241-250 (1963).

WENDAHL, R., Laryngeal analog synthesis of jitter and shimmer: Auditory parameters of harshness. *Folia phoniat.*, 18, 98-108 (1966).

YANAGIHARA, N., Hoarseness: Investigation of the physiological mechanisms. *Ann. Otol.. Rhinol. Lar.*, 76, 472-488 (1976a).

YANAGIHARA, N., Significance of harmonic change and noise components in hoarseness. *J. Speech Hearing Res.*, 10, 531-541 (1967b).

Received May 31, 1977.
Accepted September 21, 1977.

FORMANT FREQUENCY CHARACTERISTICS OF ESOPHAGEAL SPEECH

NANCY L. SISTY

Indiana University, Bloomington, Indiana

BERND WEINBERG

Indiana University Medical Center, Indianapolis, Indiana

Highly representative esophageal vowels ($N = 191$) selected from a listening experiment were subjected to formant frequency analysis. The results of this acoustic analysis showed that: (1) mean vowel formant frequencies for female esophageal speakers were higher than for males, (2) the changes in formant frequency from vowel to vowel were systematic and were essentially the same for normal and esophageal speakers, and (3) average vowel formant frequency values for esophageal speakers were consistently higher than those reported for normal speakers (Peterson and Barney, 1952). The data strongly support the hypothesis that removal of the larynx does alter vocal-cavity transmission characteristics. A reduction in effective vocal tract length for laryngectomized persons using esophageal speech is suggested.

Most of the acoustic research on esophageal speech has been concerned with the measurement of fundamental frequency. In general, the source-function characteristics of esophageal speech have been studied because investigators have assumed that the principal factors affected by laryngectomy are those of the vibratory source (Damste, 1958; and Nichols, 1968).

The literature on esophageal speech presents a contradictory picture in terms of the effects of laryngectomy on vocal-cavity transmission characteristics. For example, Damste (1958, p. 47) has suggested that "the rest of the vocal tract (the pharyngeal and oral cavities) behaves substantially the same in both normal and esophageal speech. For that reason phonetic events in this region undergo no change." His conclusions were based on studies of German- and Dutch-speaking esophageal talkers (Shilling and Binder, 1926; Beck, 1931; and Luchsinger, 1952) which, according to Damste, demonstrated little difference between the vowel formant frequencies of normal and esophageal speakers. In contrast, the more recent data of Rollin (1962) and Kytta (1964) suggest that removal of the larynx does result in altered vocal-cavity transmission characteristics. Specifically, their data show that vowel formant frequencies for esophageal speakers were generally higher than those for normal speakers.

Though experiments of esophageal vowel formant-frequencies characteristics

Reprinted by permission from *Journal of Speech and Hearing Research*, 1972, *15*, 439–448.

have been conducted, minimal effort has been made to interpret the data in terms of current acoustic theories of speech production (Fant, 1960; and Stevens and House, 1955). This situation is regrettable since information about the formant frequencies for esophageal vowels is important both in understanding the physiology of esophageal speech production and documenting changes in vocal-tract function associated with laryngectomy.

The present studies examined the vowel formant-frequency characteristics of esophageal speech produced by both male and female talkers. Comparisons were made between male and female laryngectomized talkers and between esophageal and normal talkers. A perceptual study was performed to select representative esophageal vowels and acoustic measures of the formant frequencies of these vowels were made.

METHOD

Subjects

Fourteen male and 13 female laryngectomized adults who used esophageal speech were selected for study. The speech of each subject was rated for acceptability (Shipp, 1967) and for general effectiveness (Snidecor and Curry, 1959) by two speech pathologists experienced in speech rehabilitation of the laryngectomized. All subjects were judged to have good to excellent esophageal speech and can be compared to the highly rated and excellent talkers studied by Shipp (1967) and Snidecor and Curry (1959).

Recordings and Speech Samples

High quality recordings were made of each subject producing 11 vowels in an [h-d] context prefaced by the carrier phrase, "I will say _____." The 11 vowels included /i/, /ɪ/, /ɛ/, /æ/, /ɑ/, /ʌ/, /u/, /ʊ/, /ɔ/, /o/, and /e/. The [h] V [d] words from the original recordings were spliced out, randomized, and separated by five-second intervals to form a tape for perceptual study.

Listening Procedures

Two groups of listeners were asked to evaluate the recordings to assure that vowels were phonetically representative of those intended (Peterson and Barney, 1952). One group of listeners included 44 undergraduate college students having neither formal training in phonetics nor familiarity with esophageal voice; the second group consisted of nine speech pathologists with experience in phonetics and familiarity with esophageal voices.

The listening was done in a sound-treated room with low ambient-noise characteristics. The stimuli were presented binaurally through earphones (Grason-Stadler, TDH 39) from a high quality recorder-amplifier system (Ampex 440). Listeners indicated the vowel heard on closed-set response forms.

Each listener heard two recordings. The first consisted of 50 highly representative samples of vowels selected by two experienced speech pathologists from the original recordings of esophageal speech. This training tape was used to familiarize the listeners with their task and to eliminate unreliable listeners. The second recording consisted of the 297 [h] V [d] words (11 vowels for 27 speakers) and was used to evaluate whether vowels were representative.

Listeners with the ability to identify representative esophageal vowels were first selected by examining listener responses to the 50 training-tape items. The criterion for accepting a listener was a score of 85% or better on the training-tape words. Vowel samples were selected for acoustic analysis—that is, were acceptable samples—when 80% or more of the experienced and inexperienced listeners identified them as the vowels intended by the talker. Average vowel recognition scores for the speech of normal talkers have ranged from 83% correct for /ɑ/ to 96% correct for /i/ (Peterson and Barney, 1952).

Formant Frequency Analysis

Conventional broad-band spectrograms (Sona-Graph, Model 6061-B) with a frequency display of 0-4,000 Hz were made from the high quality recordings of each of the vowels selected for analysis. The frequencies of the first three formants of each vowel were estimated directly from the broad-band spectrograms using a frequency template constructed according to a calibration spectrogram (Peterson and Barney, 1952). Formant-frequency estimates were made by measuring the mid-points of the visible dark bands of energy appropriate to the first three vowel resonances at a point within a comparatively steady-state portion of the vowel. For each vowel, the formant frequencies were measured independently by two investigators and the average of the two measurements was used to describe each formant frequency. The relative stability and linearity of the sound spectrograph was noted at the beginning and end of each analyzing session and after each hour of analysis.

RESULTS

Listener Selection and Vowel Representative Judgments

Sixteen inexperienced undergraduate listeners and seven experienced speech pathologists met the 85% correct criterion established for participation as listeners. Their responses were used to establish the acceptability of the esophageal vowels.

Of the original 297 vowels, 191 were representative according to the established criterion (Table 1). The average intelligibility for these esophageal vowels ranged from 98% correct for /ʊ/, /o/, and /e/ to 93% for /ɔ/, /u/, and /ɛ/.

Investigator Measurement and Instrumentation Error

Comparisons were made between the two investigators' measurements to determine the formant-frequency measurement error. Of the 473 measure-

TABLE 1. Number of samples accepted for each vowel.

Vowel	Male	Female	Total
o	14	13	27
e	13	12	25
i	13	9	22
ɪ	10	9	19
æ	10	8	18
u	11	6	17
ʊ	9	7	16
ʌ	10	6	16
ɛ	9	4	13
ɑ	4	9	13
ɔ	5	0	5
Total	108	83	191

ments made by each investigator, 429 (90%) differed by less than 43 Hz (± 0.5 mm); 47 (10%) differed by more than 43 Hz, but less than 86 Hz (± 1 mm); and 25 (5%) differed by more than 86 Hz. The 86-Hz difference for the latter 25 measurements exceeded the average formant-frequency error reported in a normative study by Lindblom (1962) and, consequently, they were remeasured. The majority of these large discrepancies were traced to errors in reading the template scale, to data recording mistakes, and to differences in the location at which measurements were taken.

Prior to remeasurement, the mean between-investigator differences were 32 Hz overall—19 Hz for F_1, 29 Hz for F_2, and 46 Hz for F_3. Following remeasurement, the over-all mean difference was reduced to approximately 20 Hz. In the daily measurements of the linearity of the spectrograph, the means of the 500-Hz calibration-tone segments varied between 533 and 473 Hz.

Vowel Formant Frequency Characteristics

The formant-frequency characteristics for representative esophageal vowels are summarized in Table 2. No data are shown for /o/, since it was always produced as a diphthong and no steady-state portion could be easily identified.

The first two formant frequencies of the judged vowels are plotted against each other in Figure 1; loops have been drawn to enclose most of the data points for each vowel. Considerable overlap is evident between /i/ and /ɪ/, lesser overlap between /ɪ/ and /ɛ/, minimal overlap between /æ/ and /ʌ/, /ʊ/ and /u/, and /ʊ/ and /ʌ/, and no overlap between /ɑ/ and /ɔ/. The general pattern of the plotted points in Figure 1 is similar to that found for vowels produced by normal adults (Peterson and Barney, 1952, p. 182).

The data in Table 2 permit a rapid comparison of the average formant frequencies of the men and women. In general, values for women are higher

Vowel	Frequency	Men		Women	
		Mean	Range	Mean	Range
i	F_1	401	312–537	390	312–473
	F_2	2684	2268–2935	2925	2655–3644
	F_3	3067	2752–3311	3627	3246–4525
ɪ	F_1	455	376–559	474	365–580
	F_2	2415	1881–2773	2818	2494–3747
	F_3	2866	2548–3203	3394	2967–4545
e	F_1	604	516–731	672	537–903
	F_2	2277	1892–2677	2540	2290–2752
	F_3	2835	2505–3451	3100	2870–3558
ɛ	F_1	627	580–699	645	559–731
	F_2	2308	1903–2601	2389	2290–2601
	F_3	3008	2752–3246	2980	2945–3053
æ	F_1	791	688–871	908	751–1053
	F_2	2059	1612–2569	2412	2021–3390
	F_3	2762	2365–3322	3106	2784–4121
ɑ	F_1	984	903–1075	1031	860–1215
	F_2	1357	1333–1408	1432	1247–1602
	F_3	2830	2548–3064	3012	2784–3332
ʌ	F_1	773	634–989	801	666–871
	F_2	1477	1376–1591	1657	1591–1763
	F_3	2670	2193–3064	2994	2827–3246
ɔ	F_1	709	634–774	–	–
	F_2	1081	935–1204	–	–
	F_3	2529	2257–2677	–	–
ʊ	F_1	534	451–602	587	505–666
	F_2	1179	1000–1301	1298	1150–1483
	F_3	2662	2150–2956	2872	2612–3343
u	F_1	459	387–570	435	387–473
	F_2	1213	978–1548	1134	1000–1451
	F_3	2666	2311–3203	2835	2698–3010

than for men; exceptions are seen for F_1 for /i/, F_1 and F_2 for /u/, and F_3 for /ɛ/. No comparisons are shown for /ɔ/, since no representative samples were obtained from any women. The mean formant-frequency difference between the men and women was 35 Hz for F_1, 181 Hz for F_2, and 290 Hz for F_3.

The formant frequencies for esophageal talkers are compared with those reported for normal talkers (Peterson and Barney, 1952) in Figures 2 and 3. For both groups of talkers, the systematic changes in formant frequency from vowel to vowel are markedly similar, and the mean formant frequencies of esophageal talkers are consistently higher than those of the normal group. For men, the average increases are 122 Hz for F_1, 325 Hz for F_2, and 321 Hz for F_3; for women, average increases are 76 Hz for F_1, 211 Hz for F_2, and 208 Hz for F_3.

In addition to observing formants appropriate to given vowels, unexpected

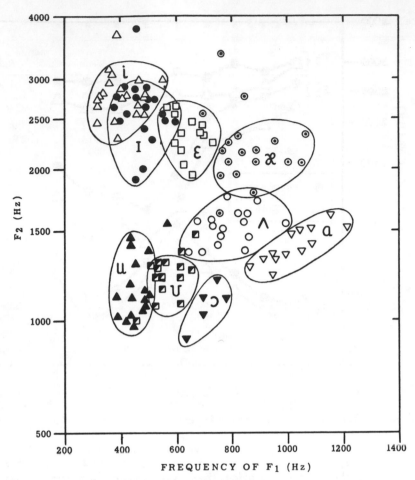

FIGURE 1. Vowel plots of representative esophageal vowels.

concentrations of energy were found in 20 (12%) of the vowel spectra examined. These energy concentrations are "formantlike" in appearance, essentially nonvarying in frequency, in frequency regions where formants are
not expected, and present throughout a major portion of the vowel. A typical
example of a vowel with an added "resonance" is shown in Figure 4. Added
resonances were observed in the vowel spectra of 10 esophageal talkers. They
were located between F_2 and F_3 for /ʊ/ and between F_1 and F_2 for the other
vowels. With the exception of Potter, Kopp, and Kopp (1966), previous
investigators have not commented about extra resonances in the vocalic portions of esophageal speech.

DISCUSSION

With respect to the measurement of esophageal vowel formant frequencies,

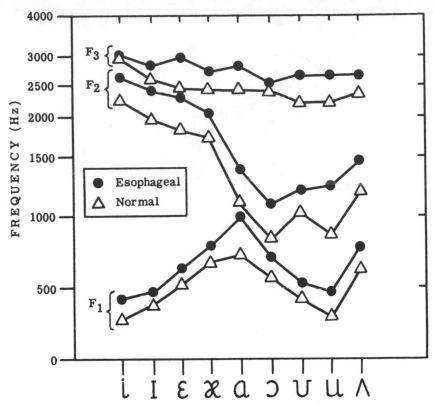

FIGURE 2. Comparison of mean vowel formant frequencies for esophageal and normal male speakers.

Rollin (1962, pp. 97-98) found that "each of the lower three formants was located, and the task of locating them was easier than that involved in locating those of normal subjects." All of the first three formants of the vowels studied in this experiment were not successfully located. Contrary to the comments made by Rollin (1962, pp. 97-98) that measurement of formants in esophageal speech was easier than in normal speech, the difficulties encountered in measurement were similar to those described by Ladefoged (1967) and Peterson and Barney (1952). Specifically, F_1 and F_2 for /ɑ/ and F_2 and F_3 for /i/, /ɪ/, /ɛ/, /æ/, and /e/ overlapped or were very close together, making precise measurements difficult. For some esophageal talkers there was an unexpectedly marked reduction in the intensity of the third formant. The presence of noise, possibly attributable to source-function characteristics of esophageal speech, tended to obscure some of the less prominent formants. In spite of these problems, the frequencies of 82% of the formants were measured.

As is the case for the normal population, these data describing esophageal speech indicate that, on the average, formant frequencies of women are higher than those of men. The average sex differences for each formant—4.5%

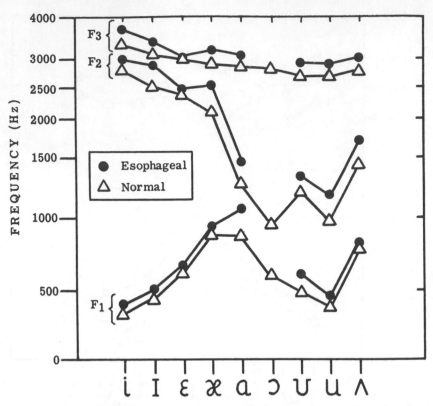

FIGURE 3. Comparison of mean vowel formant frequencies for esophageal and normal female speakers.

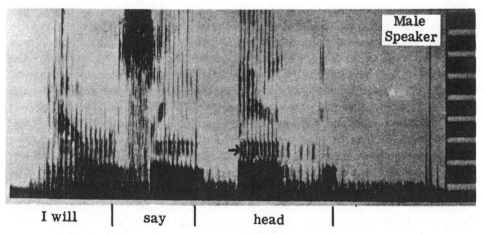

FIGURE 4. Example of extra resonance in esophageal vowel spectra.

for F_1, 12.2% for F_2 and 10.8% for F_3—were significantly less than the 17% difference reported for normal talkers (Peterson and Barney, 1952). The number of esophageal talkers and vowels, as well as the representiveness of the group, however, may not permit a firm comparison with normative vowel data. In addition, the average values for women esophageal speakers may have been lowered by the inclusion of women exhibiting highly masculine vocal characteristics. Weinberg et al. (1971) have shown recently that the sex of male and female talkers can be distinguished by both perceptual and acoustic testing procedures. Their data emphasized the need to differentiate between sex identifications based on listener judgments and those based on acoustic measurements.

Although only a limited number of representative esophageal vowels were studied ($N = 191$), the data do provide an opportunity to compare the formant-frequency characteristics of normal speech and esophageal speech. When the $F_1 - F_2$ plots of esophageal (Figure 1) and normal (Peterson and Barney, 1952, p. 182) vowels are compared, for example, for both groups adjacent vowels are observed to overlap. Considerable overlap is observed between /i/ and /ɪ/ and /ɪ/ and /ɛ/ for esophageal speech, but very little for normal speech. Conversely, there is considerable overlap between /u/ and /ʊ/ in the normal data, while little overlap is found in esophageal speech data. The contention of Rollin (1962) that the formant frequencies in esophageal speech have a larger range of variation than in normal speech is generally supported by the present data.

The finding that formant frequencies were consistently higher in esophageal speech—regardless of the sex of the talkers—than in normal speech confirms some earlier reports. Rollin (1962), in a study of English-speaking male laryngectomees, and Kytta (1964), in a study of Finnish-speaking male laryngectomees found higher-than-normal formants. The consistency of this finding across languages, sex, and vowels shows that removal of the larynx does alter vocal-cavity transmission characteristics. Differences in tongue position (Nichols, 1968) and mouth opening, per se, do not fully explain this effect (Stevens and House, 1955; and Fant, 1960); however, a reduction in the effective length of the vocal tract as a result of total laryngectomy surgery may account for these changes. The acoustically derived hypothesis that total laryngectomy results in a shortening of effective vocal tract length is compatible with existing physiologic data. Diedrich and Youngstrom (1966) obtained cinefluorograms of a patient one day prior to and 20 months following total laryngectomy. Tracings of this patient's vocal tract were made in the pre- and postoperative conditions as he produced vowels /ɪ/, /æ/, /ʌ/, and /ɑ/ (Diedrich and Youngstrom, Figures 21 and 22, pp. 93-94, 1966). For each vowel the effective vocal tract length of this patient was reduced postoperatively.

ACKNOWLEDGMENT

This research was supported in part by the National Institute of Neurological Diseases and Stroke, NS-09262-02. This article is based on a thesis submitted by Nancy Sisty to

Indiana University in partial fulfillment of the requirements for the Master of Arts degree. The authors wish to acknowledge A. S. House, M. Carpenter, and M. Schultz for their contributions. Illustrations were prepared by James Glore, Medical Illustrator, Indiana University Medical Center. Requests for reprints may be directed to Bernd Weinberg, Speech Research Laboratory, Rotary Building, Indiana University Medical Center, Indianapolis, Indiana 46202.

REFERENCES

BECK, J., Zur phonetik der stimme u. sprache laryngektomierter. *Z. Laryngol., Rhin., Oto.,* 21, 506-521 (1931).

DAMSTE, P. H. *Oesophageal Speech after Laryngectomy.* Groningen, Netherlands: Gebr. Hoitsema (1958).

DIEDRICH, W. M., and YOUNGSTROM, K. A., *Alaryngeal Speech.* Springfield: Charles C Thomas (1966).

FANT, G., *Acoustic Theory of Speech Production.* The Hague, Netherlands: Mouton, S-Gravenhage (1960).

KYTTA, J., Finnish oesophageal speech after laryngectomy: Sound spectrographic and cineradiographic studies. *Acta otolaryng.* (Stockholm), Suppl. 195, 7-91 (1964).

LADEFOGED, P., *Three Areas of Experimental Phonetics.* London: Oxford Univ. Press, 50-142 (1967).

LINDBLOM, B., Accuracy and limitations of sonograph measurements. In *Proceedings of the Fourth International Congress of Phonetic Sciences.* The Hague, Netherlands: Mouton, 188-202 (1962).

LUCHSINGER, R., Der mechanismus der sprech-u. stimmbildung bei laryngektomierten und die ubungsbehandlung. *Pract. oto-rhino-laryng.,* 14, 304-323 (1952).

NICHOLS, A. C., Loudness and quality in esophageal speech and the artificial larynx. In J. C. Snidecor (Ed.), *Speech Rehabilitation of the Laryngectomized* (2nd ed.). Illinois: Thomas, 108-127 (1968).

PETERSON, G. E., and BARNEY, H. L., Control methods used in a study of the vowels. *J. acoust. Soc. Amer.,* 24, 175-184 (1952).

POTTER, R. K., KOPP, G. A., and KOPP, H. G., *Visible Speech.* New York: Dover (1966).

ROLLIN, W. J., A comparative study of vowel formants of esophageal and normal-speaking adults. Doctoral dissertation, Wayne State Univ. (1962).

SCHILLING, R. and BINDER, H., Experimental phonetische untersuchungen uber die stimme ohne kehlkopf. *Arch. Ohr.-,Nas.-, u Kehlk Heilk.,* 115, 235 (1926).

SHIPP, T., Frequency, duration, and perceptual measures in relation to judgments of alaryngeal speech acceptability. *J. Speech Hearing Res.,* 10, 417-427 (1967).

SNIDECOR, J. C., and CURRY, E. T., Temporal and pitch aspects of superior esophageal speech. *Ann. Otol. Rhinol. Laryng.,* 68, 623-636 (1959).

STEVENS, K. N. and HOUSE, A. S., Development of a quantitative description of vowel articulation. *J. acoust. Soc. Amer.,* 27, 484-493 (1955).

WEINBERG, B., BENNETT, S., HORIE, Y., HOUSE, A. S., and HUGHES, G. W., Recognition of the sex of esophageal talkers. Paper presented at the 81st meeting of the Acoustical Society of America, Washington, D.C., April (1971).

Received September 27, 1971.

PERCEPTUAL CONFUSIONS AMONG SELECTED PHONEMES IN ESOPHAGEAL SPEECH

Pat Richard Sacco*
Mary B. Mann*
Martin C. Schultz*

Surgical removal of the larynx, from a pathological condition or trauma, requires that some procedure be undertaken to regain communicative ability. Each of the four general means,[1] available provides a vibratory pattern which is utilized in the production of speech sounds.

Since all methods of non-laryngeal voice production provide a vocalic carrier, transition from voiced to voiceless and from voiceless to voiced sounds creates special problems for the laryngectomized talker.

It seems reasonable to ask whether reduction in ability to make a rapid voicing transition, or any voicing transition, results in a significant decrease in intelligibility.

The present study was undertaken to supply information on the intelligibility of esophageal voice. The experimental design permitted evaluation of intelligibility of individual consonant phonemes and comparison of these results with data obtained on normal talkers (Miller and Nicely, 1955). Data were generated by having the esophageal talkers produce a series of syllables which served as stimuli for a recognition task accomplished by naive listeners.

The esophageal voice remains relatively constant throughout the laryngectomee's utterances, both in pitch (Tato et.al, 1954; Damste', 1958; Snidecor and Curry, 1960) and in lack of transistion from voiced to voiceless sounds (DiCarlo,

* Pat Richard Sacco, Department of Speech, Western Michigan University.
* (Mrs.) Mary B. Mann, PhD. Assistant Professor of Speech Pathology, Indiana University.
* Martin C. Schultz, PhD. Associate Professor of Speech Pathology, Indiana University.

[1] these include a mechanical larynx, an electrical larynx, esophageal speech and an electronic device inserted into the oral cavity.

Reprinted by permission from *Journal of the Indiana Speech and Hearing Association*, 1967, 26, 19–33.

Amster and Herer, 1955; Hodson, 1958). Descriptive studies, comparing esophageal talkers with users of artifical devices (Hyman, 1955; McCroskey and Mulligan, 1963) by use of comparative listener judgments, have yielded preferential judgment data but neither quantitive data on the frequency of correct identifications of a given sound, nor qualitative data identifying the specific substitutions, have appeared.

EXPERIMENTAL PROCEDURES

Subjects:

Nineteen laryngectomized subjects were used in the study: fifteen Caucasian males, three Negro males, and one Negro female. All subjects had previous instruction in the use of esophageal speech and all employed this method in daily communication.

The criterion used to determine inclusion of the esophageal speakers was that each was capable of producing specific vowel-consonant combinations in imitation. The performance of subjects was evaluated by two experienced teachers of esophageal speech. Seventeen were judged as capable of automatic fluent sentences, and two others were judged as able to utter phrases at will though not capable of performing at the greater fluency level.

Judges:

Ten undergraduate students from the Indiana University student population, majoring in Speech Pathology, were selected to serve as judges, and all met the following criteria:

1. demonstration of normal hearing (15 dB, ASA, 1951) for frequencies in the range 250-8,000 cps.

2. lack of previous clinical experience or training in listening to laryngectomized individuals using esophageal speech.

Equipment:

A clinical tape recorder (Wollensak T-1500) was used both for recording and reproducing the esophageal stimuli.

The microphone from the tape recorder was suspended at eye-level one foot from the talker, to reduce the interference of stoma breathing. All talkers were recorded in quiet surroundings.

Stimulus Materials:

Stimuli consisted of 256 consonant-vowel combinations, comprising 16 consonants each paired with the vowel /a/ 16 times. The consonants chosen were described by Miller and Nicely to "…. make up almost three-quarters of all the consonants we utter in normal speech and about 40 percent of all phonemes, vowels included" (1955, p. 338). The consonants used were: /p/, /t/, /k/, /f/, /θ/, /s/, /ʃ/, /b/, /d/, /g/ , /v/, /ʒ/, /z/, /ʒ/, /m/, and /n/. Syllable presentation order was individually randomized and each subject spoke all 256 stimuli.

Judgments:

Ten naive judges listened to the reproduction of the stored syllables of the 19 esophageal talkers, plus a second reproduction of one speaker, and identified syllables by the 16-consonant set available to them on printed sheets. The consonant-vowel combinations were presented to the judges at an average rate of one every two seconds. The 20 recorded presentations, including one subject randomly selected and presented a second time for the purpose of evaluating intra-judge reliability, were judged in seven sessions, each consisting of approximately 60 minutes.

Normative Data:

Miller and Nicely conducted a study with normal speakers which yielded data considered appropriate for comparison with those of the present study. They analyzed the identifiability of the same set of consonant phonemes through the use of a closed confusion matrix. In their study, five female subjects, trained prior to their participation, served as both talkers and listeners, in a round-robin speaking-listening experiment.

RESULTS

Master Confusion Matrix

The master confusion matrix, expressed in proportions,

Table I. Master confusion matrix for 256 syllables spoken by each of 19 subjects as judged by 10 listeners (converted to probabilities recorded as whole numbers).

RESPONSE

STIMULUS	p	t	k	f		s		b	d	g	v		z		m	n
p	39	02	02	15	01			22	02	02	09	02			03	01
t	06	39	04	07	04			03	20	03	03	05		01	01	02
k	02	02	63	02	01			01	01	25	01	01		01		01
f	10	02	01	46	06	01		10	01	01	13	04	01		02	01
θ	07	10	03	14	14	01		07	10	03	06	18	02		01	05
s	01	04	01	03	04	35	12	01	02	01	01	03	23	09		01
ʃ	01	02	01	01	01	04	43		02	03	--	01	05	37		01
b	11	02	01	08	02			40	02	01	11	05			14	04
d	06	10	02	02	02			06	52	05	01	04		01	01	08
g	01	02	20	01	01		01	01	07	53	01	02	02	05		02
v	05	02	01	15	05	01		16	04	03	24	09	02	01	09	04
ð	06	07	03	13	13	01	01	04	09	03	06	22	04	01	02	05
z	01	04	01	02	04	09	05	01	07	03	02	07	43	10		02
ʒ	01	02	01	01	03	07	10		07	05	01	05	27	28		02
m	04		01	05	01			04	01	01	05	01			66	10
n	01	02	02	01	01			01	06	02	01	02			03	76

☐ = correct identifications

is presented in Table I. Two hundred ficty-six syllables were phonated by each of 19 subjects and judged by 10 listeners for a total of 48,640 stimulus-response pairs. Table I displays the proportion of responses (columns) chosen for each stimulus consonant (rows) of the syllable. The correct identifications of a phoneme is shown as the proportion at the intersect of the column and row labelled as that phoneme, and the mean articulation score for all stimuli (obtained as the mean proportion of correct responses) was 42%.

Collapsed Matrices:

Once may combine stimuli and their corresponding responses into groups representing particular classes (e.g., voiced) according to several phoneme classification schemes. With such data, reduction schemes present smaller matrices and a new articulation score. The new score will be greater than that of the master matrix, since all responses that were originally correct remain so, and in addition, all within-group confusions become "correct" responses in the collapsed grouping. The advantage of such a smaller matrix is that it summarizes the patterns of confusion according to the phoneme classification scheme employed. The present study utilized a "linguistic features" classification grouping, to facilitate comparison with the normative data, and these results are presented in the following sections.

1. Voicing

The voiceless consonants /p/, /t/, /k/, /f/, /θ/, /s/, and /ʃ/ have been contrasted with the voiced consonants /b/, /d/, /g/, /v/, /ʒ/, /z/, /ʒ/, /m/ and /n/, to demonstrate the effect of confusion in voicing on perceptual judgements of consonants spoken by esophageal talkers.

A mean articulation score of 68% is derived from a voicing matrix, as contrasted with a score of 42% derived from the master matrix, indicating that approximately one-half (32% error as contrasted with 58% error) of all errors involved voicing confusion. Inspection of Table 2 also indicates that a listener was twice as likely to misidentify in favor of voicing (voiced for voiceless error) than toward unvoicing.

Table II. Voicing contrasts in phoneme identifications.

RESPONSE

S T I M U L U S		Voiceless[1]	Voiced
	Voiceless	60[2]	40
	Voiced	24	76

[1] See text for listing of stimuli in each category.
[2] Figures represent proportion of response.

2. Manner of Articulation

A matrix displaying a categorization of consonants by manner of articulation is shown in Table III. This matrix employs the three groups: plosives, fricatives, and nasals.

Table III. Manner of Articulation contrasts in phoneme identifications.

RESPONSE

S T I M U L U S		plosives[1]	fricatives	nasals
	plosives	77[2]	17	06
	fricatives ...	22	73	04
	nasals	13	09	78

[1] plosives include /p/, /t/, /k/, /b/, /d/, /g/; fricatives include /f/, /o/, /s/,
/ʃ/, /ʒ/, /z/, / /; nasals include /m/ and /n/.
[2] Figures represent proportion of response.

No significant differences were noted among these groups, and within-group correct identifications all approximate 75%. Listeners identified fricatives as plosives and plosives as fricatives about equally often, but seldom misidentified either as being a nasal. When a nasal was misidentified out-of-class, it was equally likely to be called a plosive or fricative.

3. Frication[1]

A matrix was constructed with the fricatives contrasted with the combined nasals and plosives, on the argument that the articulators close completely for the plosives and nasals, but are only approximated for the fricatives.

The matrix yields an average correct within-group score of approximately 80%. A fricative is almost twice as frequently called a plosive or nasal than is either of the latter groups identified as a fricative.

Table IV. Frication contrasts in phoneme identifications.

		RESPONSE	
S T I M U L U S		Fricative[1]	plosive-nasal
	fricatives	73[2]	27
	plosive-nasals	15	85

[1] See Table 3 for listing of consonants in each category.
[2] Figures represent proportion of response.

4. Duration

Four of the set of consonants /s/, / /, /z/, and / / are intense, high frequency noises of relatively long duration. These sounds were contrasted with all the other consonants and these results are displayed in Table 5. The mean articulation score for the matrix exceeds 85%. In addition, a high degree of asymmetry in incorrect identifications is apparent. The long duration sounds may be perceived (or articulated) as shorter but the reverse is not true. In general, one does not identify a consonant of an esophageal talker as being one

[1] this is the category labelled by Miller and Nicely as "affrication."

of the long duration sounds unless it is of this class, though
he may mistake a longer sound as being a shorter consonant

Table V. Duration contrasts in phoneme identifications.

		RESPONSE	
		Long[1]	Short
S **T** **I** **M** Long		76[2]	24
U **L** Short		03	97
U **S**			

[1] See text for listing of stimuli in each category.
[2] Figures represent proportion of response.

5. Place of Articulation

In their interpretation of place of articulation data,
Miller and Nicely distinguished three positions according to
the location of the major constriction of the vocal passage.
While the economy of this experimental procedure might
have made it appropriate to that study, it poses some serious problems for the phonetician. In order to effect a compromise between the demands of rigorous phonetic classification, and those of experimental economy, the following
breakdowns were made:

Miller and Nicely Classification ...... Present Study

Front /p/ /b/ /m/ .... Bilabial

/f/ /v/ .... Labio-Dental

Middle /θ / /ʒ/...................... Inter-Dental

/t/ /d/ /s/ /z/ /n/ .... Alveolar

Back /ʃ/ /ʒ/ .... Palatal

/k/ /g/ .... Volar

Table VI. Place of articulation contrasts in phoneme identifications.

		RESPONSE					
		Bil[1]	L-D	I-D	Alv	Pal	Vel
S	Bil	68[2]	17	04	08		03
T	L-D	26	49	12	10	01	03
I							
M	I-D	14	19	33	26	01	06
U							
L	Alv	07	05	07	69	07	05
U							
S	Pal	01	01	05	29	59	05
	Vel	03	02	02	09	03	81

[1] See text for listing of stimuli in each category.
[2] Figures represent proportion of response.

This grouping yielded the lowest combined mean articulation score (60%) but also has the fewest items per group.
In general, one tends to misidentify esophageal consonants, or
correctly identify misarticulated consonants, by considering
them as more anterior sounds than they are, with some pre-
dilection also to identify sounds as alveolars. This last may
represent an expectancy bias in the listener, as alveolar
sounds have a very high frequency of occurrence in American
English (Wang & Crawford, 1960).

In order to determine intra-judge reliability, one
subject was randomly selected and this recording was reproduced to the 10 judges a second time without their knowledge.
As a group, the judges performed consistently; the mean
articulation score for that subject varying only one percent
for the second evaluation.

DISCUSSION

The present study was designed to appraise intelligibility of esophageal talkers. Difficulty in understanding
esophageal speech, when syllable articulation is discrimi-

nated by naive listeners, was highlighted by an average obtained discrimination score of only 42%. No appraisal of the relationship between syllable articulation and general intelligibility was attempted. The findings that two subjects with a rating of being able to phonate phrases at will but not capable of fluent sentences achieved higher recognition scores than five subjects with the higher rating suggests that any such relationship that might exist is not simple.

An attempt was made to evaluate the phonemes which would be most often misunderstood in the esophageal talker's speech, and the phonemes that the listener would hear when he misidentified the intended stimulus. It was desirable that the listener not be biased by his knowledge of the distribution of the various phonemes in American English or by the relative familiarity of the members of any chosen population of words. A population of sixteen consonants was articulated, each in combination with the vowel /a/ in a CV combination, and each talker spoke each syllable sixteen times. The syllables were heard, in random order, by ten naive listeners and their responses were tabulated into a confusion matrix.

In addition to the generalizations about phoneme recognition behavior that can be made from observation of the confusion matrix, some information can also be obtained by contrasting these data with those obtained from normal talkers.

The contrastive data were those from an experiment by Miller and Nicely. The Miller and Nicely study utilized several experimental conditions and a confusion matrix was generated for each. The particular matrix (-6 dB, S/N; 200-6500 cps) used for comparison with the data of the present study was chosen as a wide range, flat frequency response condition with approximately the same overall discrimination score. The Miller and Nicely articulation score was 46%; that of the present study was 42%. It should be noted that the Miller and Nicely matrices demonstrate a high degree of internal consistency in that same errors are found in matrix after matrix, but under more difficult listening conditions, random error plays a progressively greater role.

The Miller and Nicely data are displayed as proportions in Table 7. The comparable table for the data of this study is Table 1. Certain differences in general patterning of responses should be observed. Perhaps the most striking con-

Table VII. Master confusion matrix determined from Miller and Nicely (1955) converted to probabilities recorded as whole numbers.

RESPONSE

STIMULUS	p	t	k	f	θ	s	ʃ	b	d	g	v	ð	z	ʒ	m	n
p	**34**	19	28	07	06	03	01									
t	29	**34**	23	02	04	01	03						01		01	01
k	23	27	**38**	04	03	03	01									
f	06	04	03	**61**	17	04		02	01		01	01				
θ	07	06	06	36	**22**	11	02	02	01	02	02	01	02			
s	03	02	02	09	02	**43**	18	02	01	01			01	01		
ʃ		02	01	02	02	12	**79**		01							
b				02	02	02		**55**	04	04	19	06	02		02	02
d							04	02	**37**	21	05	09	09	12		
g					01			01	25	**26**	01	08	15	22		01
v				01				18	02	02	**54**	17	04		01	
ð					03			13	03	07	36	**24**	09	02	03	
z								03	08	11	07	12	**39**	18		
ʒ									10	07	01	03	17	**50**		01
m								02			02		01		**75**	19
n					02				02	01		03		03	20	**69**

□ = correct identifications

trast of the two tables of proportions of response occurrence is the tight patterning of errors in the normative table and the broad scattering of errors in the responses to esophageal talkers reveal some tendency to misidentify virtually any consonant as any other consonant. The normative data show very few instances of such random guessing. One might conclude that many utterances of the esophageal talkers are so lacking in acoustic cues to the consonant "spoken" that either they are very poorly understood or the linguistic cues arising from context, during meaningful discourse, must make an extremely great contribution to word (and, perhaps, phoneme) identification.

In addition, one might question a therapy regime which rates esophageal talkers with respect to their fluency rather than their intelligibility, highlighting the need for much additional research into the therapy processes.

Note that virtually no cognate errors were obtained under the conditions of the normative study, whereas the voicing error (the misidentification of sound by substitution of another differing only in voicing) is the most frequent substitution for all the voiceless and approximately half of the voiced stimuli of the present study. It might, even more, be observed that only the nasal sounds show comparable listener behavior in the two studies. That is to say, the data of the present study, wherein esophageal talkers werc heard by normal naive listeners in the quiet, are in only superficial respects comparable to data generated by trained listeners hearing normal talkers under adverse S/N conditions.

It seemed reasonable to hypothesize, a priori, that the difficulty the esophageal talker has in producing a true voiceless sound should pre-dispose a listener to expect to hear inadequate production of voiceless phonemes, and to misidentify sounds as being voiceless more frequently than the listeners of the present study were disposed to do. Perhaps their lack of experience with esophageal talkers kept them from such a bias. Even so, Wang and Crawford have shown that the several frequency studies of English consonants all find the preponderance of voiceless sounds having higher frequencies of occurrence than their voiced cognates, which again should have predisposed any group of naive listeners to hear more voiceless sounds in misidentifying word, or syllable, utterances. Interestingly, the listeners, on the average, correctly identify the voiceless sounds slightly more frequently than they did their voiced cognates (omitting /m/ and /n/) - 40% to 37.5%, though they were much more disposed to misidentify the voiceless sound as its voiced cognate than the reverse - 23% to 13%. Obviously, there is much work to be done in evaluating the perception of the "vocal carrier" or voicing of the esophageal talker by the naive (typical) listener; specifically, the information the listener presumes to obtain which contributes to his identification of the phonemic content.

The general sequence of phonemes, when ranked from most to least intelligible, is nasals, plosives, and then fricatives. Moolenaar-Bijl (1953) and Snidecor, et.al. (1962) emphasize the use of plosives in beginning training of esophageal talkers, while Nelson (1949) emphasizes vowels, semi-vowels, and nasals. Moolenaar-Bijl, in particular, suggested the use of the voiceless plosives, indicating that the pronunciation of these made it easier to take air into the esophagus. If the immediate goal of therapy is intelligible speech, then the results of the present study would argue for the therapy sound sequence proposed by Nelson, both because of the high intelligibility of the nasals and the low intelligibility of two of the voiceless plosives. It should be stated again, however, that there was little, if any, relationship found in the present study between judgments of fluency and those of phoneme intelligibility. Patently, further study is called for before strong therapy implications will be forthcoming.

SUMMARY

Nineteen laryngectomized subjects each recorded 256 consonant-vowel combinations with esophageal voice. The recordings were evaluated by a panel of 10 naive listeners. The results of the study were compared with those obtained in a study having comparable mean articulation score achieved under adverse signal-to-noise ratio conditions by normal talkers and trained listeners.

It was found that the errors made by naive subjects listening to esophageal talkers are not comparable to those recorded for normal speakers evaluated under adverse conditions.

The findings of the present study were as follows:

1. There appears to be no relationship between the fluency of an esophageal talker and his intelligibility.

2. Approximately half of the time that a consonant phoneme is misidentified, the misidentification involves a voicing error.

3. When a misidentification involving voicing occurs, a listener tends to misidentify a voiceless sound as being voiced twice as often as he errs in the other direction.

4. Listeners tend to misidentify sounds as being shorter than those spoken (or, at least, intended) by the esophageal talker, with very few errors caused by misidentification of a sound as being longer than the intended phoneme.

5. The nasal sounds used in the study had high identifiability, which suggests that they are easy to articulate and would be appropriate sounds for starting therapy.

6. Listeners to esophageal talkers demonstrate some tendency to misidentify virtually and "intended" consonant production as any other consonant, suggesting that esophageal talkers have significant difficulty with all classes of consonants. To the extent that there is any strong relationship between phoneme and contextual intelligibility, there is significant need for articulation therapy in habilitation of esophageal speech.

BIBLIOGRAPHY

Damste', P. H., Esophageal Speech After Laryngectomy. Groningen: Boedrukkerij Voorheen Grbroeders Holtseme (1958).

DiCarlo, L. M., Amster, W. and Herer, G., Speech After Laryngectomy. Syracuse: Syracuse University Press (1955).

Hodson, J. C., and Oswald, M., Speech Recovery After Laryngectomy. London: E. & S. Livingstones, Ltd. (1958).

Hyman, M., An Experimental Study of Artificial Larynx and Esophageal Speech. J. Speech Hearing Dis., 20, 291-299 (1955).

McCroskey, R. L., and Mulligan, M., The Relative Intelligibility of Esophageal Speech and Artificial Larynx Speech. J. Speech Hearing Dis., 28, 37-41 (1963).

Miller, G., and Nicely, Patricia, An Analysis of Perceptual Confusions Among Some English Consonants. J. Acous. Soc. Amer., 27, 338-352 (1955).

Moolenaar-Bijl, Annie, The Importance of Certain Consonants in Esophageal Voice After Laryngectomy. Ann. Otol., Rhin. and Laryng., LXIII, December, (1953).

Nelson, C., Post-Laryngectomy Speech: You Can Speak Again. New York: Funk & Wagnalls Company (1949).

Snidecor, J. C., and Curry, E. T., How Effectively Can the Laryngectomee Expect to Speak? Laryngoscope, 7, 62-67 (1960).

Snidecor, J. C., et al, Speech Rehabilitation of the Laryngectomized. Springfield: Charles C. Thomas, Publishers (1962).

Tato, J., Mariani, N., DePiccoll, E. M., and Mirasov, P., Study of the Sonospectrographic Characteristics of the Voice on Laryngectomized Patients. Acta Otolaryng., 44, 431-38 (1954).

Wang, W. S-Y., and Crawford, J., Frequency Studies of English Consonants. Lang. & Speech, 31, 131-139 (1960).

INTELLIGIBILITY CHARACTERISTICS
OF SUPERIOR ESOPHAGEAL SPEECH
PRESENTED UNDER VARIOUS
LEVELS OF MASKING NOISE

YOSHIYUKI HORII *and* BERND WEINBERG

Purdue University, West Lafayette, Indiana

Broad-band masking of speech was used to assess the effects that broad-band masking noise had upon the recognition of consonants and vowels produced by esophageal speakers. Procedures were developed to compare the articulation functions of superior esophageal speech with those of normal speech under comparable levels of masking noise. Within the range of speech-to-noise ratios studied, articulation functions for vowels were essentially the same for esophageal and normal talkers (4% per dB). With respect to consonants, the intelligibility scores for esophageal speech were 12 to 14% lower than for normal speech under adverse noise conditions. Gains in the consonant articulation functions were 2.5%/dB and 4%/dB for normal and esophageal talkers, respectively. For adverse noise conditions, the lowered consonant scores for esophageal speakers were the result of poorer than normal intelligibility for liquid-glides and nasal and, secondarily, for stop consonants. Additional differences between the intelligibility characteristics of esophageal and normal speech were found in word-position and voicing features.

Broad-band masking noise is known to have a differential effect upon the recognition of speech sounds (Horii, House, and Hughes, 1971; Miller and Nicely, 1955). In this context, esophageal speakers frequently assert that the intelligibility of their speech is adversely affected by noise. The manner in which esophageal speakers raise this assertion makes it apparent that they assume (1) that their esophageal speech is different from normal speech, and (2) that, as a consequence of these physical differences, esophageal speech is more vulnerable to deterioration by noise than normal speech produced with a laryngeal sound source.

The objective of the present work was to measure the intelligibility of superior esophageal speech as a function of adverse listening conditions, that is, under various levels of masking noise. It was assumed that the broad-band masking of speech would provide an incisive approach to begin looking at how esophageal speech is different from normal speech. In addition, it was assumed that the analysis of listeners' responses to recorded esophageal speech materials being masked by continuous broad-band noise would provide an inferential asessment of the validity of the noise interference problem reported by laryngectomized patients. Thus, procedures were developed to compare

Reprinted by permission from *Journal of Speech and Hearing Research*, 1975, *18*, 413–419.

the articulation functions of superior esophageal speech with those of normal speech under comparable levels of masking noise.

METHODS

Subjects

Two superior esophageal speakers, one man and one woman, provided the speech materials used in the listening tests. The talkers were highly experienced, highly proficient esophageal speakers who had used esophageal speech as a primary method of communication for over five years. Their speech was automatic, highly intelligible, free of extraneous noises, and generally pleasant to listen to. In short, their speech was among the best alaryngeal speech the authors had ever heard.

Speech Materials and Recordings

The two talkers recorded six lists of a consonant rhyme test (House et al., 1965) and six lists of a vowel rhyme test (Horii, 1969). Each consonant list consisted of 50 monosyllabic words in which half had test consonants in the word-initial position, while the remaining half had test consonants in the word-final position. In this rhyme test, consonants appeared with frequencies approximately equal to those observed in actual English texts. On the other hand, each vowel list consisted of 24 monosyllabic words. In the vowel rhyme test, 12 different vowels appeared twice in each list.

Listeners and Listening Procedures

The listeners were 16 young adults (college students) who were paid for their services. Each listener passed a discrete frequency audiometric screening test at a hearing level of 15 dB (ANSI, 1969). Listeners were unfamiliar with alaryngeal speech and were not experienced or trained in psychoacoustic listening procedures.

The recorded word lists were delivered binaurally using a high-quality tape system and matched earphones (Grason-Stadler, Model TDH-39 with Zwislocki-type cushions). The entire experiment was conducted over a period of fifteen, 50-minute, daily sessions and all listening was done in a quiet room furnished with individual stations. In each session, 12 word lists (six consonant lists and six vowel lists) were presented at four different signal-to-noise ratios. The stimulus materials were appropriately counterbalanced with respect to list order, speaker order, and signal-to-noise ratios in order to preclude listeners from learning the order of test items and to enhance listeners' attention to the listening task.

The signal levels of each test list were determined by playing the test recordings into a Bruel and Kjaer graphic level recorder (Model 2305) and measuring the level of the vocalic maxima of each word relative to a 1000-Hz reference signal. The speech level of each word list was defined operationally as the mean level of the vocalic nuclei of the words in each list. The test tapes were prepared so that the average speech level of word lists, that is, the mean level of the vocalic nuclei of the words in each test list, was 65 dB SPL under the earphones.

For the vowel tests, the signal-to-noise ratios employed were −9 dB, −5 dB, and −1 dB. The S/N ratios for the consonant tests were −9 dB, −5 dB, −1 dB, and +3 dB. All consonant and vowel lists recorded by each of the two speakers were presented once under each S/N condition. In addition, all lists were presented in a clear condition—that is, without any masking noise. In the case of the tests administered with a masking noise, the noise was not recorded for test administration, but was produced by a standard white-noise generator (Grason-Stadler, Model 455C) and mixed with the speech at the time of testing. Thus, the esophageal speech word lists were masked by a continuous white noise. Both the noise and speech were essentially low-passed with a cutoff frequency near 8000 Hz, the upper frequency response limit of the earphones. In these tests, a S/N ratio of 0 dB was established by setting the level of the reference tone preceding each word list to a level equal to the average level of the speech. Thus, equal levels of the reference tone and the corresponding noise defined a S/N ratio of 0 dB. Other values of S/N ratio were obtained by varying the noise levels with appropriately placed attenuators.

A closed-set response strategy was used in the listening experiment (House et al., 1965). Specifically, listeners were provided answer sheets containing 50 six-word ensembles for each consonant list and 24 six-word ensembles for each vowel list. The listeners' task was to identify each stimulus word from a six-word response set appearing on his answer sheet.

The specific type of speech materials and response format was selected because it permitted the use of untrained listeners, provided stable scores after repeated exposure, reduced the effect of familiarity of test words, and substantially minimized the problems associated with an indeterminate response set (House et al., 1965). All of the S/N ratios were identical with those used by Horii et al. (1971), who recently described intelligibility functions for normal speech masked by an identical continuous noise. Because a fundamental objective of this project was to compare intelligibility functions of superior esophageal speech with those of normal speech, the test materials, response format, transmission equipment, listening conditions, levels of masking, masking signal, and nature of specifying speech levels were identical with those of Horii et al. (1971).

RESULTS AND DISCUSSION

Talker Equivalence

An initial analysis of the equivalence between the two talkers showed that there were no significant differences between the average intelligibility scores of the two talkers over the range of S/N ratios employed. By way of example, Figure 1 provides a comparison of the consonant articulation scores for each of the two talkers as a function of masking conditions and attests to the equivalence of their speech in terms of average intelligibility characteristics. Similar results were obtained when the talkers' average values for vowel test materials were compared. Thus, all information to be reported reflects the pooling of talker data.

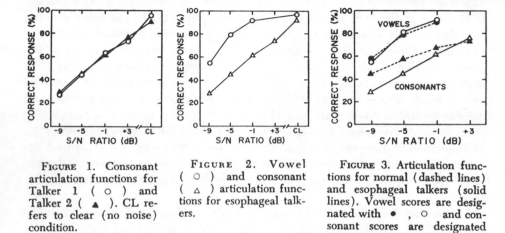

FIGURE 1. Consonant articulation functions for Talker 1 (○) and Talker 2 (▲). CL refers to clear (no noise) condition.

FIGURE 2. Vowel (○) and consonant (△) articulation functions for esophageal talkers.

FIGURE 3. Articulation functions for normal (dashed lines) and esophageal talkers (solid lines). Vowel scores are designated with ● , ○ and consonant scores are designated ▲ , △ .

Articulation Functions for Esophageal Speech

The general results of the listening tests are summarized in Figure 2, where the percentage of correct responses to the consonant and vowel test lists is plotted as a function of S/N ratio. Each data point represents an average of 9600 responses for the consonants (300 words × 2 talkers × 16 listeners) and 4600 responses for the vowels. These results show that, within the range of S/N ratios employed, the consonant functions for esophageal speech have a slope of about 5%/dB, while the vowel curves have a slope of about 4%/dB. The intelligibility of rhyme-test words heard in the quiet was high—about 98% for vowels and 94% for consonants—affirming to at least one dimension the superior proficiency of the two esophageal talkers. For each S/N condition, the intelligibility of vowels was considerably higher than that for consonants. This increase in intelligibility for vowels was expected because the S/N ratios are more realistically viewed as vowel-to-noise ratios. Since the intensity levels of consonants produced by esophageal speakers are, on the average, presumed to be considerably lower than those for vowels, consonants received more masking at a nominal S/N ratio.

Comparisons between Normal and Esophageal Speech

The intelligibility functions for esophageal speech are compared with those for normal speech in Figure 3. The data for normal talkers come from previous work obtained under identical experimental conditions (see Figure 4, Horii et al., 1971). In this figure each data point for normal speech is based on 13,200 responses for consonants (22 listeners, two talkers, and six lists of 50 words each) and 6336 responses for the vowels. Overall intelligibility functions for vowels are essentially the same for esophageal and normal speech. The vowel functions for both types of speech have a slope of 4%/dB. With respect to consonants, the intelligibility scores for esophageal speech are lower than for normal speech under the more adverse S/N conditions. The slope of the consonant function for esophageal speakers is about 5%/dB, while for normal speakers the slope is 2.5%/dB. Thus, the consonant data lend support to the clinical hypothesis that the consonant discriminability and, by inference, the intelligibility of speech produced by highly proficient esophageal speakers is reduced in adverse noise conditions. The differences in average consonant intelligibility between esophageal and normal speech were about 12 to 14% under the two (−9 and −5 dB S/N) highest noise conditions.

Additional comparisons were made to identify some of the factors that led to the reduction in esophageal consonant intelligibility under adverse noise conditions. For example, Figures 4a-d provide individual comparisons of the intelligibility scores for normal and esophageal speakers as a function of four classes of consonants: namely, liquid-glides, nasals, stops, and fricatives. Under adverse noise conditions, the lower consonant scores for esophageal speakers were largely the result of reduced intelligibility of liquid-glides, nasals, and secondarily, stops. The differences between normal and esophageal speech were particularly large for liquid-glides and nasals. Of interest was the observation that the intelligibility scores for fricatives produced by esophageal and normal talkers were nearly identical under adverse S/N conditions.

Earlier studies of the intelligibility of normal speech being masked by a continuous noise have demonstrated that the intelligibility of various classes of consonants is not equal (Miller and Nicely, 1955; Horii et al., 1971). Figure 5a illustrates the articulation functions for liquid-glides, nasal, plosive, and fricative consonants of normal speech (from Horii et al., 1971). In general, these data emphasize the inequality of intelligibility among consonants masked by a continuous noise. The rank ordering of consonants, from high to low, was liquid-glides, nasals, stops, and fricatives. By contrast, Figure 5b illustrates the articulation functions for these same four classes of consonants produced by esophageal speakers. In this case, large differences in intelligibility as function of differing consonant classes are not present. Rather, highly similar articulation functions were obtained for liquid-glides, nasal, plosive, and fricative consonants produced by esophageal speakers.

Additional comparisons uncovered other important differences between intelligibility characteristics of normal and esophageal speech. For example, the intelligibility functions for word-initial and word-final consonants of esophageal and normal speech are compared in Figure 6. For normal speech, consonants in the word-initial position were consistently more intelligible than word-final consonants. For esophageal speech, intelligibility of word-initial and word-final consonants were essentially equivalent. Secondly, voiced consonants of normal speakers were, on the average, much more intelligible than voiceless consonants (overall averages were 69 vs 47%). For esophageal speakers, the voiced consonant advantage was minimal (54 vs 51%).

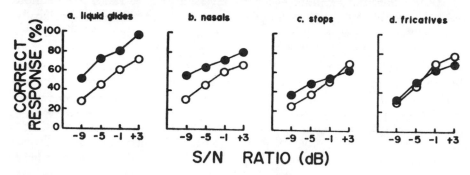

FIGURE 4 a-d. Articulation functions for liquid-glide, nasal, stop, and fricative consonants; open circles (o) represent average intelligibility scores of esophageal talkers, while closed circles (•) represent normal talkers' scores.

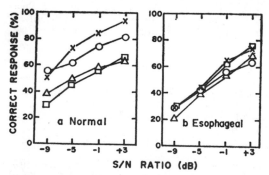

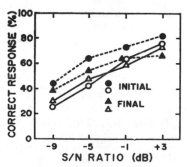

FIGURE 5a, b. Articulation functions for liquid-glide (x), nasal (o), stop (△), and fricative (□) consonants produced by normal (Figure a) and esophageal (Figure b) talkers.

FIGURE 6. Articulation functions for word-initial (open and filled circles) and word-final (open and filled triangles) consonants. Normal talkers (dashed lines) and esophageal talkers (solid lines).

In general, previous research and theory suggest that the intelligibility of consonants being masked by continuous noise varies as a function of the inherent power among the consonant sounds (see Miller and Nicely, 1955; Horii et al., 1971; and Figure 5a). If, on the other hand, a continuous noise masker did not differentially affect consonant intelligibility, one would expect the average intelligibility scores of differing classes of consonants to be homogeneous. For consonants produced by esophageal speakers, the latter appears to be the case (see Figure 5b, for example). Unfortunately, little is known about the inherent power or intensity characteristics of esophageal speech produced by laryngectomized talkers, although several authors have commented about the general restriction in intensity variation and overall reduction in average speech level associated with esophageal speech production (Drummond, 1965; Hyman, 1955; Diedrich, 1968).

Finally, it is important to note that in tests using a continuous noise masker, the intelligibility contributions of such diverse cues as consonantal spectra and vocalic transitions cannot easily be assessed as S/N ratios are manipulated (Horii et al., 1971). Unfortunately, here also little is known. Specifically, there is no information about such cues as esophageal consonant burst features, and formant transitions, and so forth. Until such information becomes available, definitive statements cannot be made about the specific factors underlying the increased vulnerability of consonant intelligibility of esophageal speech under adverse conditions. To this end, efforts are currently underway in our laboratory to obtain information about these important physical properties of esophageal speech.

ACKNOWLEDGMENT

This investigation was supported in part by research grants from the United Health Foundation, Elkhart, Indiana; Little Red Door, Inc., Marion County (Indiana) Cancer Society; and Purdue Research Foundation. We thank James C. Shanks, Indiana University Medical Center, William Cooper, and Raymond Daniloff, Purdue University, for their valuable contributions. Reprint requests should be sent to the authors, Department of Audiology and Speech Sciences, Purdue University, West Lafayette, Indiana 47907.

REFERENCES

DIEDRICH, W. M., The mechanism of esophageal speech. *Sound Production in Man*. New York: Annals of the New York Academy of Sciences, 155, 303-317 (1968).

DRUMMOND, S., The effects of environmental noise on pseudovoice after laryngectomy. *J. Laryng.*, 79, 193-202 (1965).

HORII, Y., Specifying the speech-to-noise ratio: Development and evaluation of a noise with speech-envelope characteristics. Doctoral dissertation, Purdue Univ. (1969).

HORII, Y., HOUSE, A. S., and HUGHES, G. W., A masking noise with speech envelope characteristics for studying intelligibility. *J. acoust. Soc. Amer.*, 49, 1849-1856 (1971).

HOUSE, A. S., WILLIAMS, C. E., HECKER, M. H. L., and KRYTER, K., Articulation testing methods: Consonantal differentiation with a closed-response set. *J. acoust. Soc. Amer.*, 37, 158-166 (1965).

HYMAN, M., An experimental study of artificial larynx and esophageal speech. *J. Speech Hear. Dis.*, 20, 291-299 (1955).

MILLER, G. A., and NICELY, P. E., An analysis of perceptual confusions among English consonants. *J. acoust. Soc. Amer.*, 27, 338-352 (1955).

Received March 15, 1974.
Accepted January 20, 1975.

VOWEL DURATION CHARACTERISTICS OF ESOPHAGEAL SPEECH

JOHN M. CHRISTENSEN

Idaho State University, Pocatello

BERND WEINBERG

Purdue University, West Lafayette, Indiana

The duration of a large number of representative vowels produced by 10 esophageal and nine normal speakers were measured. Overall vowel durations of esophageal speakers were consistently longer than those of normal speakers, indicating that esophageal speakers do not compensate for their striking diminution in air supply for speech by decreasing vowel duration. The differences in the vowel duration characteristics between normal and esophageal speakers were observed to vary systematically as a function of the voicing features of their consonant environments. Specifically, the durations of vowels of esophageal speakers spoken within voiceless consonant environments were consistently longer than those spoken in similar contexts by normal speakers. There were no significant differences between the average durations of vowels spoken by normal and esophageal speakers within voiced consonant environments. The observation that the durations of vowels produced by esophageal speakers differed significantly as a function of the voicing features of their consonant context was interpreted to support the belief that inherent, rule-governed durational features of English are retained following laryngeal amputation.

Until recently, most research on esophageal speech has been concerned with the measurement of acoustic and perceptual correlates of esophageal phonation. This emphasis can be attributed to the widespread assumption that the principal speech features affected by total laryngectomy surgery are those related to the vibratory source (Damste, 1958). It is now generally agreed that the average voice fundamental frequency of male esophageal speakers is about 65 Hz, that variation in average fundamental frequency among esophageal speakers is sizable, and that average fundamental frequency levels differ with the sex of esophageal speakers (Weinberg and Bennett, 1972).

The literature presents a contradictory picture regarding the effects total laryngectomy surgery have on articulatory characteristics of esophageal speakers. For example, Damste (1958, p. 3) has suggested that "the rest of the vocal tract (the pharyngeal and oral cavities) behaves substantially the same in both normal and esophageal speech. For that reason, . . . phonetic events in this region undergo no change." By contrast, the data of Diedrich and Youngstrom (1966) indicate that there are marked differences in overall vocal tract length,

---

Reprinted by permission from *Journal of Speech and Hearing Research*, 1976, *19*, 678–689.

pharyngeal cavity size and shape, and duration of articulatory motions of the tongue, lips, and velum between esophageal and normal speakers. At the acoustic level, the observation is that average vowel formant frequencies of esophageal speakers are consistently higher than those for normal speakers. This suggests that primary consequences of total laryngectomy include a shortening of the vocal tract and, by inference, altered articulatory behavior (Sisty and Weinberg, 1972). These findings, coupled with additional observations of speech intelligibility problems among esophageal speakers, suggest that total laryngectomy produces substantial changes in articulatory maneuvers in esophageal speakers.

A fundamental purpose of the present project was to explore additional dimensions of articulatory change occasioned by laryngeal amputation. Since laryngeal amputation necessitates the creation of a permanent respiratory stoma and produces a functional separation between the patient's respiratory airway and the vocal and digestive tracts, laryngectomized speakers employing esophageal speech are deprived of their normal pulmonary air supply for speech purposes. We hypothesized that esophageal speakers might compensate for their reduced respiratory supply for speech by decreasing phonetic duration. In other words, esophageal speakers were expected to decrease vowel duration in an attempt to conserve their limited esophageal air supply for speech and, thereby, maximize the efficiency of their newly modified speech production apparatus.

A second fundamental area of inquiry was to determine whether selected, inherent, rule-governed durational features of English are retained following laryngeal amputation. In this regard, it is well known that vowel durations are conditioned by the voicing features of their consonant contexts. Moreover, vowel duration lengthening in voiced consonant environments and shortening in voiceless contexts is believed to represent an inherent, rule-governed phonological feature of English (House, 1961; Stevens, House, and Paul, 1966). Accordingly, comparisons were also made of the differences in vowel durations of esophageal speakers occurring as a function of the voicing features of their consonant environment. These comparisons were completed to assess the hypothesis that important, rule-governed durational features of English are not altered by total laryngectomy.

METHOD

Subjects

Vowel duration measures were obtained from 10-adult male laryngectomized speakers who had used esophageal speech as their sole method of oral communication for more than one year. The two investigators rated each speaker in terms of speech acceptability (Shipp, 1967) and vocal effectiveness (Curry and Snidecor, 1961). All subjects were judged to have above-average to excellent esophageal speech and can be compared to highly rated speakers studied by Weinberg and Bennett (1972).

Speech Materials and Recordings

High-quality tape recordings were made of both the esophageal and normal speakers uttering vowels spoken within various consonant environments. The stimulus materials were 32 symmetric CVC syllables (for example, /pip/). The syllables were formed by combining eight consonants (/p/, /t/, /k/, /b/, /d/, /g/, /s/, /z/) with four vowels (/i/, /ɪ/, /ɑ/, /u/). The four vowels were chosen because they sample a wide range of articulatory positions within vowel space and they provide a reasonable sampling of important secondary acoustic characteristics of vowels (Peterson and Barney, 1952; House and Fairbanks, 1953; Tiffany, 1953; Stevens et al., 1966). The eight consonants were selected to provide a representative sampling for voiced-voiceless cognate pairs, varying manners of production, and three characteristic places of articulation.

The recordings were made in an anechoic chamber. The stimuli were recorded within the sentence frame "_____ is a word." The stimulus materials embedded within the sentence frame were read to each subject by the investigator from randomized lists. The lists were organized to form seven randomized repetitions for each CVC syllable. Subjects were instructed to speak each sentence frame at a conversational rate, to produce sentences in a natural manner, and to stress the initial CVC monosyllable of each sentence. Analyses of vowel durations were made on the second, third, fourth, fifth, and sixth sentence recordings. Thus, 1600 CVC utterances were available for analysis for the esophageal talkers; 1440 CVC utterances for the normal talkers.

Listening Procedures

A group of listeners was asked to evaluate the recordings of the two groups of talkers to insure that the vowels and their syllable consonant environments were phonetically representative. Ten listeners completed broad phonetic transcriptions of the recordings made by the 10 laryngectomized subjects, and five listeners transcribed the recordings made by the normal speakers. Fewer listeners were used in the latter evaluation since it was assumed that the transcription of utterances produced by normal speakers would not be as difficult. The five listeners who evaluated the recordings of the normal subjects were among the 10 listeners used to evaluate the recordings of the esophageal speakers. All listeners had extensive training in phonetics, were experienced in participating in psychoacoustic and speech perception research, and had extensive background in evaluating speech. The responses of these listeners were used to select representative vowels for durational analysis.

The stimulus materials used in the listening experiment were the high-quality recordings of each esophageal and normal speaker producing five repetitions of the 32 CVC utterances spoken within a carrier sentence. A master listening tape of these utterances was prepared by randomizing the utterances of each speaker and separating each stimulus sentence by a five-second silent interval.

Stimuli were presented by means of a loudspeaker using a high-quality tape recorder–amplifier–speaker system (TEAC A-1200U Tape Loop Repeater, Dynaco amplifier and preamplifier, and an Electro Voice Speaker Model SP-12). Signal levels were adjusted for comfortable listening conditions. The task of the listener was to phonetically transcribe the CVC elements of each sentence-initial syllable spoken within each carrier sentence on a response form. Each listener evaluated the recordings individually and was free to listen to each syllable as long as necessary by allowing any given stimulus to recur on the loop repeater.

Selection of Vowels for Duration Analysis

The selection of vowels for duration analysis was based on two criteria: (1) that 80% or more of the listeners identified a given vowel sample within a CVC utterance as the vowel intended by the talker, and (2) that 80% or more of the listeners identified both the initial syllable and final consonants surrounding a given vowel as the consonants intended by the talker.

Vowel Duration Measurements

Spectral analysis techniques were used to obtain measurements of duration of vowels selected for analysis. Specifically, broad-band spectrograms and amplitude tracings were made of each of the CVC utterances meeting representativeness criteria (Voice Print—Model 700). The symmetrical structure of the test syllables facilitated the identification of vowels and created a situation which fostered improved reliability of the durational measurements.

The specific measurement criteria used parallel those suggested by Peterson and Lehiste (1960). For example, the initiation of vowels following word-initial voiceless plosives was determined by identifying the time of voice onset, that is, the onset of phonation. In this case, the initial vertical striation present in the broad-band spectrogram was used to identify the onset of the vowel. In the case of CVC syllables containing word-initial voiced plosives, vowel measurements were made from the center of the burst spike and included the frication period as part of the vowel duration measurement. The initiation of word-final voiceless plosives was determined by observing an abrupt cessation of energy typically associated with all formants. The termination of vowels preceding word-final voiced plosives was determined by identifying the point at which this abrupt reduction in the intensity associated with the formants occurred (Peterson and Lehiste, 1960).

It is well known that the terminal boundaries of word-initial fricatives are rather easily identified on broad-band spectrograms (Peterson and Lehiste, 1960). Accordingly, the onset of the vowel following word-initial voiceless fricatives was determined by identifying the onset of phonation as reflected by the onset of periodicity, that is, by labeling the initial vertical striation in the region of the first formant. In the case of word-initial voiced fricatives the abrupt termination of the superimposed noise served to identify vowel onset. Word-final fricatives are identifiable on broad-band spectrograms by the onset of random noise. Accordingly, the termination of vowels in such environments was measured by detecting the point at which noise pattern associated with the final consonant began (Peterson and Lehiste, 1960).

RESULTS

Listener Performance and Representativeness Judgments

As indicated previously, a group of listeners was used to phonetically transcribe the recordings of both esophageal and normal speakers. The reliability of the listeners' transcription performance was assessed by requiring each listener to reevaluate a randomly selected set of 40 CVC utterances produced by one of the esophageal speakers. The percentage of agreement in phonetic transcription of both the consonant and vowel elements of the stimuli was calculated. The average percentages of agreement in phonetic transcription for the 10 listeners were 90.2% for word-initial consonants, 94.7% for word-final consonants, and 97.5% for the vowels.

The responses of these listeners were used to establish the acceptability of vowels for duration measurement. For the esophageal speakers, 931 vowels (approximately 58%) were representative according to the established criteria. For normal speakers, 1294 vowels (approximately 90%) met the two representativeness criteria.

Investigator Measurement Error

To evaluate the error in measurement of vowel duration, one of the investigators (J.C.) independently remeasured the durations of 32 randomly selected vowels produced by a normal speaker and 32 vowels spoken by one of the esophageal speakers. An analysis of the measurements for this series of vowels indicated that there were no significant differences between the repeated average values and that the average error of measurement was small ($SD = 5.57$ msec for esophageal vowels; $SD = 5.12$ msec for normal vowels). The average error values for repeated measurement were consistently smaller than both intra- and intersubject vowel duration variation values across repeated syllable productions and were well within measurement error values reported by others (Klatt, 1971). Correlation analyses were also used to assess the reliability of these repeated measurements. The correlation coefficients between the two measurement sets were $r = 0.99$ (normal speakers) and $r = 0.99$ (esophageal speakers). These observations support the assumption of adequate investigator measurement reliability for both types of speech studied.

Vowel Duration Characteristics of Normal and Esophageal Speakers

A primary hypothesis under study was that the durations of vowels pro-

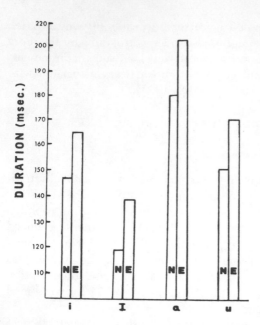

FIGURE 1. Comparison of overall mean representative vowel durations produced by esophageal (E) and normal (N) speakers.

duced by esophageal speakers would be shorter than those spoken by normal speakers. The overall average vowel duration characteristics of representative vowels /i/, /ɪ/, /ɑ/, and /u/ produced by normal and esophageal speakers are illustrated in Figure 1. These values represent vowel durations averaged across all consonant environments and subjects within each speech-type group. Overall vowel durations of esophageal speakers were consistently longer than those of normal speakers, indicating that esophageal speakers do not compensate for their loss of respiratory air supply for speech by decreasing vowel duration. Rather, it would appear that the esophageal speakers studied here increased vowel duration in the face of a diminished respiratory supply for speech.

It is important to reemphasize that the values portrayed in Figure 1 represent mean characteristics averaged across all consonant environments. Hence, any differential effect associated with such features as consonant voicing is masked. The average vowel duration properties of normal and esophageal speakers are plotted as a function of consonant voicing features in Figure 2. The differences in the vowel duration characteristics between the two speaker groups appear to vary systematically as a function of the voicing features of the consonant environment within which the vowel was spoken. Specifically, average vowel durations spoken in voiceless consonant environments were always longer for esophageal speakers. Durations were significantly ($p < 0.05$, see Table 1) longer for esophageal speakers in eight of 14 context comparisons completed. By contrast, average vowel durations spoken in voiced consonant environments appear comparable for the two speaker groups.

Analysis of variance procedures were used to test the significance of these

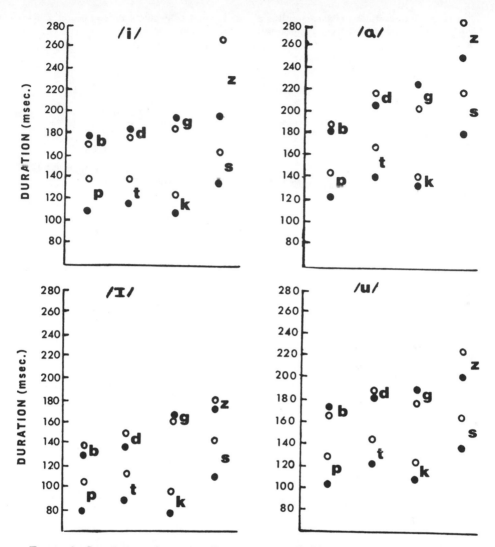

FIGURE 2. Comparison of average durations of representative vowels produced by esophageal (open circles) and normal (closed circles) speakers. Values are plotted as a function of consonant environment differences.

observations (Table 1). These results indicate that there were no significant differences in the average durations between normal and esophageal speakers for vowels spoken in voiced consonant contexts. On the other hand, significant ($p < 0.05$) F values were found in the majority of comparisons made for vowels spoken in voiceless consonant environments. Hence, the data were interpreted to support the notion that the durations of vowels of esophageal speakers spoken within voiceless consonant contexts were consistently greater than vowels spoken in similar contexts by normal speakers.

TABLE 1. Analysis of variance results (F ratios) used to evaluate differences in average duration of representative vowels produced by normal and esophageal speakers.

Phonetic Environment	df	F Ratio	p
/pip/	1/15	10.71	0.005†
/tit/	1/13	3.33	0.090
/kik/	1/13	4.73	0.048†
/bib/	1/18	0.07	0.787
/did/	1/17	0.01	0.940
/gig/	1/16	0.43	0.542
/sis/	1/18	3.03	0.087
/ziz/	1/13	1.12	0.311
/pɪp/	1/14	3.36	0.087
/tɪt/	1/14	5.43	0.034†
/kɪk/	1/15	6.83	0.019†
/bɪb/	1/18	0.34	0.572
/dɪd/	1/15	1.38	0.259
/gɪg/	1/15	0.60	0.542
/sɪs/	1/16	5.79	0.028†
/zɪz/	1/14	1.61	0.224
/pɑp/*	–	–	–
/tɑt/	1/10	2.59	0.139
/kɑk/	1/9	0.00	0.979
/bɑb/	1/17	0.39	0.548
/dɑd/	1/14	2.34	0.147
/gɑg/	1/12	0.00	0.972
/sɑs/*	–	–	–
/zɑz/	1/8	0.04	0.843
/pup/	1/11	8.07	0.016†
/tut/	1/12	4.85	0.047†
/kuk/	1/13	5.16	0.040†
/bub/	1/18	0.36	0.564
/dud/	1/16	0.05	0.818
/gug/	1/15	0.19	0.668
/sus/	1/13	3.49	0.083
/zuz/	1/13	3.18	0.096

*Insufficient data to complete analysis.
†$p < 0.05$.

THE EFFECT OF CONSONANT ENVIRONMENT VOICING FEATURES ON ESOPHAGEAL VOWEL DURATIONS

A second hypothesis under study in the present work was that the inherent relationship between vowel duration and the voicing features of the consonant environment is not altered by total laryngectomy. The average vowel durations of esophageal speakers are plotted as a function of the voicing features of their consonant environment in Figure 2. The data reveal that esophageal speakers' vowel durations in voiced consonant contexts were always longer than those uttered in voiceless consonant environments.

Analysis of variance procedures were used to test the significance of the observed differences in vowel duration occurring as a function of the voicing

TABLE 2. Analysis of variance results (F ratios) used to evaluate differences in average vowel duration of esophageal speakers occurring as a function of consonantal environment voicing features.

Comparison Stimuli		df	F Ratio	p
/pip/	vs /bib/	1/16	7.56	0.014
/tit/	vs /did/	1/13	6.55	0.023
/kik/	vs /gig/	1/7	33.14	0.001
/sis/	vs /ziz/	1/15	10.86	0.005
/pɪp/	vs /bɪb/	1/15	10.23	0.006
/tɪt/	vs /dɪd/	1/13	14.47	0.002
/kɪk/	vs /gɪg/	1/15	26.15	0.000
/sɪs/	vs /zɪz/	1/13	20.65	0.000
/pɑp/	vs /bɑb/*	–	–	–
/tɑt/	vs /dɑd/	1/8	20.76	0.003
/kɑk/	vs /gɑg/	1/5	14.34	0.020
/sɑs/	vs /zɑz/*	–	–	–
/pup/	vs /bub/	1/12	5.98	0.031
/tut/	vs /dud/	1/11	2.94	0.114
/kuk/	vs /gug/	1/12	15.32	0.002
/sus/	vs /zuz/	1/10	12.19	0.006

*Insufficient data to complete analysis.

feature of consonant contexts. These results are summarized in Table 2. With one exception (*tut* vs *dud*), esophageal speakers' vowel durations within voiced consonant environments were significantly longer than productions uttered within voiceless consonant environments. These findings provide strong support for the belief that esophageal speakers do retain the inherent relationship between vowel duration and consonantal environment voicing features.

DISCUSSION

The results of this investigation indicate that, in addition to well-established changes in phonatory characteristics, total laryngectomy may also produce changes in articulatory behavior as evidenced by altered durational characteristics of vowels. Moreover, the present results suggest that such changes may be influenced by phonetic context. Namely, the observed differences in vowel duration between normal and esophageal speakers varied systematically as a function of the voicing features of their consonant environment. Despite these differences, the present data indicate that phonological rules governing the durational properties of English vowels are preserved following laryngeal amputation.

The factors responsible for the observed increase in average esophageal vowel duration within voiceless consonant environments are not understood and their identification represents a promising area for future research. The observations made in this project suggest that the esophageal speakers studied may have initiated phonation earlier and terminated phonation later than normal speakers. It is interesting to note that a number of investigators have suggested that esophageal speakers have difficulty initiating and terminating esophageal phonation (Tikofsky, Glattke, and Perry, 1964; Sacco, Mann, and Schultz, 1967). Our current effort to obtain measurements of voice onset and offset time characteristics, syllabic durations, and relative duration measures of the consonant and vowel portions of CVC syllables of esophageal speakers are expected to provide information bearing on this question. Such analyses are also expected to be useful in identifying factors responsible for voicing feature contrast difficulties exhibited by esophageal speakers.

Altered voice onset time characteristics may provide one reasonable explanation for the observation that vowels in voiceless plosive environments were longer in esophageal speech than in normal speech. However, such an explanation does not account for the observation of vowel lengthening in voiceless fricative contexts. There are, undoubtedly, other factors responsible for vowel lengthening in these contexts. Normal speakers must satisfy two conditions to effect voicing for a vowel following a voiceless consonant: (1) there must be sufficient vocal fold adduction, and (2) there must be a sufficient transglottal pressure. The phonatory apparatus used by esophageal speakers does not have adduction-abduction capabilities. Rather, the neoglottis of esophageal speakers is in a continual state of adduction. Hence, it would seem reasonable to speculate that esophageal speakers might exhibit differences in vowel duration that reflect alterations in the time-dependent relationships necessary to effect appropriate transpseudoglottal pressure associated with voicing onset and termination.

The data of Diedrich and Youngstrom (1966) and others indicate that maximum pharyngeal expansion of esophageal speakers is larger than that observed in normals. Rothenberg (1968) has calculated normal pharyngeal expansion at 10.0 ml. He assumed that glottal pulsing would continue for an additional 10 msec for each 1.0-ml increase in pharyngeal volume. It may also be reasonable to speculate that the vocal tracts of the esophageal speakers studied are more compliant since (1) none of these speakers received radiotherapy as part of their treatment regime, and (2) their surgery might be expected to minimize substantially the stiffness normally offered by the hyoid bone, larynx, and supporting structures. Increases in pharyngeal volume and vocal tract compliance represent two factors that would permit esophageal phonation to be maintained longer. Simultaneous measurement of intraoral pressure, esophageal air pressure, and volume changes within the pharynx during appropriate utterances are expected to provide a more complete explanation of the mechanisms underlying increased esophageal vowel durations in voiceless consonant contexts.

An attractive explanation for the observed increase in vowel duration of esophageal speech within voiceless consonant environments might also be obtained by considering the relationship between articulatory maneuvers associated with the production of voiceless consonants and the behaviors required to effect voicing for the vowel during the production of voiceless CVC syllables. For example, we speculate that during such utterances esophageal speakers produce word-initial consonants principally by using lingual compression maneuvers. Stated differently, esophageal speakers might be expected to use the air within the vocal tract, that is, between the point of major articulatory constriction and the neoglottis, as the primary, if not the sole, respiratory driving force for voiceless consonant production. A reasonable response to this limited air supply within the esophageal speakers' vocal tract during such consonant compression maneuvers would be the earlier initiation of voicing for the subsequent vowel. Evidence supporting this notion could be obtained by observing shorter word-initial consonant durations together with increased vowel voicing durations.

A consideration of the relationship between articulatory maneuvers associated with the production of voiced consonants and the behaviors required to maintain voicing for the vowel during the production of voiced CVC syllables might also provide an explanation for the observed similarity in vowel durations between esophageal and normal speech within voiced consonant environments. In this circumstance, we speculate that esophageal speakers use their esophageal air supply as the primary respiratory driving force for both consonant and vowel production. If this is true, the observed comparability between vowel duration of normal and esophageal speakers in voiced consonant contexts is not surprising.

ACKNOWLEDGMENT

This research was supported in part by NDEA Fellowship Grant 5584-82-13535. This article is based on a doctoral dissertation completed by John Christensen in the Department of Audiology and Speech Sciences, Purdue University. The authors wish to acknowledge the contributions of M. A. Zlatin, R. G. Daniloff, and R. L. Ringel. Requests for reprints should be sent to John M. Christensen, Department of Speech Pathology and Audiology, Box 8116, Idaho State University, Pocatello, Idaho 83201, or Bernd Weinberg, Department of Audiology and Speech Sciences, Purdue University, West Lafayette, Indiana 47907.

REFERENCES

CURRY, E. T., and SNIDECOR, J. C., Physical measurement and pitch perception in esophageal speech. *Laryngoscope,* 71, 415-424 (1961).

DAMSTE, P. H., *Oesophageal Speech after Laryngectomy.* Groningen: Holland Boekdrukkerij Voorheen Gebroeders Hoitsema (1958).

DIEDRICH, W. M., and YOUNGSTROM, K. A., *Alaryngeal Speech.* Springfield, Ill.: Charles C Thomas (1966).

HOUSE, A. S., On vowel duration in English. *J. acoust. Soc. Am.,* 33, 1174-1178 (1961).

HOUSE, A. S., and FAIRBANKS, G., The influence of consonant environment upon the secondary acoustical characteristics of vowels. *J. acoust. Soc. Am.,* 25, 105-113 (1953).

KLATT, D. H., On predicting the duration of the phonetic segment /s/ in English. *Speech Transmission Laboratories, Quart. Prog. Rept.,* p. 130 (1971).

PETERSON, G. E., and BARNEY, H. L., Control methods used in a study of vowels. *J. acoust. Soc. Am.,* 24, 175-184 (1952).

PETERSON, G. E., and LEHISTE, J., Duration of syllable nuclei in English. *J. acoust. Soc. Am.,* 32, 693-703 (1960).

ROTHENBERG, M., *The Breath Stream Dynamics of Simple Release Plosive Production.* New York: Karger (1968).

SACCO, P. R., MANN, M. D., and SCHULTZ, M. D., Perceptual confusions of selected phonemes in esophageal speech. *Indiana Speech Hearing Ass. J.*, 6, 190-193 (1967).

SHIPP, T., Frequency, duration, and perceptual measures in relation to judgments of alaryngeal speech acceptability. *J. Speech Hearing Res.*, 10, 417-427 (1967).

SISTY, N. L., and WEINBERG, B., Formant frequency characteristics of esophageal speech. *J. Speech Hearing Res.*, 15, 439-448 (1972).

STEVENS, K. N., HOUSE, A. S., and PAUL, A. P., Acoustical description of syllabic nuclei: An interpretation in terms of a dynamic model of articulation. *J. acoust. Soc. Am.*, 40, 123-132 (1966).

TIFFANY, W. R., Vowel recognition as a function of duration, frequency modulation and phonetic context. *J. Speech Hearing Dis.*, 18, 289-301 (1953).

TIKOFSKY, R. P., GLATTKE, T. J., and PERRY, P. S., Listener identification of voiced and voiceless consonants. *Asha*, 6, 385 (1964).

WEINBERG, B., and BENNETT, S., Selected acoustic characteristics of esophageal speech produced by female laryngectomees. *J. Speech Hearing Res.*, 15, 211-216 (1972).

Received October 21, 1975.
Accepted April 14, 1976.

PRODUCTIVE VOICE
ONSET TIME CHARACTERISTICS
OF ESOPHAGEAL SPEECH

JOHN M. CHRISTENSEN

Idaho State University, Pocatello

BERND WEINBERG *and* PETER J. ALFONSO

Purdue University, West Lafayette, Indiana

The voice onset times (VOT) of a large number of stop-consonant initiated syllables produced by esophageal and normal speakers were measured. Esophageal speakers systematically varied VOT during the production of speech-sound categories with the same manner of production. Average voice onset times associated with the production of prevocalic voiceless stops of esophageal speakers were significantly shorter than those of normal speakers, while talker-group comparisons associated with the production of voiced prevocalic stops were nonsignificant. Voice onset times of both esophageal and normal speakers were differentially sensitive to place of articulation. Findings are discussed in terms of furthering current understanding of how effectively esophageal speakers achieve important phonological contrasts.

Normal speakers of English systematically vary the timing of voice onset to distinguish prevocalic stops /p, t, k/ from /b, d, g/ (Lisker and Abramson, 1964). In this context, it is now also well established that laryngectomized patients using esophageal speech have difficulty achieving voicing contrast between homorganic stop consonants (Shames, Font, and Mathews, 1963; Hyman, 1955). In a recent article we (Christensen and Weinberg, 1976) reported that the durations of vowels spoken by esophageal speakers within voiceless consonant environments were consistently longer than those spoken in similar contexts by normal speakers. It was suggested that altered timing of voice onset (VOT) might provide a partial explanation for the increase in duration of vowels observed for esophageal speakers. These observations, coupled with the view that alterations in the speech-producing systems of esophageal speakers created special problems in the initiation and termination of voicing (Sacco, Mann, and Schultz, 1968), led to an examination of variations in the timing of voice onset used by esophageal speakers. The present study obtained measurements of voice onset time to assess whether esophageal speakers systematically vary VOT during the production of speech-sound categories with the same manner of production.

Reprinted by permission from *Journal of Speech and Hearing Research*, 1978, *21*, 56–62.

METHOD

The subjects, speech materials, recordings, and listening procedures were those reported previously (Christensen and Weinberg, 1976). Briefly, 10 male esophageal and nine male normal talkers provided recordings of multiple tokens ($N = 5$) of symmetric CVC syllables created by combining six consonants /p, t, k, b, d, g/ with four vowels /ɪ, i, a, u/. The recordings were subjected to perceptual evaluation to insure that the consonant and vowel elements of the syllables were phonetically representative. Syllables were considered representative when 80% or more of the listeners correctly identified the consonantal and vowel elements of a syllable as the sounds intended by the talker. Voice onset time of prevocalic stops of representative syllables were measured using techniques described by Lisker and Abramson (1967). Measurements were completed for 931 representative syllables produced by esophageal speakers and 1294 syllables spoken by normal speakers.

RESULTS

The distributions of voice onset times associated with the production of labial, apical, and velar stops of esophageal and normal speakers are illustrated in Figures 1–3. Most voiced prevocalic stops were characterized by voicing lead. A few exhibited short voicing lag. On the other hand, prevocalic voiceless stops were characterized by relatively longer lag intervals. Study of these distributions reveals that esophageal speakers did effect systematic variation

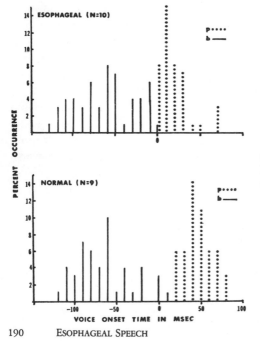

FIGURE 1. Distribution of voice onset times associated with the production of labial voiced and voiceless stops by esophageal and normal speakers.

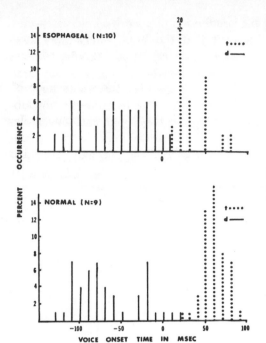

FIGURE 2. Distribution of voice onset times associated with the production of apical voiced and voiceless stops by esophageal and normal speakers.

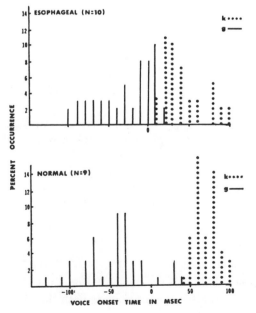

FIGURE 3. Distribution of voice onset times associated with the production of velar voiced and voiceless stops by esophageal and normal speakers.

in the timing of voice onset during the production of speech-sound categories with the same manner of production, but that the VOT values associated with the production of prevocalic voiceless stops exhibited lag intervals appreciably shorter than those used by normal speakers.

Analysis of variance procedures were used to evaluate the significance of the apparent differences in average VOT characteristics between esophageal and normal talkers. This analysis (Table 1) reveals that there were no signifi-

TABLE 1. Analysis of variance results used to compare mean voice-onset-time characteristics of normal and esophageal speakers.

Consonant Comparison	Talker Group	N	Mean VOT (msec)	SD	F-Value
/p/	Normal	9	51.75	16.71	8.15*
	Esophageal	10	28.80	18.17	
/t/	Normal	9	65.13	14.86	13.30**
	Esophageal	10	36.17	19.18	
/k/	Normal	9	75.33	14.15	10.03**
	Esophageal	10	46.02	24.31	
/b/	Normal	9	−68.01	34.91	0.01
	Esophageal	10	−66.05	36.61	
/d/	Normal	9	−71.46	39.55	0.01
	Esophageal	10	−65.66	40.67	
/g/	Normal	9	−41.80	46.29	0.29
	Esophageal	10	−31.41	37.50	

*$p < 0.05 = 4.45$ ($df = 1/17$)
**$p < 0.01 = 8.40$ ($df = 1/17$)

cant speaker group differences in average VOT for prevocalic, voiced stop comparisons. Significant F-values were obtained for all prevocalic voiceless /p, t, k/ stop comparisons, showing that esophageal speakers exhibited significantly shorter average VOT lag intervals.

Finally, the present data give evidence that the VOT characteristics of esophageal speakers were differentially sensitive to place of articulation. Lisker and Abramson (1967) noted that voice onset time increased for stops not characterized by lead, as place of articulation moved from labial to apical loci. Our results (Figures 1–3; Table 1) indicate that esophageal speakers also increased VOT as a function of moving place of articulation from labial to velar loci.

DISCUSSION

Our findings show that esophageal speakers systematically varied VOT during the production of phonetically representative speech sounds with the same manner of production and that the general pattern of these variations paralleled that observed for normal speakers. These findings are interpreted to support the belief that esophageal speakers employ variation within the voicing dimension to distinguish prevocalic stops /p, t, k/ from /b, d, g/.

Some overlap was noted in the voice onset times associated with the production of homorganic stops, emphasizing that VOT represents one, but not the sole, acoustic property normal and esophageal speakers manipulate to distinguish effectively between homorganic stop consonants (Slis, 1970; Slis and Cohen, 1969a, b; Kent and Moll, 1969; Zlatin, 1974, and others). Moreover, the observation of overlap, coupled with the disparity in absolute voice onset times between esophageal and normal speakers, particularly in prevocalic voiceless stop productions, suggests that cues to voicing such as VOT should be regarded in a relative rather than an absolute manner.

The observation that esophageal speakers effected systematic variation in VOT is intriguing because of some striking differences between the voice- and speech-producing systems of normal and esophageal speakers. For example, it can be assumed that the phonatory apparatus of esophageal speakers does not possess abductor-adductor properties. The prevailing consensus is that differences within the voicing dimension reflect temporal aspects of glottal adductor-abductor activity operating in conjunction with articulatory and aerodynamic responses, and it would be reasonable to expect that esophageal speakers might exhibit differences in VOT. Indeed, the earlier onset of esophageal voicing associated with voiceless stop productions may reflect such changes and may highlight the substantial contribution articulatory-aerodynamic responses produce in the timing of voicing onset. The earlier onset of voicing associated with prevocalic voiceless stops also serves, in part, to account for the lengthening of vowel duration observed for this group of esophageal speakers (Christensen and Weinberg, 1976).

Finally, VOT measurements were completed on phonetically representative syllables produced by both groups of speakers. In this regard, only 58% of the syllables produced by the esophageal speakers were representative, while 90% of those spoken by normal speakers met representativeness criteria. Hence, 42% of the syllables produced by esophageal speakers were not phonetically representative, and a large (approximately 25%) percentage of syllables were unacceptable because of perceived voicing contrast errors made in response to syllable-initial stops (see Christensen, 1975, for details). These observations underscore the need to verify perceptually the representativeness of utterances, particularly in experiments using talkers known to have abnormal speech production systems and articulatory difficulties. Voice onset time is known to vary as a function of such factors as voicing and place of articulation. Hence there is a need to establish independent perceptual verification of such features to insure that measurements are completed on stops with features both intended and realized.

We acknowledge that the present data delineate VOT characteristics of esophageal speakers measured from productions of representative syllables and, therefore, do not reflect variations in the timing of voice onset associated with unselected (that is, solely intended) syllable productions of esophageal speakers.

Because of the known effects such factors as place and voicing features of prevocalic stops exert on VOT, we have argued for the need to establish independent perceptual verification of such features in stimuli being evaluated. The large number of unrepresentative syllable productions of esophageal speakers merely serves to reemphasize the well-known fact that laryngectomized speakers are far less proficient in achieving important phonological feature contrasts and that they exhibit significant articulatory disturbances. On the other hand, results based on analyses of representative syllable productions were interpreted to support the view that esophageal speakers are capable of effecting systematic and linguistically appropriate variation in the timing of voicing onset. Finally, the extensive number of unrepresentative syllables uttered by esophageal speakers supports the hypothesis that they are far less consistent than normal speakers in effecting systematic manipulation of important variables underlying the perception of critical phonetic features and phonological contrasts.

ACKNOWLEDGMENT

This project was supported, in part, by a grant (PDT-69) from the American Cancer Society and by NDEA Fellowship 5584-82-13535. We acknowledge the assistance of M. Zlatin Laufer and R. Daniloff.

REFERENCES

CHRISTENSEN, J. M., Vowel durations in esophageal speech. Doctoral dissertation, Purdue Univ. (1975).

CHRISTENSEN, J. M., and WEINBERG, B., Vowel duration characteristics of esophageal speech. *J. Speech Hearing Res.*, 19, 678-689 (1976).

HYMAN, M., An experimental study of artificial larynx and esophageal speech. *J. Speech Hearing Dis.*, 20, 291-299 (1955).

KENT, R., and MOLL, K., Vocal tract characteristics of stop consonants. *J. acoust. Soc. Am.*, 46, 1549-1555 (1969).

LISKER, L., and ABRAMSON, A. S., Some effects of context on voice onset time in English stops. *Lang. Speech*, 10, 1-28 (1967).

SACCO, P. R., MANN, M. B., SCHULTZ, M. C., Perceptual confusions in selected phonemes in esophageal speech. *J. Indiana Speech Hearing Assoc.*, 6, 196-203 (1968).

SHAMES, G. H., FONT, J., and MATHEWS, J., Factors related to speech proficiency of the laryngectomized. *J. Speech Hearing Dis.*, 28, 273-278 (1963).

SLIS, I. H., Articulatory measurements on voiced, voiceless and nasal consonants. *Phonetica*, 24, 193-210 (1970).

SLIS, I. H., and COHEN, A., On the complex regulating the voiced-voiceless destruction II. *Lang. Speech*, 12, 80-102 (1969a).

SLIS, I. H., and COHEN, A., On the complex regulating the voiced-voiceless destruction I.

Lang. Speech, **12,** 141-155 (1969b).

ZLATIN, M. A., Voicing contrast: Perceptual and productive voice onset time characteristics of adults. *J. acoust. Soc. Am.,* **59,** 981-994 (1974).

Received October 28, 1976.
Accepted July 13, 1977.

THE PHARYNX AFTER LARYNGECTOMY.

Changes in Its Structure and Function.*†

JOHN A. KIRCHNER, M.D.,
JAMES H. SCATLIFF, M.D.,
FREDERICK L. DEY, M.D.,
and
DONALD P. SHEDD, M.D.,

New Haven, Conn.

What, if any, significant changes occur in the structure and function of the pharynx as the result of laryngectomy?

What are the various causes of pharyngeal dysphagia that sometimes develops after laryngectomy?

How do postoperative changes in the pharynx influence esophageal voice?

What effect has laryngectomy on the upper esophageal sphincter?

Does removal of the entire hypopharynx interfere with esophageal peristalsis?

We sought answers to these questions in data obtained from cinefluorographic examinations and intrapharyngeal and intraesophageal pressure recordings in surgical patients.

Total laryngectomy, as performed in our clinic, routinely includes the entire hyoid bone with the thyroid and cricoid cartilage. This involves detachment of the middle constrictor muscle and of the inferior constrictor and cricopharyngeus muscles. When the upper trachea is included with the specimen, the esophagus is dissected off its posterior wall. During closure, an effort is made to approximate the constrictor

*From the Divisions of Otolaryngology, Radiology, and Surgery, Yale University Medical Center.

†Supported by USPHS grants C-4435 (C1), BT 440 (C2), and A 3473 (C) and by the Norwich Chapter of the Connecticut Heart Association.

Reprinted by permission from *The Laryngoscope*, 1963, 73, 18–33.

muscles anteriorly; that this is not always successful is evidenced by cinefluorograms and by pressure recordings described below.

Other anatomical structures altered by laryngectomy include the suprahyoid muscles, which are detached surgically, and the upper portion of the infrahyoid muscles, removed with the larynx. The superior laryngeal nerve is divided near its entrance to the larynx, and the recurrent laryngeal nerve is cut alongside the trachea. The mucosa and submucosa are brought together in the midline to reconstruct the anterior wall of the cervical esophageal lumen. The closure is reinforced by the constrictor muscles, strap muscle remnants and base of tongue.

The dynamics of the normal pharynx during swallowing have been studied in experimental animals by fluoroscopy[1,2] and by electromyography.[3,4] In man, the normal act of deglutition has been demonstrated fluoroscopically and by cinefluorography[5-9] and, more recently, by intraluminal pressure recordings.[10,11] Excellent review articles have been published by Bosma[12] and Ingelfinger.[13]

The dynamics of the post-laryngectomy pharynx have received little attention except for studies of voice production. Schobinger[14] attributes post-laryngectomy dysphagia to cricopharyngeus spasm which he deduces from the prominent soft tissue mass in the cricopharyngeus region. His patients were studied by barium swallow, both pre and postoperatively. His report includes a good bibliography.

Cracovaner and Rubenstein[15] reported dilatation of the pharyngoesophagus following total laryngectomy, as a result of the removal of the intrinsic support of the pharyngoesophagus.

Since 1922, when Seeman described the X-ray appearance during esophageal speech, various observers have attempted to relate good esophageal speech to such characteristics of the pseudoglottis as its level,[16] its tonus,[16] its shape,[17-19] and the integrity of its nerve supply[18]; also to the size of the hypopharynx,[18,20] the size of the esophageal air column,[17,19] the ability to aspirate air,[21] etc.

PRESENT STUDY.

The present study, undertaken in 1959, consisted of cinefluorographic studies and intraluminal pressure recordings from the esophagus and pharynx of patients who had undergone laryngectomy, with or without radical neck dissection. Thirty-five patients were studied by cinefluorography, four months to nine years after operation. Two of these patients had also been examined within two weeks of operation, to demonstrate the origin and course of a salivary fistula. Eight of the 35 patients had preoperative cinefluorographic barium studies of the hypopharynx.

Intrapharyngeal and intraesophageal pressure recordings were made in 23 laryngectomized patients, 20 of whom were also examined cinefluorographically. The interval between operation and pressure studies varied between 28 days and six years. It was impractical to record pressures from most of these patients prior to operation because of possible trauma to the neoplasm and because of airway obstruction or dysphagia in others.

TECHNIQUES.

1. Cinefluorography. The examination consists of motion picture fluoroscopic recording of a barium mixture as it passes through the pharynx during deglutition. The Phillip's five-inch amplifier, 16 mm. Auricon camera and linograph orthofilm are used.

After development, the film is shown by a 16 mm. projector equipped with controls which allow slow motion, complete stop or reversal of direction. In this way the laryngologist can study the record in detail as often as necessary, and at his convenience.

2. Pressure Studies. The patient swallows a tube made of three polyethylene catheters that are fused together and sealed at their tip (Fig. 1). A lateral hole larger than the diameter of the catheter is situated in each of the three catheters at a distance of 0, –5, and –10 cm. respectively from a reference point. The entire tube is graduated in cm. from the 0 point or first lateral orifice.

The tube is swallowed by the patient to any desired depth. Measurements are made in centimeters from the incisor teeth

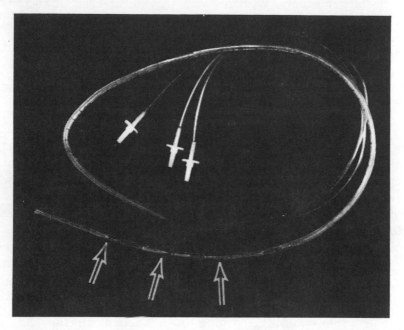

Fig. 1. Triple tube used in recording pressures inside pharynx and esophagus. The arrows mark the side openings, one in each tube, five cms. apart.

to the lateral orifices. The tubes are then filled with water so that any pressure changes within the esophagus can be transmitted through transducers and then to a Sanborn direct writing recorder. The act of swallowing is signalled on a fourth channel by a transducer connected with the accessory muscles of deglutition.

The efficacy of this system has been demonstrated by the work of Fyke and Code[10] and by Atkinson *et al.*[11]

1. Changes in Anatomy of the Pharynx.

a. Muscle Masses.

Submucosal masses can often be seen on the posterior wall of the pharynx by mirror examination and, even better, by roentgenography after barium ingestion. These masses can be mistaken for residual or recurrent neoplasm, but can be identified by their change in size or shape during deglutition. They usually occur on the posterior wall at the level of the cricopharyngeus but are sometimes seen in the region of the inferior constrictor and middle constrictor muscles, all of which have been surgically detached from their preoperative insertion into the larynx and the hyoid bone.

Lacking an anterior attachment after laryngectomy, the muscles tend to bunch up on the posterior wall when the nerve impulse reaches them, much as a biceps swells in the upper arm after its lower tendon has been severed. It seems likely that this bunching is more marked if the constrictor muscles have not been adequately approximated in the anterior midline (Fig. 2).

While the contracted belly of the cricopharyngeus may serve as a pseudoglottis, and is easily identified as such, the middle and inferior constrictor muscle masses often resemble neoplasm on routine roentographic examination. The latter muscles have been found contracting in an uncoordinated fashion in several patients who complained of dysphagia postoperatively. It seems likely that interference with the first stage of peristalsis in the pharynx has been responsible for the inability of these patients to manage solids, particularly since there was no evidence of undue narrowing of the hypopharynx.

b. Postoperative Pouches.

Thirty-five laryngectomized patients were examined by cinefluorographic visualization of a barium bolus passing through the pharynx. Thirty of these patients exhibited a pouch-like recess on the anterior wall of the pharynx at its

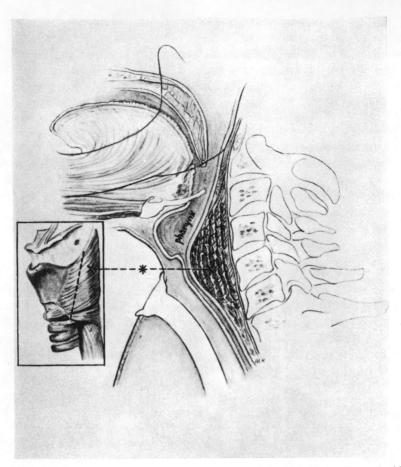

Fig. 2. After the constrictor muscles are detached from the cricoid, thyroid and hyoid framework, the cut ends are brought together in the anterior midline, but a complete closure does not usually result. This allows portions of these muscles to retract along the postero-lateral pharyngeal wall, and to produce submucosal masses visible on X-ray or on direct inspection.

junction with the base of the tongue. The pouch varied in size from a capacity of less an 1 cc. to that of about 30 cc. It was found in every patient who had developed a salivary fistula during convalescence, and in nine of the 13 patients who had not had a postoperative fistula. Five other patients exhibiting these pouches had been operated upon at other hospitals, and we could not determine whether a fistula had been present.

Symptoms resulting from these pouches have been described in a previous publication.[22] A patient operated upon more recently complained that meat frequently stuck in the throat, although a 44 F mercury dilator passed easily into the esophagus. Cinefluorography showed a moderate sized diverticulum at the base of the tongue where food fragments, pills and capsules commonly lodge.

The pouch seems to result from separation of the edges of the pharyngeal closure at the point where it joins the base of the tongue. This opening allows oral secretions and ingesta to make their way into the space under the skin flap. If the oral material reaches the skin surface by this route, a salivary fistula has occurred; if not, a permanent pouch remains (Fig. 3).

Postoperative dysphagia may occur in a patient with an adequate hypopharyngeal lumen and may be the result of regurgitation from such a pouch into the mouth or the nasopharynx. Or, it may be the result of ineffective contractions of the constrictor muscles in the pharynx, particularly with solid foods.

2. Post-Laryngectomy Speech.

Our cinefluorographic studies of esophageal speech failed to reveal significant relationships between good speech and variations in the anatomy of the laryngectomized pharynx. Pre and postoperative measurements at the cricopharyngeus level in six patients showed only that the lumen was narrower after laryngectomy (compare the report of Cracovaner and Rubenstein,[15] who described postoperative dilatation). The size of the hypopharyngeal lumen appears to have little or nothing to do with the ability to speak. The three patients with the largest hypopharyngeal lumens were our poorest speakers, while the next to smallest lumen (0.9 cm. AP, 0.6 cm. laterally) was found in the best speaker of the six.

Other factors were found to be variable among both the good and poor speakers: whether the cricopharyngeus is at C6, C5, or C4; whether the pseudoglottis consisted of a thin band or a broadly based mass; the length of the vibrating

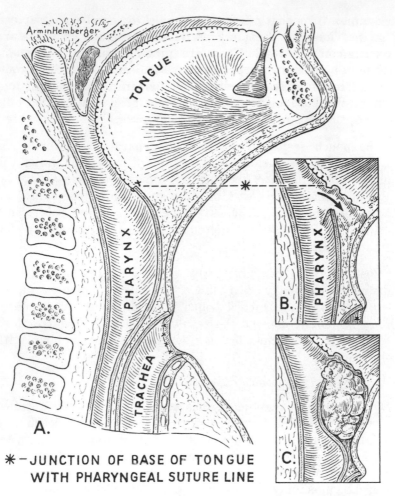

***-JUNCTION OF BASE OF TONGUE
WITH PHARYNGEAL SUTURE LINE**

Fig. 3. Mechanism of development of postoperative pouch at base of tongue. The upper end of the pharyngeal suture line separates at its junction with the base of the tongue. Oral secretions and ingesta may enter this defect and result in a permanent pouch, as shown. If the secretions reach the skin surface, a fistula is formed. Every postoperative fistula in our study had its internal origin at the tongue base as shown above.

segments; the tonus or flaccidity at the cricopharyngeus as measured by pressure studies.[24] All varieties of these were found in good and in poor speakers. Cernock and Zobril[23] reached similar conclusions in a recent report.

An interesting finding was a multiple pseudoglottis in several speakers, including one with an excellent voice and three areas of vibration, demonstrable by cinefluorography (Fig. 4). Whether these represent muscle bands or mucosal folds cannot be stated. They are probably not scar tissue, because they constantly change shape and size when observed on cinefluorography. These variations in the anatomy of laryngectomized speech are reminiscent of Kallen's observation that "Every fold of mucous membrane, every favorably

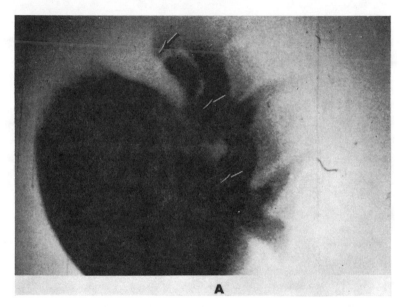

Fig. 4-a. Multiple pseudoglottis. Arrows indicate the three constrictions which were observed to vibrate simultaneously during esophageal speech.

placed cicatricial band, every muscle or muscular remnant may serve as the basis for the development of a pseudo-glottis."[21]

3. The Upper Esophageal Sphincter.

The cricopharyngeus muscle and the neighboring muscles are detached from the larynx and trachea at laryngectomy. They are usually reapproximated, in the anterior midline, and we were interested in whether a functioning sphincter usually results.

Twenty-three laryngectomized patients were studied by pressure recordings. In the normal subject, the act of swallowing is preceded by a stage of relaxation of the entire sphincter, with an abrupt fall in pressure to intraesophageal levels. The sphincter then rapidly contracts, with a rise in pressure to 10 or more mm. of mercury over resting levels. The act of swallowing then being completed, the pressure falls to previous resting levels.

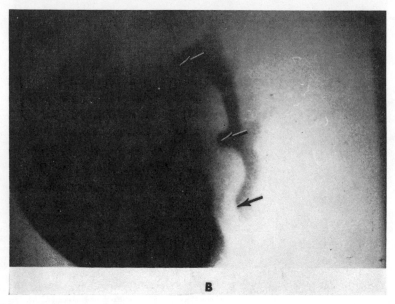

Fig. 4-b indicates the separation of these surfaces during insufflation of air just before speech.

We have found that one or more of these pressure stages are either absent or greatly altered in our laryngectomized patients. The resting pressure in four of our patients never exceeded intraesophageal levels. In 12 patients the increase in pressure was less than 5 mm. of mercury (Fig. 5).

The absence or weakening of the sphincter at this site might be expected to produce certain disorders: insufflation of air into the esophagus on inspiration; interference with

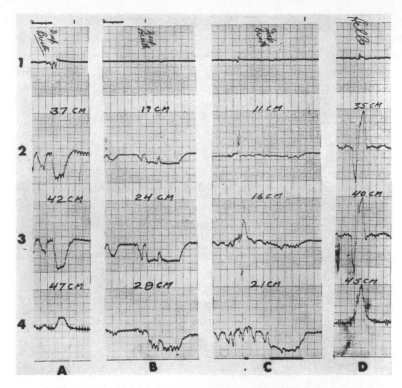

Fig. 5. Negative intraesophageal pressure on deep inspiration in a post-operative patient with no demonstrable sphincter at the esophageal inlet. Column a. Deep inspiration, signalled by deflection of electromyogram in line 1. In lines 2 and 3, the tube openings are in the esophagus, at 37 and 42 cms. from incisor teeth. A sharp, sustained drop in pressure results, so long as inspiration is maintained. The catheter on line 4, at 47 cms. is in stomach, where inspiration produces an increase in pressure. Column b. Drop in pressure in all 3 catheters, now in esophagus. Column c. Catheters represented by lines 2 and 3 are now in pharynx, and show no drop on inspiration. The lowermost catheter (line 4) is still in esophagus, and shows a drop in pressure on inspiration. Column d. Catheters on lines 2 and 3 are in esophagus, line 4 in stomach. Sudden, forced inhalation produces a drop in pressure which is not sustained, and during which the patient speaks. This negative deflection is followed quickly by an increase in pressure, as the patient continues to speak. The level of the baseline indicates resting intraluminal pressure. In this patient, there is no increase in pressure as the catheter openings pass through the upper esophageal inlet (approximately 19-22 cms. markings).

normal deglutition; and, possibly, interference with esophageal speech.

a. To test for insufflation of air, we chose a patient with no demonstrable sphincter in the upper esophagus. With the pressure recording tubes in the esophagus, the patient was instructed to take a deep breath. Tracings show that the normal drop in intraesophageal pressure was obtained and sustained during inspiration; yet, with sudden forced inspiration, the patient could aspirate air into the esophagus when he wished to speak (Fig. 5). The degree of negativity within the esophagus at these times probably assumes greater proportions than during deep breathing.[23]

b. In observing postoperative deglutition, we found that most laryngectomized patients who exhibit absence of an

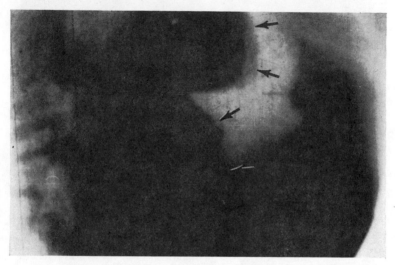

Fig. 6. Muscle masses in laryngectomized patient with dysphagia. These prominences were observed on cinefluorography to form in the region of the inferior and middle constrictor muscles. They changed size and shape during deglutition, nearly disappearing when the pharynx was at rest.

upper esophageal sphincter do not have dysphagia, but that an occasional patient complains of regurgitation into the mouth or nasopharynx. Two such patients studied by cinefluorography showed both a patulous sphincter, with barium regurgitation on repeated swallows, and muscle masses in the region of the inferior and middle constrictors. These masses contracted ineffectively, with no visible relationship to the passage of the bolus (Fig. 6).

It appears, then, that the absence of a functioning sphincter at the esophageal inlet does not, of itself, promote regurgita-

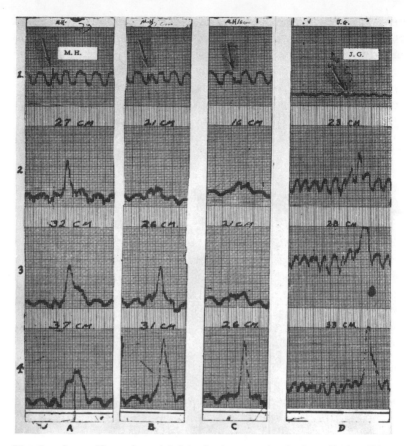

Fig. 7-a, b, c. Normal peristalsis in laryngectomized patient with no demonstrable sphincter at esophageal inlet. The base line shows no significant rise as the catheters are pulled up through the hypopharynx. Swallows are indicated by arrows on line 1. Normal peristaltic waves are seen in the recordings from the esophagus (a-2, 3, 4; b-3, 4; c-3). Absence of contraction at cricopharyngeus level, demonstrated in b-2 and c-3, is present in most laryngectomized patients. d. A 3 cm. resection of the entire circumference of the cervical esophagus, with the larynx, had been carried out in this patient eight months before this tracing was made. That this type of resection does not interfere with esophageal peristalsis is indicated by the normal recordings.

tion or produce dysphagia; coupled, however, with uncoordinate contractions of muscle masses in the inferior and middle constrictor areas, it is sometimes found in patients with dysphagia and regurgitation. The combination may represent surgical damage to the motor nerve supply of the hypopharynx, or the failure to achieve an adequate anterior midline approximation of these muscles at the suture line.

c. The third question related to non-functioning sphincter is that of esophageal speech. Our pressure studies indicate that a functioning sphincter in this area is definitely not necessary for good esophageal speech, although the bunched up cricopharyngeus may act as a pseudoglottis. Only one of our good esophageal speakers exhibited a functioning sphincter. Our best speaker had no demonstrable sphincter and could speak on both inspiration and expiration (Fig. 5).

4. Esophageal Peristalsis.

Eight of the 23 laryngectomized patients studied by intraluminal manometry demonstrated an area of decreased contractility extending for a distance of 3 to 5 cm. below the cricopharyngeus muscle. Whether this represents a denervated segment of the esophagus or whether the lumen has been weakened by closure of the anterior wall is difficult to say. It is interesting that in spite of this relatively inactive area, the peristaltic waves pass down the remainder of the esophagus in a normal fashion (Fig. 7-a, b, c).

Complete resection of the hypopharynx might conceivably interfere with the initiation of peristalsis by removing the area in which the primary peristaltic wave originates. This was investigated in a patient whose entire hypopharynx and larynx had been resected (3 cm. resection). Pressure studies showed that normal peristaltic waves pass down the esophagus (Fig. 7-d).

CONCLUSIONS.

Structural changes in the pharynx of most patients after laryngectomy include pseudodiverticulum at the base of the tongue; submucosal masses on the posterior pharyngeal wall, caused by the contractions of detached constrictor muscles or portions of them.

Postoperative dysphagia in the absence of stricture may be due to regurgitation from the pharyngeal pseudodiverticulum, or to uncoordinated contractions of the detached constrictor muscles.

Although good esophageal speakers exhibit facility in insufflating air into the upper esophagus, no other characteristics of the postoperative pharynx could be shown to affect voice production.

The normal resting tonus at the upper end of the esophagus is usually absent after laryngectomy. This, in itself, does not produce dysphagia or interfere with good esophageal voice.

The atonic condition of the upper esophagus after laryngectomy does not interfere with normal esophageal peristalsis, nor does complete resection of the cervical esophagus.

BIBLIOGRAPHY.

1. HWANG, K.: Mechanism of Transportation of the Content of the Esophagus. *Jour. Applied Physiol.*, 6:781-796, 1954.

2. HWANG, K.: Mechanism of the Functional Recovery of the Cervical Portion of the Esophagus After Bilateral Resection of the Pharyngoesophageal Nerve in the Dog. *Amer. Jour. Physiol.*, 174:231-234, 1953.

3. ANDREW, B. L.: The Nervous Control of the Cervical Esophagus of the Rat During Swallowing. *Jour. Physiol.*, 134:729-740, 1956.

4. DOTY, R. W., and BOSMA, J. F.: An Electromyographic Analysis of Reflex Deglutition. *Jour. Neurophysiol.*, 19:44-60, 1956.

5. ARDRAN, G. M., and KEMP, F. H.: The Protection of the Laryngeal Airway During Swallowing. *Brit. Jour. Radiol.*, 25:406-416, 1952.

6. RAMSEY, G. H.; WATSON, J. S.; GRAMIAK, R., and WEINBERG, S. A.: Cinefluorographic Analysis of the Mechanism of Swallowing. *Radiol.*, 64:498-518, April, 1955.

7. SAUNDERS, J. B. M.; DAVIS, C., and MILLER, E. R.: The Mechanism of Deglutition (Second Stage) as Revealed by Cine-Radiography. *Ann. Otol., Rhinol. and Laryngol.*, 60:897-916, 1951.

8. TEMPLETON, F. E., and KREDEL, R. A.: The Cricopharyngeal Sphincter, A Roentgenologic Study. THE LARYNGOSCOPE, 53:1-12, 1943.

9. ROBERTS, R. I.: A Cineradiographic Investigation of Pharyngeal Deglutition. *Brit. Jour. Radiol.*, 30:449-460, Sept., 1957.

10. FYKE, F. E., and CODE, C. F.: Resting and Deglutition Pressures in the Pharyngo-Esophageal Region. *Gastroenterology*, 29:24-35, 1955.

11. ATKINSON, M.; KRAMER, P.; WYMAN, S. M., and INGLEFINGER, F. J.: The Dynamics of Swallowing, I. Normal Pharyngeal Mechanisms. *Jour. Clin. Invest.*, 36:581-588, April, 1957.

12. BOSMA, J. F.: Deglutition: Pharyngeal Stage. *Physiol. Rev.*, 37:275-300, July, 1957.

13. INGELFINGER, FRANZ I.: Esophageal Motility. *Physiol. Rev.*, 38:533-584, Oct., 1958.

14. SCHOBINGER, R.: Spasm of the Cricopharyngeal Muscle as Cause of

Dysphagia After Total Laryngectomy. *Arch. Otolaryngol.*, 67:271-275, March, 1958.

15. CRACOVANER, A. J., and RUBENSTEIN, A. S.: Dilatation of the Pharyngoesophagus Following Total Laryngectomy. *Arch. Otolaryngol.*, 62:306-307, 1955.

16. VAN DEN BERG, J.: Röntgenfilm über Die Oesophagussprache. *Arch. Ohren-Nasen-Kehlkopfheilk.*, 169:481-483, 1956.

17. VAN DEN BERG, J., and MOOLENAAR-BIJL, A. J.: Cricopharyngeal Sphincter, Pitch, Intensity and Fluency in Oesophageal Speech. *Pract. Oto-Rhino-Laryngol.*, 21:298-315, 1959.

18. BOEHME. G., and SCHNEIDER, H. G.: The Pathophysiology of Laryngectomy in Relation to the Quality of Speech Function. *Zeitschrift fur Laryngol., Rh nol. und Otol.*, 39:512-520, Aug., 1960.

19. ROBE. E. Y.; MOORE, P.; ANDREWS, A. H., and HOLINGER, P.: A Study of the Role of Certain Factors in the Development of Speech After Laryngectomy. THE LARYNGOSCOPE, 66:382-401, 1956.

20. VANDOR, F.: X-ray Examination of the Pseudoglottis of Laryngectomized Patients. *Fortschr. Roentgenstr.*, 82:618-625, May, 1955.

21. KALLEN, L.: Vicarious Vocal Mechanisms; The Anatomy, Physiology and Development of Speech in Laryngectomized Persons. *Arch. Otolaryngol.*, 20:460-503, 1934.

22. KIRCHNER, J. A., and SCATLIFF, J. H.: Disabilities Resulting from Healed Salivary Fistula. *Arch. Otolaryngol.*, 75:46-54, Jan., 1962.

23. CERNOCH, Z., and ZOBRIL, M.: Roentgen Cinematographic Records of Esophageal Speech. *Cesk. Rentgenol.*, 15:85-92, April, 1961.

24. DEY, F. L., and KIRCHNER, J. A.: The Upper Esophageal Sphincter After Laryngectomy. THE LARYNGOSCOPE, 71:99-115, Feb., 1961.

Esophageal Determinants of Alaryngeal Speech

Charles S. Winans, MD; Elliot J. Reichbach, MD; William F. Waldrop, MA, Chicago

Techniques of intraluminal manometry were applied to the study of the esophagus and its sphincters in 20 patients following laryngectomy and in 20 control subjects. Resting cricopharyngeal sphincter pressure was found to be significantly lower in laryngectomees with fluent esophageal speech (13 mm Hg) than in those unable to develop esophageal speech after laryngectomy (30 mm Hg) and controls (39 mm Hg).

The function of the lower esophageal sphincter and the body of the esophagus was similar in all groups. Whereas the cricopharyngeal sphincter normally prevents entry of unwanted air into the digestive tract, following laryngectomy this function may be detrimental and hinder the development of useful esophageal speech.

Following total laryngectomy, the patient, though often cured of cancer, faces a formidable task in accepting his inability to speak normally and resuming a satisfying, productive role in society. The development of an effective and inoffensive alaryngeal speech is a major step in the successful rehabilitation of the laryngectomee.

Of the various alternatives, most agree that "esophageal speech"[1] is the most satisfactory method of communication for such patients. In this speech form, the laryngectomee utilizes the body of the esophagus as a reservoir for air, the eructation of which produces sound by causing vibration of a pseudoglottis. The tongue, buccal surfaces, and lips then articulate this sound into intelligible speech.

Laryngectomees vary greatly in the ease in which they acquire a useful esophageal voice. Some develop it immediately and without help,[2] while others, despite expert instruction and great perseverance, are never able to do so. Motivation[3] and personality structure[4] have been suggested as important factors in determining ability to learn esophageal speech; age, intellectual capacity, and the amount and expertness of instruction may also be important. However, none of these factors has been convincingly shown to be a major determinant of esophageal speech.

More recently, consideration has been given to the importance of anatomic and physiologic features of the postlaryngectomy esophagus[5-7] which might determine its ability to function as an effective air reservoir. The present study, performed with

Accepted for publication Dec 1, 1972.

From the Section of Gastroenterology, University of Chicago Pritzker School of Medicine, Chicago (Drs. Winans and Reichbach) and the Speech and Hearing Clinic, Rush-Presbyterian-St. Luke's Medical Center, Chicago (Mr. Waldrop).

Reprint request to Box 400, University of Chicago Hospitals, 950 E 59th St, Chicago, IL 60637 (Dr. Winans).

This study was supported in part by the National Institutes of Health Research Grant AM-2133-13.

Mrs. Rita Glass and Miss Trudy Rosenberg rated many of the patients according to speech proficiency.

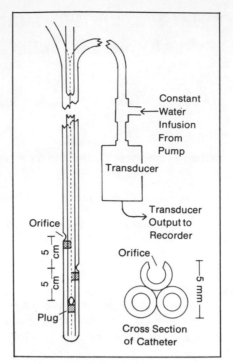

FIG 1. Essential components of recording system. Catheter constructed by bonding together three smaller polyvinyl tubes. Recording orifices were cut at 5-cm intervals near distal end of catheter. Each lumen was plugged with plastic just distal to its orifice. One of three transducers (Sanborn 267 BC) is shown. Lumens were water-filled, and constant fluid infusion entered system through sidearm adjacent to each transducer.

modern techniques of intraluminal manometry, was done to clarify the importance of these features and their relationship to the acquisition of esophageal speech.

METHODS

Twenty patients, age 50 to 82 years (mean 62), were studied 3 months to 14 years after total laryngectomy. They were referred by several speech therapists, and many were members of an esophageal voice club whose newsletter described the project and solicited volunteers. Laryngectomees were rated as to speech proficiency by the referring speech therapist on the Barton-Henja scale. This scale, described in Table 5 of Snidecor's text,[8] classifies speaking ability on an A to G scale, with A representing inability to produce sound and G representing fluent, nonhesitant speech. For purposes of comparison, 20 normal subjects, age 28 to 78 years (mean 51), without esophageal disease were also studied.

The manometric recording system (Fig. 1) used for the studies has been previously described.[9] The triple lumen, polyvinyl recording catheter was constructed by fusing together three smaller tubes (outside diameter, 2.4 mm; inside diameter, 1.4 mm). The overall diameter of the catheter was 5 mm, and it was somewhat more flexible than the standard clinical nasogastric tube. A lateral recording orifice, 1.2 mm in diameter, was cut in each tube, and these three recording orifices were spaced at 5-cm intervals near the distal end of the catheter. Proximally, each recording tube was attached to an external transducer, and during recording, each lumen was infused through a sidearm with water from an infusion pump. The infusion technique is an important modification of conventional intraluminal manometry, and pressures recorded from sphincter areas by this method correlated well with the clinical assessed competence of those sphincters.[9-11]

In the majority of the subjects, the recording catheter was passed by the nose, through the esophagus, into the stomach, although some preferred to swallow it by mouth. During recording, subjects lay in the supine position, and the external pressure transducers were leveled in the same plane as the body of the esophagus. The catheter assembly was withdrawn from the stomach, through the esophagus, into the pharynx by 1-cm increments, and both resting and postdeglutitive pressures were recorded at each station.

An illustrative pressure tracing from one of the three lumens of the recording catheter is shown in Fig. 2. The body of the esophagus is bounded at either end by a zone of elevated pressure. These high pressure zones (HPZ) are believed to be the manometric manifestations of the "squeeze" of sphincter mechanisms in these locations. The lower esophageal sphincter is intrinsic to the circular muscle of the distal esophagus,[12] while the HPZ at the upper end of the esophagus is primarily the result of contraction of the cricopharyngeus muscle.[13, 14]

Figure 2 also illustrates the method of pressure tabulation used in this study. For the stomach and esophageal body, mean (of the inspiratory and expiratory phases) resting pressures were determined. Mean maximal pressures were also determined for the two

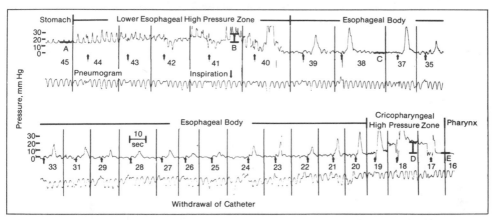

FIG 2. Pressure tracing from single lumen as catheter was withdrawn stepwise from stomach, through entire length of esophagus, into pharynx. Vertical heavy lines indicate points of 1- or 2-cm withdrawal of catheter. Large numbers indicate distance of recording point from naris. Esophageal body is separated distally from stomach by lower esophageal HPZ and proximally from pharynx by cricopharyngeal HPZ. Vertical arrows indicate swallows which are followed by pressure falls (sphincter relaxations) within HPZ's and pressure peaks (peristaltic contractions) within esophageal body. Horizontal bars A, C, and E indicate resting pressure levels in stomach, esophageal body, and pharynx, respectively. Brackets B and D indicate maximal net resting pressure within the lower esophageal HPZ and cricopharyngeal HPZ, respectively.

Table 1. Manometric comparisons of controls vs laryngectomees*

Location	Control	Laryngectomees	Significance
Stomach	11 ± 0.87	14.8 ± 1.23	P < .02
Lower sphincter	18.3 ± 2.05	18.1 ± 1.64	P > .9
Esophageal body	4.2 ± 0.81	5.6 ± 0.47	P > .1
Cricopharyngeal sphincter	39.4 ± 4.17	20.6 ± 2.80	P < .001

*Mean pressures in millimeters of mercury ± one standard error of mean.

high pressure zones. Lower esophageal sphincter pressure was taken as the difference between the maximal lower esophageal HPZ pressure and the resting gastric pressure, while cricopharyngeal sphincter pressure was measured relative to pharyngeal pressure as zero.

Although the investigator conducting the tests was unaware of the speech proficiency rating of each subject prior to the performance of the manometric study, contact with the patient necessarily resulted in some assessment of speech ability. For this reason, all pressure tracings were independently reviewed and tabulated by two other experienced investigators who had neither contact with the laryngectomees nor knowledge of their speech proficiency ratings.

RESULTS

Table 1 displays the results of the pressure measurements from the stomach, lower esophageal sphincter, esophageal body, and cricopharyngeal sphincter for both the 20 control

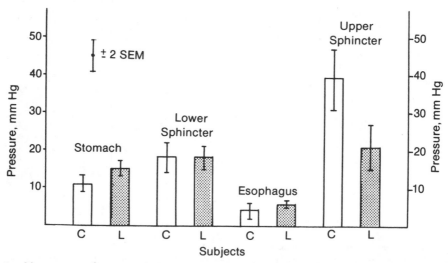

FIG 3. Mean pressures from stomach, lower esophageal sphincter, midesophagus, and cricopharyngeal sphincter of 20 control subjects (C) and 20 laryngectomees (L).

Table 2.   Manometric comparisons of good vs poor esophageal speakers*

Location	Group G good speakers	Group A poor speakers	significance
Stomach	18 ± 1.08	11 ± 2.69	$P < .05$
Lower sphincter	19.3 ± 2.84	18.3 ± 1.43	$P > .8$
Esophageal body	6.4 ± 0.67	4.4 ± 0.90	$P > .1$
Cricopharyngeal sphincter	13.1 ± 1.37	29.6 ± 6.19	$P < .05$

*Mean pressures in millimeters of mercury ± one standard error of mean.

subjects and the 20 laryngectomees. Control gastric pressures (11 mm Hg) were significantly lower ($P < .02$) than those of the laryngectomees (14.8 mm Hg), while the cricopharyngeal sphincter pressures were much higher ($P < .001$) in the normals (39.4 mm Hg) than the laryngectomees (20.6 mm Hg). Lower esophageal sphincter pressures and intraesophageal pressures were similar for the two groups. These data are shown graphically in Fig. 3.

Of the 20 laryngectomees, 7 could not speak ("A" rating), and 8 were fluent speakers ("G" rating). Manometric data from these two subgroups are shown in Table 2. Lower esophageal sphincter pressures were nearly identical in the two groups ($P > .8$), and although the good speakers had intraesophageal pressures about 2 mm Hg higher than the bad speakers, the difference was not of statistical significance ($P > .10$). On the other hand, the good speakers had significantly higher ($P < .05$) gastric pressure (18 mm Hg) and lower cricopharyngeal sphincter pressures (13.1 mm Hg) than those who had been unable to acquire esophageal speech (gastric, 11 mm Hg; cricopharyngeal, 29.6 mm Hg). These data are shown graphically in Fig. 4.

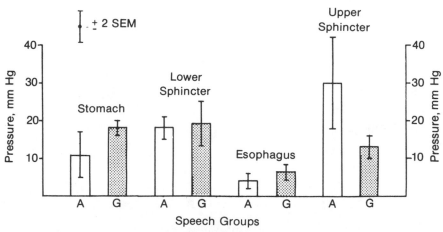

FIG 4.   Mean pressures from stomach, lower esophageal sphincter, midesophagus, and cricopharyngeal sphincter of seven laryngectomees unable to acquire esophageal speech (A) and eight with excellent esophageal voices (G).

Figure 5 illustrates the cricopharyngeal sphincter pressures of all 20 laryngectomees according to speech proficiency rating. Five of the seven group A patients had pressures higher than the highest of the proficient speakers.

The motor function of the body of the esophagus of all 20 laryngectomees was considered normal. Nearly all swallows were followed by contraction waves of normal magnitude and duration which moved distally with a peristaltic front. Failure of an esophageal motor response to occur after swallowing and the development of simultaneous, nonperistaltic contractions were only rarely seen. In three patients (two group A and one group G) the 3-cm segment of esophagus immediately distal to the cricopharyngeal sphincter displayed contractions which were substantially weaker than normal. Following a swallow, the cricopharyngeal sphincter appeared to relax normally in the majority of postlaryngectomy subjects. Figure 6 illustrates a segment of the cricopharyngeal HPZ of such a subject in whom an abrupt fall in pressure followed a swallow. In four patients (two group G, one group E, and one group A), however, the expected fall in pressure within the cricopharyngeal HPZ following a swallow was not observed. The tracing illustrated in Fig. 7 is from one of these subjects.

COMMENT

The origin of the sound utilized for the production of voice by esophageal speakers is still uncertain. Jackson and Jackson[15] and Negus[16] attributed it, however, to the cricopharyn-

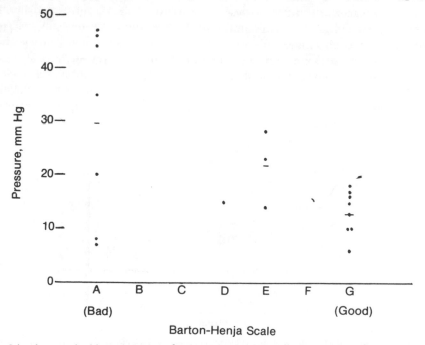

FIG 5. Cricopharyngeal sphincter pressures of 20 laryngectomees according to speech proficiency rating. Dots represent individual pressures. Horizontal lines mark means of groups.

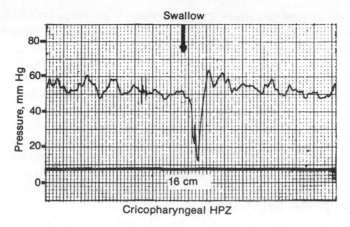

FIG 6. Maximal segment of cricopharyngeal HPZ, 16 cm from incisor teeth, of group A laryngectomee. Pressure falls normally following swallow, indicating sphincter relaxation. Horizontal line marks level of pharyngeal pressure.

geus, and Lindsay and associates[1] demonstrated, by cineradiography, vibration of this muscular fold during esophageal speech. It has seemed logical to assume, therefore, that preservation of cricopharyngeal function is an important prerequisite to esophageal speech.[17]

To perform esophageal speech, however, the patient must first master the technique of filling the esophagus with air. The cricopharyngeal sphincter normally *prevents* unwanted air from entering the digestive tract, and as Dey and Kirchner[5] have postulated, an effective cricopharyngeal sphincter following laryngectomy might act as a barrier to the entrance of air into the esophagus. Since the introduction of air into the esophagus is usually accomplished by maneuvers other than swallowing (for example, "tongue injection"), the sphincter is unlikely to be relaxed, and its resting pressure must be overcome

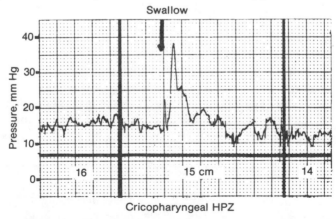

FIG 7. Maximal segment of cricopharyngeal HPZ of group G laryngectomee with fluent speech. No fall in pressure (sphincter relaxation) occurs following deglutition. Numbers indicate distance of recording point from incisor teeth. Vertical lines mark points of 1-cm withdrawal of catheter. Horizontal line is pharyngeal pressure base line.

to enable air to enter the esophagus. Dey and Kirchner[5] have presented data to show that good esophageal speech can occur in the absence of a detectable cricopharyngeal HPZ, and our data extend their findings by demonstrating that good speakers have significantly lower cricopharyngeal pressures than do poor speakers.

Further support for the role of a weakened cricopharyngeus in permitting the development of esophageal speech is found in the pressure data in the body of the esophagus and stomach. Good speakers had significantly higher gastric pressures consistent with inflation of the stomach by swallowed air, while the mean gastric pressures of the poor speakers and controls were identical. Although air reaching the stomach probably is of no use in speech production, the fact that some air does pass into the stomach of good speakers is attested to by the difficulties they experience with bloating and flatulence.[2] Although not of statistical significance, the elevated resting esophageal pressures of the good speakers as compared to both poor speakers and controls also would seem to reflect the ease of entry of air into the esophagi of good speakers.

It must be emphasized that our two laryngectomee subgroups represent the extremes of the spectrum of esophageal voice: no voice at all and fluent, *sustained* speech. These two subgroups were easily separable on the basis of cricopharyngeal pressure. However, although Fig 5 in general shows lower pressures associated with better degrees of speech, there is also considerable scatter and overlap of values. Obviously other factors must be of importance. For instance, one of the group A patients whose cricopharyngeal pressure was under 10 mm Hg was 81 years of age at the time of operation, and his senility may have adversely affected his ability to acquire esophageal speech. Furthermore, although the ability of the laryngectomee to fill his esophagus with air would be expected to correlate well with the loudness and duration of his speech, other factors such as the nature of the pseudoglottis and skill in articulating the resultant sound into speech should be more important in determining intelligibility. Bozymski and Pharr,[18] in fact, in a similar study where subjects were rated as to *intelligibility* of speech, could not demonstrate a relationship between cricopharyngeal pressure and intelligibility. Loss of cricopharyngeal sphincter function, therefore, would seem to play an important role in permitting air to be forced into the esophagus and thus allowing sound to be produced, while other factors are probably of more importance in the articulation of that sound into intelligible speech.

Incompetence of the lower esophageal sphincter has recently been described[6] as a frequent feature of laryngectomees unable to develop effective esophageal speech. Our data do not support this observation, however. Both the magnitude and function of the lower esophageal sphincter were normal in all of our laryngectomees, and the mean lower esophageal sphincter pressures of laryngectomees with both poor and good speech did not differ significantly from controls.

Could other factors explain the results of our study? The mean age of the good speakers (58 years) was somewhat less than that of the poor speakers (65 years). Although this is not a great difference, it is impossible to say what effect it might have on the ability to develop an alaryngeal voice. The poor speakers, moreover, were studied on the average much sooner after laryngectomy (16 months) than the good speakers (88 months), and this fact suggests, at least superficially, that the former simply lack experience. However, since the majority of laryngectomees who develop good esophageal speech do so within four to six weeks and since approximately 40 % of laryngectomees never learn intelligible speech regardless of the duration of their instruction,[2] this is unlikely. A more probable explanation for the discrepancy is the sources from which our subjects were obtained— speech clinics and an esophageal voice club. Successful esophageal speakers tend to remain active in such organizations, while those who cannot master the technique are embarrassed, become discouraged, and drop out. Two years have passed since the completion of the manometric tests, and all of the seven poor (group A) speakers have in fact discontinued speech instruction. None has made substantial progress in the development of an esophageal voice. Six now utilize the electrolarynx.

The results of our study invite the surgeon to cautiously alter his laryngectomy technique in favor of a looser reconstruction of the cricopharyngeus or to utilize other techniques, such as myotomy, whereby the postoperative constricting function of this muscle can be reduced. It is also conceivable that patients having difficulty mastering the technique which allows entry of air into the esophagus might benefit by mechanical dilatation of the cricopharyngeal area if manometric studies revealed an unusually high pressure.

REFERENCES

1. Lindsay JR, Morgan RH, Wepman JM: The cricopharyngeus muscle in esophageal speech. *Laryngoscope* 54:55–65, 1944.
2. Martin H: Rehabilitation of the laryngectomee. *Cancer* 16:823–841, 1963.
3. Stoll B: Psychological factors determining the success or failure of the rehabilitation program of laryngectomized patients. *Ann Otol Rhinol Laryngol* 67:550–557, 1958.
4. Schall LA: Psychology of laryngectomized patients. *Arch Otolaryngol* 28:581–584, 1938.
5. Dey FL, Kirchner JA: The upper esophageal sphincter after laryngectomy. *Laryngoscope* 71:99–115, 1961.
6. Wolfe RD, Olson JE, Goldenberg DB: Rehabilitation of the laryngectomee: The role of the distal esophageal sphincter. *Laryngoscope* 81:1971–1978, 1971.
7. Zinner EM, Fleshler B: Intraesophageal pressures during phonation in laryngectomized patients. *J Laryngol Otol* 86:129–140, 1972.
8. Snidecor JC: *Speech Rehabilitation of the Laryngectomized.* Springfield, Ill, Charles C Thomas Inc., 1968.
9. Winans CS, Harris LD: Quantitation of lower esophageal sphincter competence. *Gastroenterology* 52:773–778, 1967.
10. Pope CE II: A dynamic test of sphincter strength: Its application to the lower esophageal sphincter. *Gastroenterology* 52:779–786, 1967.
11. Haddad JK: Relation of gastroesophageal reflux to yield sphincter pressures. *Gastroenterology* 58: 175–184, 1970.
12. Fyke FE, Code CF, Schlegel JF: The gastroesophageal sphincter in healthy human beings. *Gastroenterologia* 86:135–150, 1956.
13. Atkinson M, et al: The dynamics of swallowing: I. Normal pharyngeal mechanisms. *J Clin Invest* 36:581–588, 1967.
14. Winans CS: The pharyngoesophageal closure mechanism: A manometric study. *Gastroenterology* 63:768–777, 1972.
15. Jackson C, Jackson CL: *Carcinoma of the Larynx.* Philadelphia, WB Saunders Co., 1939.

16. Negus VE: *Mechanism of the Larynx.* St. Louis, CV Mosby Co., 1929.
17. Hunt EB: Rehabilitation of the laryngectomee. *Laryngoscope* 74:382–395, 1964.
18. Bozymski RM, Pharr SY: Esophageal manometry and speech proficiency in post laryngectomy patients, abstracted. *Gastroenterology* 62:627, 1972.

EMG OF PHARYNGOESOPHAGEAL MUSCULATURE DURING ALARYNGEAL VOICE PRODUCTION

THOMAS SHIPP

Veterans Administration Hospital, San Francisco, California

EMG activity from the inferior constrictor and cricopharyngeus muscles and the voice signal were obtained from 18 laryngectomized male subjects as they produced isolated vowels using alaryngeal phonation. To inflate the esophagus prior to phonation, all subjects but one demonstrated a similar muscle pattern: either one or both muscles studied showed a burst of activity at the moment of inflation. The remaining subject had a muscle pattern during inflation that was identical to a post-laryngectomy swallowing pattern. No typical or modal muscle patterns were found for subjects during the phonatory portion of the alaryngeal voice task. Consistency of pattern within each subject was extremely high during a given procedure and on repeated procedures. The findings suggested that poor talkers had less control of differential muscle contraction than did the adequate talkers and that each laryngectomized talker adopts a phonatory method that is unique to him and consistent with his postoperative anatomy and physiology.

There has been much speculation in the last 15 years regarding the musculature involved in the production of alaryngeal voice by laryngectomized talkers. Principal interest has been focused on the pharyngoesophageal area and its role as the generator of alaryngeal voice. Radiographic studies (Diedrich and Youngstrom, 1966) show the presence of an area of constriction in the pharyngoesophageal area during alaryngeal phonation. The location of this constriction suggests that the mechanism of phonation involves the participation of several muscle groups, principally the inferior constrictor and the cricopharyngeus muscles.

Until recently the participation of these two muscles in alaryngeal phonation could only be inferred from x-ray and pressure catheter measures since direct sampling of their activity was extremely difficult.

Techniques have now been devised (Shipp et al., 1968) for direct electromyographic sampling of pharyngoesophageal muscle activity in the awake subject. Utilizing these techniques this study assessed patterns of activity by the inferior constrictor and cricopharyngeus muscles during the production of alaryngeal voice from the time of esophageal insufflation through phonation of a sustained vowel.

Reprinted by permission from *Journal of Speech and Hearing Research*, 1970, *13*, 184–192.

METHODS

Subjects for this study were 18 adult males (age range 36 to 67, mean age: 56.2 years); 14 subjects had laryngectomy surgery performed at the VA Hospital, San Francisco, and the remaining 4 underwent surgery at private hospitals in San Francisco. Twelve subjects had only laryngectomy surgery while 6 subjects had laryngectomy and unilateral neck dissection surgery. All but 1 subject received alaryngeal speech training by the clinical staff at the VA Hospital.

The equipment and the techniques employed in this study have been described in detail elsewhere (Shipp et al., 1968; 1970). Briefly, experimental procedures were conducted in a standard x-ray room at the hospital in order to utilize fluorographic and spot-film equipment. The subjects were placed supine on the x-ray table and hooked-wire electrodes threaded through hypodermic needles were inserted to the site of the inferior constrictor and cricopharyngeus muscles. The targets for the carrier needles were radiopaque McKenzie clips that were clamped and sutured to the muscles at the time of surgery. When it was observed fluoroscopically that the needle tips and the marking clips were in close proximity, the subject was asked to swallow. The resultant EMG activity pattern as monitored on a two-channel oscilloscope (Tektronix 502A) and an audio speaker usually corresponded to the differential swallowing pattern obtained during surgery when electrodes were placed in the exposed muscles. When this pattern appeared, it was felt that the wire electrodes were sampling from the target muscles. When satisfactory electrode placement was verified, the needles were withdrawn leaving the wire electrodes in place. Electrodes were connected to a junction box which led to a Honeywell EEG amplifier, a differential amplifier (Honeywell Accudata 103), and finally to a four-channel FM tape record-reproduce system (Honeywell 8100). Signals into and out of the tape system could be monitored on an oscilloscope (Tektronix 502A) and an audio amplifier-speaker. The recorded signals were subsequently played back from the tape system through an impedance-matching amplifier (Honeywell T6GA-500) to an optical oscillograph (Honeywell Visicorder 1108) equipped with galvanometers linear (± 3 dB) to 8000 Hz.

Following electrode placement the subject was placed in an unsupported sitting position and the experimental procedure commenced. The subject's head position was not limited or controlled except to prohibit exaggerated neck rotation, flexion, or extension. Since the purpose of the study was to determine how subjects used their muscles for alaryngeal voice production, it was not considered critical that some subjects may have altered somewhat their normal sitting posture to enhance their alaryngeal voice production. The high degree of intra-subject reliability in muscle pattern during voice production suggested that such an alteration was a consistent one for that subject.

The subject then produced the vowel /a/ once every 10 seconds when signalled by the experimenter. Each phonatory attempt was followed by a relaxation of the voice musculature until the experimenter signalled for the next phonation.

Only one procedure for each subject was included in the data analysis. At the time of the experimental procedure, the subject was classified by the investigators as being either an adequate talker or a poor talker, using criteria generated from a previous study (Shipp, 1967). Seven subjects were classified as adequate and 11 subjects classified as poor talkers. There were no talkers who could be classified as good or excellent.

Experimental procedures were first conducted when the subject could reliably achieve the basic alaryngeal voice maneuver: inflation of the esophagus and subsequent production of alaryngeal voice, however short the duration. Usually this first procedure was conducted approximately one month postoperatively; however, there were many subjects whose first procedure was much later than this. Experimental procedures could not be conducted at fixed time intervals since the subjects were not readily accessible either because of their medical condition or geographic distance from San Francisco. Thus, the subjects were tested when they, the otolaryngologist, the radiology facility, and the equipment were available.

Analysis of the speech data was limited principally to duration measures of the acoustic and muscle signal and to observations of muscle patterns (active or inactive muscle behavior relative to other muscle activity or to another event).

In an attempt to specify further differences between adequate and poor talkers, each record was measured for the average amplitude of the EMG signal at sequential segments during alaryngeal voice production and compared to the standard of the maximum amplitude obtained from the same muscle during the swallowing act. Each segment of the record with an interference pattern rising above baseline activity was measured and an amplitude measure derived that was a percentage of that muscle's maximum amplitude during the swallowing act. These relative amplitude measures were combined as means for each talker group. Observations were made on differences between subject groups in the patterns of signal amplitude displayed.

RESULTS

Esophageal Inflation

The moment of esophageal inflation was judged to occur at that time when the subject's microphone signal registered a short acoustic pulse, corresponding to the inflation noise noted by Berlin (1963), and Diederich and Youngstrom (1966). This acoustic signal marked the dividing line between preinjection activity and postinjection activity as shown in Figure 1. Every phonation attempt from subjects in this study was preceded by injection noise which had a corresponding short burst of activity from one or both muscles sampled. When there was no short-burst muscle activity there was neither injection noise nor subsequent phonation.

The pattern of injection noise simultaneous with a short burst of muscle activity followed by phonation was invariably the pattern displayed by the subjects

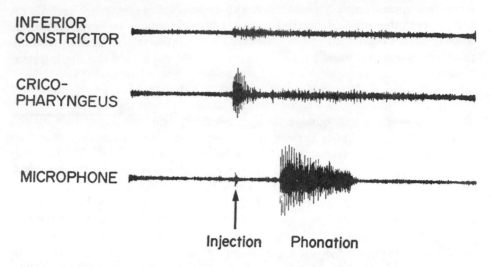

100μV ⌐
1 sec

INFERIOR
CONSTRICTOR

CRICO-
PHARYNGEUS

MICROPHONE

Injection   Phonation

FIGURE 1. EMG activity from the inferior constrictor and cricopharyngeus muscles and the acoustic signal from a subject during a single alaryngeal phonatory maneuver of esophageal inflation and subsequent sustained vowel phonation.

of this study. Occasionally, with those who had recently started speech training, the acoustic injection noise and corresponding EMG burst were not followed by a successful phonatory attempt.

The sole exception to the muscle pattern of esophageal inflation shown in Figure 1 was the one subject who received his alaryngeal speech training from a non-VA speech clinician at his home 200 miles from San Francisco. After two months of speech training he returned to San Francisco for the EMG experimental procedure. Figure 2 shows the EMG-acoustic records obtained at this time. The upper record (A) was obtained on a spontaneous swallow and was typical of what is termed the characteristic Type II swallowing pattern found in all post-laryngectomized subjects (Shipp et al., 1969). Note particularly the double burst activity pattern of the inferior constrictor muscle during swallowing. The middle tracing (B) is a representative sample of the subject's initial alaryngeal phonation efforts. The voice channel tracing shows the acoustic injection noise followed by an /a/. Coincident with the injection noise the inferior constrictor begins its double burst pattern which is similar to his swallowing pattern. The subject reported that he had been instructed to swallow the air in order to inflate the esophagus.

At this time in the procedure, the tape recorder was stopped and the subject given brief instruction and a demonstration of the glosso-pharyngeal press method of esophageal inflation. The subject adopted this method within five minutes. During this pause in the procedure, electrode position remained unchanged as did the gain settings on the EMG and voice amplifiers. Tape recordings were then made of the subject producing alaryngeal phonation using the newly learned injection method. The lowest trace (C) in Figure 2 shows two successive voice events. The most noticeable change from the other records (A and B) is in the inferior constrictor muscle channel where virtually no muscle activity occurs during injection or phonation. Cricopharyngeus activity also appears to change substantially between records B and C for the air injection moment.

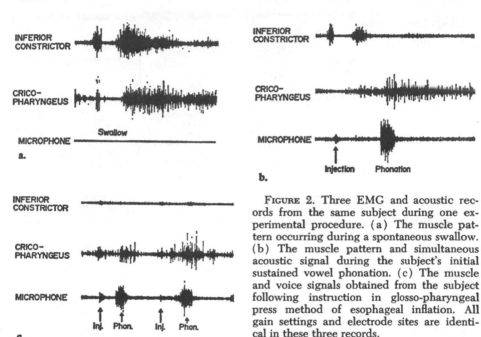

FIGURE 2. Three EMG and acoustic records from the same subject during one experimental procedure. (a) The muscle pattern occurring during a spontaneous swallow. (b) The muscle pattern and simultaneous acoustic signal during the subject's initial sustained vowel phonation. (c) The muscle and voice signals obtained from the subject following instruction in glosso-pharyngeal press method of esophageal inflation. All gain settings and electrode sites are identical in these three records.

Phonation

The most noteworthy finding of the muscle activity during the phonatory portion of alaryngeal voice was that no single type of activity emerged as the typical, average, or modal pattern of muscle behavior. The pattern variations obtained were too numerous to classify.

In contrast to the great variation between subjects, however, the intra-subject pattern reliability was extremely high during a given procedure and between successive experimental procedures. Some subjects underwent speech procedures at four different times over a two-year postoperative period. While many durational measures changed throughout this period, the intra-subject EMG pattern for phonation remained the same.

Figure 3 displays a comparison of the relative EMG amplitude in speech segments between poor and adequate talkers and shows that all talkers showed anticipatory muscle activity prior to the moment of injection. For the inferior constrictor muscle activity in adequate talkers, there was progressively decreasing EMG activity from the point of esophageal insufflation to the termination of

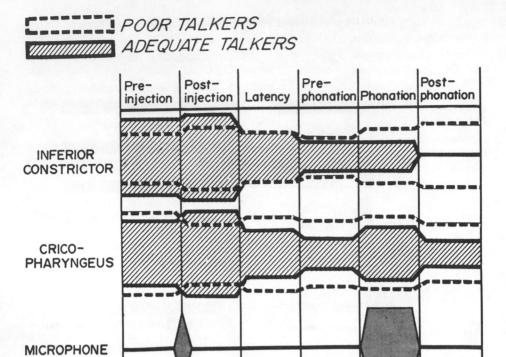

FIGURE 3. Mean relative amplitude EMG measures for the inferior constrictor and cricopharyngeus muscles during an alaryngeal voice maneuver by adequate and poor talker groups. Amplitude measures were made relative to each subject's maximum EMG signal from the muscle during a spontaneous swallow.

phonation. This trend is similar but less pronounced for the cricopharyngeus muscle activity in adequate talkers. The most noteworthy observation to be made of these data is that adequate talkers show considerable variation in muscle signal amplitude during speech, while poor talkers tend to have relatively invariant EMG amplitude measures.

The most valid and reliable estimate of EMG activity—the duration measure— was used to analyze each speech record from the onset to the termination of activity without regard to amplitude variation. Figure 4 and Table 1 present measures of activity from the preinjection segment through the pre-phonation segment. No differences were found between adequate and poor talkers in the esophageal inflation segment. Muscle activity was initiated from 72 to 107 msec before the acoustic moment of inflation and this activity continued for both muscles for approximately 320 to 370 msec after the acoustic injection point. Differences were noted between adequate and poor talkers in the pre-phonation segment where the onset of cricopharyngeus activity preceded alaryngeal pho-

Mean Duration Measures (in mscs.)

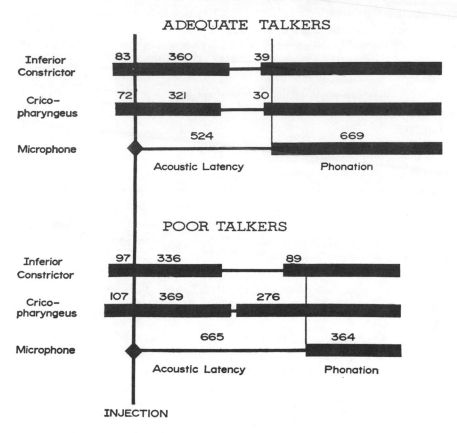

FIGURE 4. Mean EMG and acoustic duration measures (in msec) for adequate and poor alaryngeal talkers.

TABLE 1. Mean durations (in msec) of muscle activity and acoustic activity by adequate ($N = 7$) and poor ($N = 11$) talkers.

| | Muscle Activity | | | |
| | Inferior Constrictor | | Cricopharyngeus | |
	Adequate Talkers	Poor Talkers	Adequate Talkers	Poor Talkers
Pre-injection	97	83	107	72
Post-injection	336	360	369	371
Pre-phonation	89	39	276	30

| | Acoustic Activity | |
	Adequate Talkers	Poor Talkers
Latency	665	524
Phonation	669	364

nation. For the adequate talkers, the cricopharyngeus became active at a mean of 30 msec prior to the onset of phonation, whereas for poor talkers, cricopharyngeus activity was initiated at a mean of 276 msec before phonation. Also, for poor talkers the acoustic signal of voice production showed a substantially longer latency period between injection and phonation than did the acoustic latency for adequate talkers (665 vs 524 msec). Although none of the subjects was instructed to sustain phonation maximally, it was found that the adequate talkers' mean duration of alaryngeal phonation was 305 msec longer than the poor talkers' mean duration (669 vs 364 msec).

DISCUSSION

Two distinct methods of esophageal inflation were demonstrated in this study. All subjects who received training in the glosso-pharyngeal press method showed a similar muscle pattern during the esophageal insufflation or injection phase. The one subject receiving speech training elsewhere demonstrated that the so-called "swallowing" method of inflating the esophagus would most likely result in a muscle pattern similar to the Type II vegetative swallowing pattern, which was characteristic of all post-laryngectomized individuals. Undoubtedly individuals who utilize the so-called "inhalation" method of esophageal insufflation would have muscle patterns substantially different from the subjects in this study.

There are several possible explanations for the typical subject's muscle activity at the time of esophageal inflation. The burst of muscle activity coincident with inflation noise may be explained in various ways: (1) the muscles stretch as the air bolus is injected by lingual pressure into the esophagus resulting in a brief stretch reflex EMG signal indistinguishable from a short, active muscle contraction; (2) the muscles remain passive until air is injected into the esophagus then become active so that the injected air remains impounded for subsequent phonation (trap-door or valving effect); and (3) the muscles act in concert with the tongue to provide the final pressure for injecting the air bolus into the esophagus.

The appropriate explanation cannot be determined at this time since the physiologic correlate of the simultaneously produced injection noise is uncertain. Pharyngeal and esophageal air pressure data by Salmon (1965) indicated that the acoustic noise accompanying esophageal inflation or injection occurs at different times for different subjects during the inflation maneuver.

Whatever the function of the muscle activity during injection, the one subject from this study who was taught to inflate the esophagus using a swallowing maneuver demonstrated an EMG record that was quite similar to a vegetative swallowing pattern, which was in marked contrast to esophageal inflation using a glosso-pharyngeal press. The contrast in patterns indicates the dissimilarity between the two activities.

The consistency of the intra-subject muscle pattern during and between experimental procedures strongly suggests that each individual utilizes a method of alaryngeal phonation that is most efficient for him consistent with his post-operative anatomy and physiology.

The results also indicate that a subject's ability to contract the cricopharyngeus muscle differentially was more characteristic of adequate than poor talkers. Although surgery is thought to affect neither the innervation nor the blood supply of this muscle, it was apparent that a substantial difference existed among subjects in ability to control cricopharyngeus muscle activity during alaryngeal phonation.

The difference between groups in the initiation of cricopharyngeus muscle activity prior to phonation suggests that the poor talker group may not be able to activate or establish resistance to the esophageal air pressure as readily as the adequate group. This finding combined with the amplitude data lends additional support to the hypothesis that poor talkers have less voluntary control over the velocity and magnitude of pharyngoesophageal muscle contraction than do adequate talkers.

The data from this study seem to indicate that the active contraction of the inferior constrictor and cricopharyngeus musculature is not solely responsible for the pharyngoesophageal constriction during phonation noted in radiographic studies. Rather, it appears that, in addition to muscle activity, this narrowing of the tract may be a combination of factors such as the Bernoulli effect, elastic recoil of tissues, or pharyngeal wall motion secondary to movement of adjacent structures.

ACKNOWLEDGMENTS

This research was supported in part by Public Health Service Research Grant No. NB 05477 from the National Institute of Neurological Diseases and Blindness, through the Department of Otolaryngology, University of California, San Francisco Medical Center, San Francisco, California. Special acknowledgment is given to the VA Western Research Support Center for their instrumentation assistance.

REFERENCES

BERLIN, C. I., Clinical measurement of esophageal speech: 1. methodology and curves of skill acquisition. *J. Speech Hearing Dis.*, 28, 48-51 (1963).

DIEDRICH, W. M., and YOUNGSTROM, K. A., *Alaryngeal Speech*. Springfield, Ill.: Charles C Thomas (1966).

SALMON, S. J., Pressure variations in the esophagus, pharyngeal-esophageal constriction, and pharynx associated with esophageal speech production. Unpublished Ph.D. dissertation, State Univ. of Iowa (1965).

SHIPP, T., Frequency, duration, and perceptual measures in relation to judgments of alaryngeal speech acceptability. *J. Speech Hearing Res.*, 10, 417-427 (1967).

SHIPP, T., DEATSCH, W. W., and ROBERTSON, K., A technique for electromyographic assessment of deep neck muscle activity. *Laryngoscope*, 78, 418-432 (1968).

SHIPP, T., DEATSCH, W. W., and ROBERTSON, K., Pharyngoesophageal muscle activity during swallowing in man. *Laryngoscope*, 80, 1-16 (1970).

Received April 4, 1969.

Air Volume and Air Flow Relationships of Six Male Esophageal Speakers

JOHN C. SNIDECOR

NOBUHIKO ISSHIKI

Introduction

The title of this study defines its primary objectives. However, it is impossible to discuss the relationship in question without attention to historical information on these and a number of closely related topics. It is also essential that the efficiency of the speakers be defined.

The method of air intake in esophageal speech has been cause for much discussion and study. Seeman of Prague (1958) is an early proponent of the "inhalation" method of air intake in which the air is sucked into the esophagus in phase with pulmonary intake and exsufflated in phase with pulmonary exhalation. Van den Berg (1958) with Moolenaar-Bijl and Damsté has strongly supported the "plosive injection" method in which most or all of esophageal air is insufflated as a kind

of back pressure from plosive sounds or a movement akin to that made with plosive sounds.

It is our interpretation that the "injector," as described above, need not take his air into the esophagus in phase with pulmonary breath, although exsufflation would probably be assisted by outgoing pulmonary air.

Any brief historical comment is incomplete without noting that Stetson (1937) at Oberlin working early with relatively crude instrumentation but with consummate care and impeccable logic noted six important items of information in reference to esophageal speech that are of general interest and most of which are of special interest to this study. First, he noted that the plosives in a continuous series of plosives and vowels, such as pa pa pa pa, may back pressure usable air into the esophagus at about one cc per syllable. He did not speak of this as a primary method of air-charging as Moolenaar-Bijl (1953) did many years later. Second, Stetson noted synchrony between air-charging and breathing. Third, he stated that only a little air is taken into the upper part of the esophagus: from two to five cc. Fourth, he noted air in-

John C. Snidecor (Ph.D., State University of Iowa, 1940) is Professor of Speech, University of California, Santa Barbara. Nobuhiko Isshiki (M.D., The University of Kyoto, 1954) is Assistant Research Laryngologist, University of California, Los Angeles, and is on leave from his position as Dozent, University of Kyoto.

Reprinted by permission from *Journal of Speech and Hearing Disorders*, 1965, 30, 205–216.

take to be rapid and frequently fused with the movement of the consonant. Fifth, he deplored the use of large amounts of air in the stomach. Sixth, Stetson notes that a young normal speaker could insufflate 400 cc of air into the esophagus as measured by a spirometer. The air was not utilized in speech. From Stetson's viewpoint this is proof that large amounts of air can be taken, but does not constitute a recommendation to do so.

Diedrich and Youngstrom (1962) have demonstrated, with extensive X-ray studies, the validity of both inhalation and injection, but prefer to classify injection as a single method which has certain minor variations.

The actual time of air intake into the esophagus has been studied by many including Damsté (1958), Snidecor (1962), Diedrich and Youngstrom (1962), and Berlin (1963). With effective speakers these workers found the inflow to be rapid, ranging from almost instantaneous to about .75 sec. The mean time of .20 sec to .50 sec will cover most cases in most studies. Air outflow has been measured in simple time and in syllables and words per air-charge with wide ranges reported.

Superior "inhalers" studied by Snidecor (1962) have a primary outflow of air lasting mean periods of from 1.00 to 2.25 sec. According to Damsté (1958) injectors may have an outflow of air lasting a fraction of a second and then immediately charge on a plosive or simulated plosive.

Berlin (1963) has utilized the duration of phonation in early training as one of four prognostic measures. If an esophageal speaker during his first few lessons can prolong a vowel for from 2.2 to 3.6 sec the prognosis for effective speech is good. Berlin indicates that a reduction in the ability to prolong a vowel may be a signal that disease involvement has returned.

A review of the literature clearly indicates that few, if any, adequate measures of air flow in esophageal speech have been made. Such volumetric and rate measures have been limited by lack of instruments capable of recording the amount and direction of air in an act that generally uses little air and that very rapidly. The sensitivity of new instruments facilitates the study of air-flow relationships in both normal and pathological speech.

Method

The subjects were six male esophageal speakers each of whom had re-entered normal social and economic life. Each speaker was rated on a five-point scale (1 = superior, 2 = good, 3 = adequate, 4 = fair, 5 = poor) by three judges experienced with esophageal speakers. Speaker W received all "superior" ratings; speakers A and V, two "superior" and one "good" rating; speakers C and M three "good" ratings; and speaker P one "good" and two "adequate" ratings.

In descriptive terms from the five-point scale we have one superior (W), two superior-minus (A-V), two good speakers (C-M), and one adequate-plus speaker (P). All of the speakers were intelligible and even the adequate speaker was judged as belonging in the "automatic" category described by Wepman et al. (1953).

Two instructors of esophageal speech attempted to classify the speakers as to their types of air use: W is primarily an inhaler, and secondarily a "tongue pumper"; A is a "plosive injector" and

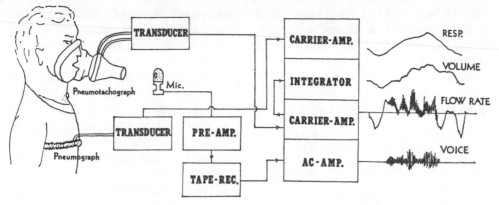

Figure 1. Diagram of the experimental arrangement.

"tongue pumper," with no "inhalation"; V appeared to use "inhalation" plus "plosive injection"; C "inhales" and "tongue-pumps"; M "tongue-pumps" and "inhales"; P "inhales" and "plosive-injects" and in fact uses every device he can.

Classification by types of air use must be approached with caution for air flow in esophageal speech appears, at least from this study, to be highly complex. Only the obvious inhaler and perhaps the pure injector can be differentiated easily by auditory and visual means and then usually in simple repetitive tasks such as contrasting time values for "ma ma ma . . ." versus "pa pa pa . . ." and in counting.

The experimental setup is illustrated in Figure 1. With this equipment simultaneous recordings were made of flow rate, air volume, thoracic movement, and voice signals. During flow measurements, the subject wore a mask against the face with extreme care so that no air should escape.

A pneumotachograph was used for measuring air-flow rate in and out of the mouth and nose during speech. The pneumotachograph was calibrated by a rotameter. The pressure-flow rate relation was linear up to 6000 cc/sec of flow rate. An integrator, to which the flow rate signals were fed, permitted direct reading of volume change as a function of time. The maximum range of possible error in reading the volume was about five per cent.

Detailed descriptions regarding the pneumotachograph, integrator, and recording system were given in previous articles by Isshiki (1964). Equipment is manufactured by Sanborn.

Movement of the thorax was recorded by means of a pneumograph. A strain gauge pressure transducer, to which the pneumograph was connected, converted the pressure change in the pneumograph into an electric signal.

Voice signals were recorded on the fourth channel of the recording system, via microphone and tape recorder. For other purposes a number of acoustical variables were explored which cannot, for lack of space, be discussed here.

While wearing the above equipment the speakers read aloud a passage of simple propositional prose. This task repeats, in large part, that used elsewhere for both normal and esophageal speakers so that direct comparisons could be made. The Rainbow Passage, as quoted by Fairbanks (1940), is a 51-word, 70-syllable "normal" reading passage widely used for a series of studies on both normal and esophageal speakers. It was presented as follows:

PLEASE READ THE PASSAGE CLEARLY AS IF TO AN AUDIENCE OF 25 PEOPLE

When the sunlight strikes raindrops in the air, they act like a prism and form a rainbow. The rainbow is a division of white light into many beautiful colors. These take the shape of a long round arch, with its path high above, and its two ends apparently beyond the horizon.

PLEASE MAINTAIN THE ESTABLISHED MICROPHONE DISTANCE

For the acoustic recording and later analysis, the esophageal voice was recorded on a tape recorder through a microphone which was placed at 25 cm distance from the mouth. Other appro-priate controls were established. Certain conventional tasks, such as prolonging vowels, and counting, were also recorded.

From the various records obtained, measures were completed to include: (1) rate of speech, (2) speech time ratio, (3) total volume of air utilized, (4) rate of volumetric change, (5) the relation between air movement and respiratory movement.

Of these, (1) and (2) are general measures of efficiency and are reported so that comparisons can be made with other studies. For example, all factors of rate and fluency define W as belonging to a superior group of speakers. The other speakers, though effective, could not be so rated. In this study we are primarily concerned with the amount of air used in esophageal speech and the rate of such use. Complex interrelationships between pulmonary and

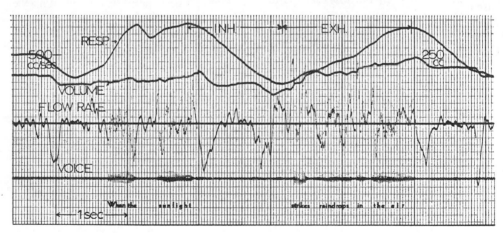

Figure 2. Recordings of the phrase, "When the sunlight strikes raindrops in the air . . . " From top to bottom the traces represent:

1. Respiration (direction only).

2. Variations in esophageal air volume (each heavy graduation, consisting of five fine graduations, corresponds to 25 cc). In both 1 and 2 incoming air is represented by the downward slope, outgoing air by the upward slope.

3. Air flow rate, line 2 from the bottom (above the baseline represents rate of outflow, below the line rate of inflow. Each heavy graduation corresponds to 50 cc/sec).

4. Voice. Example: Just after "sunlight" is phonated 50 cc of air is insufflated in 0.29 sec with a mean flow rate of 172 cc/sec. The inhalation, volume, and flow rate curves are all downward (incoming air) and synchronized. There is no voicing.

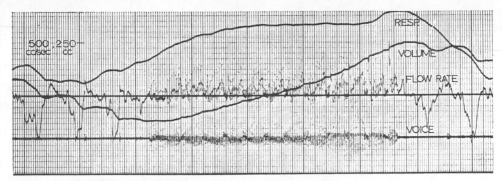

Figure 3. Simultaneous recordings of respiration, volume and flow rate of air and voice during maximum repetitions of "ba" for speaker W. Only three major intakes of air before phonation are shown here. However, two even larger insufflations were recorded prior to these three. Note that no air was insufflated in connection with the plosive "b" for this speaker. See Figure 2 for explanation of trace representations.

esophageal flow must, for lack of space, be only briefly mentioned. An example of the recording is shown in Figures 2 and 3.

Analyses were made of the recordings of the air intake and use during esophageal speech, wherein the speaker has eight possible combinations in his use of air as this act relates to the direction of pulmonary air and voicing.

(1) He can insufflate air out of phase with breathing and be silent.

(2) He duplicates this act except that he voices on out of phase inhalation.

(3) Air can be insufflated in phase with breathing, with silence.

(4) Air can be insufflated in phase with breathing with voice.

(5) Air can be exsufflated out of phase with breathing without voice.

(6) Air can be exsufflated out of phase with breathing with voice.

(7) Air can be exsufflated in phase with breathing during silence.

(8) The speaker can exsufflate in phase with voice.

Each one of the different events, referred to directly above, having to do with insufflation or exsufflation, may be continuous with another event and

fused with it to make a larger total event. For example, insufflation in preparation for a phrase might consist of intakes of air, both voiced and unvoiced, and in phase and out of phase. The voiced segment of insufflation of air can contribute to the forthcoming word or phrase. Exsufflation of air will show fewer permutations than insufflation, but even here events may fuse to make one larger event, i.e., events (6) and (8) might be utilized in speaking one continuous phrase. Thus, examples of each parameter do not necessarily bear a direct relationship to syllables, words, or phrases. In general, previous studies have emphasized the larger units of performance as these relate to the production of certain numbers of syllables, words, and length of phrases.

Results and Discussion

One of the useful measures of efficiency in speech is rate in words per minute. Darley (1940) has established rate norms of normal speakers for a passage similar in contextual level and

TABLE 1. General temporal relationships.

Rank Order of Speakers	Esophageal Speakers						Normal Speaker
	1* W	2 A	2 V	3 C	3 M	4 P	
Words/Minute	153	128	122	80	122	96	140-185
Syllables/Minute	210	183	168	117	168	147	203-265
Ratio of Phonated to Total Time	.51	.47	.57	.40	.38	.44	.60-.75

*This and other following numerals on the horizontal represent the average rating of the esophageal speakers, 1 represents the best performance, 4 the poorest.

word length to The Rainbow Passage which was used here. His zero percentile was represented by 129 words per minute, the fiftieth percentile by 166 words per minute and the one hundredth percentile by 222 words per minute. Of especial importance to this present study is Franke's (1939) investigation of judgment of rate which determined that critical listeners judge rate too rapid if it exceeds 185 words per minute, and too slow if it is less than 140 words per minute. A previous study of rate in superior esophageal speech by Snidecor (1962) indicated a range of from 108-137 words per minute with a median rate of 122.5 for The Rainbow Passage. Lower rates for other performances are reported in this same study. In this earlier report, no speaker exceeded Darley's fifth percentile and no speaker would be judged as adequately rapid by Franke's norms.

Table 1 summarizes information on rate. Only W exceeds previously reported norms and he does so by a substantial margin. W is exceptionally rapid for an esophageal speaker. One feels no impatience in listening to his flow of speech. As indicated in Table 1, his rate of 153 words per minute is at Darley's fifteenth percentile for normal

speakers and within the limits of satisfactory rate for normal speakers as defined by Franke. No other effective esophageal speaker in this study or the Snidecor study is closely competitive (see Table 1, columns A, C, M, P, V as regards performance in rate). It is of incidental interest that W can speak even more rapidly, but vocal quality deteriorates with increased rate. Speakers A, M, P, and V have normal rates as esophageal speakers, speaker C is a slow and deliberate, but acceptable speaker. Within reasonable limits of efficiency, rapid rate in itself does not make for effective speech.

The ratio of phonated time to total time gives some measure of vocal efficiency. If the esophageal speaker has many or long pauses, his effective total rate will be reduced. Moreover, his speech will be either unduly staccato or hesitant thus distracting from the meaning of his speech. According to Black (1942), Hanley (1951), and Snidecor (1951), normal speakers phonate from 60 to 75% of the time during continuous speech.

Table 1, item 3, indicates a range of phonated time from 38.4% to 57.4% for esophageal speakers, figures below those for the normal speaker. The poor

TABLE 2. Gross measures of air volume, cc 51 words of continuous speech.

| | | | Esophageal Speakers | | | | |
	W	A	V	C	M	P	Normal*
Air in	948	1118	888	987	1189	335	2830
Air out†	984	1115	871	887	1085	372	3020
Air per word	19.3	21.9	17.1	17.4	20.9	7.3	59.2
Air per syllable	14.1	15.9	12.4	12.7	15.5	5.0	43.1

*Normal speakers also speaking as if to an audience of 25 people.
†Air out is, of course, the best measure of air used in speech. Discrepancies between air in and air out can run as high as 600 cc if the subject is an inhaler and fills before speaking.

esophageal speaker has badly broken rhythm, and is hesitant, whereas the effective esophageal speaker is rhythmical but more staccato than the effective normal speaker.

Table 2 shows gross measures of air volume in continuous speech. The values contained therein are much higher than the values reported by Stetson (1937) of from 2-5 cc, by Howie (1947) of 1 cc per syllable, and Snidecor (1962) of 9.5 cc per word. However, Kaiser (1926) studied one superior speaker who frequently insufflated a little less than 100 cc before beginning to speak. She does not discuss air volume per word, but if we assume, for the sake of an estimate, that her speaker can speak as many as five words per

charge, and superior "inhalers" can (Snidecor 1962), then he uses 20 cc per word or substantially the same amount of air used by speakers in this study (Table 2). It must be remembered that these quoted values are estimates based on early spirometric measuring methods, inspection of X-ray plates, etc. Modern electronic air-flow meters are highly sensitive and react instantaneously to air flow in either direction.

Subjects W, A, V, C, and M use from 12.4 to 15.9 cc per syllable, figures much higher than generally reported. Even subject P, our poorest speaker, at 5.0 cc per syllable uses more air than usual in past reports. It is of especial interest to note that subject A, who is clearly an "injector," uses as much air as subject

TABLE 3. Mean flow rate, cc/sec, for four types of air intake during continuous speech.*

	W	A	V	C	M	P	Normal
Out of phase, unvoiced	62	96	83	64	46	57	
Out of phase, voiced	50	118	71	45	56	33	
In phase, unvoiced	94	58	135	95	73	39	976
In phase, voiced	40		123		77	30	

*Numerals in italics represent dominant use.

W, who is principally an "inhaler." Five out of six of the esophageal speakers used approximately one-third the air used by the normal speaker. Here it must be recalled that the accrued volume for the esophageal speaker represented many air-charges whereas for the normal speaker, only a few breaths were needed for the same oral reading performance.

Table 3, mean flow rate cc/sec, represents a simplification of highly complex data in that only the dominant type of air flow in cc/sec is shown. Of the eight combinations of air use previously mentioned, only two speakers failed to use them all. Speakers A and C did not voice insufflated air synchronously with inhalation, all other speakers did, but not frequently. To put this in positive terms, speakers W, V, M, and P took in air during both silence and voicing and did so both in and out of phase with pulmonary action. All of the speakers exsufflated some air in silence as well as during voicing and in and out of phase with pulmonary action.

However, each speaker has a dominant manner of air intake. Speakers A and P were initially rated as injectors and we note that their dominant mode

of air intake is out of phase with pulmonary action and at the rate of 118 cc/sec and 33 cc/sec. Speaker W was judged principally an inhaler, V, C, and M were judged combination air-users. These speakers dominantly take in air at rates of from 73-135 cc/sec, and in phase with pulmonary action. Most, but not all of the air that goes out is used in speech, it should be stressed that such air is dominantly in phase with pulmonary action no matter what the type of speaker. (Figures 2 and 3.)

Air is taken in faster than it is utilized for speech as it is with normal speakers. The normal speaker has a much more rapid flow of air per second, and he uses much more air. Of course the term "phase" is not applicable to his air use, and he does not voice on inhalation as do some esophageal speakers.

Mean flow rate of normal adults has been studied by Isshiki (1964) and Isshiki and von Leden (in press) who found that it ranges from about 70-180 cc for the most comfortable sustained phonation of the vowel /ɑ/. Esophageal speakers, excepting our superior speaker, ranged from 27 to 49 cc/sec. The corresponding value for our best speaker was 72 cc/sec. From these data

TABLE 4. Mean flow rate cc/sec for four types of air expulsion during speech.*

	W	A	V	C	M	P	Normal
Out of phase, unvoiced	26	60	63	43	84	36	
Out of phase, voiced	112	57	88	53	137	55	
In phase, unvoiced	39	84	73	41	83	43	
In phase, voiced	69	97	56	45	66	25	219

*Air outflow from the esophagus is dominantly in phase with pulmonary exhalation.

it appears that only W reaches the lower limit of air flow for normal speakers.

A previous report with respect to flow rate in esophageal speech made by van den Berg, Moolenaar-Bijl and Damsté (1958) deduced the mean-flow rate as about 40 cc/sec from spirometric measurement of air intake and the maximum-phonation time. With the exception of our superior speaker, these data and ours are in essential agreement.

The superior speaker in this present study deserves special mention because of his use of an air reservoir.

The maximum capacity of the esophagus and/or stomach as an air reservoir has been of great interest and controversy in esophageal speech. Voorhoeve (1926) and Kaiser (1926) observed roentgenographically that the stomach contains the air during speech. Beck (1956) stated that the stomach is not used as an air reservoir in trained speakers but only occasionally in beginners. Van den Berg and Moolenaar-Bijl (1959) wrote that they had never seen an esophageal speaker who fills the stomach with air.

In W, the total air volume expelled continuously from the mouth and nose, without any directional reversals, was measured ten times while he sustained the vowel /ɑ/ as long as he could. It ranged from 78 to 253 cc. These values were surprisingly great, as compared with those for the other esophageal speakers tested (mostly below 50 cc).

However, to our further surprise, once when he attempted to count as far as he could with one breath, the amount of air expelled during that period (6.26 sec) reached the value of 615 cc. The rate of flow was 98 cc/sec.

The capacity of the esophagus was evaluated as about 80 cc by van den Berg and Moolenaar-Bijl (1959). From these data, it seems obvious that W is using or can use the stomach as an air reservoir.

However, attention should be directed to the fact that this enormous amount of air is not usually utilized during conversation or reading. It simply indicates the possibility of his skill.

In reading the propositional prose passage the mean-flow rate of outgoing air during vocal utterance ranged from 25 to 97 cc/sec for the present subjects. The corresponding value for a normal male was 219 cc/sec or three times over that for the esophageal speaker. The flow rate for normal speakers in continuous speech is generally higher than that for easy sustained vowel phonation.

Summary

Six effective esophageal speakers, ranging from superior to adequate-plus, were subjected to simultaneous air-volume, air-flow, pulmonary, and acoustical recording of a standard reading passage, vowel prolongation, etc. Computations were made relative to speaking rate and ratio of phonated time to total time as general measures of efficiency. Specific to the primary goals of this study, computations of air volume, rate of air flow, and phase relationships were completed.

Within the limits of the experiment and summary statement the results were as follows:

(1) Speaking rate ranged from 80 to 153 w.p.m., indicating that the speakers were in general efficient, with the best speaker within the limits of acceptable rate for normal speakers.

(2) Ratio of phonated time to total time ranges from .38 to .57 which is below mean figures of .60 to .75 reported for normal speakers, but which, nevertheless, indicates a good level of efficiency.

(3) Total air volume used for a 51-word passage ranged from 372 cc to 1115 cc in contrast to a normal speaker who used 3020 cc. The poorest speaker used the least air. Air volume is not related to the type of speaker in continuous speech. Volume per syllable ranged from 5 cc to 16 cc, figures substantially higher than previously reported. A normal speaker used 43 cc per syllable.

(4) Air-flow rate for air intake ranges from 33 cc/sec to 135 cc/sec. The poorest speaker ("adequate-plus") had substantially slower air-flow rate on intake than did the more effective speakers. The speaker who is primarily an inhaler insufflates in phase with pulmonary intake whereas the "plosive-injector" dominantly insufflates out of phase with pulmonary intake. All speakers have some out of phase relationships. A normal speaker had an air-intake rate of 976 cc/sec or about ten times that of an esophageal speaker.

(5) Air-flow rate for exsufflation during speech ranged from 25 cc/sec to 97 cc/sec. All speakers used air at a slower rate in speech than the rate for intake. The poorest speaker is slow in air use. Air-flow rates as well as volumes of air used are, in general, substantially higher than previously reported. A normal speaker used air in speech at the rate of 219 cc/sec or about three times faster than esophageal speakers.

(6) The superior speaker (W), mentioned in some detail, could use 615 cc of air, in counting to 14, at the rate of 98 cc/sec, with no air reversals whatsoever. He is an inhaler and uses the stomach as a reservoir. In normal continuous speech, he is a heavy air user, but amount and rate decline. The excellence of this speaker does not constitute proof that his methods are necessarily those to be taught to others.

Clinical Interpretations

The objective results of this study, viewed also with some historical perspective, allow for certain clinical interpretations that may serve as guide lines to esophageal speakers and those who teach them.

1. The speaking rate of speaker W at 153 w.p.m. is unrealistically rapid for almost all esophageal speakers. The range of the other speakers (80-128 w.p.m.) is in keeping with previous information on rate for superior esophageal speakers. Clarity and smoothness of speech often contribute to the rating given a speaker even though his speaking rate is slow.

2. The ratio of phonated time to total speaking time should be only a little lower than that of the normal speaker. The relatively legato esophageal speaker will, other factors being equal, sound superior to the staccato speaker.

3. Good effective air flow with a high rate of flow is to be encouraged. The rate of flow for insufflation must be rapid and under complete voluntary control. The rate of outward flow may approximate as high as one-third that of the normal speaker.

4. One speaker used very large amounts of air (615 cc) in one count from 1-14 with no air reversals. But

in normal conversation he does not ever speak in such long phrases. The clinician should beware of relating certain "acrobatic" performances such as this with good continuous esophageal speech.

5. By far the most important clinical interpretation of this study is that all of the effective esophageal speakers studied used a combination of methods of air intake during continuous speech. The clinician who arbitrarily insists upon any one method of air intake should probably revise his methodology in the direction of eclecticism. The eclectic view would not preclude starting with a single method that seemed best for a particular individual, but even here variety and versatility should be encouraged as soon as moderately fluent speech has been attained.

Acknowledgments

This study was completed at the Voice Research Laboratory, U.C.L.A., Hans von Leden, M.D., Coordinator, and supported by USPHS Research Grant NB-04430-03 from the National Institute of Neurological Diseases and Blindness. The subjects were nominated by Robert Harrington and Morton Cooper, both of whom are experienced teachers of esophageal speech. Dr. Cooper was available for judging and gave valuable assistance in rating the speakers.

References

BECK, J., Substitute esophageal voice in laryngectomized. *Rev. Laryng.* (Bordeaux), 77, 1956, 729-739.

BERG, J. VAN DEN, MOOLENAAR-BIJL, A. J., and DAMSTÉ, P. H., Oesophageal speech. *Folia Phoniat.*, Basel, 10, 1958, 65-84.

BERG, J. VAN DEN and MOOLENAAR-BIJL, A. J., Crico-pharyngeal sphincter, pitch, intensity and fluency in oesophageal speech. *Pract. Oto-Rhino-Laryng.*, Basel, 21, 1959, 298-315.

BERLIN, C. I., Clinical measurement of esophageal speech: I. Methodology and curves of skill acquisition. *J. Speech Hearing Dis.*, 28, 1963, 42-51.

BERLIN, C. I. and ZOBELL, D. H., Clinical measurement during the acquisition of esophageal speech: II. An unexpected dividend. *J. Speech Hearing Dis.*, 28, 1963, 389-392.

BLACK, J. W., A study of voice merit. *O.J.S.*, 28, 1942, 67-74.

CURRY, E. T. and SNIDECOR, J. C., Physical measurement and pitch perception in esophageal speech. *Laryngoscope*, 71, 1961, 3-11.

DAMSTÉ, P. H., *Oesophageal speech after laryngectomy*. Groningen, 1958.

DARLEY, F. L., A normative study of oral reading rate. M. A. thesis, State Univ. Iowa, 1940.

DIEDRICH, W. M. and YOUNGSTROM, K., An investigation of speech after laryngectomy. Office of Vocational Rehabilitation Summary Report, Project No. 337, 1962.

FAIRBANKS, G., *Voice and Articulation Drillbook*. New York: Harper & Bros., 1940.

FRANKE, P., A preliminary study validating the measurement of oral reading rate in words per minute. M. A. thesis, State Univ. Iowa, 1939.

HANLEY, T. D., An analysis of vocal frequency and duration characteristics of selected samples of speech from three American dialects. *Sp. Monogr.*, 18, 1951, 78-93.

HOWIE, T. O., Rehabilitation of the patient after laryngectomy. *Occup. Ther.*, 26, 1947, 372-383.

ISSHIKI, N., Regulatory mechanism of voice intensity variation. *J. Speech Hearing Res.*, 7, 1964, 17-29.

ISSHIKI, N. and VON LEDEN, H., Hoarseness-aerodynamic studies. *Arch. Otolaryng.*, (in press).

KAISER, L., Examen phonétique experimental d'un sujet privé de larynx. *Arch. neerl Physiol.*, 10, 1926, 468-480.

MOOLENAAR-BIJL, A. J., Connection between consonant articulation and the intake of air in oesophageal speech. *Folia Phoniat.*, Basel, 5, 1953, 212-215.

SEEMAN, M., Zur pathologie der oesophagus-stimme. *Folia Phoniat.*, Basel, 10, 1958, 44-50.

SNIDECOR, J. C., The pitch and duration characteristics of superior female speakers during oral reading. *J. Speech Hearing Dis.*, 16, 1951, 44-52.

SNIDECOR, J. C., *Speech Rehabilitation of the Laryngectomized*. Springfield, Ill.: Charles C. Thomas, 1962.

STETSON, R. H., Esophageal speech for any laryngectomized patient, *Arch. Otolaryng.*, Chicago, 26, 1937, 132-142.

VOORHOEVE, N., Der magen als vikariierender luftkessel nach laryngektomie. *Acta. Radiol.*, *Stockh*, 7, 1926, 587-594.

WEPMAN, J. M., MACGAHAN, J. A., RICKARD, J. C., and SHELTON, N. W., The objective measurement of progressive esophageal speech development. *J. Speech Hearing Dis.*, 18, 1953, 247-251.

Received June 26, 1964

The Objective Measurement Of Progressive Esophageal Speech Development

Joseph M. Wepman

John A. MacGahan

Joseph C. Rickard

Neil W. Shelton

THE PHENOMENON known as esophageal speech was first reported about a hundred years ago (4). It has been used extensively in the rehabilitation of laryngectomized patients, however, for only a little more than the past ten years (1). The literature of the last decade has dealt widely with the subject. By and large these articles have concerned the results of therapy and recommended techniques of therapy. Only a very few of them have been of a research nature and most of these have been concerned with the physiological mechanisms of sound production. The others have been largely discursive without research data or findings. It appears to the present writers that a sufficient number of patients have now received the benefits of therapy and are successfully using esophageal speech to make further subjective analysis of methodology only minimally beneficial. It is held

that emphasis should now be placed on such aspects as scientific evaluation of methods used, prediction of success in therapy, and recognition of the psychological problems faced by the laryngectomized patient. The present article deals with the first two of these problems; a later one will deal with the third.

It has been established, to the satisfaction of the writers, that the site of sound production used by most laryngectomized patients is the cricopharyngeus sphincter at the head of the esophagus, while the source of air supply is most probably the upper esophagus (3, 5, 7, 8). Beyond the research data establishing these vital mechanical factors, however, almost no objective data has been reported in the field. Several articles have dealt with estimates of success in therapy. Notable among these is the study reported by Jackson (2). Using a self-evaluation technique, he reports that 50 per cent of his cases achieved 'good voice.' This can be compared with the 80 per cent achieving successful voice estimated by Martin (6) and the 70 per cent judged as 'doing well' by Gardner (1). In all of these studies the evaluations were made subjectively either by the patients themselves or by observ-

Joseph M. Wepman (Ph.D., Chicago, 1948) is Lecturer in Psychology and Clinical Instructor in Otolaryngology, and John A. MacGahan (M.A., Chicago, 1950), Joseph C. Rickard, and Neil W. Shelton (M.A., Cincinnati, 1950) are graduate students, University of Chicago. This study is from the V.A. Hospital, Hines, Illinois, and the Departments of Otolaryngology and Psychology, University of Chicago.

Reprinted by permission from *Journal of Speech and Hearing Disorders*, 1953, *18*, 247–251.

ers. Since no objective measuring rod was available the percentages reported must be considered as being relative to the individual criteria of success and therefore are not comparable.

In consequence, the writers propose a rating scale of esophageal speech which will permit objective reporting. It has been formulated in such a way that it should be equally useful for self-evaluation and for observation. Additional values should accrue from a widespread use of the scale. For example, the therapist should be able to judge the stage of recovery for his patients at any given time; the patient should be able to visualize his progress and foresee the stages through which he must go before success is achieved, and outside observers, such as the families of patients and the interested physicians and surgeons, should be able to support the patient's efforts more realistically. In addition to other values, then, the scale offers a real motivating device which recognizes the need of every patient to gauge his own speech recovery as well as to see the sub-goals which lead to normal communication.

The rating scale shown in Table 1 is felt to be more than simply a logical tool comprised of arbitrary levels established by the writers. Rather, it is an explicit statement of observations made over many years of studying the development of speech after laryngectomy. While several different therapies were used in this work, which has spanned more than a decade, the findings indicate that most if not all laryngectomized patients go through these stages in a natural progression on their path to normal speech development. The scale was derived by itemizing the stages of this progression and then establishing arbitrary limits for each separate level. The result is not felt to be an artificial or unique way of observing esophageal speech, nor does it lead to the forcing of the observations into unwieldly categories.

One salient feature of the scale should be noted. It has long been recognized that the essential problem in producing useful, audible speech after laryngectomy lies in developing for automatic use a new source of sound production. Despite this recognition there has been an almost universal tendency to consider recovery solely on the basis of speech production. It should be unnecessary to point out that speech is rarely affected by laryngectomy. Only the ability to produce sound is affected by removal of the source of sound production, the

TABLE 1. A rating scale for esophageal speech.

Level	Esophageal Sound Production	Speech Proficiency
7	None	No speech
6	Involuntary only	No speech
5	Voluntary part of the time	No speech
4	Voluntary most of the time	Vowel sounds differentiated Monosyllabic speech
3	At will	Single word speech
2	At will with continuity	Word grouping
1	Automatic	Esophageal speech

larynx, producing thereby a lack of communication between the body of air in the lungs and the articulators. This focus of attention upon speech production in therapy rather than upon the more basic problem of sound production has tended to instill in many patients an unwarranted negative evaluation of progress. It is felt that many patients discontinue their efforts to obtain satisfactory esophageal speech because they cannot visualize their progress, since sound production itself is only vaguely dealt with in the recovery program. In consequence, the scale takes into consideration the dual nature of the recovery process. First, and most important, is the progression of esophageal sound production; second, and correlated with the first, is that of speech proficiency. The scale establishes the primary importance of the esophageal mechanism and its function. There may be some observed variations in the development of speech proficiency; however, the basic function, sound production, is established in such a way that accurate observations can be recorded by any observer, trained or untrained.

Levels of the Scale

Level 7. No esophageal sound production; no speech. At this level there is usually little or no attempt at verbal communication. Patients frequently write any questions they may have or when they do attempt speech it is of the 'pseudo-whispered' type. The rating is given when the patient is unable to produce esophageal sound, either involuntarily or voluntarily.

(Note: Some patients whose operations have been extensive are incapable of making sound at the esophagus because of damage to that structure. These patients should be given a short trial at esophageal speech, but if it is not easily achieved they should be advised to use an artificial larynx.)

Level 6. Involuntary esophageal sound production; no speech. Here the patient demonstrates the ability to produce an esophageal sound. This is accomplished involuntarily, that is, not as the direct result of willing it, but as the indirect result of swallowing air. The sound produced is uncontrolled, is produced without effort, and is nothing more than the common eructation or 'belch' that is produced involuntarily by anyone. Its value lies in the recognition by both the therapist and the patient that the production of sound at the esophagus is possible. The mechanism for esophageal speech, then, is known to be intact and must be brought under voluntary control. Many patients come to therapy at this level.

Level 5. Voluntary sound production part of the time; no speech. At this stage the patient demonstrates his ability to produce esophageal sound voluntarily. The production is limited in both amount and quantity, considerable effort is expended and the effort is only infrequently rewarded. Therapy sessions may result in no more than one or two voluntary sounds. During the later aspects of this stage some sounds may be produced which contain modulation and some simple differentiation of vowels. The level is largely characterized by the inconsistency of esophageal sound production with the involuntary sounds appearing more frequently than the voluntary.

The achievement of voluntary sound production, the basic criterion of this level, is felt to be exceedingly important from a prognostic viewpoint. This accomplishment not only indicates that the musculature for sound production is present and capable of functioning, but also that voluntary control is possible. It is felt that progress beyond this point is largely the product of practice and motivation.

(Note: When there is great delay reaching this level, special problems frequently occur. Patients often inadvertently discover the phenomenon of 'buccal speech' or 'pseudo-whispered voice.' The product here is a crude whisper, rarely intelligible and hardly useful for communication. While it is known that some writers propose such a technique as a serious alternative to esophageal speech, the present writers consider it a deterrent to maximally effective speech and discourage its practice.)

Level 4. Voluntary sound production most of the time; vowel sounds differentiated, monsyllabic speech. At this point muscular control for sound production is close to being satisfactory. The patient begins this level with the ability to produce voluntary sounds in an undifferentiated way. He then starts to make the vowel sounds differentially. With this accomplishment comes the ability to produce several short words of a single syllable. Many failures are experienced, but success is increasing and involuntary eructation is decreasing.

(Note: The tendency is present at this level for the patient to hurry his production. When this occurs the amount of intelligible sound production is decreased. Constant admonition to 'go slowly' is necessary. The emphasis must still be on sound production with speech attempts kept to a minimum.)

Level 3. Esophageal sound produced at will; single word speech. Here the patient is able to produce esophageal sound whenever he wishes. The effort is almost always rewarded. The attempts have little or no continuity,

but single words, especially short ones, are easily distinguishable by the listener.

Level 2. Esophageal sound produced at will with continuity; word grouping. At this stage the elongation of sound production that permits words to be grouped in short phrases is present. The sounds follow definite swallowing effort and there is still a tendency to hurry the production in order to produce more sounds and more words on each attempt. This produces an occasional failure. The major aspect of the level, however, is the continuity of production even though it takes constant conscious effort.

Level 1. A u t o m a t i c esophageal speech. Here the patient speaks with continuity. One aspect more than any other characterizes his efforts, he is now able to speak without thinking of swallowing or of eructation. His speech is effortless and, while hoarse-sounding and somewhat lacking in volume, it is naturally and easily produced. The tendency to speak without preparatory thought or effort is easily observed. Speech is rapid and automatic.

Discussion

Experience with this scale has shown it to be useful in many ways. Administratively, it has permitted the keeping of rather complete records of progress for each patient with a minimum of time and effort. It has provided a common frame of reference for discussions relative to prognosis and to progress with interested families and physicians. Therapeutically, it has proven its value many times in demonstrating progress to the patients. This has resulted in improved motivation and increased stimulation to the degree that far fewer patients are disturbed by the length of the therapy and the slowness of the process. In addition, there has accrued the very real value of placing the emphasis more squarely upon the basic function of sound production and only secondarily upon speech proficiency. Finally, there are the advantages of an objective scale for research that have already been commented upon.

The extensive literature on speech after laryngectomy has raised many questions. Most of these have not received valid and demonstrable answers because there has been no way for true comparisons to be made on an objective basis. Some of the problems raised and unanswered which might be resolved by the use of the suggested scale are:

1. Are there demonstrable values to pre-operative orientation to speech recovery?

2. Do patients trained in a hospital setting do better than those trained outside a hospital?

3. Are artificial aids for eructation useful in the early stages of therapy?

4. Are previously operated laryngectomized patients who are now esophageal speakers the best therapists?

5. Are particular personality characteristics related to the development of esophageal speech?

6. Is the use of 'pseudo-whispered voice' detrimental to the eventual development of esophageal speech?

7. Is there a significant difference in the development of speech depending upon the economic-cultural pattern of the patient?

8. Is the use of an artificial larynx during the early stages of therapy a detriment to successful esophageal speech?

9. Are age, sex, and intelligence of the patient correlated positively with both rate of esophageal speech development and level of eventual success?

All of the above questions if answered objectively would make recovery of satisfactory communication a more positive and predictable process than it is today. It is felt that only by objective research design can these questions be answered.

Summary

An objective scale following the natural progression of the development of esophageal speech has been presented. The levels used, while arbitrarily set, are believed to be mutually exclusive. The scale points out the very essential role of esophageal sound production and the secondary nature of speech proficiency as related to it. The values of the scale in research, in therapy, and in administration have been pointed out. It is hoped that the field of esophageal speech after laryngectomy will be stimulated toward further research through the effort presented here.

References

1. GARDNER, W. Rehabilitation after laryngectomy. *Publ. Hlth Nurs.*, 43, 1951, 612-615.

2. JACKSON, C. L. Voice after direct laryngoscopic operation: Laryngofissure and laryngectomy. *Arch. Otolaryng., Chicago*, 31, 1940, 23-37.

3. LINDSAY, J., MORGAN, R. AND WEPMAN, J. The cricopharyngeus muscle in esophageal speech. *Laryngoscope*, 54, 1944, 1-10.

4. McCALL, J. Preoperative training of the esophageal voice in laryngectomized patients. *Ann. Otol., etc.*, 52, 1943, 364-371.

5. MARTIN, H. Esophageal speech. *Ann. Otol., etc.*, 59, 1950, 687-689.

6. ———. Rehabilitation of the laryngectomee. *Bull. cancer Prog.*, 1, 1951, 147-152.

7. NEGUS, V. Affections of the cricopharyngeal fold. *Laryngoscope*, 48, 1938, 827-858.

8. TEMPLETON, F. AND KREDEL, R. The cricopharyngeal sphincter: A roentgenologic study. *Laryngoscope*, 52, 1943, 1-12.

Clinical Measurement of Esophageal Speech:
I. Methodology and Curves of Skill Acquisition

CHARLES I. BERLIN

The importance of measuring a patient's progress in treatment need not be stressed again. Regardless of the pathology the patient presents, both he and the clinician need simple, valid, and reliable feedback on how well they are both progressing. In dealing specifically with laryngectomees, Wepman, et al. (9), described the benefits accruable from being able to measure the progressive development of esophageal speech:

> . . . the writers propose a rating scale of esophageal speech which will permit . . . [the clinician] to judge the stage of recovery for his patients . . . ; the patient . . . to visualize his progress and foresee the stages through which he must go before success is achieved. . . . the scale [to offer] a real motivating device which recognizes the need of every patient to gauge his own speech recovery as well as to see the sub-goals which lead to normal communication.

Charles I. Berlin (Ph.D., University of Pittsburgh, 1958) is a National Institute of Neurological Diseases and Blindness Post-doctoral Fellow in Medical Audiology, Johns Hopkins Hospital, Baltimore, Maryland. The patient material for this study was collected while the author was on the staff of the United States Veterans' Administration Hospital in San Francisco. The completion of the study was supported by NINDB grant-BT-856 while the author was at the Johns Hopkins Medical Institutions. Parts of this paper were presented at the 1961 and 1962 conventions of the American Speech and Hearing Association.

Both Wepman's work (9), and that of Hyman (5), describe verbal rating or reporting scales. However, the measurements described in the present paper were used to quantify, rather than describe qualitatively, the learning of four specific skills taught to laryngectomees as part of their general acquisition of esophageal speech.

Description and Rationale for Face Validity

The following four skills appeared to the author to have a face validity relationship to adequate esophageal speech:

a. Ability to phonate reliably on demand.

b. Maintenance of a short latency between inflation of the esophagus and vocalization.

c. Maintenance of an adequate duration of phonation.

d. Ability to sustain phonation during articulation.

The following clinical measures were devised to assess the four skills mentioned above. Materials used initially to take the measures included a stop watch, a pencil, and paper.

Per Cent Vocalization in Twenty Trials. The patient was asked to make a single inflation and to follow it by

Reprinted by permission from *Journal of Speech and Hearing Disorders*, 1963, 28, 42–51.

the phonation of [ɑ]. Twenty trials were given and scores were tabulated and translated into percentages. To be considered successful, a vocalization had to last for 0.4 secs or longer. Since normal speakers can usually phonate on demand, similar skills were expected of laryngectomees who had achieved adequate speech.

Latency between Inflation and Phonations of [ɑ]. Compared with the normal speaker, the laryngectomee has far less air to use for phonatory purposes (*8*, p. 118). It should be expected, and has been observed (*8*, pp. 71-78, *3*, pp. 71-72, *1*), that the laryngectomee must reinflate his phonating system much more often in the course of ordinary conversation than must the normal speaker. The speed and ease with which the laryngectomee can accomplish this feat should be reflected in the smoothness and continuity of his connected speech.

To measure this skill, the patient was asked to phonate as quickly as possible after an inflation. The examiner activated his stop watch at a signal from the patient that he was beginning to inflate his esophagus. The watch was stopped as soon as the examiner perceived vocalization. The patient was given 10 trials, and the mean time was recorded. The same 0.4 secs criterion, as above, was used to denote a successful phonation.

Maximum Possible Duration of Vowel [ɑ] *on One Inflation.* Normal speakers usually have air available for at least the duration of individual phrases. We might wish good esophageal speakers to do nearly as well so that they might present an adequate facsimile of connected speech. Anderson (*1*), in fact, felt that high intelligibility of esophageal speech is linked to the patient's ability to sustain a lengthy phonation of [ɑ].

The patient was asked to phonate a single vowel [ɑ] and to sustain it for as long as possible. He was permitted only one inflation per trial. Ten trials were made, and the mean duration was recorded.

Although the author decided to use this measure as one dimension of esophageal speech development, he does not suggest that the longer a laryngectomee can sustain an [ɑ] the better esophageal speaker he will be. The data to be discussed later indicate that such a conclusion is not entirely justified. The sustained phonation of the vowel [ɑ] was used because the author felt the task would be most wasteful of air and would deny the laryngectomee the chance to reinflate his esophagus subtly with consonant articulations (*6*).

Number of [dɑ] *Syllables per Inflation.* The patient was asked to use only one inflation in repeating [dɑ] as many times as he could without consciously reinflating. He was given five trials. The examiner noted each [dɑ] which he perceived, and the mean number produced in five trials was recorded.

The author felt that skill in this latter area would relate significantly to the laryngectomee's ability to coordinate phonation with articulation and to reinflate his esophagus with a plosive consonant. Diedrich (*4*), Snidecor (*8*, Chap. 7), and Moolenaar-Bijl (*6*), have discussed in detail the importance of reinflation of the esophagus by plosive consonants.

Accuracy of the Measures

The first sample patient to be studied was a 48-year-old male laryngectomee who was four months postoperative. He was asked to make a recording of the four skills described above. This recording was played through a Brujl and Kjaer octave band analyzer, model 2107, which was adjusted to make intensity level recordings. Paper speed was 30 mm/sec and pen speed was 500 mm/sec. Figure 1 and Figure 2 are representations of the graphic recordings obtained.

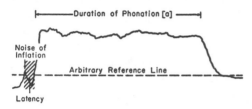

FIGURE 1. B&K recording of phonation of [ɑ].

Figure 1 shows the graphic record of a sustained phonation of [ɑ]. The pip at the beginning of the recording represents the sound of the inflation of the esophagus. Latency (skill *b*) can be measured from this point to the onset of vocalization. The onset of vocalization was considered to be that point at which the tracing rose at an 80 degree or greater angle from the reference line. The cessation of vocalization, for the purpose of this paper, was considered to be the point at which the tracing dropped below the reference line for 0.2 secs or more.

Figure 2 is the graphic record of one inflation followed by a series of repetitions of the syllable [dɑ]. A syllable was considered successfully articulated when the graphic representation of its

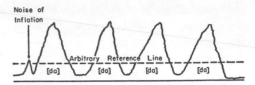

FIGURE 2. B&K recording of four syllables per inflation.

recording had a parabolic shape, with slopes of 80 degrees or more on the leading edge and 110 degrees or less on the trailing edge. These acoustic recordings were then used as 'true values' with which to assess how accurately clinicians could measure these skills without the instrumentation. The results are reported in Tables 1 and 2.

Six judges[1] took measures *c* and *d*, (see paragraph 2), from the tape recording. The 'Author' columns of Tables 1 and 2 show my estimates made at the time of recording. Columns 2 through 7 of Table 1 are the judges' estimates of the duration of the vowel [ɑ] sustained by the patient. The judges used stop watches to make these estimates. The column labeled 'B&K' shows the 'true values' with which these were compared. The tracings which were used to get 'true values' were read by both the author and an independent observer, with a correlation of agreement at 0.98. A simple analysis of variance yielded an F ratio of 2.66 which showed that there were no statistically significant differences between the values reported by the judges, and the 'true values.'

Table 2 shows the agreement of the judges with the B&K tracings on the

[1]All held M.A. or Ph.D. degrees in Audiology and Speech Pathology and were full-time employees of the Veterans' Administration.

TABLE 1. Agreement of judges with B&K recorder on duration of [ɑ] prolonged by esophageal speaker.

Vowel Sample	AUTHOR	2	3	4	Judges 5	6	7	MEAN	B&K
1	4.0	4.0	3.6	3.5	3.4	4.1	4.2	3.8	4.2
2	4.8	4.2	4.4	4.0	4.2	4.3	4.5	4.3	4.6
3	5.0	5.0	4.8	4.4	4.4	5.1	5.2	4.8	5.0
4	5.0	4.6	4.0	4.5	4.4	4.9	5.0	4.6	5.2
5	5.4	5.0	4.8	4.8	4.8	5.2	5.2	5.1	5.4
6	5.0	4.6	4.8	5.0	4.6	4.9	5.2	4.9	4.8
7	4.6	4.4	4.0	4.4	4.9	5.0	4.6	4.6	4.6
8	4.8	4.8	4.4	4.2	4.6	5.1	5.6	4.8	4.9
9	4.0	3.8	3.6	3.8	4.4	4.1	4.4	4.0	4.2
10	4.4	3.8	4.8	4.2	4.0	4.3	4.6	4.3	4.2
Mean	4.7	4.4	4.3	4.3	4.4	4.7	4.9	4.5	4.7

number of syllables the speaker produced on one inflation. The same type of analysis of variance yielded an F ratio of 2.87, which again indicated no statistical differences between the measures. These preliminary data showed that clinical observers could take the measures accurately in relation to a criterion for accuracy (B&K analyzer).

The judges were not asked to assess skills a and b. Measure a (number of successful vocalizations) would be indirectly recorded each time a judge made an estimate of phonatory duration in excess of 0.4 secs. In order to take measure b, the judges would have had to have been present during the making of the recording. This was not feasible. However, the author's measurements of latency, which were taken at the time the tape recording was made, agreed well with an independent observer's reading of latency from the B&K tracings.

Test-retest Reliability of the Measures

One week later, three of the judges were asked to repeat their measure-

TABLE 2. Agreement of judges with B&K recorder on number of syllables per inflation of air by esophageal speaker.

Syllable Sample	AUTHOR	2	3	4	Judges 5	6	7	MEAN	B&K
1	7	6	6	6	7	8	8	6.9	7
2	10	10	10	9	10	10	10	9.9	10
3	12	11	11	10	11	11	11	11.0	11
4	10	9	8	9	8	10	8	8.9	9
5	12	12	10	10	10	11	10	10.7	11
Total	51	48	45	44	46	50	47	47.4	48

ments of skills *c* and *d*. Three Pearson Product Moment correlations of 0.99 supported the conclusion that these measures were made quite reliably by the judges.

Procedure with Experimental Subjects

When it was observed that clinicians could use both a stop watch and their own observations to record such measures accurately and reliably, the measures were used routinely in the clinic. Skills *a* and *b* were measured in the early stages of the development of esophageal speech, while attempts were made to measure skills *c* and *d* only after a patient demonstrated good success in the two basic skills. It became evident that it was more difficult to obtain these measures accurately with very poor speakers. They often tried to make two or more inflations before phonation and seemed to need more instruction before they comprehended the tasks. However, the curves of skill development of 38 patients were ultimately recorded.

Subjects. These 38 male patients were seen at the San Francisco Veterans' Administration Hospital from March 1960 to December 1961. After final data collection, the patients were divided into good-speaker (N = 28) and poor-speaker (N = 10) groups on the basis of recordings of their responses to a TAT picture and to a short standard interview, adapted from the work of Schaef (7). The TAT picture was used only as a stimulus to elicit connected speech. The recordings to be used for speech rating purposes were made on the last day of treatment. The grouping was done by three experienced speech pathologists and two otolaryngologists at separate sittings. The judges were asked to rate the esophageal speakers on a five-point scale, where 1 represented excellent esophageal speech and 5 represented very poor esophageal speech. Subjects whose mean ratings were 2.8 or better were put in the good-speaker group. Subjects whose mean ratings were 4 or worse were put in the poor-speaker group. Four ratings fell initially between 3.0 and 3.9. These recordings were rerated, but could not be fit into either group definitively. The subjects were therefore dropped from the study. In addition, one patient with a stenosis of the esophagus did not make any esophageal sounds during therapy hours. Since he could not perform on any of the measures, he was also dropped from the study. Thus, a total of 43 patients was evaluated, but only 38 were retained for the study. Twenty-six of these patients were seen three times a day for two individual half-hour meetings, separated by one half-hour group meeting. Twelve of the patients were seen only twice a day because group meetings were not possible. All the patients but one started as in-patients and left after an average stay of 32 days of speech practice. Fourteen continued their out-patient visits.

The mean age of this group was 62.5 with a range of from 32 years to 83 years. The mean age of the 28 good-speaking laryngectomees was approximately 56, and the mean age of the poor speakers was approximately 69. Nineteen of the good-speaking laryngectomees and six of the poor-speaking patients had either unilateral or bilateral neck dissections. Six of the good-speaking and four of the poor-speaking laryngectomees had significant bilateral sensori-neural hearing losses, (SRT greater than 20 db and discrimination of 88 per cent or less). One of the poor-speaking laryngectomees had a total hearing loss in one ear, and both facial and glosso-pharyngeal pareses.

Eight laryngectomees (seven poor speakers) were seen by the hospital's psychological rehabilitation team for problems relating to alcoholism. Twenty-four other patients (22 good speakers) also admitted to problems with alcohol, but did not request or show emergent need for treatment. All patients with squamous cell carcinoma revealed a history of smoking one or more packs of cigarettes per day, for a period of 20 years or longer.

Problems of Measurements. The examiner took the measures in the same way they were taken from the sample patient. A periodic check of the recordings of every five patients, using the B&K sound level recorder as an external validity criteria, revealed that the examiner continued to make accurate measurements. The routine use of the B&K recorder was not feasible since it was not clinic property.

An attempt was made to keep a patient working at the first two skills until he maintained 100 per cent success on measure *b* for two days. However, when some of the beginning patients learned that their more advanced ward mates were practicing other skills, the beginners wanted to try skills *c* and *d*. Since a few showed measurable success with these skills, despite their failure to score consistently well on measures *a* and *b*, their progress on measures *c* and *d* was recorded from the date of

256   ESOPHAGEAL SPEECH

their first success. Measures *c* and *d* were taken until dismissal from therapy. Weekly rechecks of skills *a* and *b* revealed their stability (particularly of skill *b*) once acquired.

The appropriate measures were taken daily at the beginning of the last therapy session. The raw data are not complete for each therapy day since I missed six meetings due to illness or due to administrative necessity, and eight patients missed a total of 29 more meetings. For each two half-hour meetings missed, a 'therapy day' was subtracted from the patient's record.

Results

The means, ranges, and standard deviations which will be reported for all skills are for the twentieth day. In addition, since the patients were seen as often as three times daily in an in-patient setting, caution should be used in trying to generalize about the speed with which patients in other settings should acquire esophageal speech.

Figure 3 describes the 'therapy days' it took for the good and poor speakers

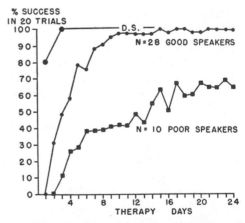

FIGURE 3. Per cent successful phonation of [a] in 20 trials.

to master the skill of phonating on demand. The line labeled D.S. describes the performance of a speaker who learned exceptionally fast. It should be noted that all the good speakers acquired and maintained this skill at virtually the 100 per cent level of success by 10 to 14 days. In skill *a*, the good speakers showed a mean of 100 per cent and, of course, no range or standard deviation. The poor speakers showed a mean of 68 per cent, a range of 15 per cent to 100 per cent and a standard deviation of 22 per cent.

Figure 4 shows the development of 0.2 secs latency by the good speakers.

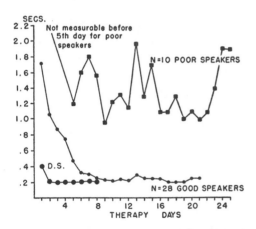

FIGURE 4. Latency between inflation and phonation [ɑ].

This agrees with the findings of Damste' (2) and Snidecor (8, pp. 77), who report 0.17 secs and 0.45 secs, respectively. Two of the poor speakers were able to get rapid inflation only by preceding the vowel with an audible plosive consonant. However, their durations for [ɑ] were less than 1.2 secs. At the twentieth day, the good speakers showed a mean latency of

0.24 secs, with almost no range or variablity (r = 0.2 - 0.6 secs, s.d. = .03 secs). In contrast, poor speakers had a mean latency of as high as 1.3 secs, a range of from 0.2-2.0 secs, and a standard deviation of 0.88 secs.

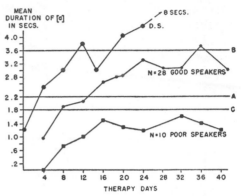

FIGURE 5. Sustained duration of vowel [ɑ] per inflation.

Figure 5 shows the development of the skill of the good and the poor speakers in sustaining the duration of the vowel [ɑ]. Note that the range of duration for the good speakers is between 2.2 secs (Line A) and 3.6 secs (Line B) and a longer duration did not appear to be necessary for good speech. Once a patient surpassed 1.8 secs (Line C), it seemed to prognosticate well for his ultimate development of good esophageal speech. The good speakers presented a mean duration of [ɑ] of 2.8 secs, a range of from 1.8-4.0 secs and an SD of .52 secs. In contrast the poor speakers showed a mean of 1.3 secs, a range of from 0.4-1.6 secs, and a standard deviation of 0.8 secs. Patient D.S., the exceptionally fast learner, ultimately could prolong [ɑ] for up to 8 secs. However, the author did not see this patient speak in phrases that lasted for more than three or four secs without using some form of overt re-inflation.

Figure 6 shows the number of plosive syllables spoken by patients using only

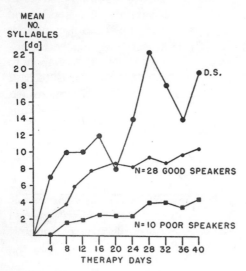

FIGURE 6. Number of syllables [dɑ] per overt inflation.

one overt inflation. For most patients, the duration of [ɑ], per inflation, was less than the elapsed time of repeated syllable articulation, per inflation. This agrees with the observations of Diedrich[2] and Moolenaar-Bijl (6) that some form of air conservation or reinjection is accomplished through the use of a plosive consonant. The measurements from which the latter observations were made may prove to be fruitful enough to merit a separate report. In this final skill the good speakers produced a mean of 8.6 syllables, with a range of from 4-14 syllables and a

standard deviation of 2.24 syllables. The poor speakers showed a mean of only 2.3 syllables, with a range of 0-5 syllables and a standard deviation of 0.8.

Sixteen patients were selected to check the stability of the skills themselves within a given therapy day. The measurements on these patients were taken twice instead of once at the last meeting of the day. These were called the A and B measurements. One three-minute rest period was allowed between the taking of the A and B measures. At the end of the patient's stay, all the data for the A and B trials were plotted and the curves appeared to agree well for 14 of these patients. Two patients showed divergent curves, where the B measures were consistently poorer than the A measures. These were both poor-speaking patients who complained often of fatigue.

Discussion

These measures were designed to chart progress in the early stages of development of esophageal speech. They were not intended to rank or rate adequacy of communication via esophageal speech. The measures are too artificial for such purposes since they do not consider dimensions such as fundamental pitch, articulation, inflection, rate, phrasing, language structure, gestures, facial expressions, stoma noise, etc. On the other hand, taking these measures at each therapy session seemed to clarify for the patients some of the dimensions needed for esophageal speech, (9). In addition, the measures were helpful in reinforcing laryngectomees for very small gains. The early graphic successes, which

[2]Personal communication with the author by Dr. William Diedrich, University of Kansas Medical Center, Kansas City, Kansas, 1962.

usually followed even the briefest practice at a skill, seemed to keep the patients from striving for complete communication prematurely. Such early reinforcement appeared to reduce the frustrations of patients who may ordinarily have had to work toward a remote, sometimes obscure, set of goals without being rewarded for daily and intermediate successes.

It should be noted that, with certain laryngectomees, inflation and articulation seemed to occur almost simultaneously. Such patients seemed to use plosive consonants to inflate and to reinflate the esophagus via the backpressure of the consonant as described by Moolenaar-Bijl (6). The author believes that the smoothest esophageal speakers he has seen have used a combination of one initial major inflation followed by a series of small consonant-linked reinflations to maintain the smooth flow of speech. With these patients, a large reservoir of air did not appear to be necessary. They needed only to make the initial investment of air and to replenish it during speech. Such patients usually found it difficult to phonate [ɑ] alone without preceding it with some form of plosive consonant. If they were good speakers, they also showed moderate durations (2½-3½ secs) for the phonation of [ɑ] in isolation.

An unexpected dividend was also realized. While most of the patients maintained or improved their skills after discharge, three patients who came in for follow-up showed a marked reduction in skill c. They maintained [ɑ] about half as long as before. Two of these patients were later found to have a recurrence of Ca. in the region of the esophagus and the third had an acute exacerbation of alcoholism followed by pneumonia. This finding will be the subject of a later report.

To the author, the essentials of these findings are that a good esophageal speaker learns to get his air charges in quickly, (in roughly 0.2 secs), and can sustain his phonation for periods of at least 2.2 secs. In connected discourse, he may not be called upon to use this much skill but he seems to have it available on demand. Furthermore, those patients who did well at the four skills were judged to have good esophageal speech.

Summary

The skills of 38 laryngectomees (28 good speakers and 10 poor speakers) were measured in these dimensions:

a. Ability to phonate reliably on demand.

b. Maintenance of a short latency between inflation of the esophagus and vocalization.

c. Maintenance of an adequate duration of phonation.

d. Ability to sustain phonation during articulation.

It was shown that performance on these skills could be measured accurately and reliably by a clinician using a stop watch and a marker.

It should be noted that patients were seen two to three times daily, for half-hour meetings. Those patients who developed into good speakers could:

a. Phonate virtually 100 per cent of the time on demand, after 10 to 14 days.

b. Maintain a latency of approximately 0.2-0.6 secs between inflation and phonation, by the eighteenth day.

c. Sustain the vowel [ɑ] for 2.2 secs

to 3.6 secs, by the twenty-fourth day.

d. Phonate eight to 10 plosive syllables per overt inflation after 25 days.

Two patients who returned for follow-up, and showed marked reduction in skill c, had recurrences of Ca. in the esophageal area. A third patient also showed sharp reduction of skill c and was found to be suffering from acute alcoholism and pneumonia.

The limitations of these measurements for rating and ranking esophageal speakers were also discussed.

Acknowledgments

The author is indebted to Dr. Mark Ross for the suggestion of using the B&K analyzer as an external criterion and for the acquisition of some of the records. Thanks are also due to Drs. Lyman Barrett, Joseph Chaiklin, Ira Ventry, Bob R. Alford and Elias Adamopoulos, and to Fred Garbee, Jeanette Filbert, Josephine Wilson, John Carter and Eolin Kuper, all of whom acted as judges. The author also acknowledges the courtesy of the Stanford University Department of Audiology and Speech Pathology in making B&K recorder time available.

References

1. ANDERSON, J. O., A descriptive study of elements of esophageal speech. Unpub. Ph.D. dissertation, Ohio State Univ., 1951.

2. DAMSTE', P. H., Oesophageal speech. Ned T. Geneesk., 101, 1957, 1784-1786.

3. DI CARLO, L., AMSTER, W., and HERER, G., Speech After Laryngectomy. Syracuse, New York: Syracuse Univ. Press, 1956.

4. DIEDRICH, W., and YOUNGSTROM, K., A cineradiographic study of the pseudoglottis in laryngectomized patients. American Speech and Hearing Association Convention paper, Los Angeles, 1960.

5. HYMAN, M., A rating scale for esophageal speech. Presented at the Sixth Postgraduate Course in Disorders of Voice and Speech and Esophageal Speech, Miami, Florida, June 20-24, 1960.

6. MOOLENAAR-BIJL, ANNIE, The importance of certain consonants in esophageal voice after laryngectomy. Ann. Otol., Rhin. and Laryng., 1953, 62, 979-989.

7. SCHAEF, R., The use of questions to elicit stuttering adaptation. J. Speech Hearing Dis., 20, 1955, 262-265.

8. SNIDECOR, J., Speech Rehabilitation of the Laryngectomized. Springfield, Ill.: American Lecture Series, Charles C. Thomas, 1962.

9. WEPMAN, J. M., MacGAHAN, J. A., RICKARD, J. C., and SHELTON, N. W., The objective measurement of progressive esophageal speech development. J. Speech Hearing Dis., 18, 1953, 247-251.

Clinical Measurement During the Acquisition of Esophageal Speech:

II. An Unexpected Dividend

Charles I. Berlin

Dean H. Zo Bell

Valid and reliable techniques have been reported (Berlin, 1963) with which a clinician can measure a patient's progress in certain specific skills related to esophageal speech. This report is being presented because three patients presented an unexpected change in their performance of one of the skills, and it was subsequently observed that this change may have been an early sign of recurrence of cancer in the hypopharyngeal area.

Review of Measures. In the study cited above, 38 laryngectomees (28 good speakers, 10 poor speakers) were followed during their inpatient experience with esophageal speech training. The patients were studied as they developed the following four skills:

a. Ability to phonate reliably on demand.

b. Ability to demonstrate short latency between inflation of the esophagus and vocalization.

c. Ability to maintain an adequate duration of phonation on [a].

d. Ability to sustain phonation during articulation.

The three subjects of this report showed marked changes only on Skill C. Therefore, the method of measurement of that particular skill is presented: Each patient was asked to phonate a single vowel, [a], and to sustain it for as long as possible. He was permitted only one inflation per trial. Ten trials were made, and the mean duration was recorded by the examiner using a stopwatch. Accuracy of this method of recording was verified by the use of a high quality sound level recorder.

Observations. Table 1 is presented to indicate the progress of three patients in whom cancer recurred at or near the esophagus. Their progress is compared with the progress of three other subjects roughly matched on the basis of age, and matched for speech proficiency scores and use of an artificial larynx. This table shows that the three patients in question presented a marked and, at the time, unexplained decrement in their ability to sustain [a][1], while the performance of the comparison subjects remained stable.

---

[1] The use of the electrolarynx should not be held exclusively responsible for the loss of Skill C since two of the comparison patients used electrolarynges but were able to maintain their limited abilities to phonate and sustain [a]. In addition, the ability to sustain an [a] (at approximate levels attained by the time of hospital discharge) was maintained by six other patients who used electrolarynges.

Reprinted by permission from *Journal of Speech and Hearing Disorders*, 1963, *28*, 389–392.

TABLE 1. Duration of [a] in seconds for the three patients with recurrences and three other patients selected from the parent population of 38 (Berlin, 1963) for purposes of comparison.

	Patient	Age	Speaker Group	El Larynx	10th Day	20th Day	1st Follow-up	2nd Follow-up	3rd Follow-up	4th Follow-up
			Inpatient				*Outpatient*			
Subjects	S.O.N.	47	Poor	Yes	0.8	1.0	1.4	1.2	0.4	...
	A.H.	46	Poor	Yes	1.0	1.8	2.2	0.8	...	...
	A.R.L.	55	Good	No	1.4	2.8	3.0	3.2	3.0	0.8
Comparison Subjects	D.P.	50	Poor	Yes	0.8	2.0	1.6	1.4	1.6	1.4
	J.R.	49	Poor	Yes	0.6	0.8	0.8	1.0	1.0	1.2
	J.H.	48	Good	No	2.2	2.0	2.0	2.4	2.6	2.8

Patient S.O.N., a 47-year-old white male fireman, was first seen 10-8-59 with a history of onset of hoarseness 10 months prior. Two months after the onset of hoarseness he had been seen by a private otolaryngologist who made the diagnosis of carcinoma of the larynx, involving the right vocal cord. The patient was treated with 5000 r. x ray to the larynx. There were no symptoms, until he had recurrence of hoarseness one month prior to this admission. Examination revealed an ulcerated area involving the anterior portion of both vocal cords. Biopsy showed squamous cell carcinoma.

The patient had a laryngectomy and left radical neck dissection on 10-27-59 with a smooth postoperative course. On 12-5-59, a right radical neck dissection was performed. Healing was as before, but the patient was troubled with more than usual postoperative edema of the face.

The patient developed his own buccal speech following the laryngectomy. On approximately 1-1-60, he was started on esophageal speech training, and progressed rather slowly, with frequent mental depression. On a routine check,

4-28-60, he showed a marked loss of his already limited facility with Skill C (see Table 1). Subsequently, on 5-6-60, the patient was readmitted to the hospital with a one-week history of a nodule which was on the posterior tracheal wall, approximately 1 cm from the skin junction. Biopsy showed cells related to chronic inflammation.

On 7-2-60, the patient was readmitted with a tracheo-esophageal fistula, passing through a mass on the right side of the tracheal stoma, approximately 1 cm from the cutaneous border. Biopsy showed squamous cell carcinoma.

The patient was then in and out of the hospital several times with continuous enlargement of this tumor mass. He expired at home due to hemorrhage from the tumor.

Patient A. H., a 46-year-old white male, was first admitted on 7-7-60, with a history of increasing hoarseness for two years. Two weeks prior to admission, he began having shortness of breath and difficulty swallowing solid foods. Examination revealed a large lesion of the left vocal cord with extension to the false cord, subglottic, and to the right cord. Biopsy showed squamous cell carcinoma.

On 7-19-60, a laryngectomy and left radical neck dissection was performed. The postoperative course was complicated by the development of an esophageal-cutaneous fistula and infection requiring isolation technique treatment for one month. On 11-1-60, a right radical neck dissection was performed.

The patient continued to follow up on an outpatient basis in the Ear, Nose, and Throat and the Speech Pathology Clinics. On 2-17-61, he showed marked reduction in Skill C, but would not stay for additional study. His speech had been poor from the start.

On 3-15-61, the patient was readmitted for 3 days because of hemoptysis. Examination revealed a friable tumor mass 4-5 cm from the tracheo-cutaneous border on the left. The patient was treated with 1600 r x ray in an attempt to shrink the tumor mass.

On 4-4-61, the patient developed a tracheo-esophageal fistula. He expired 5-1-61 with bleeding from the tumor mass into the trachea.

Patient A.R.L., a 55-year-old white male builder, was admitted on 11-16-59, with a history of progressive hoarseness and pain in the throat of four months duration. Examination revealed a tumor mass of the left aryepiglottic fold and pyriform sinus, with a 1.5 cm node in the left submaxillary region. Biopsy of the larynx showed a squamous cell carcinoma.

On 11-16-59, a laryngectomy and left radical neck dissection was done. The postoperative course was complicated by the development of a pharyngo-cutaneous fistula which

healed after five days. Pathology study showed probable transection of tumor in the inferior pharyngeal region.

The patient was readmitted to the hospital on 1-4-60 and received x-ray therapy to the hypo-pharyngeal region, with a 4400 r. tumor dose. During this time, he also attended daily speech meetings and learned easily and well.

On 6-6-60, he was found to have a marked reduction of speech ability and Skill C. Therefore, the patient was readmitted for further intensive speech training because of this recent decline in ability. Chest x ray on 6-29-60 revealed a left pleural effusion with subsequent cytology and bronchoscopic studies unrevealing. Shortly thereafter, the patient became markedly depressed and disoriented, presumably due to diffuse metastatic disease. On 9-30-60 biopsy of the left eighth rib revealed squamous cell carcinoma. The patient continued to decline gradually and expired on 11-1-60.

Discussion. These were not the only laryngectomized patients in our caseload who expired during the period that this study was being carried out (January, 1960-December, 1961). However, to the best of our knowledge, no other patients suffered disease processes which affected control of the pseudoglottis; and no other patients showed loss of Skill C.

It would seem that, since Skill C is related to speech, the clinician could simply watch for changes in speech during followup meetings. However, although many patients did not have sufficient esophageal speech to evaluate, they were able to sustain [a] for as long as 1.0 to 1.5 secs. Therefore, Skill

C could be tested even in those patients who were not speaking.

BERLIN, C. I., Clinical measurement during the acquisition of esophageal speech: I. Methodology and curves of skill acquisition. *J. Speech Hearing Dis.*, 1, 1963, 42-51.

*Johns Hopkins Hospital
    and
Naval Hospital, Key West*

Clinical Measurement of Esophageal Speech:
III. Performance of Non-Biased Groups

CHARLES I. BERLIN

A specific thesis has been proposed throughout this series of studies: Berlin, 1963a; Berlin and Zo Bell, 1963. Those who ultimately become good-speaking laryngectomees identify themselves early in treatment by successfully performing the following skills:

1. Phonating reliably on demand.

2. Maintaining a short latency between inflation of the esophagus and vocalization.

3. Maintaining an adequate duration of phonation.

4. Sustaining phonation during articulation.

In our experience, the daily measurements of these skills have reinforced small gains made by the patients and reduced the frustrations of working toward remote, sometimes obscure, goals; however, most of our experience, including that reported in the preceding two studies of this series (Berlin, 1963a; Berlin and Zo Bell, 1963) were with the author's own cases. This relationship could have been a source of bias. For example, we might unconsciously have positively reinforced patients who did well on the measures and negatively reinforced patients who did poorly. The present experiments study patients not trained by the author, in an effort to study further the predictive efficiency of the above skills and to assess the possibility that selective reinforcement was responsible for the results obtained in the earlier studies.

Two unique subgroups of laryngectomized patients became available for study. Members of the first group were laryngectomees who had problems ranging from tic douloureux to hearing loss, and data on these subjects are presented at the end of the first experiment. The second experiment studied subjects who used consonant-linked re-inflations to replenish their esophageal air supply during connected speech (van den Berg, 1958).

Three purposes, then, motivated this work.

1. To study esophageal speech skill performances in a group of subjects unbiased by having been the author's patients.

2. To study the effects of complicating problems (that is, dysarthria, hear-

Charles I. Berlin (Ph.D., University of Pittsburgh, 1958) is Assistant Professor of Otolaryngology at the Johns Hopkins Hospital of Baltimore, Maryland. The completion of this study was supported by NINDB Research Career Development Award 1-K3-NB-19488-01. Parts of this paper were presented at the 1964 Convention of the American Speech and Hearing Association.

Reprinted by permission from *Journal of Speech and Hearing Disorders*, 1965, *30*, 174–183.

ing loss, tic douloureux, etc.) on speech acceptability scores and the performance of the four basic skills.

3. To study these skills in speakers who used consonant-linked re-inflations.

EXPERIMENT 1

Procedure

Subjects. Sixty-two laryngectomees attending the 1961 convention of the International Association of Laryngectomees, volunteered to act as subjects. The 51 males reported a mean age of 58, and the 11 females reported a mean age of 53. The sampling was somewhat restricted since these people had been chosen to attend the convention by their respective lost-chord clubs, or had been sufficiently motivated and funded to attend at their own expense.

Subject Classification. Each subject's speech was rated on the basis of recordings made in response to a standardized interview (Schaef, 1955) and a TAT picture (Berlin, 1963a). Twenty-five speech and hearing students in training rated the samples on a seven-point scale. The students were told to use a rating of one to represent "highly acceptable esophageal speech," and to use a rating of seven to mean "unacceptable esophageal speech." At the close of the rating sessions the students were asked to list the qualities on which they based their ratings. The qualities reported most often were:

1. Intelligibility and clarity of articulation.
2. Lack of air (stoma) noise.
3. Relaxed sound, no strain in voice.
4. Fluency in going from phrase to phrase.

Four classes of subjects were obtained from these ratings: (1) Very good speakers (N=30) were operationally defined as those who were rated from one to 2.5; (2) adequate speakers (N=14) who were operationally defined as those rated from 2.6 to 4; (3) very poor speakers (N=12) who were defined as those rated from 5 to 7; and (4) six speakers with special problems. The criteria for separating the fourth group will be discussed in a later section.

Twenty-four of the very good speakers were male and six were female. These subjects ranged in age from 39 to 73 years, with a mean of 50, and a standard deviation of 9.86 years. They were 5.5 years postoperative (Range= 1.5-16, SD=4.41) at the time of the study (August 1961).

The acceptable speakers (12 males, 2 females) averaged 54.5 years old (Range=40-70, SD=9.24), and were five years postoperative (Range=0.2-11.3, SD=3.8).

The poor speakers (ten males, two females) averaged 57.8 years old, (Range=49-72, SD=15.95) and were 1.8 years postoperative (Range=0.5-4.0, SD=1.23).

The good speakers had spent significantly more postoperative years than had the poor speakers ($t=6.53$), but the mean ages of the group did not differ significantly.

Rater Reliability. Test-retest rater reliability could not be assessed. However, the samples were rerated by 19 judges (three experienced speech pathologists, two otolaryngologists, and 14 laryngectomees). The Pearson r correlation of the latter ratings with the student ratings was 0.84.

Data Collection. A Wollensak T-1500 tape recorder, at 7½ ips, was used to make the recordings in two carpeted and draped rooms of the Jack Tar Hotel. The tip of the standard crystal microphone was held at the zygomatic bone since perceptibly less stoma noise is recorded with the microphone in this position than if the microphone is placed in line with the stoma blast. The subjects were interviewed, asked to respond to the TAT pictures, and then, after a brief rest, were asked to perform these tasks:

1. Phonate /ɑ/ and hold it as long as possible. Twenty trials were given.

2. Repeat /dɑ/ as many times as possible without consciously re-inflating the esophagus. Ten trials were given.

An analysis of the importance of consonant-linked re-inflation can be found in the works of van den Berg et al. (1958), while rationale for the choice of these skills to obtain the measurements can be found in the first work of this series (Berlin, 1963a).

Data Extraction. A Brujl and Kjaer octave band analyzer, Model 2107, adjusted to make intensity level recordings, with paper speed of 30 mm per second and pen speed at 500 mm per second, was used to study the tape recordings. Illustrations of the graphic recordings, criteria for measuring onset and cessation of syllables, vocalization, etc., were presented earlier (Berlin, 1963a).

Data on duration of /ɑ/, number of syllables of /dɑ/, latency between inflation and vocalization, and number of successful vocalizations, were extracted from graphic records by the experimenter and an independent observer. Since time data were recorded only to the tenth of a second, no disagreement between readers of greater than 0.2 secs was tolerated. Nine conditions arose where the two readers disagreed by 0.2

secs or more, and a mean time was recorded in these cases. In contrast, the number of syllables was recorded in whole numbers. Since very strict acoustic criteria were set for a successfully articulated syllable, there were only two disagreements between the readers, and these were resolved by listening to the tapes. It was then agreed that the subjects had articulated the syllables in question, but they had done so voicelessly. Here, the human ear was a better judge of whether a syllable was both articulated and phonated than was the B&K instrument set as a broad band level recorder.

The following measures were obtained for each subject:

1. His mean percent of successful vocalization of /ɑ/ in 20 trials.

2. His mean latency between inflation and phonation of /ɑ/.

3. His mean duration of /ɑ/ over 20 trials.

4. His mean number of /dɑ/ syllables per overt inflation.

Problems of Measurement of Latency

In the first work of this series, the author measured latency crudely with a stop watch, and reported that good speakers had latencies of roughly 0.2 secs. Since Snidecor had reported latencies of 0.4 secs (1962, p. 77), the author tried to use the presumably greater accuracy of the B&K recorder to resolve the latency differences between his own work and Snidecor's work. Unfortunately, in this experiment, latency measurements could not be made from all the subjects' charts. First, many patients made no audible inflation noise; therefore, the records

TABLE 1. Means, ranges, and standard deviations of the performance of three esophageal speech groups on the four measures of esophageal speech skill.

Skill	Speaker Groups		
	Very Good (N=30)	Adequate (N=14)	Poor (N=12)
Mean per cent vocalization in 20 trials	100	100	88.1
Range			75-100
SD			8.03
Mean latency between inflation and vocalization	0.46*	0.40*	0.47*
Range	0.23-1.01	0.27-0.74	0.31-0.73
SD	0.24	0.13	0.13
Mean duration of /ɑ/	2.37	1.93	0.98
Range	1.30-5.53	1.31-4.63	0.42-1.61
SD	1.08	0.34	0.37
No. syllables of /dɑ/ per single overt inflation	10.52	7.88	3.99
Range	5.6-23.1	5.4-14	1.8-6.4
SD	3.69	3.53	1.40

*Mean latencies for very good, adequate, and poor speakers are based upon Ns of 13, 11, and 7 respectively.

of their phonations showed no activity just prior to vocalization. Other patients had such long latencies that extraneous sounds contaminated the records and a reader couldn't tell which marks on the record referred to inflation noise, or which charted unrelated signals. The experimenter and the independent judge clearly agree on which prephonation mark represented the noise of inflation by listening to the recordings while watching reruns on the level recorder. For some patients, of course, latency data could not be extracted; therefore, an entry was made in the latency category of Table 1 to show the number of subjects on whom latency data could be measured from the charts.

Results

The mean scores of three of the groups on the measures of esophageal speech skill are reported in Table 1. The adequate speakers and the very good speakers performed as a homogeneous group on these measures. No statistically significant differences were found.[1] Thus, skills which separate an adequate speaker from a very good speaker were not the four skills studied in this work.

The poor speakers were significantly poorer than either the good speakers or the adequate speakers on the skills measuring ability to phonate reliably, sustain phonation, and maintain articulation

[1] All results reported were obtained at the one per cent level of confidence by two types of t tests. The test used most commonly was designed for groups which have different variances and Ns and was described by Li (1957, p. 128); he presents a special technique for assessing the degrees of freedom at which one should enter the t distribution. The more conventional t test was used where groups had similar Ns and homogeneous variance.

during phonation. However, all of the groups scored alike on the measures of latency between inflation and vocalization. This was the only observation not consistent with the previous work.

Agreement with Previous Work. The subjects' performances of skills 1, 3, and 4 agreed well with the measurements done on the esophageal speech of the author's own patients (Berlin, 1963a). But the values for latency did not agree well with those of the first work, since both the good speakers and the poor speakers in the present study showed roughly 0.4 secs latencies between inflation and vocalization, while latency in poor speakers was first reported as 1.3 secs with a range from 0.2 to 2.0 secs, and a standard deviation of 0.88 secs. The problems of latency measurement described earlier may account for some of the differences between the works. Further error may have been introduced in the first study by including some very long latencies produced by patients who were just learning to phonate. Third, subjects of this study were not the author's pa-

tients and some may have learned esophageal speech by using small latencies between inflation and phonation from the very beginning of their training (van den Berg et al., 1958). In sum, the latencies found agree more with Snidecor's work than with the author's earlier work.

Clinical Implications

Good esophageal speakers, not biased by training with the author, phonated reliably on demand. They sustained the vowel /ɑ/ for roughly two seconds and repeated approximately ten syllables per inflation. This suggests that these skills are basic to any form of esophageal speech and should be taught to, or at least learned by, beginning laryngectomees. Although maintaining a short latency between inflation and phonation is probably important to good esophageal speech, it was not a skill found exclusively in the good esophageal speakers of this study.

TABLE 2. Performance of special group on esophageal speech skills. All were rated as poor speakers, and all had 100% vocalization-on-demand scores.

Problem	Age	Sex	Years Post Op.	Means*	Mean duration /ɑ/	Mean duration /dɑ/
Dialect, hearing loss	63	M	9	0.36	3.15	10.00
Dialect, hearing loss	49	M	3	†	1.52	4.2
Hearing loss	56	M	2	0.61	2.63	10.06
Dysarthria	64	M	1.3	0.47	2.73	8.3
Tic douloureux	72	M	9	0.53	2.08	8.1
Infant. artic.	5	F	1	0.60	1.20	3.0

*In seconds.
†Not measurable.

The Laryngectomees with Special Problems

This group was composed of a five-year-old girl[2] with articulatory errors (/θ/ for /s/ and /w/ for /r/ substitutions, /w/ for /l/ substitutions, and misarticulation of most blends), a seventy-two-year-old male with a history of tic douloureux, one man with bilateral sensory-neural hearing loss, two men with foreign accents and hearing losses, and one man with both facial and palatal pareses and concomitant dysarthria.

The mean scores obtained by each of these subjects on the skills are shown in Table 2. The performance skills for these subjects appear to be those of good speakers, but these laryngectomees were all rated by listeners as poor speakers. This observation points to the limited relationship the four skills have to the adequacy of esophageal speech, as a global skill. Good speakers all performed well on these skills, but good performance on the skills did not guarantee that their esophageal speech would be rated high. The author's clinical observation suggests that additional measures of articulation, phrasing, range of inflection, linguistic structure, and fundamental frequency may serve as parameters on which to base predictions of esophageal speech success.

EXPERIMENT 2

Esophageal speakers do not either need or use a major air reservoir for speech in the way that normal speakers do; certain patients apparently can re-inflate the esophagus with small charges of air during connected speech (Berlin, 1963a; Berlin, 1963b; Diedrich, 1960; Snidecor, pp. 115-116, 1962; Moolenaar-Bijl, 1953; McClear, 1963; van den Berg, 1958). The purpose of this experiment was to investigate the ability of such patients to maintain articulation without stopping for repeated overt re-inflations.

Procedure

Subjects. Ten very good speakers in the first study appeared to the author to use consonant-linked re-inflations.[3] The data from these subjects were reanalyzed in two dimensions:

1. The duration during which the speakers had sustained /ɑ/ while they had no chance to re-inflate.

2. The elapsed time during which the speakers maintained the repetitive articulation of /dɑ/. The subjects were asked to repeat as many /dɑ/s as possible on one inflation, at maximum rate.

The scores on the first measure were subtracted from the scores on the second measure to get an estimate of the talking time gained by the use of a plosive syllable.

These data were compared with scores taken from ten other good speakers who appeared to use a major air reservoir which they filled once,

---

[2] Her larynx was taken because of rhabdomyosarcoma.

[3] These speakers were chosen on the basis of the author's observation of their connected speech, some of their teaching methods (eight of the ten multiple-inflation subjects are esophageal speech instructors while only two of the single-inflation speakers are professional instructors), and the repeated appearance of an air sac in the upper esophageal area during articulation of consonants.

TABLE 3. Comparison of multiple-inflation with single-inflation speakers.

Speaker	Sex	Mean duration /a/	Mean duration /da/	/da/—/a/
		Multiple Inflation Group		
W.W.*	M	1.80	2.54	0.74
E.McQ.*	F	5.53	76.35†	>2.00
A.L.*	F	1.59	2.54	0.95
J.H.*	M	1.78	3.23	1.45
E.W.*	F	1.39	1.71	0.32
E.T.	M	1.29	1.83	0.54
J.McC.*	M	2.96	4.20	1.24
A.R.*	M	1.43	2.13	0.70
W.P.	M	4.36	7.45	3.09
H.W.*	F	2.74	3.60	0.86
Means		2.49	3.69	1.19
		Single Inflation Group		
T.T.	F	2.34	2.50	0.16
M.H.*	M	2.62	2.97	0.35
E.W.	M	3.40	3.77	0.37
D.S.	M	3.50	3.45	−0.05
V.P.	M	1.71	1.87	0.16
J.F.	M	2.22	2.27	0.05
E.F.	M	2.14	2.16	0.02
B.H.	M	2.18	2.20	0.02
B.W.	M	2.34	2.44	0.10
J.McK*	M	2.34	2.19	−0.15
Means		2.48	2.58	0.10

*Esophageal speech instructor.

†Patient could have continued—was stopped by experimenter. She used no major inflation—just started talking. Her score of 76.35 secs was scored as simply 7.63 seconds to keep from skewing the multiple inflation speaker data.

appeared to exhaust, and then filled again when necessary. (These subjects will be called "single-inflation speakers" while those in the first group will be called "multiple-inflation speakers".)

Results

Table 3 shows that the multiple-inflation speakers maintained /da/ repetitions for a longer period of time than did the single-inflation speakers. A small time difference in favor of the duration of the repetition of /da/ was to be ex-pected, since during the repetition there were brief silent periods between syllables. However, note the exceptional performance of multiple-inflation subject E. McQ. who simply began to repeat /da/ with no apparent major inflation, and could have repeated /da/ far past the 75 secs recorded had the examiner not stopped her. She was scored as having a /da/ vs. /a/ difference time of "greater than two seconds" to prevent undue skewing of the multiple inflation speaker data. Inspection of the raw /da/ vs. /a/ times shows far more than common statistical analysis could transmit. Speaker E. W. had the smallest /dɑ/ vs. /ɑ/ time difference shown by a subject of the multiple-inflation group (0.32 secs), but his score is almost as large as the greatest difference shown by any subject in the single-inflation group (M.H. 0.35, E.W. 0.37, and B.W. 0.10). In addition, multiple-inflation speaker E. W. had increased his phonation time by 23% using the consonant-linked syllable, while the best single-inflation speakers increased their phonation times by only 13% using /dɑ/.

Discussion

Cinefluorographic techniques offer a more direct measurement of the effect of consonant-linked re-inflations; however, this /dɑ/ vs. /ɑ/ timing method offers easily obtainable but indirect evidence of the extent to which a laryngectomee can use consonant-linked re-inflations to prolong his talking time. Other consonants, such as /s/, /tʃ/, /dʒ/, /t/, /p/, /k/, and particularly the /st/ blends have been used for the purposes of re-inflation (Berlin, 1963b) and must be studied in more detail.

Clinicians should note that multiple inflation may be one secret underlying the ease with which some laryngectomees talk for long periods of time, free from symptoms of hyperventilation and apparently free from fatigue. Normal speakers use a single reservoir of air until it runs out; some laryngectomees replenish their air supply for speech by the act of speech itself. Such inflation during speech is a skill foreign to speakers with a normal larynx and must be taught to, or at least explained to, patients who may have difficulty in ac-

quiring adequate duration of phonation by the more "logical" methods based on the major reservoir principle. Teaching a patient to take a single inflation for each cycle of phonation, and to use all his esophageal air before he re-inflates, is probably not as conducive to fluent esophageal speech as has been suggested (Di Carlo et al., 1955, p. 164). It is quite probable that many good esophageal speakers use two or three methods of air intake during any given speaking period, depending upon the context during which it becomes necessary to have more air for speech. Clinicians interested in esophageal speech technique should be willing to positively re-inforce those air-intake methods which lead to smooth, uninterrupted, effortless esophageal speech.

Good clinical management requires consideration of many other special problems of the laryngectomee. For example, hearing is one of the least studied yet most crucial factors in the acquisition of esophageal speech (Berlin, 1964). In the present studies, the hearing of the subjects could not be tested; however, in the first work of the series (Berlin, 1963a) it was noted that four out of ten poor-speaking laryngectomees had significant hearing losses (SRT greater than 20 dB and discrimination of 88% or less) and Shames et al. (1963) reported that 17% of their poor speakers believed they had hearing losses.

The effects of a hearing loss on learning and monitoring esophageal speech need not be stressed here. Speech clinicians are especially aware that a high tone sensory-neural loss with reduced discrimination is one of the most common audiograms seen in older patients. A patient with such a loss might complain that he has difficulty understanding rapidly shifting conversations in group situations or in noisy environments. If such a recent laryngectomee is to be taught esophageal speech in a group, he is already at a disadvantage compared to a normal-hearing contemporary. Laryngectomized patients with hearing losses, dysarthrias, personal problems relating to alcoholism and financial catastrophes, need professional services of people working in, or affiliated with, medical and social agencies. It follows that physicians and hearing and speech specialists should meet their clinical and scientific responsibilities to the laryngectomized by helping any lay teachers in the community to identify and compensate for such problems. Further discussion of these complications, directed. primarily toward the physician, may be found elsewhere (Berlin, 1964).

Summary

Studies of 62 laryngectomees (30 very good speakers, 14 adequate speakers, 12 poor speakers, and 6 speakers with special problems) non-biased by any clinical training administered by the author, showed that:

1. Good and adequate speakers phonated virtually 100% of the time on demand; poor speakers could not always phonate on demand.

2. Good speakers sustained the vowel /a/ for an average of 2.37 secs. Adequate speakers showed similar skills, but poor speakers had significantly poorer phonation times (M=0.98 secs).

3. Very good speakers averaged over ten syllables of /a/ on a single inflation, adequate speakers nearly eight, while poor speakers could repeat less than four syllables.

4. All the groups had latency times between inflation of the esophagus and phonation of from 0.4 to 0.5 secs, although the author's earlier work had suggested that poor speakers would show 1.3 secs latencies.

5. Six laryngectomees with special problems, including a five-year-old girl, three patients with significant hearing losses (two of whom also had foreign accents), one with dysarthria and facial pareses, and one with tic douloureux, received poor speech ratings, even though they performed well on the skills. These examples showed the skills described here are limited in their ability to predict esophageal speech success.

A second experiment showed that ten speakers who used consonant-linked inflation during connected speech showed remarkably extended times of phonation, compared with patients who used the single air reservoir until it was exhausted. It was suggested that consonant-linked re-inflations may permit laryngectomees to speak for long periods of time, free from symptoms of hyperventilation and apparently free from fatigue.

Acknowledgment

I am indebted to Messrs. Jack Ross, Jack Ranney, and John McClear for their help in collecting data and acquiring subjects for this study. Thanks are due to Drs. William Castle, Clara Busch, and Dorothy Huntington, for help in processing some of the records and getting judgments on the adequacy of the esophageal speech. Appreciation is expressed to Drs. Bob R. Alford, Elias Adamopoulis, and to John Carter and Eolin Kuper, all of whom acted as judges. Special thanks go to Lowell

Kallen who helped to analyze the data records. Finally, my gratitude goes to those laryngectomees at the 1961 IAL Convention who gave of their time so that this work could be completed.

References

BERG, J. VAN DEN, MOOLENAAR-BIJL, A. J., and DAMSTÉ, P. H., Oesophageal speech. *Folia Phoniat., Basel*, 10, 2, 1958, 65-84.

BERLIN, C. I., Clinical measurement of esophageal speech, I. Methodology and curves of skill acquisition. *J. Speech Hearing Dis.*, 28, 1963a, 42-51.

BERLIN, C. I., On the use of /s/ in esophageal inflation, Letter, *J. Speech Hearing Dis.*, 28, 1963b, 208.

BERLIN, C. I., Hearing loss, palatal function and other factors in post-laryngectomy rehabilitation, *J. Chronic Dis.*, 17, 1964, 677-684.

BERLIN, C. I. and Zo BELL, D. H., Clinical measurement during the acquisition of esophageal speech: II. An unexpected dividend. *J. Speech Hearing Dis.*, 28, 1963, 389-392.

DI CARLO, L. M., AMSTER, W., and HERER, G., *Speech after Laryngectomy*. Syracuse: Syracuse Univ. Press, 1955.

DIEDRICH, W. and YOUNGSTROM, K., A cineradiographic study of the pseudo-glottis in laryngectomized patients. Paper presented at American Speech and Hearing Association convention, Los Angeles, 1960.

LI, J. C. R., *Introduction to Statistical Inference*. Ann Arbor, Mich.: Edwards Bros., 1957.

McCLEAR, J., Clinical approaches to the production of esophageal voice. Lecture presented at IAL voice institute, San Francisco, 1961.

MOOLENAAR-BIJL, A. J., Connection between consonant articulation and the intake of air in oesophageal speech. *Folia Phoniat., Basel*, 5, 1953, 212-215.

SCHAEF, R. A., The use of questions to elicit stuttering adaptation, *J. Speech Hearing Dis.*, 20, 1955, 262-265.

SHAMES, G. H., FONT, J., and MATTHEWS, J., Factors related to speech proficiency of the laryngectomized. *J. Speech Hearing Dis.*, 28, 1963, 273-287.

SNIDECOR, J., *Speech Rehabilitation of the Laryngectomized*. Springfield, Ill.: American Lecture Series, Charles C. Thomas, 1962.

Received April 13, 1964

EVALUATING ESOPHAGEAL SPEECH

Henry B. Creech

Of the several methods of communication available for the laryngectomee, esophageal speech is the most desirable method. Yet, relatively little attention has been directed to measuring the intelligibility of esophageal speech other than by subjective opinions. Subjective opinions do not yield useful measures of the speech and have been criticized by many authors, the most recent was Berlin (1963) who commented on the lack of quantification of esophageal speech.

Wepman and others (1953) rated esophageal speech on a seven-point descriptive scale from *no speech* to *automatic esophageal speech*. This scale has been found satisfactory in clinical use to indicate to the patient his progress from time to time. However, it does not provide useful samples of esophageal speech which can be used to quantify, or illustrate the various levels of proficiency of speaking.

Snidecor and Curry (1960) reported "suitable and attainable" goals for esophageal speakers. Various qualities demonstrated by superior esophageal speakers are again described, but not illustrated nor quantified.

Variables in speech proficiency of the laryngectomized were studied by Shames, Font, and Mathews (1963). The results of this study demonstrated the superiority of esophageal speech over other methods and the variables which appear to lead toward better esophageal speech are described. Although measured, the intelligibility of their speakers was not reported.

Excellent clinical studies have been reported recently by Berlin (1965) and Snidecor and Isshiki (1965) both of whom objectively measure various important aspects of esophageal speech by using equipment not generally available to the speech clinician. Unfortunately these techniques of measurement cannot be duplicated or used in everyday practice by most of the speech clinicians working with the laryngectomized.

Henry B. Creech (Ph.D., Ohio State University, 1962) is Chief, Audiology and Speech Pathology, Veterans Administration Hospital, Richmond, Virginia. This research was supported in part by a grant from the Ohio Division, American Cancer Society.

Reprinted by permission from *Journal of the Speech and Hearing Association of Virginia*, 1966, 7, 13–19.

Four specific skills of "good" esophageal speakers were quantified by Berlin (1963). As a result of his study a speech clinician can, with a minimum of equipment, measure a patient's progress and somewhat predict his ability to acquire esophageal speech. The intelligibility of his speakers was not reported, nor was it reported in his later studies: Berlin and ZoBell (1963); Berlin (1965).

There are several methods available for the quantification of speech intelligibility. Of these methods, two are in general use and are available for clinical application. One method is a scale of judgments of how intelligible a person speaks. Observers listen to selected samples of speech and assign a rating to the over-all speaking intelligibility. The judgments are then pooled to obtain an intelligibility score for each speaker. The other method is a measure of actual speaking efficiency whereby a count is made of the number of words understood by observers as compared to the total number spoken. Thus a percent intelligibility score is derived for each speaker. In this study both methods of measuring speaker intelligibility were used to quantify esophageal speech and the effectiveness of the two methods were compared.

RATINGS OF INTELLIGIBILITY

From time to time, laryngectomees enrolled in speech therapy should be made aware of their progress. A recorded scale of esophageal speech which illustrates various levels of performance, from good to poor, would be both practical and useful to demonstrate as well as measure this progress.

A scale of the auditory characteristics of esophageal speech has many applications, for example, to acquaint and train medical personnel, speech clinicians, rehabilitation workers, and experimental personnel to recognize various qualitative levels of esophageal speech. The scale can also be used to obtain criterion measures for evaluating different clinical techniques, to demonstrate individual progress in therapy, and to demonstrate, auditorily, levels of esophageal speech beyond that presently attained by the patient in therapy.

The present study employed the psychophysical method of equal-appearing intervals to scale the auditory characteristics of esophageal speech. This scaling method has been found to be reliable in rating selected aspects of speech and has been used for this purpose by experimenters to rate stuttering (Lewis and Sherman,

1951), articulation (Morrison, 1955), nasality (Sherman and Goodwin, 1954), and cleft palate speech (Spriestersbach, 1955).

Procedure. To obtain the stimulus material 48 laryngectomized esophageal speakers from various regions of Ohio read 48 speaker-lists of multiple-choice intelligibility tests, Forms A and B (Black, 1957) and the alternative Forms A'_1 and B'_1 (Black and Haagen, 1963).

Ten-second segments of the recorded material were extracted from the tapes and randomly spliced, two seconds apart. Four 10-second segments were taken from each speaker's recording.

The recorded segments of esophageal speech were played free-field to observers in a quiet classroom. The observers were 34 undergraduate students enrolled in an elementary speech course at Ohio Wesleyan University. All had only a layman's familiarity with speech problems and no experience in clinical diagnosing or therapy.

At the outset of the experimental listening session, the observers were instructed to rate the segments of speech on the nine-point equal-appearing intervals scale with *one* representing the best speech, that is the speech which is most fluent, has the best quality, and is most understandable, and *nine* representing the speech which has the poorest quality, is least fluent, and is least understandable.

Immediately following the training session, the 192 experimental segments of esophageal speech were presented in random order to the observers for rating.

Results. To evaluate the reliability of observer ratings, the intraclass correlation procedure described by Ebel (1951) was applied to the scale values. The analysis of variance indicates that observers differ significantly in their general level of rating. Thus, the between-observers variance was removed. The resulting intraclass correlation coefficient was .72. A coefficient of this magnitude is evident that values obtained by this method are quite reliable.

As a means of determining the reliability of the ratings of the segments, a split-half correlation was computed between the median values of 25 individuals who had one segment rated in the first half of the listening session, and another segment rated in the last half of the listening session. The obtained Pearson r was .97. A correlation of this magnitude would indicate that, (1) the observers were consistent in their ratings, and (2) the stimulus materials from a single source were equated in general level of merit. Thus, it is apparent that reliable estimates of esophageal speech may be obtained from sample to sample in a study of this type.

The median scale values and Q-value were computed for each segment as described by Thurston and Chave (1929). On the basis of the lowest Q-value at each nine levels, segments were selected to represent the levels on demonstration and training tapes.

These recordings have been used to demonstrate the various levels of proficiency of esophageal speakers to beginning speech clinicians and new esophageal speech patients. The recordings have been well received by both groups. The better speakers not only demonstrate higher levels of speaker proficiency but also tend to motivate the person in therapy since many recent post-laryngectomy patients have not had the opportunity to hear esophageal speech other than their own attempts or that of their speech clinician's.

TESTS OF INTELLIGIBILITY

The multiple-choice intelligibility tests, since their introduction in 1944 (Black and Haagen, 1963) have been widely used to measure speaker intelligibility. Some authors have used these tests to measure the intelligibility of esophageal speakers, the latest being McCroskey and Mulligan (1963).

The purpose of this part of the study was to see how well measures of actual speaking intelligibility compared to the ratings assigned the speakers on the equal-appearing intervals scale.

Procedure. Eleven observers, again students with only a layman's familiarity with speech problems listened to the 48 esophageal speakers read an entire list of 24 multiple-choice intelligibility test words. (The recording and listener procedures have been described previously.) Intelligibility scores were assigned to each speaker and then compared to the mean score of the rating scale values.

Results. A Kendall Rank Correlation procedure (Siegel, 1956, pp. 213-223) was used to test the relationship of the two values. A summary of the mean scale values and measures of intelligibility are shown in Table 1. An inspection of these values reveal a significant relationship between the two methods used to evaluate esophageal speech. The distribution of scale values and corresponding intelligibility scores are shown in Table 2.

TABLE 1. Comparison by test forms of mean intelligibility scores and rating scale values of 48 esophageal speakers.

	Form A	Form A$_1$	Form B	Form B$_1$
Percent Intelligibility	61.40	64.84	63.42	59.30
	r = .29**	r = .56*	r = .67*	r = .49*
Scales Ratings	3.87	4.30	4.91	3.94

**Significant beyond .06
*Significant beyond .01

TABLE 2. Distribution of rating scale values and corresponding intelligibility test scores for 48 esophageal speakers.

Rating Scale Values	Mean % Intelligibility Scores	N = 48
1	82	2
2	67	2
3	64	4
4	60	6
5	54	9
6	52	8
7	49	8
8	44	4
9	31	5

DISCUSSION

A clinician can easily determine a speaker's intelligibility by applying either of the above procedures. The patient may read a standardized list of the multiple-choice intelligibility tests (Black,

1957; Black and Haagen, 1963) and a percentage score can be obtained by comparing the words understood to those spoken. A recording made of the esophageal speech and then played to a panel of judges to obtain intelligibility scores would yield an objective measure of the speech. The recordings could then be judged for over-all intelligibility and rated on a 1-9 scale. Since the two methods are highly correlated, either method may be used. Judges of esophageal speech should be laymen since the greatest percentage of the laryngectomee's speaking time will be directed to that type of listener. Professional clinicians should be available for any critical analysis of the speech.

The mean intelligibility scores obtained in this study of 61.4, 64.8, 63.4, and 59.3 per cent compare very favorably with those obtained by McCroskey and Mulligan (1963), for student listeners of 62.9 per cent and naive listeners of 58.2 per cent.

These are very respectible intelligibility scores for the esophageal speakers when compared to the mean range of scores obtained for normal speaking persons of between 64.2 and 65.5 per cent (Black and Haagen, 1963). Apparently the over-all intelligibility for esophageal speakers is very close to 60 per cent with a mean score for excellent speakers of around 82 per cent. As an esophageal speaker approaches 60 per cent intelligibility, serious consideration should be given to dismissing him from therapy since only a small percentage of those who have successfully learned esophageal speech can ever hope to attain higher intelligibility of speech.

The results of this study can also be applied to the problem of therapists with respect to communicating with each other about the efficiency of esophageal speakers. Subjective terms such as *good, poor,* etc. are not useful measures of esophageal speech. Quantitative measures of intelligibility are professional measures and should be used as such. If one therapist judges a certain segment of speech an "8" on a nine-point scale or that a speaker is 40 per cent intelligible, the other therapists understand this value. This value does not diminish in time. The same sample of speech when quantified today will be rated, or be measured, just as intelligible a year from now. Therefore, scaled ratings of over-all intelligibility or actual percent intelligibility scores obtained by multiple-choice tests are quite meaningful and are good prefessional measures of esophageal speech.

SUMMARY

The purposes of the study were: (1) to devise a scale based upon judgments of over-all intelligibility to illustrate, auditorily, various levels of esophageal speech, and (2) to compare these scale values with measures of actual speaker intelligibility as determined by multiple-choice tests. The two methods used in this study were well correlated. This indicates that either method may be used by professional people, not only to quantify esophageal speech, but for training and clinical use as well. A mean intelligibilty score of 62.24 per cent was obtained by the esophageal speakers in this study.

REFERENCES

Berlin, C. I., Clinical measurement of esophageal speech: I. methodology and curves of skill acquisition. *J. Speech Hearing Dis.*, 20, 42-51 (1063).

Berlin, C. I., Clinical measurement of esophageal speech: III. performance of non-biased groups. *J. Speech and Hearing Dis.*, 30, 174-183 (1965).

Berlin, C. I. and ZoBell, D. H., Clinical measurement during the acquisition of esophageal speech: II. an unexpected dividend. *J. Speech Hearing Dis.*, 28, 389-392 (1963).

Black, J. W., Multiple-choice intelligibility tests. *J. Speech Hearing Dis.*, 22, 213-235 (1957).

Black, J. W. and Haagen, C. H., Multiple-choice intelligibility tests, Forms A and B. *J. Speech Hearing Dis.*, 28, 77-86 (1963).

Ebel, R. L., Estimation of the reliability of ratings. *Psychometrika*, 16 407-424 (1951).

Lewis, D. and Sherman, D., Measuring the severity of stuttering. *J. Speech Hearing Dis.*, 16, 320-326 (1951).

McCroskey, R. L. and Mulligan, M., the relative intelligibility of esophageal speech and artificial-larynx speech. *J. Speech Hearing Dis.*, 28, 37-41 (1963).

Morrison, S., Measuring the severity of articulation defectiveness. *J. Speech Hearing Dis.*, 20, 347-351 (1955)

Shames, G. H., Font, J., and Mathews, J., Factors related to speech proficiency of the laryngectomized. *J. Speech Hearing Dis.*, 28, 273-287 (1963).

Sherman, D. and Goodwin, F., Pitch Level and Nasality. *J. Speech Hearing Dis.*, 19, 423-428 (1954).

Siegel, S., Nonparametric Statistics for the Behavioral Sciences. New York: McGraw-Hill, (1956).

Snidecor, J. C. and Curry, E. T., How effectively can the laryngectomee expect to speak? Norms for effective esophageal speech. *Laryngoscope*, LXX 62-67 (1960).

Snidecor, J. C. and Isshiki, N., Air volume and air flow relationships of six male esophageal speakers. *J. Speech Hearing Dis.*, 30, 205-216 (1965).

Spriestersbach, D. C., Assessing nasal quality in cleft palate speech of children. *J. Speech Hearing Dis.*, 20, 266-270 (1955).

Thurstone, L. L. and Chave, E. J., *The Measurement of Attitude*. Chicago: (1929).

Wepman, J. M., MacGahan, J. A., Richard, J. C., and Shelton, N. W., The objective measurement of progressive esophageal speech development. *J. Speech Hearing Dis.*, 18, 247-251 (1963).

A Comparison of the Intelligibility of
Esophageal and Normal Speakers

By R. S. TIKOFSKY

Studies of the intelligibility of populations of esophageal speakers
have been reported [1, 5, 6, 7, 12]. However, these investigations do
not report direct comparisons between esophageal and normal speakers. Such comparisons might provide useful information concerning
the similarities and differences between the two populations. In addition, objective measures of intelligibility when taken with data
from acoustic phonetic analyses should afford more accurate descriptions of esophageal speech.

The most obvious difference between the two populations is in
the structures available for the phonatory act. It can be assumed
that the articulatory mechanism is not markedly altered in the
laryngectomized subject, although the interaction of the articulatory and phonatory mechanisms may differ. The effects produced by these interactions may, in part, establish the limits of
maximum proficiency for an esophageal speaker. The limits of intelligibility are also influenced by the speaker's ability to learn the skills
necessary to produce esophageal voice. Research by *Van den Berg*
[2, 3], *Damsté* [4], *Perry* [10], and others has attempted to define the
acoustic and physiologic parameters of the esophageal voice. However, it is possible to attempt to describe esophageal speech output
in terms of a listener's ability to recognize the speech signal produced
by the esophageal speaker.

Most of the studies of esophageal intelligibility cited earlier tend
to divide their populations into discrete groups: good speakers –
poor speakers. Although such an approach is useful for some analyses of intelligibility, it seems more reasonable to expect that
there will be a more continuous distribution of speakers in terms
of intelligibility and that this distribution should be normal if a

Reprinted by permission from *Folia Phoniatrica*, 1965, *17*, 19–32.

large enough population of subjects is studied. It might also be expected that there would be some, if not considerable overlap between the distributions of esophageal and normal speakers at the upper end of the esophageal curve. Casual observation of highly proficient esophageal speakers would suggest that this is in fact the case. If it is possible to define the esophageal intelligibility distribution then it should also be possible to establish a given speaker's intelligibility relative to other esophageal speakers. Establishing such a distribution would enable the therapist to estimate the extent of improvement a given subject makes as he acquires the techniques of esophageal speech.

The research reported in this paper is concerned with gross comparisons of intelligibility between esophageal and normal speakers. This study is part of a more extensive investigation of the phonetic and intelligibility characteristics of esophageal speech. The research design is similar to that employed by *Tikofsky and Tikofsky* [13] in their studies of dysarthria.

One of the primary aims of this study was to compare the intelligibility of a population of esophageal and normal speakers. Intelligibility was determined by the number of correct responses made by a group of listeners to recorded speech samples. These responses were also analyzed to determine whether there were significant differences in intelligibility between the word lists and the order in which the lists were heard by the listeners. The position of a given speaker on a particular list relative to the other speakers in the population was compared across lists in terms of his intelligibility scores. Listener responses to each word on a given list were combined to yield the total list intelligibility score. These scores were employed in the statistical analysis. Single word intelligibility analyses will be reported in a subsequent paper.

Methods

Word lists. Three word lists were recorded by each of the speakers in addition to other material to be used in other experiments. The lists were composed of 50 CNC (Consonant-Syllable Nucleus-Consonant) words; 60 monosyllabic words containing initial and/or final consonant clusters; and a set of 50 randomly selected spondee words. These lists had been previously employed by the author in studies of dysarthric intelligibility [13]. The CNC words were taken from the *Lehiste and Peterson* lists [8]. The cluster words were monosyllabic and all demanded complex consonant articulation in either the initial or final positions. In all, 160 words were used for this research.

Speakers. Nine esophageal and ten normal speakers provided the recorded material which was audited by the listeners. The esophageal speakers were selected from a larger population who were participating in other studies on esophageal speech. However, the larger group of speakers could not meet the criteria for inclusion in the intelligibility study. Only speakers who were native to the middle west or who had lived in that area prior to the time they might have established a fixed dialect pattern were included in this study. In addition, no member of either population exhibited a hearing loss as determined by audiometric screening examinations. No speech proficiency criteria were established. The nine esophageal speakers ranged in age from 38 to 65 years with a mean age of 50. All of the speakers had received instruction in esophageal speech, and had been recruited from the University of Michigan Speech Clinic's current and past patient files and through Mr. *Max Freed*, esophageal speech instructor of the Michigan Cancer Foundation. The ten normal speakers met the dialect criteria established for the esophageal speakers and were matched with them in terms of age, sex and education. Their ages ranged from 37 to 60 years with a mean age of 49.2 years.

Recording Conditions. Subjects were recorded in the recording studios of the Communication Sciences Laboratory at the University of Michigan or at the Rehabilitation Institute of Metropolitan, Detroit. The recordings were made on an Ampex 350 full track tape recorder using a 633A Altec microphone, or an Ampex 351 full track tape recorder with an Electro voice 655c microphone. Each speaker was instructed to repeat the word spoken by one of the experimenter's assistants. The recordings obtained were then used to construct the tapes for the listening experiments.

Experimental procedures. A set of three listening tapes were made for each speaker from the original master tapes. Each tape contained instructions for the listeners and the three word lists. The order in which the lists appeared on these tapes was varied so that each list appeared only once in each of three positions; initial, middle, and final. None of the words spoken by the experimenter appeared on the listening tapes. An interval of 5 to 10 seconds followed each stimulus word to allow the listener time to write his response. The listening tapes were played to the listeners through a single TDH-39 earphone on an Ampex PR-10 tape recorder with a laboratory-constructed amplifier. A dummy earphone was placed on the opposite ear. The stimuli were presented to the listeners at a comfortable intensity level above normal threshold. Five hundred and seventy listeners participated in this experiment. The listeners were all students in Speech courses at the University of Michigan. None of the listeners had a history of any hearing loss. Ten listeners audited each of the listening tapes and a total of 30 listeners were used for each speaker.

The following instructions were presented to the listeners: "You are about to hear three lists of words. Please write down the word you think you hear on the sheets provided. If you do not understand a word, draw a line in the space alongside the appropriate number. Ready? List number 1." At the end of each list and before the onset of the next list the following instructions were heard: "list number... Remember, if you do not understand the word, draw a line in the space opposite the appropriate number. Ready? List number..." Listeners recorded their responses on answer forms designed for this purpose. At no time prior to the listening session were they told whether they were to listen to a normal or esophageal speaker.

Scoring Procedures. A listener's response was scored as correct if it was the word that was to have been produced by the speaker. In some instances a response was scored as correct if the word written could only be pronounced as the word which was intended as the stimulus. (E. g. one of the stimulus words was "size", if either "size" or "sighs" was written, the response was scored as correct.)

Intelligibility was measured in terms of the number of words correctly identified by listeners. Four separate intelligibility scores were computed for each speaker and for each population of speakers. The four intelligibility scores were: (a) total intelligibility, the total number of correct responses; (b) total list intelligibility, the total number of correct responses made by all of the listeners for a given speaker for a given word list without regard to the position of the list on the listening tape; (c) total order intelligibility, the total number of correct responses made by all of the listeners for a given order (e. g. CNC-Clusters-Spondees); and (d) a list by order intelligibility score, the total number of correct responses made by all of the listeners for a given speaker for a given list in a given position on the listening tapes.

TABLE I

Correct Response Totals for Thirty Listeners to Each of Nine Esophageal and Ten Normal Speakers on the CNC, Cluster and Spondee Word Lists

Subject	CNC	Cl.	Sp.	Total
E-1	1,073	1,282	1,411	3,766
E-2	1,825	1,181	1,244	3,251
E-3	810	994	1,357	3,161
E-4	921	1,329	1,371	3,621
E-5	541	911	1,064	2,507
E-6	728	847	1,257	2,832
E-7	395	709	1,074	2,178
E-8	417	436	889	1,742
E-9	1,003	1,196	1,347	3,546
Total	6,713	8,885	11,014	26,603
N-1	1,284	1,672	1,476	4,432
N-2	1,427	1,642	1,489	4,558
N-3	1,265	1,462	1,478	4,205
N-4	1,464	1,778	1,486	4,728
N-5	1,446	1,754	1,494	4,694
N-6	1,418	1,692	1,494	4,604
N-7	1,059	1,637	1,390	4,086
N-8	1,112	1,410	1,395	3,917
N-9	1,472	1,769	1,489	4,730
N-10	1,414	1,659	1,489	4,562
Total	13,361	16,475	14,680	44,516

Results

A summary of the total number of correct responses made by the listeners for each of the three lists and for each subject is presented in Table I. The means and standard deviations based on these data is presented in Table II. Although there was one more speaker in the normal group compared to the esophageal population, the differences between the two groups still appears to be quite large. On the whole, the means obtained for the normals were considerably greater than those obtained for the esophageal speakers and could not be accounted for by the difference in the total number of responses available for each population. The esophageal speakers appeared to reflect greater

TABLE II

Means and Standard Deviations for the Nine Esophageal and Ten Normal Speakers Derived from the Total Scores for CNC, Cl. and Sp. Word Lists

Subject Group	CNC	Cl.	Sp.	Total
Esophageals				
Mean	24.86	32.91	40.79	98.53
S. D.	8.66	10.23	6.69	23.17
Normals				
Mean	44.54	54.92	48.93	148.39
S. D.	5.27	4.44	1.87	10.02

variation in terms of intelligibility than normals as is seen by comparing the standard deviations for both groups. Inspection of these data strongly suggests that there were significant differences between the two populations of speakers in terms of intelligibility as measured in this research. Statistical analyses were carried out to determine the significance of these differences. To account for differences in length between lists the raw scores were converted to standard scores. These scores were used in all of the statistical analyses.

In order to compare the intelligibility of esophageal and normal speakers the hypothesis of a significant difference between the mean standard scores for the two populations was tested. The hypothesis was tested for the three list (CNC, Cluster and Spondee) scores and the total intelligibility score. The results of the statistical treatment of the data support the hypothesis in every case.

The t-ratio computed for the lists and for the total intelligibility scores were all significant beyond the 0.001 level of confidence. A t-ratio of 32.28 was obtained for the CNC's, 32.64 for clusters, 19.28 for spondees and 32.01 for total intelligibility (a t-ratio of 3.291 is significant at the 0.001 level). These results indicate that there was essentially no overlap between the populations studied in this research. It is possible, however, that the differences between normals and esophageal speakers may be somewhat reduced or even be made negligible if only esophageal speakers judged to be highly intelligible using some other criterion were compared to normals. However, since the esophageal population employed in this research was not selected on this basis, the findings reported above required that scores obtained on the two populations be subjected to independent statistical analyses.

The stability of a given speaker's position across lists in terms of intelligibility relative to other speakers in the population is of interest and clinical import. *Kendall's* coefficients of concordance [11] were employed to compare speaker ranking on the word lists and total intelligibility score for the three orders of presentation. This procedure was also employed to compare the ranks across the three lists and across the lists plus total score without considering the order of presentation. These statistical procedures were carried out on both the normal and esophageal populations.

The coefficients of concordance and the significance levels for both populations are presented in Tables III and IV. Coefficients which

TABLE III

Kendall Coefficients for CNC, Cl., Sp. and Total Intelligibility Scores across Three Orders of Presentation for Esophageal and Normal Speakers

List	W	P
Esophageals		
CNC	0.956	>0.001
Cl.	0.944	>0.005
Sp.	0.949	>0.005
Total	0.952	>0.005
Normals		
CNC	0.903	>0.005
Cl.	0.939	>0.005
Sp.	0.760	>0.025
Total	0.957	>0.005

were at, or beyond the 0.01 level of confidence were considered as significant. In no instance was there a coefficient obtained for the esophageal population which could not be considered as significant. All but one of the coefficients was significant at or beyond the 0.005 level. These results indicate that the rank of a given esophageal speaker's intelligibility score will remain the same across lists and total score. The highly significant coefficients suggest that the stabi-

TABLE IV

Kendall Coefficients across the CNC, Cl., and Sp. Lists and across the CNC, Cl., Sp. and Total Intelligibility for Esophageal and Normal Speakers

Lists	W	P
Esophageals		
With totals	0.927	>0.005
Without totals	0.907	>0.010
Normals		
With totals	0.854	>0.005
Without totals	0.823	>0.010

lity of ranking could be extrapolated to the general population of esophageal speakers. Thus, if a given esophageal speaker's rank in terms of intelligibility for one of the indices employed in this study is known, it should be possible to accurately predict his rank on any of the other indices. The coefficients and significance levels obtained for normals were similar to those obtained for esophageal speakers. The only coefficient not significant was the one obtained for the spondee list (W = 0.760, sig >0.025). This lower coefficient was due to the large number rank ties between normal speakers as might have been predicted on the basis of the high mean number of correct judgments ($\bar{X}$ = 48.93) and low standard deviation (S. D. = 1.87). The variance in intelligibility scores for the normals on this list was far less than for the other list or for the esophageal speakers across all lists. Although corrections for ties were made in the computations of the coefficients, the narrow range of spondee intelligibility scores for the normals was not offset, partially accounting for the lower coefficient. Except for spondee intelligibility, the comments concerning the esophageal speakers' stability also hold for normal speakers.

Analysis of variance techniques were employed to test hypotheses relevant to determining the significance of the differences in intelligibility scores between subjects, word lists, and order of presentation for each population. Examination of the raw data suggested that there might be significant interactions between subjects and lists as well as order and lists. A treatment by levels analysis of variance design [9] was employed to determine the significance of the observations based on the raw scores. An F ratio was considered significant if it was at or beyond the 0.01 level of confidence.

The results of the analysis carried out on the normal population is presented in Table V. The subject main effect was significant at the 0.001 level. Main effect for list and order were not significant. These findings indicate that normal speakers differ significantly from each other in intelligibility, and that it is possible to define quantitatively a scale of intelligibility for this population. List and order of pre-

TABLE V

Summary of Analysis of Variance for the Standard Intelligibility Scores for Esophageal Speakers (N = 9)

Source	df	ms	F	P
Subjects (Sub.)	8	5568.08	300.17	0.001
Lists (Lst.)	2	216.85	0.83	NS
Order (Ord.)	2	56.29	1.14	NS
Sub. Lst.	16	259.91	14.01	0.001
Sub. Ord.	16	49.30	2.66	0.001
Lst. Ord.	4	383.61	30.35	0.001
Sub. Lst. Ord.	32	12.64	0.68	NS
Within	729	18.55		
Total	809			

sentation do not appear to make a significant and independent contribution to the listener's determination of a speaker's intelligibility. This is a somewhat surprising finding in view of the differences between list means. Apparently the lists and the orders of presentation are of equal difficulty. However the subject x list and list x order interactions were significant. The F ratio of 1.65 for subject x order at the 0.025 level was not considered as significant. The significant interactions suggest that for some speakers some lists are not as difficult as others and that the order of presentation does have some effect on the resultant intelligibility scores for the individual lists. The significance of the list x order interaction could be partially accounted for by a differential practice effect produced by the three lists.

The summary of the analysis of variance results for the esophageal speakers is given in Table VI. Inspection of the table reveals that there is only a significant main effect for subjects. This finding is analogous to the results obtained for normal speakers. Apparently

TABLE VI

Summary of Analysis of Variance for the Standard Intelligibility Scores for Normal Speakers (N = 10)

Source	df	ms	F	P
Subjects (Sub.)	9	771.17	197.74	0.001
Lists (Lst.)	2	193.85	1.84	NS
Order (Ord.)	2	6.28	0.97	NS
Sub. Lst.	18	105.73	27.11	0.001
Sub. Ord.	18	6.45	1.65	0.025 (NS)
Lst. Ord.	4	16.61	3.78	0.01
Sub. Lst. Ord.	36	4.39	1.13	NS
Within	810	3.90		
Total	899			

the variance for lists and orders does not make an independent and significant contribution to the evaluation of intelligibility. The low F-ratio for lists (F = 0.834) indicates that there is no one list that will produce a significant difference in intelligibility scores for the population of esophageal speakers. This is also true for order of presentation. The order in which the lists are presented to listeners will not significantly affect their intelligibility scores when the population as a whole is considered. However, all of the second order interactions were significant at the 0.001 level of confidence. The significant interactions indicate that only when considered with differences between individual subjects does the variance for lists and orders have some influence on the listener's judgment of intelligibility. The variance for order will also have some effect on the listener's judgment of intelligibility when considered with differences between lists as well as subjects.

Discussion

The results of this investigation indicate that there are significant differences between normal and esophageal speakers in terms of listener judgments of intelligibility. These differences appeared in every comparison made between the two groups of speakers. The intelligibility scores of the esophageal population employed in this investigation were significantly lower than those of a matched population of normal speakers. In view of the highly significant t-ratio, we would predict that these differences would obtain if the comparisons were replicated on other relatively unbiased samples of esophageal and normal speakers. We further suggest that there would be only minimal overlap between the two populations, and that probability of such overlap occurring would be quite low. Thus, for all practical purposes it would be best to treat the esophageal and normal speakers as two independent populations.

The results of the statistical treatment coupled with an examination of the data suggest that the intelligibility scores for normals tend to be close together and not vary from speaker to speaker as do the scores for esophageal speakers. This implies that if larger samples of both populations were studied in the manner described above, the resulting distributions would not be parallel. The distribution of intelligibility scores for normals would probably be somewhat narrower than for esophageals and be somewhat skewed in the direction of the higher intelligibility scores. On the other hand, the frequency distribution for esophageal speakers would probably be wide and skewed in the direction of the lower intelligibility scores. We would expect that this distribution would hold for a population of esophageal speakers who had achieved maximum benefit from training.

Changes in the speech signals produced by esophageal speakers which effect a reduction in intelligibility appear to result from modifications of production other than just those introduced by the use of a different sound producing mechanism. Apparently the activity necessary to produce esophageal voice affects the esophageal speaker's ability to exercise the same degree of control over the articulatory, phonatory, and resonating systems as is available to the normal speaker. It is beyond the scope of this paper to attempt an anatomic or physiologic explanation of the modifications. However, whatever changes must be effected by the speaker to produce speech signals, they appear to be relatively stable in terms of their effect on a speaker's intelligibility. The significant coefficients of concordance obtained for the esophageal speakers lends support to this argument. If this were not the case, one would expect to find that a given esophageal speaker's rank relative to other speakers in the population would shift much more than it does.

There is another and perhaps an even more important inference to be derived from the comparison of the speakers' rankings. The fact that all of the obtained coefficients were highly significant indicates that a given speaker's ranking on a list, order, or total score can be predicted from his ranking on any one of these measures. This holds for both the normal and esophageal speakers. This means that it is probably not necessary to obtain many listener judgments on a large number of lists to determine a speaker's ranking in terms of intelligibility. Failure to obtain a significant main effect for lists or orders in the analysis of variance is evidence in support of the inference. Since the lists themselves do not differ significantly from each other, they would not need to be retained as they are presently constituted for further research on esophageal intelligibility. Failure to obtain a significant main effect for order indicates that there probably is no great practice effect when the populations are considered. This is not the case for individual subjects or lists as seen by the significant second order interactions. However, it seems that a more efficient instrument could be constructed by creating a new list based on a combined analysis of the three lists. Inspection of the intelligibility scores for each of the words on the lists reveals that some words are poor discriminators, while others discriminate quite well between speakers. An item analysis of all the words would indicate which words serve to permit the best distinctions to be made between speakers in terms of intelligibility. Such an analysis is now being made for the esophageal speakers and the results will be reported in a subsequent publication.

The research reported in this paper only attempted to explore one means of assessing and comparing the intelligibility of esophageal and normal speakers. The results of this study indicate that the esophageal and normals do differ significantly from each other in terms of intelligibility. However, independent analyses of the populations suggest that it should be possible to develop instruments which will permit accurate and quantitative evaluations of intelligibility. Construction of such instruments should include estimates of intelligibility based on sentences and other forms of connected speech as well as single words. If instruments of this sort are developed, they will provide the clinician with a powerful tool for his assessment of the esophageal speaker's intelligibility.

Summary

A comparison of esophageal and normal speaker intelligibility based on listener responses to CNC (Consonant-Syllable Nucleus), Cluster and Spondee word lists was conducted. Statistical analyses reveals that the esophageal and normal populations were significantly different from each other on all measures of intelligibility used in this study. Speakers in both groups maintained the same rank with respect to each other across lists and orders of presentation. There were significant differences between subjects in both groups, but not between word lists or order of presentation. Significant interactions between subject, lists, and orders were obtained for both populations. The results of this study indicate that it should be possible to devise objective measures of esophageal intelligibility based on listener responses to single words.

Zusammenfassung

Der Verfasser hat einen Vergleich der Verständlichkeit Normalsprechender und von Laryngektomierten mittels spezieller Wortlisten (Konsonant-Silben-Kerne) durchgeführt. Statistische Auswertungen ergaben, daß normale Sprecher und Laryngektomierte sich deutlich von einander unterschieden in bezug auf alle Maßstäbe der Verständlichkeit. Es waren signifikante Unterschiede zwischen Vp. beider Gruppen, aber nicht zwischen Wortlisten oder der Art der Anbietung. Die Ergebnisse dieser Untersuchungen rufen nach objektiven Meßgeräten für die Verständlichkeit der Oesophagussprache, die auf der Beantwortung der Zuhörer für Einzelworte aufgebaut sind.

Résumé

L'auteur établit une comparaison entre l'intelligibilité de la voix œsophagienne et de la voix normale basée sur les réponses d'auditeurs, ceci en utilisant certaines listes de mots. Les analyses statistiques montrent une différence importante entre les deux groupes. Le résultat de cette étude indique qu'il doit être possible de trouver des mesures objectives de l'intelligibilité œsophagienne basées sur les réponses d'auditeurs à des mots simples.

Acknowledgements

This research was supported by a PHS research grant, number NB-03064 from the National Institute of Neurological Diseases and Blindness. The author wishes to thank *Peter S. Perry*, *Gale L. Reynolds*, *Charles E. Speaks* and *Rita P. Tikofsky* for their assistance in collecting and analyzing the data.

References

1. *Anderson, J. O. D.:* Study of some factors concerning esophageal speech. Unpublished diss. (Ohio State Univ. 1951).
2. *Berg, J. van den; Moolenaar-Bijl, A.* and *Damsté, P.:* Oesophageal speech. Folia phoniat. *10:* 65–84 (1958).
3. *Berg, J. van den* and *Moolenaar-Bijl, A.:* Crico-pharyngeal sphincter, pitch, intensity, and fluency in esophageal speech. Pract. oto-rhino-laryng. *21:* 298–315 (1959).
4. *Damsté, P. H.:* Oesophageal speech after laryngectomy (Hoitsema, Groningen 1958).
5. *DiCarlo, L. M.; Amster, W. W.* and *Herer, G. R.:* Speech after laryngectomy (Syracuse University Press, Syracuse 1955).
6. *Hyman, M.:* An experimental study of the relative pressure, duration, intelligibility and esthetic aspects of the speech of artificial larynx, esophageal and normal speakers. Unpublished diss. (Ohio State Univ. 1953).
7. *Hyman, M.:* An experimental study of artificial larynx and esophageal speech. J. Speech Dis. *20:* 291–299 (1955).
8. *Lehiste, I.* and *Peterson, G. E.:* Linguistic considerations in the study of speech intelligibility. J. acoust. Soc. Amer. *131:* 250–286 (1959).
9. *Lindquist, E. F.:* Design and analysis of experiments (Houghton Mifflin, Boston 1953).
10. *Perry, P. S.:* An investigation of the lowest frequency in the integral harmonic series of normal and esophageal phonation. Unpublished diss. (Univ. Mich. 1964).
11. *Siegel, S.:* Nonparametric statistics (McGraw-Hill, New York 1956).
12. *Snidecore, J.* and *Curry, E. T.:* Temporal and pitch aspects of superior esophageal speech. Ann. Otol. Rhinol. Laryng. *68:* 623–626 (1959).
13. *Tikofsky, R. S.* and *Tikofsky, R. P.:* Intelligibility of dysarthric speech (in press).

Author's address: Dr. Ph. D. Ronald S. Tikofsky, Speech Clinic the University of Michigan, *Ann Arbor*, Michigan (USA)

FREQUENCY, DURATION, AND PERCEPTUAL MEASURES IN RELATION TO JUDGMENTS OF ALARYNGEAL SPEECH ACCEPTABILITY

THOMAS SHIPP

Veterans Administration Hospital, San Francisco, California

Thirty-three recordings of laryngectomized speakers reading a standard passage were subjected to two separate perceptual evaluations and to fundamental frequency and durational analysis. Factors related to higher speech acceptability ratings include: (1) a rapid rate of speech production, (2) little perception of respiratory noise, and (3) a relatively higher mean fundamental frequency. The most invariant of the factors measured were respiratory noise prominence and fundamental frequency *SD*. It was apparent that naive listeners tended to rate alaryngeal speakers higher as the speaker approached the norms for normal laryngeal speakers.

In the reporting of normative data on factors associated with the speech of laryngectomized individuals, most studies have failed to correlate their findings with any meaningful perceptual attribute of the speech production. Several problems have been manifest in conducting cross-parametric studies of the speech skill of laryngectomized subjects. A major difficulty has been the lack of a reliable method for classifying laryngectomee speech. Some studies have described alaryngeal[1] speaker samples as "good" or "poor" according to unstated criteria, while others have used a five- and seven-point designation with the classification done by the investigator. Such methods are sufficiently imprecise and unreliable as to prevent their use by other investigators studying acoustic or physiologic factors.

Other difficulties encountered in establishing normative data on alaryngeal voice have been caused by the differences in the speech stimulus analyzed as well as in the equipment and techniques for acoustic analysis used. For instance, Tato et al. (1954), using 12 randomly selected subjects, Damste (1958), using 20 randomly selected subjects, and Kytta (1964), using 18 "good" speakers, all used the Kay Sonograph for acoustic analysis. Tato and Kytta examined only sustained vowels while Damste's subjects read a four-word sentence. Fundamental frequency data were obtained by averaging the vertical striations on the Sonogram.

---

[1]The term "alaryngeal" will be used throughout this report to include both the terms "esophageal" and "pharyngeal" as adjectives describing the voice of the laryngectomized patients.

Reprinted by permission from *Journal of Speech and Hearing Research*, 1967, *10*, 417–427.

In the most complete investigation of fundamental frequency characteristics of laryngectomized speakers, Curry and Snidecor (1961) selected the six best speakers from an original sample of 50 good speakers. These six highly selected speakers were termed "Superior Esophageal Speakers" by the authors. These six subjects were recorded reading the first paragraph from Fairbanks' "Rainbow Passage" (1960). To obtain the fundamental frequency data, Curry and Snidecor used the phono-photographic technique described in detail by Cowan (1936).

Although the investigations cited above have provided some information on several acoustic factors of alaryngeal speech, their relationship to a listener's impression of the speaker's acceptability can only be conjectured.

It was the purpose of this study to measure a number of phonatory variables in the speech of laryngectomized patients and relate these findings to the acceptability of alaryngeal voice as perceived by naive listeners.

METHODS

Subject Selection

High fidelity tape recordings were made of subjects selected from the population of laryngectomized individuals in the Los Angeles and San Francisco area. An attempt was made to control selection bias by using in the study each subject who appeared for the recording session. It was expected that the subjects would fall along the full continuum of alaryngeal speech skill. Thirty-three recordings were made in which each subject read the first paragraph of "The Rainbow Passage." One subject who volunteered for the study demonstrated what was judged perceptually and later verified acoustically, to be two distinct alaryngeal voices. The experimenter used both voice productions in the study.

The second sentence from the full paragraph reading was extracted for the perceptual evaluations and acoustic analysis. The sentence was selected because of the amount of analysis anticipated and also because it had been previously demonstrated that measures of fundamental frequency, mean, and standard deviation correlated 0.99 with the same measures for the full paragraph.[2] Each single-sentence recording was duplicated and the 66 speech samples were randomly spliced into an experimental tape for the judging sessions.

Judgments

The judges were 116 students from three colleges in the San Francisco area. More than 100 judges were used so that the mean ratings could be carried out to two decimal places. Six judging sessions were conducted in college

---

[2]Unpublished study by the Stanford Speech Research Laboratory, 1959

classrooms where there was a minimum of ambient noise. Various high fidelity tape recorders were used to feed the same speaker system, which was placed in the front of the classroom. The judges' task was to rate each of the 66 speech samples on the acceptability of the speech production. No specific definition was given for the term "acceptability." A five-point rating scale was used in which "one" was defined as the least acceptable and "five" defined as the most acceptable speech production. Ten samples of the single-sentence utterance were selected at random and used prior to the presentation of the experimental tape as practice items for the judges' rating task. The 66 speech samples were presented to the judges with a three-second pause between stimuli. Three weeks later, 21 of the judges were asked to rate the 66 speech samples for prominence of respiratory noise using the same five-point scale. To identify respiratory noise, a number of words such as "wheezing" and "stoma noise" were used in the instructions. Recorded samples selected by the experimenter were used to demonstrate this acoustic parameter. The same ten samples that were used in the acceptability rating were then presented for practice prior to the beginning of the test tape. Subject order and between-stimuli intervals were the same as for the previous rating task.

A mean rating for each subject was computed for acceptability and for respiratory noise prominence. Intrajudge reliability was computed by correlating each judge's two ratings of the same speech sample from each of the 33 subjects.

Acoustic Analysis

In order to determine the variability of the optical oscillograph write-out system, a 1,000 pulse per second timing signal was recorded on the second track of each speech sample. The periodic signal was measured and from this it was determined that the overall time resolution of the write-out and data reduction system was 0.025 msecs.

The two-track recording was played from an Ampex 351-2 tape recorder to a Honeywell Visicorder, Model 1108, operating at a chart speed of 2,000 mm/sec. The mirror galvanometers in the Visicorder were type M-1000.

The fundamental frequency record of each speaker was edited by the experimenter and segmented so that the signal was categorized as (1) quasi-periodic phonation, (2) unmeasurable phonation, or (3) silence. Each wave of a segment designated as quasi-periodic was marked for measurement. The records were then measured using a Benson-Lehner Oscar N-2 data reduction system. In this manner each wave within a quasi-periodic segment as well as segments categorized as silence or unmeasurable phonation were measured.

From the measurements the following statistics were computed: Mean, standard deviation, and 90% range of fundamental frequency; total duration; and percentage of entire utterance spent in periodic (measurable) phonation, aperiodic (unmeasurable) phonation, and silence. Intercorrelations among all of the physical and perceptual data were performed as well as multiple correlations to determine the contribution of each measure to the rating of speech acceptability.

RESULTS AND DISCUSSION

Judgments

The tabulation of the two ratings showed that the means of 2.94 for acceptability and 2.89 for respiratory noise are close to the desirable mid-point mean of 3.00.

The intrajudge reliability figures were remarkably similar for the two rating tasks: 0.75 for acceptability and 0.73 for respiratory noise. This order of reliability was felt to be satisfactory considering the lack of sophistication among the judges in the task of perceptual rating.

The apparent success of the naive judges in the present study to rate in a reliable fashion a large group of alaryngeal speakers on the parameter of speech acceptability suggests that this technique may be used in studies that attempt to relate psychological, physiological, or acoustic parameters to perceptual factors in the voice of laryngectomized speakers. In future studies, a measure of acceptability in combination with intelligibility scores such as those obtained by Tikofsky (1965) would provide a strong perceptual specification of alaryngeal speech instead of the current practice of using labels such as "good" or "fair."

Table 1 shows the tabulation of the measures for the 17 speakers whose mean acceptability ratings were above 3.0 and 16 speakers whose ratings were below 3.0 on the five-point scale. It also shows the three measures of fundamental frequency for the six speakers discussed by Curry and Snidecor in their

TABLE 1. Mean and median fundamental frequency and duration measures obtained on low and high-rated speakers from the present study and Curry and Snidecor's six superior speakers.

Physical Measures	Mean Acceptability Rating			Curry & Snidecor Superior Speakers (N = 6)
	Below 3.0 (N = 16)	Above 3.0 (N = 17)	Six Best Speakers	
Fundamental Frequency				
Mean (Hz)	64.74	84.4	94.38 (mdn:86.1)	62.8
SD (Tones)	2.49	2.27	2.56	2.30
90% Range (Tones)	8.00	7.60	8.25	6.5
Total Duration (Secs)	7.92	5.54	4.39 (mdn:5.03)	6.01
Proportion of Utterance				
Periodic	37.8%	48.3%	53.6%	°
Aperiodic	16.4%	13.1%	8.7%	°
Silence	45.8%	38.6%	37.7%	46.3%

°Unable to measure accurately.

published material (1961). Their measures of total duration for the single sentence and the proportion of silence within the sentence were obtained by playing a dubbed recording of their six speakers through the instrumentation used in this study. The quality of the dubbed recording was not adequate for measures of periodic and aperiodic phonation.

Table 1 shows that factors coincident with above-average acceptability ratings include a higher mean fundamental frequency, a more rapid utterance of the test sentence, a greater proportion of periodic phonation, and a lesser proportion of both aperiodic phonation and silence.

The increase in mean fundamental frequency coinciding with the progressively higher rating for acceptability is notable in that nowhere in the literature are there indications that this is an important alaryngeal speech variable. The references to the level of fundamental frequency by Curry and Snidecor (1961) and by Kytta (1964) remark only on the coincidence that the mean fundamental is approximately one octave below that of normal, laryngeal male voice. It would appear that there is great variability among alaryngeal speakers as to their average frequency level and that the higher mean level is a desirable trait. It should be noted, however, that the method used for extracting the fundamental frequency on a wave-by-wave basis used in the present study differs from the techniques and instrumentation used by previous investigators. Studies using an averaging procedure will tend to mask short periods of high frequency phonation since these short periods will be averaged in with low frequency waves occurring within the averaged segment. However, at the other end of the frequency scale, a single low frequency period from 25 to 50 Hz occupies a major portion of a 50-msec averaging segment, and is essentially measured on a wave-by-wave basis. Hence, the resulting frequency distribution will be attenuated only at the high frequency end. The measures reported by investigators using the averaging procedure will have lower mean and median fundamental frequencies and, further, the standard deviation and 90%-range figures will be diminished as compared with the wave-by-wave analysis conducted in the present study.

Since it has been demonstrated that alaryngeal speakers may have mean fundamental frequencies in the range from 40 Hz to 185 Hz, then it would seem logical to hypothesize a physiologic basis for such frequency variance. Snidecor[3] has postulated that mean fundamental frequencies in the range from 50 Hz to approximately 100 Hz are produced when the neoglottis is located at the entrance to the esophagus. A mean fundamental frequency above 100 Hz occurs when the speaker utilizes to a great extent neoglottis constriction above the level of the cricopharyngeus muscle. Another possible explanation for the observed frequency variation might be the selective control over whatever muscle group is the principal participator in forming the neoglottis. If the laryngectomized individual is capable of highly selective contractions of this muscle group, he may well be able to achieve the necessary muscle-tension

---

[3]Telephone conversation, June, 1965.

balance against the air pressure below the neoglottis to achieve a higher voice frequency.

The standard deviation of fundamental frequency shows little variability between the two groups of speakers in the present study or in comparison to Curry and Snidecor's speakers. It has been assumed by previous investigators that the measure of standard deviation is not truly descriptive of voice-frequency variability. The preferred measure is that of the mid-90% range of frequencies, termed the "effective range" (Curry, 1940). On this parameter no significant trends were noted between the two groups in this study as shown in Table 1, but there is a marked difference for Curry and Snidecor's six superior speakers. The greater 90% range for both groups from the present study is probably best explained by the different methods used in each study for fundamental frequency analysis.

It was surprising to find that the measures of fundamental frequency standard deviation and 90% range did not differentiate between high- and low-rated speakers. Perhaps the frequency variation in and of itself is unimportant but the location within the frequency spectrum where the variation takes place may weigh heavily in the listener's evaluation of speech acceptability.

The difference in scores between the higher rated and lower rated speakers of the present study is quite pronounced in the time domain. Those speakers rated below average took 2⅓ seconds longer (7.92 vs 5.54 seconds) than the above-average speakers to read the 12-word test sentence. The six best speakers from the present study had a mean of 4.39 seconds and a median of 5.03 seconds duration, while Curry and Snidecor's six subjects had a mean duration of 6.01 seconds. Normal duration for this sentence was available to the author from another study and was found to be 4.16 seconds. It is apparent that the above-average and six best speakers from the present study more closely approximate the normal rate while speakers rated below average take almost twice the time of normal speakers to read the sentence. The difference of approximately 0.5 seconds between the speakers rated above average from the present study and the six superior speakers from the Curry and Snidecor study may reflect real differences in the skill of the two speaker groups.

With respect to the proportion of the utterance classified as periodic and aperiodic, the tendency is for the better speakers to spend about 50% of the total duration of the test sentence in periodic phonation while the low-rated speakers spend only 38%. For the proportion of aperiodic phonation, the difference between the low-rated speakers of 16.4% and the high-rated speakers of 13.1% is small. This means that the better speakers tend to put out a vocal signal that is somewhat less noisy than lower rated speakers.

For the lower-rated speakers the proportion of the utterance classified as silence is 45.8% while the higher-rated speakers had 38.6% silence during the reading of the test sentence. These two figures are almost the inverse of the proportion of periodic phonation for the two speaker groups. The 46.3% of silence for Curry and Snidecor's six speakers is a higher proportion than the low-rated speakers from the present study. It seems that the previously noted difference in total duration between the high-rated speakers in the present study and Curry and Snidecor's subjects is accounted for by the greater periods of silence measured in the latter speakers.

The findings from the present study indicate the importance of rate of speech to the acceptability of the alaryngeal voice production. Further, it appears that the principal method of speeding up speech is to lessen the amount of silence within an utterance. It was apparent from the records of the speakers in the present study, that the majority of the silence time was devoted to recharging the air supply in the esophagus.

Intercorrelations

The results of the intercorrelations among the nine variables is shown in Table 2. Although the correlations are not at all an exact test of the existing relationships, it was found that five of the eight measures were significantly correlated with the judgment of speech acceptability. Significant correlations with speech acceptability included the mean fundamental frequency, duration, the respiratory noise rating,[3] the percentage of periodic phonation, and the percentage of silence measures.

Examination of other correlations in the table shows that significant inter-relationships exist between total duration and the measures of respiratory noise prominence, percentage of measurable phonation, and percentage of silence. Apparently the speakers who were able to utter the test sentence in a shorter time did so while producing more measurable phonatory periods and by attenuating the moments of silence during the utterance. Accompanying these traits was the ability to inhibit the prominence of respiratory noise.

TABLE 2. Intercorrelations among the nine physical and perceptual measures obtained on 33 alaryngeal recordings.

Measures	Fundamental Frequency			Total Dura.	Resp. Noise Rating	% of Per. Phon.	% of Aper. Phon.	% of Silence	Accept. Rating
	Mean	SD	90% Range						
Fundamental Frequency									
Mean	1.00	0.18	−0.07	−0.25	0.14	0.33	−0.18	−0.26	0.35°
SD		1.00	0.81°	−0.04	0.05	−0.23	0.13	0.16	−0.27
90% Range			1.00	−0.01	0.07	−0.36°	0.30	0.17	−0.20
Total Duration				1.00	−0.56°	−0.43°	−0.01	0.61°	−0.65°
Resp. Noise Rtng.					1.00	0.39°	−0.34°	−0.15	0.73°
% Periodic Phon.						1.00	−0.72°	−0.58°	0.56°
% Aperiodic Phon.							1.00	−0.15	−0.28
% of Silence								1.00	−0.46°
Acceptability Rating									1.00

°Significant at 0.05 level.

[3]The more prominent the respiratory noise, the lower the rating.

The prominence of respiratory noise also coincided with an increase of aperiodic phonation. This statistic indicates, perhaps, that portions of the aperiodic speech wave were unmeasurable because of the overriding respiratory noise masking the voice signal.

The significant intercorrelation between the percentage of periodic phonation and aperiodic phonation is a natural result of the measurement technique used. An increase in one category resulted in a decrease in the other. However, the negative correlation between periodic phonation and percentage of silence implies that speakers producing clear acoustic wave forms tend to have less silent time within the utterance. They are apparently more skilled speakers.

These data suggest that alaryngeal speech will be rated as more acceptable when the mean fundamental frequency is higher, the duration of the utterance is shorter, the utterance is perceived as having less respiratory noise, and the voice has a higher percentage of measurable phonation with a smaller percentage of silence within the utterance.

Further, these data appear to verify the notion that the more an alaryngeal speaker approximates the characteristics of the normal speaker, the more highly he is rated on acceptability. This judging characteristic applies even to the voice fundamental frequency as was noted before. The speaker who is able to complete an utterance in a short time does so by increasing the percentage of the utterance spent in periodic phonation with a reduction in the percentage of silence. Furthermore, the combination of these two factors appears to coexist with the speaker's ability to inhibit the respiratory noise from the tracheostoma.

Multiple Correlations

The data from the intercorrelations point up the importance of certain factors in the alaryngeal speaker's output that act strongly to influence the listener's judgment of speech acceptability. In order to assess the relative importance of these factors, multiple correlations were run on the eight dependent variables with the independent variable of speech acceptability.

Fifteen multiple correlations were run of the eight variables, deleting each variable singly and in combination to determine their interaction and the resultant influence on the rating of acceptability. Table 3 shows the results of the fifteen multiple correlations arranged in order of the decreasing value of the coefficient of determination.

When all of the variables are included in the multiple correlation (multiple R Column 1) all but 19% of the variance in the speech acceptability rating is accounted for. The measure of total duration is the most heavily weighted factor since it explains 32% of the variance. Respiratory noise rating is second in importance, contributing 19% to the acceptability rating variance.

In multiple correlations 2 through 10, one or two of the variables are deleted with little resultant effect upon the judgment of acceptability as shown by the small shift in the coefficient of determination. However, as more of the critical

TABLE 3. Proportion of variance in rating acceptability accounted for by the physical and perceptual measures obtained. X's denote variables deleted. (Numbers are rounded to two decimal places.) Multiple correlation columns arranged in order of decreasing value of the coefficient of determination.

Measures	1	2	3	4	5	6	7	8	9	10	11	12	13	14	15
							Multiple Correlation								
Fundamental Frequency															
Mean	0.12	0.12	0.12	0.12	0.12	0.12	0.12	0.12	XX	XX	0.12	XX	0.12	0.12	0.12
SD	0.11	0.11	0.11	0.11	0.11	0.11	0.11	0.11	0.07	0.07	XX	XX	0.11	0.11	0.11
90% Range	0.04	0.04	0.04	0.04	0.04	0.04	XX	0.04	0.00	0.00	0.03	XX	0.04	0.04	0.04
Total Duration	0.32	0.32	0.32	0.32	0.32	0.32	0.33	XX	0.44	XX	0.34	0.42	0.32	0.32	XX
Respiratory Noise	0.19	0.18	0.18	0.18	0.19	0.18	0.20	0.45	0.20	0.55	0.20	0.19	XX	XX	XX
% Periodic Phon.	0.01	XX	0.01	XX	XX	0.01	0.00	0.02	0.03	0.06	0.01	0.05	0.04	0.05	XX
% Aperiodic Phon.	0.00	0.00	XX	XX	0.00	0.00	0.01	0.03	0.00	0.04	0.01	0.01	0.02	XX	XX
% Silence	0.00	0.01	0.00	0.00	XX	XX	0.00	0.00	0.04	0.04	0.00	0.00	0.01	0.02	XX
Coef. of Determination	0.81	0.80	0.80	0.80	0.80	0.80	0.79	0.79	0.78	0.76	0.73	0.69	0.68	0.67	0.28

variables are deleted in multiple correlations 11 through 15, the coefficient of determination is decreased until it reaches the low point of 0.28.

It is apparent that the most independent factor in the speech acceptability judgment is the rating of respiratory noise prominence. When this variable is deleted singly (multiple R Column 13), there is little compensatory increase in the contribution of any of the other variables. This deletion results in decreasing the coefficient of determination from 0.81 to 0.68. Although the measure of total duration is weighted more heavily when all of the variables are present (multiple R Column 1), when this variable is deleted (multiple R, Column 8) the majority of its variance was taken up by an increase from 19% to 44% in the respiratory noise measurement. It is apparent that total duration and respiratory noise rating had variation in common (−0.55) but not with the other measures. The interaction between respiratory noise and other major variables is even more dramatic in multiple R Column 10. In this case the respiratory noise contribution jumped from 0.19 when all of the variables were present to 0.55 when both the mean fundamental frequency and total duration variables were deleted. This shift in respiratory noise contribution almost completely compensated completely for the deletion of the two variables since the coefficient of determination only decreased from 0.81 to 0.76.

One further interaction among the variables appears important. All three of the fundamental frequency measures remain quite stable and are uninfluenced by deletion of any one or all of the five remaining variables. The deletion of the mean fundamental frequency's 12% contribution to acceptability ratings is almost totally compensated for by the increase in the contribution of the total duration measure. But the standard deviation measure interacts very little with the other measures when deleted, as in multiple R Column 11, wherein the coefficient of determination is reduced proportionally.

The data from the multiple correlation table seem to suggest that of the eight measures taken in the present study, the variables of fundamental frequency standard deviation and the rating of respiratory noise prominence are the two best predictors of alaryngeal speech acceptability.

The data processing for this study was performed by the Veterans Administration Western Research Support Center. Special acknowledgement is made to Patti Grubb and Dorothy Huntington for their assistance on instrumentation, and to the late Grant Fairbanks who consulted on the study during its inception.

REFERENCES

Cowan, M., Pitch and intensity characteristics of stage speech. *Arch. Speech*, Supplement (1936).

Curry, E. T., The pitch characteristics of the adolescent male voice. *Speech Monogr.*, 7, 48-62 (1940).

Curry, E. T., and Snidecor, J. C., Physical measurement and pitch perception in esophageal speech. *Laryngoscope*, 71, 415-424 (1961).

Damste, P. H., *Oesophageal Speech After Laryngectomy*. Univ. of Groningen, Netherlands (1958).

FAIRBANKS, G., *Voice and Articulation Drillbook*. (2nd ed.) New York: Harper and Brothers (1960).

KYTTA, J., Spectrographic studies of the sound quality of oesophageal speech. *Acta Otolaryng.*, Supplement 188 (1964).

TATO, J. M., MARIANI, N., DePICCOLI, E. M. W., and MIRASOV, P., Study of the soma spectrographic characteristics of the voice in laryngectomized patients. *Acta Otolaryngol.*, **44**, 431-438 (1954).

TIKOFSKY, R. S., A comparison of the intelligibility of esophageal and normal speakers. *Folia Phoniat.*, **17**, 1-18 (1965).

Received for publication December 1966

RELATIONSHIP OF SELECTED ACOUSTIC VARIABLES
TO JUDGMENTS OF ESOPHAGEAL SPEECH

H. Ray HOOPS

Department of Speech, Speech and Hearing Center,
Wayne State University, Detroit, Michigan, USA

and

J. Douglas NOLL

Department of Audiology and Speech Sciences,
Purdue University, Lafayette, Indiana, USA

The relationship between selected acoustic attributes of esophageal speech and listener judgments of laryngectomized speakers was investigated. The twenty-two laryngectomees in the study were filmed and recorded reading the first paragraph of the Rainbow Passage and these films were judged by sixty judges. Frequency, intensity and rate analyses were performed. Relationships between the acoustic variables and listener judgments were investigated.

The following conclusions were drawn: (1) Mean vocal fundamental frequency, fundamental frequency variation and degree of wave-to-wave consistency are not significantly related to speech proficiency. (2) Vocal sound pressure level and sound pressure variation are not related to esophageal speech proficiency and (3) Speaking rate is related to speech proficiency. Better speakers speak at a significantly faster rate.

Introduction

As Moore et al. (1959) observed, the acoustic description of the esophageal voice cannot be considered complete. It is of obvious importance that the acoustic characteristics of the substitute voice of the laryngectomee be carefully described and that the relationship of the acoustic parameters to overall speaking ability be established. While a large number of studies have dealt with this area, few of them have been of sufficient scope to be considered definitive. With few exceptions, the studies concerned with the acoustic aspects of esophageal speech have used small subject samples, usually from two to six, and have analyzed relatively short speech samples. Further research is indicated in this area using larger subject numbers, analyzing larger speech samples, and employing modern instrumental techniques to effect such analysis. Features which would seem to merit further investigation are the fundamental frequency, intensity and rate aspects of esophageal voice. A number of studies have been concerned with the mean fundamental frequency of esophageal voice and with the variability of

Reprinted by permission from *Journal of Communication Disorders*, 1969, *2*, 1–13. Copyright North-Holland, Amsterdam.

fundamental frequency. However, as Lieberman (1963) and Perry (1963), observed, these two meaures actually give a minimum of information about the vocal source. Risberg (1962), Saito, Kato and Teranishi (1958), Sugimoto and Hiki (1962) and Koshikawa (1962) have indicated that valuable information concerning vocal output can be obtained from studies of pitch perturbations; that is, the small but rapid variations in fundamental frequency measured during sustained phonation. Lieberman (1962) applied this technique in a comparative investigation of normal and pathological laryngees. The technique would seem to be of considerable merit in description and analysis of esophageal voice.

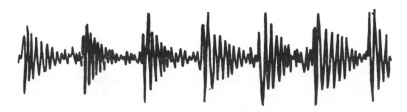

A. Record of periodic esophageal vocal signal

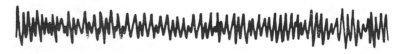

B. Record of noise

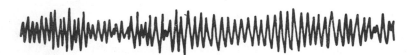

C. Record of stomal sound

Fig. 1. Characteristic traces seen in visicorder records of esophageal voice.

Very little attention has been given, experimentally, to the intensity aspects of esophageal voice. The clinical literature is in general agreement that average intensity level as well as the laryngectomized speaker's ability to vary intensity is an important consideration but other than a cursory investigation by Anderson (1950), little in the way of empiric data has been reported.

Purpose

It was the purpose of the present study to investigate the acoustic characteristics of the esophageal speaker and the relationship of speaking ability to these characteristics. The hypotheses of the study stated in the null form are:

There is no significant relation between judged ratings of esophageal speakers and any of the following parameters of speech: (1) Mean vocal fundamental frequency, (2) standard deviation of vocal fundamental frequency, (3) perturbation of vocal fundamental frequency, (4) mean vocal sound pressure level, (5) standard deviation of vocal sound pressure level, (6) mean word-per-minute rate, and (7) mean word-per-minute-per-sentence rate.

Method

Subjects

Subjects of the present study were twenty-two male laryngectomees chosen from among seventy-seven available subjects in a major metropolitan treatment center. Subject selection criteria included: (1) no foreign accent or dialect other than general American, (2) the use of esophageal speech as the primary method of communication, (3) the ability to complete the ninety-seven word first paragraph of the Rainbow Passage. The twenty-two subjects were chosen using a stratified randon selection procedure designed to insure a wide range of speaking ability. The subjects selected were twenty-two caucasian males ranging in age from thirty-six to eighty-one years with a mean age of fifty-eight years. The interval of time since therapy ranged from some individuals who were still actively engaged in therapy to sixteen years since the termination of active therapy.

Data collection

Each subject was recorded on color motion picture film including an optical sound track and on magnetic tape. The subject was seated in front of a neutral background and dressed in a white laboratory coat so that visual conditions would be as consistent as possible from subject to subject. The subject was asked to assume a comfortable position and a dental head positioner was adjusted to this "comfortable position" so that the head would remain stabilized.

In order to provide a reference level for later sound pressure level analysis, a pure tone of known intensity was recorded on the tape recorder with the record level set at the same point as for data collection. The pure tone was produced by a signal generator and sent through a speaker into a sound field situation. The tone was then calibrated to 80 dB SPL with a General Radio sound level meter, model 1551-B, at a speaker to microphone distance of twelve inches. This tone was then recorded on the tape recorder maintaining the speaker to microphone distance of twelve inches.

The subject was given a practice period and was then asked to read the ninety-seven word first paragraph of the rainbow passage to the examiner who was seated facing him at a distance of three feet. The subject's reading of the passage was recorded at 15 ips with a mouth to microphone distance of twelve inches on a Nagra III tape recorder and simultaneously filmed and recorded by an Auricon 16 mm sound on film camera. The subject's head, neck and trunk was filmed in a three quarter profile.

Judges

The judges who participated in the study consisted of two groups of thirty individuals. One group, considered to be sophisticated judges, were speech therapists at a graduate level who had had extensive listening or therapy experience with the laryngectomee. The other group, considered to be unsophisticated judges, was composed of thirty individuals who reported never having heard an esophageal speaker.

Judgment sessions were conducted in a sound treated projection room with good acoustic qualities. Judges were asked to rate each subject on a seven point equal appearing intervals scale permitting successive approximations. Judges were instructed to rate the subject on the basis of general communicative effectiveness. Overall mean rating was considered to be the measure of speaker ability for each subject.

Frequency analysis

The frequency analysis consisted of wave-by-wave measurement of the Oscillographic record of the recorded esophageal speech sample of each subject. The speech sample was supplied by a Honeywell Visacorder Oscillograph Model 1508. The sample, which had been recorded at fifteen inches per second was played into the Visicorder at a tape speed of 375 inches per second. The paper speed of the Visicorder was 250 millimeters per second. A time line consisted of a 50.1 Hz sinusoidal wave produced by the pulse wave generator and counted by a Beckman Frequency Counter Model 523. This time line was plotted on the Visicorder trace and since it was of known frequency, it made possible the compensation in later computations for the discrepancies in paper speed or galvanometer reproduction.

Fundamental frequency analysis

The period value for each wave of each subject's speech sample for the entire passage was measured. The first step in measurement was the determination as to whether or not a given portion of the trace was to be considered a periodic wave. Exploratory work had indicated that the characteristic wave of the esophageal speaker exhibits an abrupt onset and a highly damped waveform. (See Fig. 1A). Other forms sometimes seen in the esophageal trace were those considered to be noise (Fig. 1B), whose origin could not be determined and a third type of wave (Fig. 1C) which seemed to have some periodic characteristics but did not display the characteristic of a highly damped waveform. These waves, though quasi-periodic, did not seem to be a part of speech production. Pilot work, in which stomal noise* alone was reproduced on the Visicorder, indicated that this

---

* The sample of stomal noise was obtained by splicing from the experimental tape, a sample of sound from a subject who demonstrated a clearly audible escape of air past the stoma.

periodic form tended to be present in certain parts of the trace of stomal noise. Only those waves having the highly damped form described above were considered to be periodic waves representative of esophageal speech for the purposes of the present study. When decisions had been made concerning the presence of a wave, the period length of the wave was measured. Since the study was concerned with frequency perturbations and the perturbation factor involves the subtraction of each period value from the period value of the wave immediately preceding it, only waves occurring in groups of three or more were measured. The period value of each wave was obtained by measuring, under magnification, the distance from a portion of one wave to a corresponding portion of the following wave. For measurement purposes, the general configuration of the wave as well as the points of maximum amplitude were used to determine that constituted corresponding points in subsequent waves. An attempt was made, in instances where it was deemed feasible, to measure from the point of maximum amplitude in one wave to the corresponding point of maximum amplitude in the following wave. This was possible at most times except when this portion of the wave form was undergoing a major transition. When this circumstance occurred, which was rare, another equivalent portion which did not appear to be in a state of transition was selected for purposes of measurement. The period values were measured to the nearest one-tenth millimeter. These period values provided the basis for all subsequent analysis of vocal frequency. The values were supplied to a computer programmed to compute the following functions for each subject:

1. Mean of fundamental frequency or period values.
2. Standard deviation of fundamental frequency or period values.
3. Perturbation factors of the period values.

Analysis of vocal sound pressure level

The vocal sound pressure level of the subjects was analyzed using a Bruel and Kjaer Power Level Recorder model 2305 and a Bruel and Kjaer Statistical distribution analyzer model 4420.The speech samples were supplied to the power level recorder, which had been calibrated using the 80 dB test tone, by the tape recorder. The power level recorder activated the statistical distribution analyzer which sampled pen position on the power level recorder at a sampling rate of ten per second, thus producing a frequency distribution of sound pressure level for each subject's reading of the rainbow passage. From this frequency distribution, the following values were computed for each subject: (1) Mean vocal sound pressure level and (2) standard deviation of sound pressure level.

Rate analysis

The rate analysis was performed from the graphic power level trace obtained during the sound pressure level analysis previously described. When the sample had been supplied to the power level recorder and displayed graphically, the length of the trace was measured for each sentence and for the entire passage.

After these measurements were converted to time values, computations of the following values were made: (*1) Total reading time for the ninety-seven word passage, (2) reading time for each sentence, (3) overall word-per-minute reading rate, and (4) word-per-minute per sentence reading rate.

Results

Analysis of vocal fundamental frequency

The period measurements obtained in the fundamental frequency analysis were supplied to a computer which converted the measured period values to fundamental frequency values for each subject. A perturbation factor was also computed. The value for this factor was obtained by subtracting the period value of each wave from the preceding wave in a segment of consecutive phonation. The perturbation factor represents the percent of the time this value exceeded plus or minus one millisecond (msec). The one msec value differs from the value set for perturbations in the initial work of Liberman (1963) who used a .5 msec criterion for perturbation analysis of the vocal fundamental frequency of normal and pathological laryngees. The value of .5 msec, however, was inappropriate for the present data because the vocal fundamental frequency of the esophageal speakers of the study was so variable on a wave-to-wave basis that most subjects would have approached or possibly reached a perturbation factor of one hundred per cent. The one msec value resulted in a range of perturbation factors for the twenty-two subjects of 8.9 per cent to 66.8 per cent and a mean factor of 41.1 per cent. Mean vocal fundamental frequency varied from 42.92 cycles per second (Hz) to 85.81 Hz with an average mean fundamental frequency for the group of 65.59 Hz. The standard deviation of fundamental frequency for the group ranged from 7.79 Hz to 25.00 Hz with a mean standard deviation of 14.66 Hz.

The results of the present study are comparable to the Curry and Snidecor (1961) and Martin (1966) studies. The former study reported a mean fundamental frequency of 65 cps for six laryngectomized subjects considered to be superior speakers. Martin (1966) reported a mean fundamental frequency of 65 cps for a subgroup considered to be good esophageal speakers. However, he found higher fundamental frequency values for his groups of average and poor speakers though the differences were not statistically significant. The mean fundamental frequency of the subject group of the present study was 65.59 Hz and is in close agreement with the figures cited for superior speakers but not with the subgroups of poorer speakers.

The vocal fundamental frequency perturbation data are not readily amenable to comparisons with previous research since, on the basis of an extensive review of the literature, no investigation of this factor of esophageal speech is in evidence. Lieberman (1962) found that laryngeal subjects with hoarse voices differed from normals in that they demonstrated greater perturbation factors. Although Lieberman (1963) used .5 msec as the criterion for a perturbation and 1.0 msec was considered to be a perturbation in the present study, it is obvious that the esophageal speakers demonstrated, as a group, greater perturbations than did either Lieberman's normal or pathological subjects.

Mean vocal sound pressure level measurements

Mean vocal sound pressure level measurements for the twenty-two subjects ranged from 57.02 dB SPL to 67.57 dB SPL. The average mean vocal sound pressure level was 62.40 dB SPL. The variability of vocal SPL of the twenty-two laryngectomized subjects as measured by the standard deviation of the SPL values ranged from 2.55 dB SPL to 5.17 dB SPL with a mean standard deviation for the group of 3.60 dB SPL. This information is not comparable to earlier studies. The results of the studies cited were not reported in terms of sound pressure level but were equated in terms of other reference levels. Some comparison, however, will be possible in later analysis of the relation of such measures to the judged rating of the esophageal speakers.

Rate analysis

The rate analysis of the twenty-two esophageal speakers indicated a mean word per minute rate (wpm) for the entire passage of 114.3 wpm. The wpm values ranged from 65.4 wpm to 169.0 wpm. The mean of the average word per minute per sentence rate was 131.8 wpm per sentence. This value was obtained by adding the wpm rate for each of the seven sentences in the passage and dividing by the number of sentences. The mean wpm values for each sentence ranged from 113,6 wpm for the twenty-two word third sentence to 154.3 wpm for the seven word fifth sentence. The seventeen word first sentence had a mean wpm rate for all speakers of 124.2 wpm; the twelve word second sentence, 121.9 wpm; the thirteen word fourth sentence, 128.1 wpm; and the twenty-six word sixth sentence yielded a mean wpm score of 149.7 wpm.

The rate data of the present study are quite comparable to the Snidecor and Curry (1959 and 1960) finfing that esophageal speakers averaged 113 words per minute. The values obtained also generally fell within the range of 80 to 153 wpm reported by Snidecor and Isshiki (1965) with only two subjects falling below the range and none exceeding it.

Relation of acoustic measures to judgments of communicative effectiveness

In order to determine the existence of relationships between judgments of communicative effectiveness and the acoustic measurements, a multiple correlation analysis was performed. The mean judged ratings of communicative effectiveness were considered to be the dependent variable in all subsequent analyses. In other words, the ratings under this condition were considered to be the criterion measurements of relative acceptability of each speaker. Seven independent variables were investigated in the analysis procedure: Mean vocal fundamental frequency, perturbation factor of vocal fundamental frequency, standard deviation of vocal fundamental frequency, mean vocal sound pressure level, standard deviation of vocal sound pressure, overall word per minute rate, and word per minute per sentence rate. Because of the earlier finding (Hoops, 1967) that the judgments of communicative effectiveness differed significantly depending on the sophistication level of the two judge groups, two multiple correlation procedures were performed using the set of seven independent variables.

The first analysis, illustrated in table 1, was based upon the ratings made by the sophisticated judges as the dependent variable. The technique permits the analysis of not only the correlation of each independent variable with the dependent variable, but also each independent variable with each other independent variable. As table 1 indicates, variables two through six were not correlated to variable one to a degree significantly different, at the .01 level of confidence, from a zero order correlation. Variables seven and eight were correlated to

Table 1

Matrix of multiple correlation analysis between ratings
by sophisticated judges and acoustic measures

		Variable number						
		2	3	4	5	6	7	8
Variable number	1	.162	.220	.268	.099	−.182	−.691 *	−.736 *
	2		−.267	.484	.538 *	.323	−.175	−.160
	3			.479	.036	−.062	−.195	−.230
	4				.439	.141	−.245	−.261
	5					−.205	.069	.035
	6						.008	.057
	7							.989 *

Critical value at .01 = .537

Variable number	Description
1	Mean judged rating
2	Mean vocal fundamental frequency
3	Perturbation of vocal fundamental frequency
4	Standard deviation of vocal fundamental frequency
5	Mean vocal sound pressure level
6	Standard deviation of vocal sound pressure level
7	Overall word per minute rate
8	Word per minute per sentence rate

judged communicative effectiveness to a degree significantly different from zero at the .01 level of confidence. The r values for these two factors are: Overall word per minute rate, -.691 and word per minute per sentence rate, -.756. It will be noted that since a high rating value on the scale of communicative effectiveness indicated a poorer judgment of a subject in terms of his communicative effectiveness, and vice versa, those correlation indexes with a positive sign indicate that the better the individual was judged in terms of his communicative effectiveness, the smaller the value of the given acoustic measurement. If the sign of the r value is negative, it indicates that better ratings of communicative effectiveness accompanied larger values of the respective variables. The positive signs of variables two through five indicated that they varied in an inverse rating of esophageal communicative effectiveness, while variables six through eight varied in a direct relationship. However, as was indicated earlier, only variables seven and eight produced statistically significant values and only these can be considered to represent relationships not due to chance. The results indicate that, of the seven acoustic variables measured, only overall word per minute rate and word per minute per sentence rate can be considered to be significantly related to judged ratings of communicative effectiveness. In other words, the faster a given speaker's rate, the better he was judged by the group of sophisticated judges. In view of the r values for these two variables and the fact that the

Table 2

Matrix of multiple correlations between ratings by unsophisticated judges and acoustic measures

		Variable number						
		2	3	4	5	6	7	8
Variable number	1	.122	.346	.349	.028	−.139	−.738 *	−.780 *
	2			−.267	.484	.538 *	.323	−.175
	3			.479	.036	−.062	−.195	−.230
	4				.439	.141	−.245	−.261
	5					−.025	.069	.035
	6						.008	.057
	7							.989 *

Critical value at .08 = .537

Variable number	Description
1	Mean judged rating
2	Mean vocal fundamental frequency
3	Perturbation of vocal fundamental frequency
4	Standard deviation of vocal fundamental frequency
5	Mean vocal sound pressure level
6	Standard deviation of vocal sound pressure level
7	Overall word per minute rate
8	Word per minute per sentence rate

coefficient of determination was .986, the relation between the measures on the two rate variables and the measure of speaker proficiency must be considered quite strong.

A significant intercorrelation was found between variables seven and eight, the overall mean word per minute rate and the word per minute rate. The correlation between these two variables was .989, which was statistically significantly different from a zero order correlation at the .01 level of confidence. A significant intercorrelation was also found between factors two and five, mean vocal fundamental frequency level and mean vocal sound pressure level. The r value for these two variables was .538 which significantly differed from zero order correlation at the .01 level of confidence.

As table 2 illustrates, the results of the multiple correlation analysis of the relation of the same independent variables as those reported in the preceding paragraphs with the dependent variable of unsophisticated judge ratings of communicative effectiveness yielded essentially the same findings as those reported in table 1. The independent variables of mean vocal fundamental frequency, standard deviation of fundamental frequency, perturbation factor of fundamental frequency, mean vocal sound pressure level, and standard deviation of vocal sound pressure level, were not significantly different from a zero correlation at the .01 level of confidence. The variables of overall word per minute rate and word per minute per sentence rate were significantly correlated with judgments of general communicative effectiveness. The overall word per minute rate and the word per minute per sentence rate yielded r values of -.738 and -.780 respectively. The coeffecient of determination for the independent variables to the judgments of unsophisticated judges was .987.

The intercorrelation between overall word per minute rate and the word per minute per sentence rate was .989, and between mean vocal fundamental frequency and mean vocal sound pressure level was .538, both of these values were significantly different from a zero order correlation at the .01 level of confidence.

Since the results of the two analyses of intercorrelation yielded essentially identical results, some general discussion will be presented applying equally to both analyses. The results must be considered to be in conflict with those studies indicating that pitch level and intensity level are significantly related to esophageal speaking ability. Although the present study concerned itself with the physical measurement of voice characteristics, the data must be considered to be related to the observations made by other investigators about the perceptual aspects as well as to those who also performed physical analyses of various vocal parameters. Anderson (1950), Nichols (1964), Rickenberg (1953) and Hyman(1955) indicated that intensity factors are related to esophageal speech proficiency. The present study found no significant relation between vocal sound pressure and judgments of speech success. The results must also be considered to be in conflict with the studies of Snidecor and Curry (1959). Tato et al. (1954), and Shipp (1967) who found that fundamental frequency was

318   ESOPHAGEAL SPEECH

positively related to speech proficiency. The results of the present study agree with those of Martin (1965) which indicated no statistically significant relationship between speech proficiency and fundamental frequency. The r value of .537 between mean vocal fundamental frequency and mean vocal sound pressure level tend to lend support to the observation by Berg and Moolenaar Bijl (1959) that pitch and intensity are correlated to each other.

The results must be considered to be in close agreement with the indications of Svane-Knudsen (1960), Snidecor and Curry (1959) and Snidecor and Isshiki (1965) that the better speaker tends to have faster rate. The results tend to refute the finding by Anderson (1950) that rate of speaking is not significantly related to speech proficiency.

Summary and conclusions

It was the purpose of the present study to investigate selected acoustic attributes of esophageal speech and the relationship of these attributes to listener judgments of esophageal speech.

A subject sample of twenty-two laryngectomized individuals representing a wide range of speaker ability was selected and recorded on magnetic tape and sound on motion picture film while reading the Rainbow Passage and judged by listeners in terms of overall speech proficiency.

Each speaker's recorded production was analyzed to provide acoustic data concerning vocal fundamental frequency vocal sound pressure level, and reading rate. The vocal fundamental frequency analysis was performed by displaying a continuous oscillographic trace on chart paper and subsequently measuring the period value of each wave of the speech sample. The period values were used to compute mean fundamental frequency values, vocal fundamental frequency perturbation values, and standard deviation values of vocal fundamental frequency.

The vocal sound pressure level analysis was performed by supplying the recorded speech sample for each subject to a Power Level Recorder and analysing the graphic output of the recorder with a Statistical Distribution Analyzer. This analysis permitted the computation of values for mean vocal sound pressure level and standard deviation of vocal sound pressure level.

The rate analysis procedure consisted of the measurement of elapsed time for each speaker's production of the passage and for each sentence in the passage. Overall word per minute rates and word per minute per sentence rates were then obtained from the data.

Correlations between judged ratings of communicative effectiveness of the esophageal speakers and the above measures of acoustic factors of speech were investigated.

Under the limitations of subject sample, experimental design, and statistical technique, the following conclusions are presented:

1. Mean vocal fundamental frequency, fundamental frequency variation, and

degree of wave-to-wave frequency consistency are not significantly related to speech proficiency.

2. Vocal sound pressure level and sound pressure variation are not related to esophageal speaker proficiency.

3. Speaking rate is related to speech proficiency. Better speakers speak at a significantly faster rate.

References

Anderson, J.O., 1950, A descriptive study of the elements of esophageal speech. Unpublished Ph. D. Dissertation, Ohio State University.

Berg, J. Van Den, A.Moolenaar-Bijl and P.H.Damste, 1958, Oesophageal speech. *Folia Phoniat.*, 10, 65–84.

Hoops, H.R., 1967, Listener sophistication in relation to acoustic measures of esophageal speech. Ph. D. Dissertation, Purdue University.

Hyman, M., 1955, An experimental study of artificial larynx and esophageal speech. *J. Speech Hearing Dis.*, 20, 291–299.

Isshiki, N. and J.C.Snidecor, 1962, Air intake and usage in esophageal speech. *Acta Oto-Laryng.*, 59, 559–574.

Koshikawa, T. and T.Sugimoto, 1962, The information rate of the pitch signal in speech. In: *Proceedings of the Stockholm Speech Communication Seminar*, Speech Transmission Laboratory, Royal Institute of Technology, Stockholm.

Kytta, Jyrki, 1964, Finnish esophageal speech after laryngectomy: sound spectrographic and cineradiographic studies. *Acta-Oto-Laryngologica Supplementum*, 195.

Liberman, P. 1963, Some acoustic measures of the fundamental periodicity of normal and pathologic larynges. *J. Acoust. Soc. Amer.*, 35, 344–353.

Martin, D.E., 1966, A photo-phono-phonellegraphic study of various frequency measures of esophageal speech samples representing a range of listener acceptability. Master's Thesis, Purdue University.

Moore, P., (chairman), V.Anderson, J.Irwin and W.Waldrop, 1959, Report of subcommittee on problems of voice and speech problems associated with laryngectomy. ASHA Convention, 1958, *J. Speech Hearing Dis., Monograph Supplement Number 5*, 18–25.

Nichols, A.C., 1964, Loudness and quality in esophageal speech and the artificial larynx. In: J.C.Snidecor et al., *Speech Rhabilitation of the Laryngectomized*. Springfield, Ill.: C.C.Thomas.

Perry, P.S., 1963, An investigation of the lowest frequency in normal and esophageal voice production. Ph. D. Dissertation, the University of Michigan.

Risberg, A., 1962, Statistical studies of fundamental frequency range and rate of change. Speech Transmission Laboratory, *Quaterly Progress and Status Report.* Royal Institute of Technology, Stockholm, 7–8.

Siato, S., K.Kato and N.Teranishi, 1958, Statistical properties of the fundamental frequencies of Japanese speech voices. *J. Acoust. Soc. Japan*, 14, 111–119.

Shipp, T., 1967, Frequency, duration and perceptual measures in relation to judgments of alaryngeal speech acceptability. *J. Speech Hearing Res.*, 10, 417–427.

Snidecor, J.C. and E.T.Curry, 1959, Temporal and pitch aspects of superior esophageal speech. *Ann. Otol. Rhinol. Laryng.*, 68, 623–629.

Snidecor, J.C. and E.T.Curry, 1960, How effectively can the laryngectomy expect to speak? *Laryngoscope*, 70, 62–67.

Snidecor, J.C. and N.Isshiki, 1965, Air volume and air flow relationships of six male esophageal speakers. *J. Speech Hearing Dis.*, 30, 205–216.

Sugimoto, T. and S.Hiki, 1962, On the extraction of the pitch signal using the body wall vibration at the throat of the talker. In: *Proceedings of the Stockholm Speech Communication Seminar.* Speech Transmission Laboratory, Royal Institute of Technology, Stockholm.

Tato, J.M., N.Mariana, E.De Picolli and P.Mirasov, 1954, Study of the sonospectrographic characteristics of the voice in laryngectomized patients. *Acta-Oto-Laryng.,* 44, 431–438.

Factors Related to Speech Proficiency of the Laryngectomized

GEORGE H. SHAMES

JOHN FONT

JACK MATTHEWS

Success in learning to communicate following a laryngectomy has been variable. For the most part, explanations of success and failure have been based on casual impressions of clinicians. The study by Robe, Moore, Holzinger, and Andrews in 1956 represents a major research attempt to identify factors associated with the successful learning of esophageal speech. They found that better esophageal speakers had narrow fields of surgery. However, there is still very little understanding of the reasons for success or failure in learning to communicate following a laryngectomy.

The primary purpose of this project was to study variables which might be related to the learning of speech by laryngectomized patients. Specifically, biographical, medical, personality-social, communication and speech training variables were studied as correlates of speech proficiency.

Descriptions of speech training procedures were also obtained and correlated with measures of speech proficiency. In addition, a group of esophageal speakers was compared with a group of artificial appliance users on several measures of speech proficiency, as well as on variables associated with speech proficiency.

Research Procedures

Subjects and Sampling Procedures. The data for this study were obtained from 153 laryngectomized subjects. One hundred subjects made tape recordings of samples of their speech and were interviewed at the annual meeting of the International Association of Laryngectomees. In addition, university speech and hearing clinics and Lost Chord Clubs in Pennsylvania, Ohio, New York, and Texas were contacted for subjects.

No attempt was made to restrict the size of the research population. How-

George H. Shames (Ph.D., University of Pittsburgh, 1952) is Associate Professor of Speech and Psychology and Associate Director of the Speech Clinic at the University of Pittsburgh. John Font (Ph.D., University of Pittsburgh, 1960) is Assistant Professor and Supervisor, Training Clinic, Division of Speech Pathology and Audiology, Stanford Medical Center, Stanford University. Jack Matthews (Ph.D., Ohio State University, 1946) is Professor of Speech and Chairman of the Department of Speech and Theatre Arts at the University of Pittsburgh. This study was partially supported by funds provided by the Office of Vocational Rehabilitation (Project Number 465) and the National Science Foundation (Grant Number G-14594).

Reprinted by permission from *Journal of Speech and Hearing Disorders*, 1963, *28*, 273–287.

ever, an attempt was made to obtain a wide range of speaker proficiency to enable correlation analyses and to justify limited generalizations. The only criterion for inclusion in the study was that the laryngectomee's vocal training was terminated.

The esophageal speakers ranged in age from 26 years to 80 years with a mean age of 58 years. There were nine women and 109 men in this group. The age at which the laryngectomy was performed ranged from 16 years to 72 years with a mean age of 58 years.

The artificial appliance group was composed mainly of users of the 'Electrolarynx' instrument. Two of the subjects used the Western Electric 'artificial larynx' and one subject used the Cooper Rand instrument. There were two women and 33 men in this group. Their ages ranged from 38 years to 76 years with a mean age of 61 years. The age at the time of surgery ranged from 34 years to 75 years with a mean age of 56 years.

Method of Gathering the Data. Each subject who agreed to participate in this study was given a questionnaire, a self-administered personality test, and several forms for describing esophageal speech teaching to complete at his leisure. In addition, each subject made a tape recording of a phonetically balanced word list and a 101 word paragraph. Because of time limitations, only every third subject recorded one of the Harvard Sentence Intelligibility lists.

The speech recordings of these subjects were made in various locations and varying recording conditions. In Pittsburgh, during the annual meeting

of the International Association of Laryngectomees the recordings were made in five of the hotel rooms of the Penn-Sheraton Hotel, which were located high above the street level. The conditions were good for recording and reasonably constant from room to room. However, the greatest variability in the testing situations occurred during the field trips. In Cleveland, Erie, and Buffalo, all of the recordings were in the homes of the individual participants or at places of business. In New York, the recordings were made at the Park Sheraton Hotel, while at Bowling Green State University, Kent State University, and the Youngstown Hearing and Speech Center the recordings were made in partially sound-treated rooms. In Texas, the recordings were made at the Houston Hearing and Speech Center.

Description of Measurements. The Questionnaire. A questionnaire containing 45 items (See Appendix) was designed to provide information about the following: biographical variables, medical variables, personality and social behavior, and communication and speech training variables. The medical information was provided by the laryngectomized subject's physician. All other questionnaire data were provided by the laryngectomized subjects.

Personality Needs. The Edwards Personal Preference Schedule (Edwards, 1959) was used to assess the personality needs of the subjects. This test evaluates 15 relatively independent normal personality variables, based on the concept of manifest needs developed by Murray, et al. (1938, pp. 36-242). These personality needs, as defined by Edwards, are: achievement, deference, order, exhibition, autonomy, affiliation, intraception, succorance, dominance, abasement, nurturance, change, endurance, heterosexuality, and aggression.

Word Intelligibility. The Harvard Phonetically Balanced word lists (Egan, 1948) were utilized for measuring word intelligibility. There are 20 equivalent lists available, with each list containing 50 monosyllabic words.

Five undergraduate students at the University of Pittsburgh were used as auditors for judging word intelligibility. They listened to the tape recordings of the laryngectomized subjects and wrote the words they heard.

The reliabilities of the word intelligibility measures were determined by Ebel's adaptation (1951) of Fisher's intraclass formula for analysis of variance. The reliability of the five judges of word intelligibility for the esophageal group was .94 and for the artificial appliance group .98, indicating that the PB word intelligibility measure was a reliable method for assessing the intelligibility of laryngectomized speakers.

Sentence Intelligibility. The Harvard Sentence Intelligibility lists (Abrams, et al., 1944) were used for measuring sentence intelligibility. Each list contains 20 sentences. Scoring was based on whether five key words in each sentence were heard and written correctly by five auditors, in the proper sequence. The highest possible score was 100. The same auditors were given instructions and practice sessions similar to those used in their auditing of word intelligibility. Sentence intelligibility measures were obtained for 31 of the esophageal subjects and 12 of the artificial appliance users. Ebel's an-

alysis of variance technique was employed for estimating the reliabilities of the sentence intelligibility measures. For both the esophageal and artificial appliance group listener reliability was .99.

Time. The present study employed as a time measure the total time consumed during a reading task. A paragraph from Fairbanks' *Voice and Articulation Drillbook* (1940, p. 154) was selected for this purpose. The paragraph contained 101 words and was composed of five sentences. Each sentence was timed separately by two observers with a stopwatch. These measures were obtained on 110 esophageal subjects and on 33 artificial appliance subjects. Pearson product moment correlations were computed between the results of the two timers. Both correlations were .99, indicating high reliability of the simple timing measure.

Articulation and Surd-Sonant Errors. The phonetically balanced word lists used for assessing word intelligibility were analyzed for accuracy of production of initial and final sounds in each word. In addition to an articulation score based on the total number of correctly produced sounds, specific instances of surd-sonant substitutions were separately analyzed. For these analyses, three different auditors competent in phonetic transcription were utilized. Each auditor's task was to judge the correctness of articulation and to describe the articulation error which may have occurred. For sound substitutions they also described the substitution.

For the esophageal group, all three judges agreed on 71.8 per cent of the sounds (whether the sound was correct or incorrect and the nature of the articulation error). At least two judges agreed on 97.3 per cent of the sounds. On 2.7 per cent of the sounds there was complete disagreement among the judges. For the artificial appliance group, all three judges agreed on 59.9 per cent of the sounds. At least two judges agreed on 94.8 per cent of the sounds. On 5.2 per cent of the sounds there was c o m p l e t e disagreement among the judges. Only those data on which two of the three judges agreed were used in the later analyses of surd-sonant errors and articulation.

Descriptions of Speech Teaching Procedures. The c r i t i c a l incident method developed by Flanagan (1954) was employed for obtaining descriptions of speech training procedures from the laryngectomized subjects.

The subjects were asked to write out, in narrative form, specific descriptions of episodes during which effective and ineffective behaviors by their speech teacher were observed. They were asked to report in detail what their speech teacher did that they thought was helpful or a hindrance in learning esophageal speech. The behaviors reported by the subjects were later extracted from these narratives and independently sorted into categories of teaching behavior by two observers.

Frequency tabulations were made for each behavior. In addition, each subject was catalogued with reference to the behaviors he reported, enabling these data to be correlated with the speech proficiency data available to him.

A reliability check was made of the categorizations of teaching procedures by comparing the sortings of the two observers. The teaching behavior was

placed in the same categories by the two observers 82 per cent of the time.

Results

Correlations Among Measures of Speech Proficiency. Tables 1 and 2 show the product-moment correlations among the various measures of speech proficiency for the esophageal and artificial appliance groups. For both groups of laryngectomized subjects, the correlations among articulation, word intelligibility, and sentence intelligibility ranged from .80 to .86 and were statistically significant. The correlations involving surd-sonant errors and time were somewhat smaller, but still statistically significant for the esophageal group. These correlations ranged from .38 to .58. For the artificial appliance group, none of the correlations involving time was significant. This may have been due to the clustering of time scores at the faster end of the continuum. Some of the correlations involving surd-sonant errors for this group were as high as .66 and were statistically significant.

Relations Between M e a s u r e s of Speech Proficiency and Biographical, Medical, Personality-Social, Communication and Speech Training Variables. Fifty-nine variables were analyzed for their relations with each of the five measures of speech proficiency for each group. Nineteen significant variables were identified for the esophageal group while 13 significant variables were identified for the artificial appliance group. Tables 3 and 4 summarize these data. Seven variables (education, age at surgery intact cricopharyngeous muscle, the exhibition scale of the Edwards personality inventory, the length

TABLE 1. Pearson product-moment correlations among measures of speech proficiency for the esophageal group.

	Time (N=110)	Articulation (N=107)	Word Intelligibility (N=118)	Surd-Sonant Error (N=28)	Sentence Intelligibility (N=31)
Time		−.54†	−.47†	−.38*	−.51†
Articulation			.86†	−.58†	.83†
Word Intelligibility				−.38†	.85†
Surd-Sonant Error					−.18

*Significant at 5 per cent level of confidence.
†Significant at 1 per cent level of confidence.

TABLE 2. Pearson product-moment correlations among measures of speech proficiency for the artificial appliance group.

	Time (N=33)	Articulation (N=35)	Word Intelligibility (N=35)	Surd-Sonant Error (N=27)	Sentence Intelligibility (N=12)
Time		−.10	−.04	−.04	−.31
Articulation			.81*	−.66*	.80*
Word Intelligibility				−.63*	.86*
Surd-Sonant Error					−.45

*Significant at 1 per cent of confidence.

of time using his first method of communicating, the length of time between surgery and being understood, and the length of time in speech training) were significantly correlated to measures of speech proficiency for both groups. However, some of these correlations were unaccountably negative in direction. Twelve factors were significantly correlated to measures of speech proficiency for the esophageal group only. These were: age, removal of strap muscles, presurgical knowledge of voice problem, the number of speech lessons, and to nine of the Edwards personality scales (See Table 3). For the artificial appliance group only seven variables were significantly correlated with measures of speech proficiency. These

were: the presence of a fistula, the report of a difficult adjustment for the family, the duration of social withdrawal, the report that the problem was a source of embarrassment, the nurturance scale of the Edwards inventory, the length of time between surgery and speech training. Generally for both groups higher speech proficiency scores were related to being younger, more educated, less surgically involved, and to receiving speech training soon after surgery.

Of special interest are two variables that emerged after surgery which were significant for the artificial group but not significant for the esophageal group. These were: reported difficulty of adjustment for the family and the

TABLE 3. Summary of significant correlations* between measures of speech proficiency and biographical, medical, personality-social, communication, and speech training variables for esophageal group.

Variables	Time r N	Articulation r N	PB Word Intellig. r N	Surd-Sonant r N	Sentence Intelligibility r N
Biographical					
Age			−.40† 118		−.51† 31
Education		.21 107			
Age at Surgery			−.46† 118		−.53† 31
Medical*					
Intact cricopharyngeous		.27 95			
Removal of Strap muscles	−.26 110				
Presurgical knowledge of resulting voice problem				.41 28	
Edwards Personal Preference Schedule					
Achievement					−.51† 31
Deference			−.34† 75		
Order	.24 75	−.28 75			
Exhibition	.38† 75				
Affiliation		.54† 75			
Intraception			−.37† 75		−.45 31
Abasement					−.43 31
Heterosexuality			.31† 75		
Aggression					.42 31
Communication and Speech Training					
Length of time using first communication method	.32† 106		−.25 106		
Time between surgery and being understood	.26† 117	−.22 107	−.22 117		
Length of time in speech training	.23 97				.38 31
Number of speech lessons					.39 31

*Correlations with medical variables are biserial correlations. Others are product-moment correlations. All correlations given are significant at or beyond the 5 per cent level of confidence.

†Significant at or beyond the 1 per cent level. All others significant between 5 per cent and 1 per cent level of confidence.

subject's assessment of his speech problem as a s o u r c e of embarrassment. These two variables suggest the presence of speech and social contingencies for the artificial appliance users that were present to a lesser extent for the esophageal speakers. Such contingencies might well have been important in electing to use an artificial appliance instead of learning the more difficult and time-consuming esophageal speech.

Comparisons of Esophageal and Artificial Appliance Groups. Chi-square analyses and *t* tests of significance of difference revealed that the esophageal and artificial appliance groups were significantly different from one another on 12 of the 64 variables studied in this project. The *t* test results appear in Table 5. Although the artificial appliance group had significantly faster reading times than the esophageal group, the esophageal group was superior on all other dimensions of speech proficiency. The esophageal group has significantly higher mean articulation and word intelligibility scores and a significantly lower mean number of surd-sonant errors. These results do not support Hyman's findings (1955) that esophageal speakers and artificial appliance users are not significantly different in intelligibility. Hyman's small sample and his use of only good speakers as subjects may explain this disagreement between the two studies.

In terms of the Edwards scale measures the artificial a p p l i a n c e group showed greater need to avoid conformity, while the esophageal group showed less need to stick to a task but greater need to influence others. Because speech training had already been terminated prior to this project, it is difficult to in-terpret these personality differences between the groups. They may reflect presurgical personality status, but may just as easily reflect the results of therapy.

In addition to those items listed in Table 5, chi-square analyses revealed that the two groups were significantly different from each other in their reported preference for their present method of communicating, their difficulty in learning esophageal speech, and their report that esophageal speech was undesirable. However, the differences between the groups on these variables as well as the significantly greater time interval between surgery and being understood by the artificial appliance group may also be a reflection of therapeutic results.

Over 90 per cent of both groups reported that they used writing as their first method of communicating. However, the esophageal group discontinued such writing after less than three months, while the artificial appliance group continued writing on the average for 11 months. It cannot be stated whether the persistent use of writing was the result or the cause of not learning esophageal speech. However, this factor not only differentiated the two groups but was related to measures of speech proficiency for both groups, and suggests its importance during the course of treatment.

Procedures for Teaching Esophageal Speech. Through the critical incident method, 63 esophageal subjects reported 184 effective speech teaching incidents and 28 ineffective speech teaching incidents. These incidents were classified into categories of teaching behavior. They are listed in Table 6 with

TABLE 4. Summary of significant correlations* between measures of speech proficiency and biographical, medical, personality-social, communication, and speech training variables for artificial appliance group.

| | Measures of Speech Proficiency | | | | | | | | | |
| Variables | Time | | Articulation | | PB Word Intellig. | | Surd-Sonant | | Sentence Intelligibility | |
	r	N	r	N	r	N	r	N	r	N
Biographical										
Education	−.41	'33	.47†	35	.45†	35				
Age at Surgery			−.52†	35	.51†	35				
Medical*										
Presence of fistula									−.61	12
Intact cricopharyngeous									.68	12
Personality-Social										
Difficult adjustment for family									.58†	12
Length of time of social withdrawal	−.94†	6								
Speech problem as a source of embarrassment					.39†	35				
Edwards Personal Preference Schedule										
Exhibition	−.44	27					.47	27		
Nurturance					−.39	28				
Communication and Speech Training										
Time between surgery and speech training					−.37	28	.42	27		
Time using first method of communicating			.35	33	.41	33				
Time between surgery and being understood			.48†	29	.45	29				
Time in speech training			.45	24	.49	27				

*Correlations with medical variables are biserial correlations. Others are product-moment correlations. All correlations given are significant at or beyond the 5 per cent level of confidence.

†Significant at or beyond the 1 per cent level. All others significant between 5 per cent and 1 per cent level of confidence.

the frequency with which each was reported.

The most frequently reported effective speech therapy behavior was that of the therapist verbally motivating the laryngectomee by giving encouragement support, prodding, and criticism. This was closely followed by explanation of therapy procedures which focused on developing phonation, such as trapping the air or swallowing. The least frequently reported behavior was

TABLE 5. Variables for which esophageal group was statistically different from artificial appliance group.

Variables	Esophageal Group N	Mean	Artificial Appliance Group N	Mean	t
Time reading a paragraph (in seconds)	110	60.40	33	42.03	6.44*
Number of correctly articulated consonants in PB words	107	66.30	35	58.03	3.09*
Number of correct PB words	118	54.90	35	35.50	5.51*
Surd-sonant errors (per cent)	28	5.61	27	8.54	2.33**
Edwards Personal Preference Schedule					
Need for autonomy	75	13.30	27	16.04	3.70*
Need for dominance	74	15.60	28	12.82	2.55†
Need for endurance	74	15.30	28	17.75	2.15**
Length of time using first method of communicating (in days)	106	84.00	33	342.90	4.21*
Length of time between surgery and being understood (in days)	117	105.80	29	227.90	2.45†

*Significant at the .01 level of confidence.
†Significant at the .02 level of confidence.
**Significant at the .05 level of confidence.

the use of extrinsic motivational devices such as use of speech games and tape recorders. Because of the sparseness of these data, this phase of the project must be considered exploratory and the findings only tentative.

Biserial correlation analyses revealed that none of these categories of teaching behavior was significantly related to the speech proficiency scores of the subjects reporting the behavior. Also, t test analyses revealed that no particular method for developing phonation was demonstrated as being better than another by virtue of the speech proficiency scores of the subjects reporting the use of that method.

Finally, t test analyses showed that there were no significant differences in speech proficiency scores between subjects taught by speech therapists and subjects taught by other laryngectomees. It was revealed that speech therapists and laryngectomees did similar things in teaching esophageal speech, with speech therapists emphasizing phonation procedures to a significantly lesser extent than laryngectomized teachers.

General Interpretations

It is of interest that many of the commonly held ideas about what is good for the laryngectomized patient were not supported by this study. For example, such things as presurgical

TABLE 6. Frequency with which effective and ineffective speech training procedures were listed by 63 esophageal speakers.

Effective Categories	Frequency
Teacher provided verbal motivation	43
Phonation procedures	36
Explanations	20
Shaping of behavior through successive approximations	19
Teacher demonstrated with own esophageal speech	18
Outside practice activities	15
Breathing, rhythm and rate	14
Visual stimuli of speech production	11
Use of extrinsic motivational devices and aids	9

Ineffective Categories	Frequency
Poor motivational techniques	10
Unsuccessful phonation procedures	4
Poor explanations	4
Failed to shape behavior through successive approximations	4
Ineffective practice schedules	3
Not enough time for lesson	3

speech training and presurgical ability to belch voluntarily were not related to proficiency as an esophageal speaker. As revealed by these data, the subjects' source of speech training was also not a factor in his esophageal proficiency; nor were various medical and surgical factors, such as removal of certain muscles and structures, found to be associated with proficiency. Some of these negative findings suggest that some of our current speech therapeutic procedures may be inefficient and can be eliminated. It is possible that a clinician's time and effort may be directed toward more critical problems prior to and following surgery, such as counseling with the patient and family, rather than attempting to teach speech to a presurgical patient, whose current anxieties about his impending surgery may limit the values of such teaching.

Emerging from this study is a sharper picture of the patient who becomes a proficient esophageal speaker, and of the factors associated with this proficiency. The results demonstrate the superiority of esophageal speech over that produced with an artificial appliance, in terms of articulation, phonation, and intelligibility. As such, esophageal speech should be considered the method of choice for communication for the laryngectomized.

An examination of their responses to the questionnaire (see Appendix) shows that the esophageal and artificial appliance groups were similar in their biographical and surgical histories. It would seem that their selection of either the esophageal method or the artificial appliance method of communicating after their laryngectomy cannot be attributed to variables in these two areas. Such results logically lead us to consider further such things as presurgical personality and social variables which may affect the patient's motivation and postsurgical management variables, such as family relations, occupational and financial pressures, counseling and speech training.

There is reason to believe that the younger and more educated laryngectomee will become the better esophageal speaker. The same thing can be said for the better artificial appliance user. It is also felt that a more favorable prognosis might be made for the patient whose strap muscles and cricopharyngeous muscles are preserved. When possible, the time interval between surgery and the initiation of speech training should be short. The role of the family also seems important to the laryngectomee's rehabilitation. Pressures for immediate speech by the laryngectomees should be kept to a minimum, whether the pressures be from the family or from the laryngectomee. This suggests the need for the competent counseling of both the family and the patient so that he will have optimum conditions for trying to learn esophageal speech. With an accepting and understanding family, and a laryngectomee who is not under pressure to communicate immediately, poor communication habits such as persistent writing can give way to his emerging skills as an esophageal speaker. Finally, the laryngectomee needs a competent teacher who is proficient in esophageal speech processes,

general learning processes, and who can provide proper motivation.

Summary

This project studied the relationships between several measures of speech proficiency and a number of biographical, medical, personality, social, and speech training variables in a population of 153 laryngectomized patients. In addition, comparisons were made between a group of 118 esophageal speakers and a group of 35 users of artificial appliances.

The results revealed:

1. The artificial appliance group read a paragraph significantly faster than the esophageal group. The esophageal group had significantly better mean articulation, word intelligibility, and surd-sonant scores. There were no significant differences in mean sentence intelligibility scores.

2. Both groups showed high and statistically significant c o r r e l a tions among a number of measures of speech proficiency.

3. Both groups showed a wide range of significant correlations between measures of speech proficiency and the variables studied. For both the esophageal and artificial appliance group these variables included: (a) education, (b) age at surgery, (c) an intact cricopharyngeous muscle, (d) length of time using the first postoperative method of communicating, (e) length of time between surgery and being understood, (f) length of time in speech training, and (g) several personality variables measured by the Edwards Personal Preference Schedule.

For the esophageal group there were several additional significant variables.

These were: (a) age, (b) removal of strap muscles, (c) presurgical knowledge of a resulting voice problem, and (d) number of speech lessons.

For the artificial appliance group there were several additional significant variables. These were: (a) presence of a fistula, (b) reporting of difficult family adjustment, (c) length of time of social withdrawal, (d) reporting of embarrassment about the speech problem, and (e) length of time between surgery and the beginning of speech training.

4. Nine categories of teaching procedures were identified through the critical incident method. Good esophageal speakers were not differentiated from poor esophageal speakers by (a) any one or combination of these teaching procedures, (b) the method of teaching phonation, (c) the source of esophageal speech teaching (speech therapist, another laryngectomee, self-taught). Speech therapists and laryngectomees do similar things in teaching esophageal speech.

Acknowledgement

Acknowledgement is made of the following individuals and agencies who assisted in this research by providing laryngectomized subjects and making their facilities available: Dr. Jack Bangs, Houston Hearing and Speech Center, Houston, Texas; Frances Beyers, Buffalo, New York; William Bolger, Cleveland, Ohio; Mrs. Sondra Hill, Youngstown Hearing and Speech Center, Youngstown, Ohio; Arthur Kaltenborn, Kent State University, Kent, Ohio; Oscar Lueders, New York, New York; Jack Ranney, Executive Secretary, International Association of Laryngectomees; Management of the Penn-Sheraton Hotel, Pittsburgh, Pennsylvania; and National Hospital for Speech Disorders, New York, New York.

References

ABRAMS, M. H., GOFFARD, S. J., KRYTER, K. D., MILLER, G. A., MILLER, J., and SANFORD, F. H., Speech in noise: a study of the factors determining its intelligibility. Psycho-Acoustic Laboratory, Harvard Univ., OSRD Report No. 4023 (PB 19805), Sept. 1, 1944.

EBEL, R. L., Estimation of the reliability of ratings. Psychometrika, 16, 1951, 407-424.

EDWARDS, A. L., Edwards Personal Preference Schedule. New York: Psychological Corp. 1959.

EGAN, J. P., Articulation testing methods. Laryngoscope, 58, 1948, 955-991.

FAIRBANKS, G., Voice and Articulation Drillbook. New York and London: Harper and Bros., 1940.

Flanagan, J. C., The critical incident technique. Psych. Bull., 51, 1954, 327-358.

HYMAN, M., An experimental study of artificial-larynx and esophageal speech. J. Speech Hearing Dis., 20, 1955, 291-299.

MURRAY, H. A., and others, Explorations in Personality. New York: Oxford Univ. Press, 1938.

ROBE, E. Y., MOORE, P., ANDREWS, A. H., JR., and HOLINGER, P. H., A study of the role of certain factors in the development of speech after laryngectomy, 1. Type of operation. Laryngoscope, 66, 1956, 173-186.

Appendix

Questionnaire for biographical, medical, social, communication, and speech training variables. Response mean scores or totals are given where appropriate.

Item		Response Esophageal Group (N=118)	Artificial Appliance Group (N=35)
1. Birthdate	mean age (years)	57.7	60.5
2. Sex	number of males	109	33
	number of females	9	2
3. Education	mean number of years of education	11.1	10.5
4. Age at time of operation	mean age of surgery (years)	52.4	55.6
5. Is your hearing normal?	yes	101	30
	no	17	5
6. Is your health generally good?	yes	116	33
	no	2	2
Name of surgeon for laryngectomy			
Date of operation			
Hospital where surgery took place			
7. Length of time in hospital	mean number of days	24.9	23.3
8. How soon after operation were you able to return to work?	mean number of days	87.2	93.1
9. How soon after operation did you begin speech training?	mean number of days	54.7	67.6
10. How did you communicate immediately after the operation?	writing	114[1]	33
	artificial larynx	3	2
	other (specify)	0	0
11. How long did you use this method?	mean number of days	84	342.8
12. Is your present method of communicating the method you prefer?	yes	115	27
	no	2	7
	no response	1	1
13. If you do not use esophageal speech, is it because you:	were unable to learn it		15
	never tried it		4
	do not like it		8
	prefer other speaking methods		1
	were advised not to use it		2
	other		3
14. Do people have difficulty understanding you?	yes	3	11
	no	31	107
15. How long after the operation was it before you could be reasonably well understood when speaking to others?	mean number of days	105.8	227.9

[1]The totals for the responses do not always add up to 118 for the esophageal group and to 35 for the artificial appliance group because all of the questions were not answered by some of the subjects.

16. Is a foreign language spoken in the home?	yes no	8 110	3 31
17. Did you have speech difficulties of any nature prior to the operation?	yes no	5 113	0 35
18. Were you able to voluntarily belch before the operation?	yes no	68 39	17 18
19. Are you usually able to make yourself heard when speaking?	yes no	111 6	32 1
20. Did you know before surgery that you would be unable to speak after the operation?	yes no	101 15	25 9
21. Did you find adjusting to not having your voice difficult?	yes no	66 51	24 10
22. Was it difficult for your family?	yes no	64 53	21 14
23. Do these difficulties exist now?	yes no	6 103	3 32
24. Has the removal of your larynx ever caused you to withdraw from social activities?	yes no	39 77	9 25
25. If you withdrew from social activities, for how long?	mean number of days	82.4	229.3
26. Do you engage in as many social activities now as you would had you never had the operation?	yes no	92 26	22 12
27. Is your condition ever a source of embarrassment to you?	yes no	25 92	10 25
28. Length of time of speech training	mean number of days	101.2	155.3
29. Approximate number of lessons	mean number of lessons	19.4	19.9
30. Did you attend instructions:	regularly occasionally infrequently hardly at all no response	86 3 0 5 24	20 3 0 3 9
31. Did you have any speech training prior to surgery?	yes no	4 112	1 30
32. Were you ever advised not to use or try to use esophageal speech?	yes no	3 112	5 28
33. Was learning esophageal speech difficult for you?	yes no	43 74	22 5
34. Did you find esophageal speech undesirable?	yes no	19 95	13 12
35. If you have had speech training, was it from:	speech therapist another laryngectomee family self taught	66 28 1 22	23 1 1 5
36. Was there a postoperative fistula?	yes no	19 77	5 23

37. Was any portion of the esophagus resected?	yes	14	3
	no	81	25
38. Was the cricopharyngeous muscle left essentially intact?	yes	69	20
	no	26	8
39. Was the epiglottis removed?	yes	82	26
	no	12	2
40. Was any portion of the tongue removed? If so, which?	yes	6	1
	no	87	26
41. Was a radical neck dissection also done?	yes	18	7
	no	76	21
42. Were the strap muscles removed?	yes	55	19
	no	37	9
43. Was the hyoid bone removed?	yes	62	17
	no	29	11
44. Did you consider the person a good candidate for learning esophageal speech?	yes	86	23
	no	2	3
45. Was there any x-ray therapy prior to or following surgery?	yes	14	2
	no	79	25

Preoperative Ideas of
Speech After Laryngectomy

MARSHALL J. DUGUAY, MS, BUFFALO, NY

PHYSICIANS and surgeons are becoming more and more aware of the need to treat the "whole person." This is particularly true in laryngectomy, where satisfactory results involve an essential overlapping of physiology and psychology. Ideally the rehabilitation of a laryngectomy patient should begin as soon as he is informed of the possibility that he may have to undergo laryngectomy. Of course, he ordinarily cannot be expected to understand all of the details, but certainly he ought to be aware, in general, of what is going to happen to him and how he will be able to keep the consequent limitations to a minimum. ·Such knowledge is especially important to the psychological well-being of the laryngectomy patient.

The present study was undertaken in an effort to find out what sorts of ideas laryngectomy candidates have concerning postoperative speech. On the basis of such ideas, it is more or less apparent what some of the problems facing laryngectomy patients actually are, and it is possible to make a few tentative suggestions as to how the patients can best be helped in providing those problems with satisfactory solutions.

Problems of Laryngectomy Patients

"Cancer of the larynx," say Holinger and his associates [1] "is one of the most curable

Submitted for publication Oct 26, 1965.
From the Speech Therapy Clinic, Roswell Park Memorial Institute, New York State Department of Health, Buffalo, NY.
Reprint requests to 1300 Elmwood Ave, Buffalo, NY 14222.

of all malignancies." Adequate treatment for advanced laryngeal cancer usually involves surgical removal of the entire larynx together with as much of the surrounding tissue as must also be excised in order to provide a reasonable margin of safety. In many cases, the only important anatomical structure sacrificed is the larynx itself.

According to Gardner,[2] "Early removal of the cancerous growth gives greater assurance of survival and indeed permits large numbers of persons to resume normal lives." Under the circumstances, the best interests of the patient ordinarily require that appropriate surgery be performed as soon as possible after it has been established that he has laryngeal cancer.

"Probably the most serious blow to the patient," Laguaite [3] points out, "is the fact that he will be deprived of the normal voice mechanism." Speech is the principal human means of communication,[4] and thus is essential to human activities in general.[5] It follows that the patient can hardly be expected to maintain his psychological well-being unless he is suitably informed concerning the extent to which he is likely to recover his ability to speak.

As Williams [4] puts it:

The rehabilitation of the laryngectomy patient should start before surgery. I am sorry to say that this is not always the case. In this day and age of modern surgery and knowledge of the social-emotional factors involved in the total rehabilitation of a patient, we still have patients who have their larynx removed without pre-surgical consultation in regard to the fact that they will be voiceless after surgery, or that a means of talking can be developed. Consequently, many never completely recover from the psychological shock of being voiceless, develop habits that retard the development of esophageal speech, or even refuse to have surgery at the last moment.

From what has been said, it is evident that the problems facing laryngectomy patients deserve a good deal more attention than they have received in the past. Before much progress can be made in solving those problems, however, it is first necessary to determine exactly what those problems are.

Procedure

Every patient included in the present study had been referred to Roswell Park Memorial Institute by his family physician because of a diagnosis of possible cancer of the larynx. At Roswell Park, the patient had undergone an extensive medical examination, including a biopsy of the laryngeal tissue. The surgeon in charge of the case had informed the patient of the presence of malignant tissue in the biopsy specimen, had advised him to undergo laryngectomy as the most effective treatment for his laryngeal cancer, and had explained to him that he would presumably be able to learn how to speak without a larynx. The surgeon's remarks varied somewhat in detail from one surgeon to another, depending on such factors as the individual surgeon's medical training and philosophy and the exact nature and extent of the individual patient's cancer, but always included the pathological findings, the advisability of laryngectomy, and the possibility of postoperative speech.

After the surgeon had completed his preoperative consultation with the patient, the speech clinician was free to proceed with an interview to obtain data for the present study. A conventional questionnaire, with its paper-and-pencil approach, would have tended to distort material of the kind that was wanted for the study, and hence a tape recorder was set up in the interview room. Then the speech clinician brought the patient in, introduced himself, and proceeded with the interview. The recorder and microphone were neither concealed from the patient nor called to his attention. If he asked about the

recorder, he was told, "We always use it." Considering the value of a tape recorder in various aspects of speech therapy, this explanation was as true as any generalization of the same type could possibly be.

The speech clinician began the interview with a couple of sentences like the following: "I know the doctor has told you that you are to have surgery and that your voice box has to be removed. After your voice box is gone, how do you think that you will be able to talk?" The patient was then encouraged to verbalize his feelings.

Whenever the patient tended to digress from the topic under study, an attempt was made to bring him back to it. In the great majority of instances, this proved no easy task; most patients seemed ready to talk about anything that they could think of, other than postoperative speech. Perhaps some felt that they knew too little about the subject to be able to say anything worthwhile; no doubt many were largely inhibited by the emotion-laden preoperative situation. In any event, it is certainly not very hard to understand why a laryngectomy candidate might have difficulties in talking at any length about oral communication.

The interview room was relatively quiet, and hence the recordings are generally free from excessive background noise. In preparing material for analysis, the speech clinician replayed each tape a number of times, for the purpose of selecting key sentences that he felt were representative of the patient's preoperative concepts regarding postoperative speech.

Results

The results of the present study are too varied for any kind of tabulation to be really meaningful. In fact, the nature of the results is such that it even seems best just to let some of the patient's own comments during their interviews speak for themselves.

These comments were, of course, chosen so as to provide a cross section of the almost innumerably many that were heard during the entire series of interviews, but they will come simply in the order in which they were obtained; the multiplicity of ideas represented in individual comments makes completely impracticable any attempt to organize the comments according to type. At the beginning of each interview excerpt, however, the patient will be identified as to age, sex, and occupation.

CASE 1.—This 43-year-old furniture salesman stated: "I know it's going to be quite a struggle to learn speech all over again. It would be, I assume, much harder than teaching a child how to talk, because the air is then shut off somewhere at the nose and mouth. There is no air intake there, only through the aperture, which I must use for speech and for breathing. I imagine I'll have to take a deep breath, and when I let it out, that's when I form the speech-talk through the opening in my neck."

CASE 2.—This 62-year-old housewife said: "When they operate, they put in a switch. I don't know—like a little box. I never saw it."

CASE 3.—This 57-year-old housewife stated: "I haven't figured out whether it will or won't affect the way I talk. Something with the tube in my neck—you put your finger over that tube and talk. A woman in my room talks like that."

CASE 4.—This 42-year-old male postal worker said: "I'll use the diaphragm method to talk. I saw a man talk like that. He was breathing heavy and talking out of the hole in his throat. Sound will come out of the hole in my neck. I'll breathe air in. The sound's made there by cartilage moving on cartilage or flesh on cartilage. Something must already be there. I don't think they'll put anything in."

CASE 5.—This 73-year-old retired farmer stated: "If I can't learn to talk with therapy, I could get a voice box. I don't know if they have to put this in or not."

CASE 6.—This 63-year-old retired steel-plant foreman said: "They put something in there, don't they? You draw breath in some way into your lungs—develop some kind of pressure. The sound comes from your lungs. The words are formed down there, too."

CASE 7.—This 62-year-old millwright stated: "I haven't the least idea of how I can talk with no voice box."

CASE 8.—This 59-year-old automobile-factory foreman said: "You can talk from the stomach. It comes all the way up—take a deep breath."

CASE 9.—This 63-year-old mechanic stated: "I'll have to learn to speak from my diaphragm. To be honest, I'm not sure—from the stomach or something. Down here, I guess."

CASE 10.—This 56-year-old farmer said: "They claim that after a while you can get to whisper a bit. They have some of these other things you put up there and then throw your voice some way. There's a fellow back home who had it. He talks just the same as I do now, only it's all messed up—

hoarse and sounds as if his mouth were full of water. He gets by with it."

CASE 11.—This 61-year-old retired carpenter stated: "I don't know how it's gonna be. Air will come up from my stomach. It will get into my stomach, I guess, through this hole in my neck."

CASE 12.—This 58-year-old club steward said: "I have no idea. There was one man at home—he had a little tube that fit in his mouth and in the hole there. He spoke well. Of course, he died in Florida a few years later. He carried this tube in his pocket and you could understand him. I don't know—that's what worries me. What in the world will I do?"

CASE 13.—This 54-year-old painter stated: "I read something here one time not too long ago about that movie actor—what's his name?—William Gargan. He said they swallow their breath or something and then they control it."

CASE 14.—This 60-year-old security guard said: "I don't know. I'll try any system. I did meet a man today who had the operation. He doesn't put wind down in his stomach—he just keeps right on going. He can count to 500 without stopping. He must breathe through here some way and still keep right on talking. I don't know how it is."

CASE 15.—This 59-year-old chef stated: "My sister-in-law has no voice box. It was an accident. They cut her vocal cords out when they took her tonsils out. She talks from her stomach. They wanted her to go to a clinic in Cleveland and explain how she does it. She learned herself. That's just one idea of mine. I suppose they have electronic devices now, too. I was never in a hospital before, so I don't know too much about it."

CASE 16.—This 66-year-old retired railroad worker said: "They got, I guess like a little box in there that they give you, and then you get it up from your stomach."

CASE 17.—This 75-year-old steam fitter stated: "He says he may be able to replace it. There's a possibility he can put it back in. I know two fellows—two pals of mine—they have them battery larynxes they put here and talk through the batteries."

Comment

On the basis of many interviews like the ones from which the preceding excerpts were drawn, it is obvious that laryngectomy candidates' preoperative ideas concerning postoperative speech are generally unrealistic, and are often completely contrary to fact. Certain misconceptions were very common among the laryngectomy candidates in the present study.

They would have to swallow air all the way down into the stomach in order to talk.

They would talk from the stomach.

They would talk from the diaphragm.

They would talk from the lungs.

They would talk through the hole in the neck (ie, the tracheal stoma).

They would have to cover the hole in the neck in order to talk.

They would talk from some kind of voice box "put in" by the surgeons.

Most of the patients had one or another of these seven common misconceptions. At the one extreme were patients who did not actually verbalize any misconceptions, but did express complete ignorance in relation to postlaryngectomy speech. At the other extreme were patients who verbalized two or more misconceptions, frequently misconceptions that were anatomically incompatible not only with fact, but also with one another!

Since laryngectomy candidates' misconceptions regarding postoperative speech are mostly due to ignorance of the anatomy involved, the logical thing to do would be to provide the candidates with appropriate knowledge concerning the anatomical structures that are affected by laryngectomy and associated procedures, how these structures are affected, and what compensations have to be made. In particular, it might be valuable to utilize a simplified "before and after" diagram in connection with preoperative counseling. An explanation of the difference between a temporary tracheotomy and a permanent tracheostomy would presumably be helpful. The patient should be informed that esophageal speech can be accomplished by at least two different methods, neither of which requires actual swallowing of air. To protect against erroneous ideas in relation to artificial larynxes, there should be some discussion of what can and cannot be done with such devices.

Summary

Tape recordings were made of preoperative interviews with laryngectomy candidates who had been counseled by their surgeons in regard to their impending surgery. In each interview, the patient was encouraged to verbalize his own ideas concerning how he would be able to talk without a larynx. Some patients expressed complete ignorance of any mechanism for speaking after laryngectomy, but most made comments that indicated one or another of various misconceptions of nonlaryngeal speech. In order to avert the psychological trauma that such misconceptions might contribute to, subsequent to surgery, laryngectomy candidates should be provided with much more complete knowledge of what is going to happen to them and how they will be able to cope with it.

REFERENCES

1. Holinger, P.H.; Johnston, K.C.; and Mansueto, M.D.: Cancer of the Larynx, *Amer J Nurs* 57:738-743, 1957.

2. Gardner, W.H.: Problems of Laryngectomees, *Rehab Rec* Jan-Feb 1961, pp 15-18.

3. Laguaite, J.K.: Psychological and Social Problems of the Laryngectomized Individual, American Speech and Hearing Association Short Course on Esophageal Speech, New York, 1962.

4. Williams, N.H.: Speech Rehabilitation of the Laryngectomized Patient, *CA* 11:126-130, 1961.

5. Division of Vocational Rehabilitation, abstracts of the Third Postoperative Course in Esophageal Speech and Organic Voice Problems, Miami, Fla, June 17-28, 1957, p 21.

Adjustment Problems of
Laryngectomized Women

WARREN H. GARDNER, PhD, CLEVELAND

THE PROBLEMS of women who have undergone laryngectomy have not been discussed previously in the literature. At the convention of the International Association of Laryngectomees in Indianapolis in 1963, the female members gave a style show. The display of formal gowns, hostess and breakfast costumes, and attractive recreational attire demonstrated that the woman who has had a laryngectomy can be well dressed without attracting attention to the surgical scars in the neck. Year after year, the IAL programs have listed speakers who gave advice on how wives can ease the adjustments of their laryngectomized husbands and never on how husbands can ease the problems of their laryngectomized wives. In this paper the psychological and adjustment problems of female laryngectomees are considered.

Names of 625 laryngectomized women were obtained from the secretaries of local Lost Chord Clubs of the IAL. The names and addresses of the patients were obtained through special permission of the officers of the clubs. Their use was limited specifically and only to this survey. Three pages of questions were sent to these women. They were urged to be frank and honest in their answers, and they were assured that no one but the author would have access to their replies. They were also told that no quotations by name would be given without permission. Many of the women answered with

revealing statements about the problems that they had in facing surgery and in making adjustments after surgery. Hence, the results of this survey should be regarded as indicative of the reactions of the general population of female laryngectomees. The sults of this survey should be regarded as tabulation of more than 10,000 items.

Replies were received from 240 women in 35 states, the Virgin Islands, and Canada. Included were 178 married and 62 single women. All 240 women are not included in every category considered because of omission of replies on numerous issues.

The ages of the patients at the time of the laryngectomy ranged from 21 to 80 years (Table 1). The largest number of patients, 84, were from 51 to 60 years of age. Eighty-eight or 37% of the 237 women (Table 2) had survived five years or longer. One woman was alive 29 years after operation for cancer of the larynx.

Three fourths of the women were married at the time of surgery, but seven were sepa-

Submitted for publication June 8, 1965.

From the Department of Otolaryngology, Cleveland Clinic, Cleveland.

Reprint requests to Editorial Department, Cleveland Clinic, 2020 E 93rd St, Cleveland, Ohio 44106.

TABLE 1.—*Ages of 237 Women at Time of Laryngectomy*

Age Range, Years	Married	Single	Total
		No. of Patients	
21-30	4	1	5
31-40	22	3	25
41-50	63	11	74
51-60	60	24	84
61-70	24	20	44
71-80	4	1	5
Total	177	60	237

TABLE 2.—*Duration of Survival After Laryngectomy in 237 Women*

Duration, Years	Married	Single	Total
	No. of Patients		
1 or less	41	19	60
2	37	12	49
3	18	8	26
4	11	3	14
5	10	2	12
6-10	35	9	44
11-15	16	5	21
16-20	6	2	8
21-29	3	0	3
Total	177	60	237

TABLE 3.—*Duration of Cigarette Smoking by Married and Single Women*

Duration, Years	Married	Single	Total
	No. of Patients		
0-5	4	5	9
6-10	12	10	22
11-15	14	2	16
16-20	35	10	45
21-25	21	5	26
26-30	23	4	27
31-35	7	3	10
36-40	4	3	7
41-	3	—	3
Total	123	42	165

rated, six by mutual consent and one by illness. Of the single women, 11 were divorced, 34 were widows, and 15 had never married. Families that had children living at home totaled 86. More than one half of the single women and one third of the married women were working before surgery.

Table 3 shows that 165 or 70% of the women had been smoking up to the date of surgery. The largest number had smoked for between 16 and 20 years; but 44% had smoked over 20 years; 3 had smoked for more than 41 years; and only 9 had smoked five years or less. Table 4 shows that about the same percentage of patients (26.6%, 27.3%, 28.5%) began smoking in each of the three decades from 11 to 40 years of age. The percentage of married women who began smoking in their teens was almost three times as great (31.7% vs 11.9%) as that of single patients. Also, most of the single patients started smoking one decade later than the married women. The cause of this interesting difference requires further analysis, but a guess might point to the possibility that the married women were more sociable and, hence, had more contacts with smokers at an earlier age.

From 20 to 59 cigarettes were smoked daily by 84% of the smokers before laryngectomy. One patient was smoking four packs (80 cigarettes) a day, having started smoking 35 years before, at the age of 11 years (Table 5).

Fifty percent of the single women and 53% of the married women had a simple laryngectomy. The others had radical neck dissection or plastic surgery or both. One patient had five surgical procedures; and another patient had six plastic repairs within a period of two years. Some of the patients had the upper third of the esophagus re-

TABLE 4.—*Ages of Married and Single Women at Time of Laryngectomy and Start of Smoking*

Age at Surgery, Years	Total	Married	Single	Age at Start of Smoking, Years											
				1 to 10		11 to 20		21 to 30		31 to 40		41 to 50		50 —	
	No. of Patients			M	S	M	S	M	S	M	S	M	S	M	S
20 to 30	2	1	1	—	—	1	—	—	1	—	—	—	—	—	—
31 to 40	15	12	3	1	—	7	1	4	2	—	—	—	—	—	—
41 to 50	62	52	10	1	—	24	2	13	2	11	5	3	1	—	—
51 to 60	60	43	17	—	—	5	2	11	5	21	4	5	4	1	2
61 to 70	25	15	10	—	—	2	—	4	3	4	2	5	3	—	2
71 to 80	1	—	1	—	—	—	—	—	—	—	—	—	—	—	1
Total	165	123	42	2	—	39	5	32	13	36	11	13	8	1	5
				2		44		45		47		21		6	
Percent each age, single at time of operation						11.9		31.0		26.2		19.0		11.9	
Percent each age, married at time of operation				1.6		31.7		26.2		29.2		10.5		0.8	
Percent each age, all patients at time of operation				1.2		26.6		27.3		28.5		12.8		3.6	

moved, others had portions of the pharynx or of the tongue excised.

The Preoperative Period

Reactions to the Diagnosis of Cancer.— The patients were asked to describe their thoughts when the surgeon told them that they had cancer of the larynx. Three women thought of suicide; one of them begged the surgeon to give her poison. Thirty women wept, but ten of them were so ill that they didn't care what happened to them. Fright and speechlessness were the reactions of 80 women who also worried about leaving their families and their babies without a mother. They thought: "This is the end, why has this happened to me?" Twenty rejected the news; they wanted to be able to talk, to sing, to keep their jobs; and they objected to the expense. The remainder calmly accepted the news because many of them had anticipated it; others had had radiation or had had cancer previously, and they all believed they had nothing to lose.

More than three fourths of the married women were bolstered by the presence of their husbands when the report of cancer was given them. The other wives were alone because of illness, estrangement, or urgency of their husbands' businesses. Two thirds of the single women had someone with them in the physician's office at the time they heard the diagnosis.

Reactions of the Husbands to News of Cancer.—The emotional reaction to news of cancer in their wives so disturbed one third of the husbands that they were unable to talk. Another one third questioned the surgeons: "Will it save her life? Will she talk? Will she be able to care for the children?" They protested: "We can't afford it," or "We will have to think it over." Another third calmly said: "If you can cure her, go ahead and operate." One husband spoke warmly: "She's helped others all of her life; now you can help her, Doc."

Eighty-nine of the wives reported the remarks of their husbands during that time that they were deciding whether or not to undergo surgery. One chronically ill husband asked: "What will me and the dog do?" Two husbands asked for a divorce.

TABLE 5.—*Number of Cigarettes Smoked Daily by Women Before Laryngectomy*

No. of Cigarettes Smoked Daily	Married	Single	Total
	No. of Patients		
1-20	14	8	22
20-39	74	27	101
40-59	32	6	38
60	2	1	3
80	1	0	1
Total	123	42	165

One of them emphatically insisted that his professional standing would be jeopardized if he had a wife with a hole in her neck. The other husband blurted out: "The strain is too great. I can't take it." Faced with these attitudes, one half of the wives made up their own minds. Another third of the husbands held their wives' hands as they assured them that they loved them. One husband was reported as saying: "As long as you are with me, that is all that counts. Your love is my strength." Other couples prayed together and asked for strength for the wife to endure surgery and to be able to return to her husband and children.

Only one quarter of the single women reported reactions of relatives and friends; half of these relatives calmly gave practical advice, and the other half were so shocked that they were neither decisive nor encouraging. Consequently more than 85% of all single women were forced to make their own decisions to accept or to reject surgery.

The Waiting Period.—The hours and days of waiting for the removal of their larynx were not happy ones for all of the wives. One husband was so antagonistic that he canceled his hospitalization insurance so that his wife could not use it. All discussion was avoided by 17 husbands who avoided their wives as much as they could. Nine wives were alone in the hospital during the waiting period. However, almost 75% of the husbands were assuring and optimistic, attentive, protective, and affectionate. One husband gave his wife ". . . as gay a time as they ever had during the waiting period." In two instances, the wives had to bolster the morale of their husbands!

Seventy percent of the single women either refrained from reporting on this question or had no moral support from relatives and friends during the waiting period. The other women wrote that kind and understanding persons had expressed optimism and confidence that all would be well in the future days.

The Postoperative Period

The postoperative days in the hospital were not pleasant for some of the wives. Five wives had infrequent visits from their husbands, and 22 wives refrained from describing their hospital days. However, 75% of the wives reported that husbands were most attentive and came as often as their businesses permitted them. One husband kept insisting: "You're as pretty as a picture." Slightly more than 50% of the single women were visited by relatives and friends. One blind patient had original surgery and five plastic revisions within five months during which time not one person visited her.

Visitation by Other Laryngectomees.— One of the principal activities of the Lost Chord Clubs is the visitation program. Upon request of the surgeon, one to three persons who have undergone laryngectomy, who have good speech, and who are well adjusted are asked to call upon the patient at the hospital. The visit is usually made on the sixth day after surgery, when the patient is beginning to feel better physically, but emotionally she realizes that she cannot talk and may never speak another word. Forty-five percent of the married women and 62% of the single women had visitors from the Lost Chord Clubs; 48 were men and 69 were women; 82% of the visits were made after surgery.

Reactions to the First View of the Stoma.—What does a laryngectomized woman think when she gets her first view of the stoma and scars of surgery? More than 48% of them reacted unfavorably; 60 patients were horrified and shocked at their appearance; 28 were disgusted and regarded themselves as being repulsive; 14 of them had difficulty with reviving any enthusiasm for living; and 4 fainted. Some of the remarks contributed were: "A blow to my vanity." "I've lost the best part of my life." "I'm a scarecrow." "I wish I was dead."

However, others looked at their scars and said, "Just what the doctor said it would be." "What a wonderful job of sewing me up." "Not as bad as I thought it would be." "Thank God I can breathe again."

Only 23% of the patients said that they believed that surgery had made them less feminine. Less than 35% thought that the scars and stoma made them less attractive to others. About 16% thought that they would not be able to display affection as zealously as they had done before surgery.

The Return to Their Homes.—The return home was a pleasant experience for some wives and most unpleasant for others. Sixty-five wives refrained from discussing the attitudes of their husbands. Forty-six percent of the reporting wives stated that their husbands avoided them, showed too much pity, babied them too much, or did not show enough interest in and sympathy for their efforts to adjust to personal and emotional problems and to regain health and happiness. However, 54% of the reporting wives gladly wrote stories about their loyal husbands who displayed optimism and confidence that their wives would succeed in returning to their domestic and social lives.

Depressing experiences were reported by 60% of the single women because neither relatives nor friends called upon them to have courage, nor inspired them to return to their normal routine.

Reactions to the First Sounds of Their New Voices.—The first esophageal speech sound that the women made evoked varied emotional responses from pessimism to optimism; the pessimists' first impressions were described as feeling embarrassed, frustrated, pitiful, terrible, awful. They thought that they faced a hopeless, unhappy, sad, and doubtful future because they were "petrified" by the frog-croaking, hoarse, male voice. The optimistic group were happy, hopeful, thrilled, proud, and confident; they laughed at the funny voice. It was music to their ears and a sign that they would talk. Altogether 61% of the women had a favorable impression, and 39% had an unfavorable impression of their first esophageal voice sounds. More single women

(42.6%) than married women (38.6%) had unfavorable impressions.

Eighty-two percent of the patients who had a favorable reaction to their first speech attempts were successful in attaining esophageal speech compared with only 64.1% of those who had an unfavorable impression. Likewise, 91% of the patients who were determined to talk were successful in regaining their speech compared with 40% of those who dejectedly decided that they would not be able to talk.

Hearing the substitute voice so depressed 30% of the patients that they vowed they would henceforth avoid their friends; however, 70% were confident that their friends would not forsake them. These first impressions did have some influence on the number of friends that stayed with them. All of their friends stayed with 56% of the pessimistic group and with 83% of the optimistic group. Also, 20% of the pessimistic group and only 6% of the optimistic group lost all of their friends.

The impulsive decisions and later experiences of the two groups seem to be related to the ultimate recovery of their speech. Speech was regained by 75.7% of the patients who sought to avoid their friends and by 89.6% of those who refused to shed their friends. More married patients, 92%, than single patients, 81.5%, who sought out their friends, regained speech. Finally, there was a consistent relationship between the extent to which patients kept their friends and the ability to talk. Speech was regained by 83.4% of the patients who actually kept all of their friends; and speech was regained by only 30% of those who lost all of their friends. It thus appears that successful speech was an important asset in retaining friends, and some patients regained speech in spite of their efforts to avoid their friends. However, it is seen also that the sheer experience of keeping their friends was an important factor in regaining speech.

Problems in Learning Esophageal Speech.
Forty-four percent of the wives reported that husbands were indifferent to or disliked or ridiculed the beginning speech sounds. They complained that their husbands did not encourage them to learn speech, nor did they show sympathy or understanding of their speech problems. Two thirds of the lonely single women struggled to conquer new voice without advice and encouragement. Husbands, friends, and relatives expressed dislike of their efforts to talk or walked away from them. They reported that "People were ashamed of me." "They were afraid of hurting my feelings." "People throw up when I try to talk to them." "They think I am deaf." "They are afraid of catching cancer." People did not listen to them, became impatient, and often filled in with words that were not fitting to the thought that they were trying to express.

One hundred fifteen or 66% of the wives reported that their husbands were kind and patient and gave them inspiration and encouragement to start learning esophageal speech. Some husbands took them to speech classes; others brought visitors into the home to give the wives opportunity to talk. Still others insisted that their wives use voice instead of whisper. One third of the single women stated that friends and relatives could not have helped them more than they did by encouraging them to talk and by listening patiently. However, some determined laryngectomees ignored unfavorable attitudes and remarks and made their friends listen. They asked for no sympathy and wanted no pity. They remarked that their "real friends stayed with them and joked with them in the right way."

The most common complaint was that esophageal speech was not easily understood. This was especially true when it was noisy or when the auditors were hard of hearing. The laryngectomized women were often mistaken for men over the telephone. Related to the difficulty in being understood was inability to compress air and to sustain enough vocal tone to say two or more syllables. Others complained of tightening up and being short of breath when they talked.

The laryngectomized women gave important advice on problems associated with learning esophageal speech. (1) Every patient must be informed on the ways and means of learning to communicate. (2) Patients should be taught only by trained teachers. (3) The patient must completely accept the new voice. (4) The patient must be determined to learn, have patience, and practice frequently while learning; she should continually strive to improve her speech. (5) Practice in exaggerating the consonants improves clarity and eases the strain of communicating. (6) Affection, confidence, and encouragement from the husband and friends are important factors in regaining speech. (7) Motivation and self-discipline are other requisites. For example, one woman, mother of five sons and grandmother to eight children, vowed that she would learn to talk to all of them. She gave them her new voice as a Christmas present. Another wife who raised dogs made herself talk to them until they understood her commands. (8) Instead of worrying about misunderstandings or being called "Sir" over the telephone, the speaker should identify herself and always put a smile in her voice. (9) Working women should return to the job early because their speech will improve rapidly by talking to other personnel.

Intelligibility of Esophageal Speech.— Two criteria were given to the patients to evaluate the intelligibility of their own esophageal speech: (1) Is your speech understood over the telephone? (2) Is your speech understood in person-to-person conversation? When the auditor is face to face with the esophageal speaker, visual cues enable the listener to understand speech that is not so precise as that required to communicate by telephone. Hence, the larger percentage of speakers (77%) was understood in person-to-person conversation, and 66% were understood over the telephone. More married women (71%) than single women (54%) were understandable over the telephone, and 81% of the married women and 66% of the single women could communicate satisfactorily in close conversation. An artificial larynx was used by only 14 of the 41 married nonspeakers and only by 4 of the 21 single nonspeakers. Some of the wives who used an artificial larynx recommended that all laryngectomized women be informed of its value and urged nonspeakers to use it everywhere without fear or embarrassment.

Problems in Reemployment.—More than 55% of the laryngectomized women, 58% of the married and 50% of the single women, who had worked before surgery returned to the same jobs after surgery. The return to work was closely related to the ability of the patients to regain speech. Good speech was regained by 84% of all patients who returned to work, and by 66% of those who did not return. Good speech was regained by 90% of the married women who returned to work and by 73% of the single women who returned to work. Good speech was regained by only 64% of the married women and by only 68% of the single women who did not return to work.

Although significantly fewer patients who did not return to work had acquired speech than those who returned to work; speech ability was not the sole criterion for regaining or losing one's job. For example, seven of nine salespersons and five of six factory workers lost their jobs; however, three of eight teachers and four of 11 secretaries lost their jobs. It is noteworthy that all six bookkeepers retained their jobs; speech was not too important for them to keep books. The same salaries were retained by 15 of the 17 women who reported on this question; the other two received increases in salaries.

The reemployed laryngectomees gave some practical advice to those who wish to return to work. (1) Dress neatly. (2) Cover the stoma with attractive scarves, bibs, or lacy material. (3) Return to work as soon as possible after operation because work provides excellent stimulation for improving speech. (4) If one has good speech there should be no employment problem. However, a person who does not talk need not have a problem with fellow workers if she is natural, dresses neatly, and keeps busy on the job. Most fellow employees accept the laryngectomized women with understanding and great consideration for their comfort, in spite of their inability to communicate well. The co-workers encouraged the patients to talk and praised them when they tried to express themselves. These pleasant relationships reduced tension and worry. (5) Emotional stability, success to social adjustments, and determination to overcome speech handicaps are additional factors in enabling the laryngectomized persons to retain their jobs.

Methods of Covering the Stoma.—The laryngectomized women were clever in devising ways and means of concealing the stoma. Hygiene and unobtrusive neatness were the goals: to keep the stoma covered with material that permitted adequate air exchange and yet would not attract attention. They used layers of gauze or sponges or cleverly designed gold, stainless steel, or aluminum screens, or cardboard medallions with designs of gold and silver thread or jeweled stones. Others used crocheted or knitted bibs of cotton or nylon threads. Solid material such as nylon, organdy, or curtain goods were used to cover the stoma; also dickies made of nylon and woolen materials; scarves of chiffon, tulle, net, rayon, and silk; different colors were used to match the dresses. High-necked dresses and shirtwaists, and turtle-necked sweaters were also preferred. The collars were closed by jeweled pins and brooches. For formal occasions, they wore necklaces, brooches, pendants or pins of openwork filigree to conceal the stoma. Three to five strands of beads, pearls or popbeads were sewn to a cloth backing. Husbands and wives designed discs and openwork medallions that were fashioned by jewelers from white gold, stainless steel, or aluminum.

Family and Social Adjustments

Husband and Wife Relations: The Husband's Role.—The following statement is a condensation of voluminous bits of advice that laryngectomized wives gave on the subject of husband and wife relations. Misunderstanding and tension will be avoided if, before surgery, the husband and other members of the family are adequately informed on details such as loss of voice, the hole in the neck, the probability of bitterness and depression in the first weeks after surgery and later on, if the wife does not regain her voice. The husband must understand a woman's fears that she may be less wanted and her bewilderment by the change in her life. Hhe should reassure her frequently that the operation has made no difference between them. He should help to maintain the same relationship that they had before surgery. He should plan for her comfort, making adjustments for suitable humidity and temperature and do some of the dusty chores that might make her cough excessively.

Inadequate communication leads to serious difficulties and frustrations. The husband should let the wife complete her sentence rather than interrupt and fill in a word that may be inappropriate. He should not nod his head that he understands before she is through expressing herself, nor should he walk away from her if she cannot convey her thought clearly. The husband should display strong interest in her speech development by taking her to speech classes until she has acquired good speech. He should realize that esophageal speech is not heard well in noise or in a crowd. If he turns down the radio or television, he can understand her more easily. If the couple plan to attend a party, the husband should inform the hostess about the wife's weak voice in order to anticipate and avoid problems in conversation.

Husband and Wife Relations: The Laryngectomized Wife's Role.—The laryngectomized wife should not feel sorry for herself, nor should she exaggerate her misfortune. She should realize that many other physical handicaps are much worse than hers, whereas she can do practically everything that she did formerly except to swim. If she must weep, she should do it in private. (Several wives reported that they wept every night for a year.) She should realize that this behavior is hard on the family and delays her return to a healthy attitude.

The wife should make the husband's role as easy as possible, and she should show him that she is really trying to make good for his sake. She should thank God she has a second voice and that she has a chance to be with and to help her husband and children. She should be neat around the neck and shoulders. "Nothing cheers a man so much as a happy, smiling, lovely wife."

It is wise for the wife to welcome visitors in the home just as cheerfully as she did in the past. She should get out of the house and widen her activities so that she must talk with people.

The wife should not be impatient if the husband does not answer quickly. It is just as hard for the husband to understand as it is for her to talk clearly. Hence, she should control her temper over frustration because anger inhibits natural fluency. Both husband and wife should understand that no one ever learns speech by being alone. On the other hand, the husband should not push his wife onto friends against her wishes; rather, he should wait until she is ready to meet others.

Does Surgery Bring Husband and Wife Closer Together?—Seventy-three percent of the wives reported with three different answers: farther apart, same as before, and closer. Twenty-three wives reported that tensions and misunderstandings were aggravated by the laryngectomy. Some husbands avoided their wives. Others refused to understand the wives' problems and to offer sympathy; this behavior caused the couples to grow apart. Strained finances, resulting from large surgical and hospital bills, were a source of irritation. The elderly hard-of-hearing husbands were irritated because they did not understand the wife's early efforts to talk. Wives who cried a lot, who thought it was a disgrace to have a hole in the neck, and to have poor speech, were not of much help to their husbands; they experienced lonely heartbreak.

Sixty-one women reported that their relationship with their husbands had become closer after the operation. Husbands were more patient, more considerate, more thoughtful, and more protective. Several husbands took over homemaking responsibilities, especially where there were children. Wives became less dependent as their speech improved. Women who did not return to work tried harder to please their husbands; hence, they enjoyed many happy times together. "Life became exciting and each of us is a better person," commented one wife.

Forty-five women said that their closeness with their husbands was the same before and after surgery. The husbands never treated the wives as oddities nor teased them because of speech errors. They listened at-

tentively to conversation. One husband demonstrated his morale-building activity by frequently saying to his wife, "You sure look nice." That true love endures was proved by several couples who had babies after the laryngectomy.

How Does Laryngectomy Change the Life of a Woman?—Only nine laryngectomized wives wrote frankly about the depressive aspect of their lives. One wife said that all she does is to take the family dog for a drive. Another wife has given up all social activity and feels old at 45 years of age. Another one covers her emotions in the daytime but weeps copiously all night. Another lives day by day and sees no future. Still another is "marking time 'till I go." One wife says she is "living only one-half of a life and that is down to zero." Another said, "Only Christian beliefs keep me from ending it all." One wife wrote: "It's a lousy deal for anyone." A wife bitterly protested: "I sang for a living; now I can't even baby sit—I can't control children."

Optimism was voiced by more than the majority of wives who expressed two views: some had made no marked change; others had changed for the better. More than 50% of the wives said that they had not changed in their domestic or social activities; they did everything they had done before surgery, except to swim. They lead normal lives as housewives, mothers, grandmothers, and even great-grandmothers.

The other group of wives were happy because they had "changed for the better." Their health was improved; they were physically stronger and could work harder and longer than before surgery. They had become closer to their families and had received gratitude and affection in return. They gained many new friends as they became more active socially. Their activities were as varied as any unselected group of women. They worked at their former jobs with greater enthusiasm. Many of their activities gave excellent speech stimulation. One wife and mother was depressed, shunned people, and was afraid to go back to work. She realized her actions were hurting her family. She faced about, returned to work, and later got a raise in salary.

Laryngectomized women who worked had contrary opinions about the difficulties (or ease) of adjustment. One fifth of them stated that their problems were multiplied because the wife had to work, to face financial problems, and do housework. She works all day as a breadwinner, and then manages the home at night. She has a hundred daily incidents that "drive her to distraction." Another fifth of the women stated that work keeps the mind off of the physical problem. They learn to talk because they have to communicate; competition is a challenge to the working women. They fight hard to regain their social and economic status.

The women also disagreed on adjustment problems of laryngectomized housewives. One quarter of the women stated that the housewife's work is never ended; she has to keep managing the home until she dies. Confinement to the home prevents her from meeting people; hence, she is embarrassed when she does meet them. Thus, she is doubly handicapped in regaining speech. One half of the women gave a different view. The home situation is more favorable to working out the laryngectomized wife's problem, provided she has the incentive. She has no economic worries and does not have to meet people; her difficulties are lessened if she keeps busy·as a housewife, mother, or grandmother. She has no time to worry and forgets about her problem. Furthermore, she has ample time for the practicing that is so essential to good speech.

Successful adjustment depends on the nature and temperament of the patient. The women reported that those who are easily upset cannot take the stares and crude remarks of strangers and even friends. Those who are vain worry about their personal appearances, especially about their scars. The masculine esophageal voice attracts attention; it is not acceptable to the public. She advertises her misfortune the moment the female laryngectomee opens her mouth. She is reluctant to use her masculine voice for fear of losing her position in the relationship with the other sex.

TABLE 6.—*Unfavorable Reactions of Laryngectomized Women to Their First Views of Their Surgical Scars*

Type of Reaction	Visited Patients		Patients Not Visited	
	Married, %	Single, %	Married, %	Single, %
Unfavorable reaction	55	38	46	44
Made less feminine	29	30	17	22
Marred for life	42	40	30	30
Made less attractive	30	20	25	34
Made less affectionate	20	10	16	12

She instinctively feels that she has become unattractive and fears that her husband will look toward other women.

Other wives reported that emotionally stable persons, on the other hand, adjust more easily. Older couples accept changes more readily than do younger couples; they have become toughened by life to accept hardships. Furthermore, an older woman has less worry and less responsibility than a younger mother of children.

Finally, the family's understanding is essential to successful change. If the father and children encourage and praise her success in talking, the wife will try harder to overcome all the difficulties that a laryngectomy caused.

Problems of the Single Laryngectomized Women.—Single laryngectomized women were more outspoken on their physical and speech handicaps; they narrated more depressing experiences than the married laryngectomees. One patient said that surgery took from her all alertness and happiness. Another one who formerly had many friends now shuns everyone because one half of her tongue was removed; she cannot eat or swallow well, let alone talk. Another woman withdrew from, and felt inferior to, others because the second of two operations deprived her of speech. Surgery took all of the happiness and interest in life from a lonely widow. Still another widow has been rebuffed by people so frequently that she never goes out. Another widow says that no one should ever accept surgery because it leaves one dependent on others.

Many of the single women's difficulties arose from speech problems. A single switchboard operator had indescribable fears not only because she lost her means of earning a living, but because neither she nor her family were informed of the problems they would face. A waitress has "gone through living hell because I can't talk or get work." A widow was embittered when she heard "people say horrible things about me." A spinster heard such "awful speech at the Lost Chord Club meeting that I went into a depression and lost my voice." Still another was "nagged to speak" by so many wives of laryngectomees at the club that she never returned and still cannot talk. One widow had no speech for three years because she had never met another laryngectomee. Another one used an artificial larynx ten years before she met a laryngectomee who talked spontaneously. Women who lived alone seldom acquired esophageal speech.

More than 50% of the laryngectomized single women made satisfactory adjustments to problems that were related to deprivation of voice. They transferred liability to an asset; have more friends than before surgery and have had many pleasant experiences; hence, they no longer think of themselves as being handicapped. One widow had always taken life for granted. "Now I know it is a gift." New and wonderful friends were the reward for her new outlook on life. After surgery, a widow became more tolerant: "I had a ball listening to remarks of people who thought I was deaf." Another widow went out and visited people daily. "I talked like a frog and laughed about it."

Reactions and Adjustments of Married vs Single Women.—A. Reactions to their scars.—Table 6 shows that in four of five types of reaction to their scars by the patients who had been visited by another laryngectomized person, the married patients reacted unfavorably in greater numbers than did the single women. Likewise, among the unvisited groups, more married women than single women reacted unfavorably in two categories: (1) to their first views of the stoma and (2) with the belief that they would be able to show less affection to their families. It is difficult to evaluate the significance of the greater incidence of unfavorable reactions of the married patients

than of the single. By viewing the table as a whole, the impression is gained that the married women had certain values which were threatened by disfigurement, whereas the single women may not have appreciated their significance as being less threatening to them.

(B). Reaction to the first sounds of their new voices. Fewer married patients (38.6%) than single patients (42.6%) had an unfavorable reaction to the first sounds of their esophageal voices. More married patients (65%) than single patients (57%) who were visited by laryngectomized persons had a favorable impression of their new voices. There was no difference between the married and single patients who were not visited. Within this same group, more married (76%) than single patients (57%) decided to keep their friends, and more married patients (93%) than single patients (86%) succeeded in talking.

Value of the Visitation Program.—The women laryngectomees were asked if there was any value in having laryngectomized persons visit them in the hospital. Sixty-one percent (146) of the patients reported that the visitors had not only inspired them to get well but had given them the impression that they would be able to talk again. No response was given by 21% of the patients, and 18% said that there was no value to such a visit.

The same percentage of patients (61%) stated that a visit by a husband who had already faced a similar situation, having a laryngectomized wife, would be a source of inspiration to the husband of a newly laryngectomized woman. Such a call would forestall misunderstandings, worries, and emotional conflicts, and would give the couple an earlier and better approach to rehabilitation.

The women who opposed visitations did so because they had had unpleasant experiences with visitors. They told of male laryngectomees who entered their rooms and made grimaces and clicking sounds in their efforts to talk. Others were depressed when they saw the male visitor's scars and breathing tube. The women were unanimous in the advice that only a woman should visit a laryngectomized woman. Such a person should be dressed attractively, have a good voice, and should display a wholesome attitude toward her own limitations.

The effectiveness of the visitation program can also be evaluated by comparing the reactions of the visited and unvisited patients to their new voice sounds. More patients who were visited (63%) than patients who were not visited (60%) had a favorable reaction. Likewise, more patients who were visited (86%) than those who were not visited (84.6%) were determined to talk. Also, 78.6% of visited patients who had a favorable reaction to their voices regained speech, whereas 66.7% who had an unfavorable reaction regained speech. These figures show how important it is to forestall an unfavorable response when the patient first hears her new voice.

Suggestions That Laryngectomized Women Believe Would Be Helpful to Future Laryngectomees

1. Never put off surgery if you have cancer of the larynx.
2. Become busy with activities both in the home and outside the home.
3. Think of, and take care of others; your own problems will dwindle away.
4. Dress neatly from the first day that you return home. Some husbands have never seen the stomas of their wives.
5. If you want friends, be pleasant and you will have them.
6. Communication is a two-way affair. Be patient when people do not understand or interrupt what you are trying to convey. Do not let an embarrassing situation become a catastrophe; and do not be irritated if someone says "Yes, sir" to you in a telephone conversation.
7. "Cope, not mope" with your problems. Do not cast gloom over the family or group; rather, return a stare with a smile.
8. Be thrilled if a stranger's telephone voice replies, "Have you a cold?"
9. Faith and prayer will keep one carrying on despite obstacles, real or imaginary; make up your mind to overcome your handicap; overcome self-pity.
10. Take advantage of educational material that will help you and your husband to understand each other's problems. The family should be informed of the loss of voice, problems of adjustment, possibilities of bitterness and depression, and the need for cooperation of everyone to insure successful adjustment. If all of those involved can be patient for six months, they will have solved their problems.

How Can the Lost Chord Clubs Help the Laryngectomees?

The laryngectomized women were unanimous in recommending that the Lost Chord Clubs maintain a dual program: services to the patients and public education. They were very insistent that either the surgeon or a visitor tell the patient and her relatives that she will lose her natural voice, but that she should talk again in a new manner or that she can always talk with an artificial larynx. A motion picture was regarded as a most useful device for preoperative orientation. The club should have a trained person, such as a social worker, to give personal counsel to the female laryngectomee when she comes to the club in order to prevent depression and discouragement.

They also urged that a close follow-up of patients be made after they leave the hospital, because they often forget advice that was given at a time when the news about cancer prevented comprehension and retention of important suggestions. They must be befriended and brought to the club where they can see and hear about how others have conquered fear and embarrassment. Club members should be assigned as sponsors to new patients in order to insure a successful adjustment and continuous attendance.

The women emphasized that only female laryngectomees call on newly laryngectomized women. They should be dressed neatly; have a good personality and be well adjusted—and have good speech. If there is no female laryngectomee in the vicinity, the club should give names and addresses of laryngectomized women to whom the new patients could write.

Club activities should be pointed to the interests and welfare of both women and men. They wish that the one or two women members could be treated more delicately by the predominating male members. They dislike seeing the men parading with wide-open shirts and exposed stomas from which they breathe noisily and blow out beer-laden air. They resent being pressed to talk when they haven't had sufficient training and practice. They dislike being told that all they need to do is to drink ginger ale and belch it up. The men shouldn't walk away from a new member if they don't understand her, nor should they treat the women as freaks. The club members should give as much advice to the laryngectomized women as they make available to laryngectomized men.

Individual speech instruction should precede group instruction until the patients gain more confidence. This should include advice on dressing and personal appearance. The women want ideas on the neatest and safest hygiene of the stoma, on methods that will conceal the stoma and protect them from embarrassing coughing. The thought that dominates the women patients is their personal appearance and their urgent desire to present as good images as they had before surgery. They want advice on soaps, liquids, and makeup that will cover scars. (No-mark is recommended by some surgeons and skin specialists.) They seek ideas for using jewelry and other materials that women have found successful in adorning their scarred necks.

The other part of the club program should be public education. The public should be told that cancer is not contagious, that a laryngectomee can talk, that she is not deaf, and that it is not necessary to whisper or yell in conversation. The public should see more laryngectomized persons, and the laryngectomee should be before the public more often. This may be accomplished by informative radio and television programs, first aid and rescue demonstrations aided by pamphlets, and newspaper publicity. Employers should be informed that a laryngectomee need not be regarded as a handicapped person; hence, she should be reemployed on the same job she had before surgery. Patients who lost their jobs should be informed about advisory and retraining facilities that are available.

Summary

Confidential questions were answered by 240 laryngectomized women from 36 states and Canada. Thirty-seven percent were operated on between the ages of 51 and 60 years; 37% had survived more than five years. Seventy percent had been smokers; and 44% had smoked more than 20 years. Former patients visited 46% of the women in the hospitals; 65% of the patients had depressing experiences at home; and 40% received little inspiration from relatives in regaining speech. Fifty percent were horrified at their surgical scars; 83% of those who kept all of their friends and 10% of those who lost all of their friends regained speech. Speech was intelligible among 77% in close, and among 66% in telephone, conversation. Lives of the majority were the same or better after surgery, although more married than single women adjusted successfully.

This study was supported by a grant from the Cleveland Clinic Foundation, Cleveland.

PSYCHOSOCIAL FACTORS AND SPEECH AFTER LARYNGECTOMY

Walter W. AMSTER, Russell J. LOVE*, Otto J. MENZEL,
Jack SANDLER**, William B. SCULTHORPE, Florence M. GROSS

*Veterans Administration Hospital,
Miami, Fla.*

Phase I of this investigation involved thirty-eight male veterans (twenty laryngecto-mized speakers, ten with surgery for non-laryngeal malignancy and eight without history of malignancy). The subjects received a series of tests investigating intelligence, anxiety level, achievement motive, aspiration level, frustration tolerance and hearing. Each subject was also seen for social service interviewing. Speech intelligibility scores (PB and sentences) and history information were obtained for the laryngectomized. Phase II initiated after a three year interval specifically evaluated the variable months after surgery and its relationship to speech intelligibility and social adjustment. Speech samples and social adjustment data were secured for eighteen laryngectomized speakers previously evaluated. Phase I results revealed that none of the psychosocial variables, including the social adjustment data, clearly differentiated the three groups, or the laryngectomized subjects with respect to speech intelligibility. Within the laryngectomized group, achievement motive, anxiety level, months after surgery, years of education and verbal intelligence revealed low positive correlations with speech intelligibility. Phase II results continued to suggest only a moderate relationship between months after surgery and speech intelligibility. No significant gains in speech intelligibility were noted after a twenty-four month postoperative period. Social adjustment data revealed no marked changes between Phase I and II.

Problem

During the past century there has been a paucity of investigative effort specifically concerned with the relationships between psychosocial variables and the acquisition of intelligible speech after laryngectomy. This dearth of research with respect to psychosocial parameters is indicative of the prevailing

* Now at Vanderbilt University Medical School, Nashville, Tenn.
** Now at University of South Florida, Tampa, Fla.

Reprinted by permission from *Journal of Communication Disorders*, 1972, 5, 1–18. Copyright North-Holland.

interest in such primary areas as the diagnosis of laryngeal malignancy, surgical techniques for laryngectomy, physiological determinants of voice production, speech intelligibility factors and speech rehabilitation procedures.

Consequently, considerable information, primarily descriptive in nature, is currently available regarding the communication process after laryngectomy. Despite this fund of data, no appropriate rationale to account for the disparity noted among the laryngectomized in acquiring adequate communication skills has yet evolved.

The psychological concomitants of laryngectomy, however, have not been entirely ignored. A number of authors have discussed reaction to laryngeal malignancy and subsequent surgery, emphasizing the anxieties and fears prior to surgery as well as the emotional trauma following laryngectomy. The resultant inability to use speech for communication, altered physical appearance and related medical and social problems provide a basis for catastrophic behavior (Schall 1939; Greene 1947; Pitkin 1953; Moses 1958; Stoll 1958; Heaver and Arnold 1962; Webb and Irving 1964; Locke 1966).

Medical and paramedical personnel involved in rehabilitation programs for the laryngectomized have indicated that psychological variables such as motivation, favorable attitude, pre-morbid verbal ability, adequate personality adjustment and average intellectual status appear to be related to the successful acquisition of speech after laryngectomy (Levin 1940; Morrison 1941; McCall 1943; Gardner 1951; Heaver et al. 1955; Putney 1958; Fontaine and Mitchell 1960; Svane-Knudson 1960).

Relationships between the speech intelligibility of the laryngectomized and the factors of age, educational level, hearing status, postoperative time and the amount and frequency of speech therapy have specifically been investigated.

Beamer (1954) and Damsté (1958) discussed the adverse influence of advanced age on the development of intelligible speech. Shames, Font and Matthews (1963) reported a significant correlation for age at surgery and speech intelligibility. Hudson (1965) indicated that the variable of age significantly differentiated the good and poor laryngectomized speakers in her investigation. In contrast, DiCarlo, Amster and Herer (1955), Berlin (1965), Diedrich and Youngstrom (1966), and Snidecor (1968) did not find significant relationships between age and speech intelligibility for their laryngectomized subjects.

With respect to educational level, Shames, Font and Matthews (1963) reported a significant correlation for speech intelligibility and years of education. This finding was not supported by Hudson (1965) who indicated that the factor of education did not significantly differentiate her good and poor speakers.

In evaluating the relationship of hearing to speech proficiency, Berlin (1963) observed that four of the ten poor speaking laryngectomee subjects in his investigation had significant hearing losses. Shames, Font and Matthews (1963) noted that of 153 laryngectomized subjects replying to a questionnaire, 22 reported difficulty in hearing. In this regard, Diedrich and Youngstrom (1966) reported a significant correlation between hearing loss and speech intelligibility for their sample. Hudson (1965), however, noted that hearing loss was not a differentiating factor with respect to the speech intelligibility of her subjects.

Postoperative time and speech proficiency were not found to be related by Damsté (1958) who observed that subjects receiving intensive speech therapy evidenced primary gains during the first year, while those who were self-taught reported continued improvement during a two year period. Conversely, Berlin (1965) and Diedrich and Youngstrom (1966) reported postoperative time and speech intelligibility to be significantly correlated. A tendency for speech abilities to plateau at the two year postoperative level for subjects receiving speech therapy was observed by Diedrich and Youngstrom (1966). In a questionnaire phase of their investigation, 45 of 87 laryngectomees indicated reaching maximum improvement during the first postoperative year, while others noted gains for as long as two years after surgery. Interestingly, several subjects reported deterioration of speech with the passage of time.

Robe et al. (1956) found no apparent relationship between the number of therapy sessions and speech proficiency. Shames, Font and Matthews (1963), however, reported length of time in therapy and speech intelligibility to be significantly correlated.

Only minimal attention has been devoted to personality variables and speech after laryngectomy. Beamer (1954) employing the Minnesota Multiphasic Personality Inventory (MMPI) with eight laryngectomized subjects reported no typical profile for the laryngectomized. Selected items of the MMPI indicated best adjustment for vocational factors and general mental health and least adjustment for self-concept and general physical health. The investigator further noted that the ability to use speech after laryngectomy does not necessarily guarantee adequate adjustment. Shames, Font and Matthews (1963) in administering the Edwards Personal Preference Schedule reported significant relationships for speech intelligibility and the factors of exhibition (attention seeking), aggression and achievement.

It would seem apparent that the experimental data concerning relationships between psychosocial variables and speech after laryngectomy are limited and somewhat equivocal. Further investigation of a more definitive nature appears warranted. Therefore, the present study was designed to:

1. Determine whether laryngectomized subjects differ significantly from subjects with non-laryngeal surgery for malignancy and subjects with no history of malignancy, on the variables of age, hearing, social adjustment, intelligence, anxiety level, achievement motive, aspiration level and frustration tolerance (Phase I).

2. Investigate relationships between the speech intelligibility of the laryngectomized and the variables of age, hearing, social adjustment, years of education, pre-surgical occupation, postoperative time, amount and frequency of speech therapy, intelligence, anxiety level, achievement motive, aspiration level and frustration tolerance (Phase I).
3. Investigate on a longitudinal basis relationships between the speech intelligibility of the laryngectomized and the variables of postoperative time and social adjustment (Phase II).
4. Determine whether a discrete cut-off point in speech improvement is evident for the laryngectomized subjects (Phase II).

Method

Phase I

Subjects

The subjects, thirty-eight male veterans receiving outpatient services at the Veterans Administration Hospital in Coral Gables, Fla., were divided into three groups for the purpose of this investigation:

Group A. Twenty subjects with total laryngectomy who were using speech for communication.

Group B. Ten subjects who had surgery for malignancy which did not involve the larynx, oral region, neck or central nervous system.

Group C. Eight subjects who had no history of malignancy.

The age range for Group A was 43–75 with a mean age of 62.1 yr and a median age of 65 yr. Group B's range was 38–72 with a mean age of 57.7 yr and a median age of 55 yr. Group C had an age range of 48–83 with a mean age of 64.8 yr and a median age of 65.5 yr. The mean ages for the three groups were not significantly different.

Procedure

All subjects were seen individually for social service interviewing, psychological testing and audiological evaluation. In addition, speech intelligibility materials were recorded and audited and history information was obtained for the laryngectomized subjects.

Social adjustment evaluation

The social service interview specifically structured for this investigation examined factors of marital, social and vocational adjustment (Barrabee, Barrabee and Finesinger 1955; Pinchek and Rollins 1960). Pre- and post-surgical adjustment factors were explored for subjects in Groups A and B. Interviews for each subject were conducted by a staff member of the Social Work

Service. The social adjustment data were evaluated by the interviewer and an additional staff member of the Social Work Service who was not involved in the interviewing process.

Psychological evaluation

The psychological instruments selected were performance in nature to avoid undue penalty for the laryngectomized subjects with respect to communication. The battery included the following tests:

1. Performance scale of the Wechsler adult intelligence scale (Wechsler 1955).
2. Full-range picture vocabulary test (Ammons and Ammons 1948).
3. Manifest anxiety scale (Taylor 1953).
4. Achievement motive test. Four cards (13B, 8BM, 2 and 17BM) from the Thematic apperception test (Murray 1943) were presented to subjects in that order. The written responses were analyzed and scored by the examiner and an independent judge in accordance with procedures described by McClelland et al. (1953). The Pearson product-moment correlation between the two evaluations for the total n Achievement score for each subject was 0.97.
5. Level of aspiration task. This task involved matching of numbers and symbols (Bayton 1943). Each of the 12 trials involved 25 matchings. Following the first practice trial, 7 more preliminary trials were administered. At the completion of each trial, the subject was given fictitious scores in a standardized order. After trial 8, the subjects were asked to estimate the best score, the lowest score and the exact score they would achieve. For each of the remaining trials, the time in seconds was recorded without the subjects being aware of their true values. The critical trials for determining the level of aspiration were trials 10, 11 and 12. Using the actual time on trial 9 and the estimated performance, a difference between the two scores was obtained for the remaining 3 trials. The mean of the difference for these trials was calculated and this score constituted the degree of over or under aspiration.
6. Frustration tolerance task. Two mirror tracing tasks were employed to determine the degree of frustration tolerance (Ellis, Barnett and Pryer 1957). The first task enabled the subject to practice tracing a six-pointed star and the second task required the tracing of a more complex figure. No subject was able to complete the second task in the required time. An error was defined as any crossing of the tracing guidelines. After the time limit elapsed, the complex figure was removed and another star was placed in front of the subject, who was then requested to trace one more design. A score was obtained by determining the difference in number of errors on the last star trial prior to the complex design and the final star tracing task.

Audiological evaluation

Audiometric testing consisted of a conventional air conduction pure tone audiogram covering the range of frequencies from 125 Hz to 8000 Hz in octave intervals, a speech reception threshold, and a PB max score for W-22 recorded word lists. Calibration for pure tones was based on ASA-1951 reference levels. Speech reception thresholds were based on a reference level of 29 dB.

All testing was done in a two-room IAC suite. A Beltone 15C audiometer was used for pure tone testing. Speech testing was done with a Grason-Stadler speech audiometer, Model 162.

History information

Information regarding age, education, pre-surgical occupation, and duration of speech therapy was obtained from the laryngectomized subjects by means of a questionnaire. The pre-surgical occupation was ranked in accordance with the Dictionary of Occupational Titles (United States Department of Labor 1949).

Speech intelligibility recording

Speech intelligibility recordings were completed for the twenty laryngectomized subjects. The materials utilized were ten lists of 50 phonetically balanced words (Egan 1948) and ten lists of 10 sentences each, representing "everyday American speech" prepared at Central Institute for the Deaf (Davis and Silverman 1960). A two-room IAC suite was used for both recording and auditing purposes. A Magnecord Model PT 6 was employed for tape recording of the speech samples. The subject stood while speaking into a Turner Dynamic Model 51A microphone placed at a distance of 12 inch from the speaker's mouth. A technician in the control room monitored the recording level by means of a VU meter. The subjects were given an opportunity to become familiar with the speech materials and recording procedures.

Auditing and scoring of speech intelligibility materials

Two groups of undergraduate students majoring in speech pathology and audiology at the University of Miami in Coral Gables served as auditors. Samples of recorded laryngectomized speech (PB words and sentences) were presented for orientation purposes. The auditors wrote on scoring sheets the words and sentences that were spoken by the laryngectomized subjects. Each group consisting of five students audited the speech intelligibility recordings of ten laryngectomized subjects. The tape recordings were played back on the Magnecord model PT 6, employed for original taping, through a 15 inch high-fidelity speaker at comfortable loudness levels.

The fifty phonetically balanced words were scored according to the percentage of words correctly understood. The sentences were scored similarly in percent correctly understood. Minor variations (omissions, additions or substitutions) which did not affect basic meaning were scored correct. The maximum intelligibility score for each criterion was 100%.

An index of reliability of judgements of intelligibility for Phase I was determined by interclass correlation described by Ebel (1951). For word intelligibility, the first group of auditors obtained a correlation of 0.94 while the other group obtained 0.92. The correlation for sentence intelligibility for the first group was 0.83 and for the second 0.87.

Phase II

Of the twenty laryngectomized subjects who participated in Phase I, eighteen were available for re-evaluation in Phase II. This second phase of the investigation which involved only the laryngectomized subjects was initiated three years after the completion of Phase I.

Speech intelligibility recordings were repeated for the eighteen laryngectomized subjects using the identical PB and sentence materials, recording equipment, and experimental conditions employed for each subject in Phase I. The speech intelligibility materials were audited by two groups of 5 auditors each who did not participate in auditing activities in Phase I. Interclass correlation (Ebel 1951) for word intelligibility for the two auditing groups was 0.93 and 0.94, and for sentence intelligibility 0.93 and 0.85.

Each subject was seen individually for social service re-evaluation of marital, social and vocational adjustment. In addition, the subjects were requested to indicate whether their speech had improved, regressed or remained essentially the same during the preceding three year period.

Results

Phase I

Intergroup analysis

The first series of statistical analyses which concerned intergroup comparisons were undertaken to determine whether Group A (laryngectomy) differed significantly from Group B (non-laryngeal surgery) and Group C (no history of malignancy) on the variables investigated. Analyses of variance were applied to data concerning: (a) age, (b) intelligence, (c) anxiety level, (d) achievement motive, (e) frustration tolerance, (f) aspiration level and (g) hearing (Table 1).

Only one variable, frustration tolerance, appeared to distinguish the three groups ($F = 7.67$, $df = 2$ and 36, $p < 0.01$). The contribution of each group to the significant F was evaluated by t tests, none of which proved to be signifi-

Table 1

Means, standard deviations, and F ratios for Group A (laryngectomy), Group B (non-laryngeal surgery) and Group C (no history of malignancy) on age, hearing, and psychological measures

Measure	Mean	Standard deviation	F ratio
Age in years			
Group A	62.1	9.4	
Group B	57.7	10.9	1.16
Group C	64.9	8.8	
Hearing in better ear			
PTA (dB)			
Group A	8.9	38.9	
Group B	8.7	15.4	3.38
Group C	22.7	63.8	
SRT (dB)			
Group A	7.1	10.0	
Group B	10.0	31.5	2.38
Group C	18.5	33.2	
PB (%)			
Group A	93.8	408.7	
Group B	95.2	285.5	3.46
Group C	86.0	226.6	
FRPV			
Group A	101.0	12.6	
Group B	99.2	16.6	0.07
Group C	101.4	12.4	
WAIS performance scale			
Group A	107.8	10.9	
Group B	103.8	9.0	0.64
Group C	105.8	6.9	
Manifest anxiety			
Group A	11.7	7.4	
Group B	13.0	6.0	0.64
Group C	15.7	11.8	
n Achievement			
Group A	+0.3	6.4	
Group B	−0.4	38.5	0.26
Group C	+1.0	5.3	
Level of aspiration			
Group A	−0.5	2.3	
Group B	−0.3	2.0	0.26
Group C	−0.9	2.0	
Frustration tolerance [†]			
Group A	5.5	8.9	
Group B	1.4	3.0	7.67**
Group C	17.3	16.0	

** Significant at the 0.01 level.

[†] Frustration tolerance with data transformed (Bartlett, 1947): $F = 4.87$, significant at 0.05 level.

cant. Transformation of the data (Bartlett 1947) and reapplication of analysis of variance again revealed a significant F ratio. (F = 4.87, df = 2 and 36, $p < 0.05$.)

Intragroup analyses

Relationships between the speech intelligibility of the laryngectomized subjects and the variables studied were evaluated by means of Pearson product-moment and Spearman rank correlations. The results in Table 2 indicate that the relationships for the most part are low or negative. Only eight of the thirty-two correlations were significant at or beyond the 0.05 level of confidence. Intelligence, as measured by the Full Range Picture Vocabulary Test (FRPV), n Achievement, and months after surgery correlated significantly with both indices of intelligibility. The highest correlation, 0.63, significant beyond the 0.01 level, was between the FRPV and sentence intelligibility. Low but significant correlations were present between the FRPV and word intelligibility (0.39), performance IQ on the WAIS and sentence intelligibility (0.42), anxiety level and word intelligibility (0.37), and n Achievement with word and sentence intelligibility (0.40) and (0.44) respectively.

Table 2

Correlations between speech indices and variables investigated for the laryngectomy group

Variable	Word intelligibility	Sentence intelligibility
Age in years	−0.14	−0.27
Hearing in better ear		
PTA	−0.20	0.07
SRT	0.33	0.11
PB	0.32	0.19
2K	−0.11	0.18
4K	−0.05	0.08
X: 2K, 4K	−0.07	0.17
FRPV	0.39*	0.63**
WAIS performance scale	0.22	0.42*
Manifest anxiety	0.37*	0.13
n Achievement	0.40*	0.44*
Level of aspiration	−0.14	−0.29
Frustration tolerance	−0.11	−0.31
Months after surgery	0.54*	0.46*
Years of education	0.12	0.28
Pre-surgical occupational status†	−0.07	−0.12

* Significant at 0.05 level.
** Significant at 0.01 level.
† Spearman rank correlation.

Speech intelligibility

The laryngectomy group (N = 20) was divided on the basis of speech intelligibility scores (PB and sentences). Those subjects falling above the median intelligibility score on each of the intelligibility measures were designated as "high" intelligibility speakers, and those below the median score as "low" intelligibility speakers.

The series of t tests (Table 3) comparing high and low intelligibility speakers in word intelligibility on the several variables investigated revealed significantly greater scores for the high intelligibility speakers only with respect to anxiety level (t = 2.33, df = 18, $p<0.05$). In sentence intelligibility the scores for the high intelligibility speakers were significantly greater than those for the low intelligibility speakers in n Achievement (t = 2.27, df = 18, $p<0.05$) and years of education (t = 2.17, df = 18, $p<0.05$).

To eliminate possible overlapping of scores that might have obscured clear-cut differences when the group was halved, the five most intelligible speakers, designated as the "high five" and the five least intelligible speakers, as the "low five", were compared on the variables under investigation. Results of t tests (Table 4) revealed no significant differences for the psychological variables when the criterion of word intelligibility was used.

When the two subgroups of extremes in sentence intelligibility were compared, however, the scores for the "high five" were significantly greater than those for the "low five" in intelligence as measured by the Performance Scale of the Wechsler Adult Intelligence Scale and the Ammons and Ammons Full Range Picture Vocabulary Test (WAIS: t = 2.54, df = 8, $p<0.05$; FRPV: t = 3.31, df = 8, $p<0.05$).

Table 3

Summary of t tests results on variables investigated between laryngectomees with high (N = 10) and low (N = 10) scores on speech intelligibility measures.

Variable	Word intelligibility	Sentence intelligibility
Age in years	0.442	1.288
Hearing in better ear		
PTA	0.149	0.585
SRT	0.604	0.338
PB	0.512	1.160
FRPV	1.546	1.542
WAIS performance scale	0.432	1.145
Manifest anxiety	2.329*	1.419
n Achievement	1.681	2.274*
Level of aspiration	0.071	0.626
Frustration tolerance	0.047	0.060
Months after surgery	1.616	1.112
Years of education	1.175	2.174*

* Significant at the 0.05 level.

Table 4.
Summary of *t* tests results on variables investigated between laryngectomees with highest
(*N* = 5) and lowest (*N* = 5) scores on speech intelligibility measures

Variable	Word intelligibility	Sentence intelligibility
Age in years	0.761	0.245
Hearing in better ear		
PTA	1.195	0.502
SRT	0.659	0.242
PB	1.213	1.072
FRPV	0.538	3.307*
WAIS performance scale	0.550	2.544*
Manifest anxiety	1.612	1.519
n Achievement	1.556	1.711
Level of aspiration	0.554	1.616
Frustration tolerance	0.715	1.437
Months after surgery	1.909	1.979
Years of education	1.405	1.489

* Significant at the 0.05 level.

Social adjustment

Evaluation of the social adjustment data revealed no marked differences among the three groups of subjects with respect to marital, social and vocational adjustment. The laryngectomized subjects (Group A) and the subjects in Group C (no history of malignancy) were judged to be most similar in their adjustment patterns. Subjects in Group B (surgery for malignancy which did not involve the larynx) differed specifically from the laryngectomized subjects in their less positive adjustment to the concept of malignancy and the concomitant medical and social problems.

Attempts to accurately differentiate speech intelligibility levels for the laryngectomized subjects on the basis of the social adjustment data were not successful.

History information

Examination of the questionnaire responses revealed the mean number of years of education for the laryngectomized subjects to be 9.5 years with a range of 0—14. Pre-surgical occupations were generally skilled or semi-skilled in nature with respect to the guidelines established by the United States Department of Labor (Dictionary of Occupational Titles).

Duration of speech therapy averaged 7.5 months, with a range of 2—24. The mean number of therapy sessions was 40.4 with a range of 10—144. Inspection of the data revealed no apparent relationship between speech intelligibility and the number of months in therapy or the number of therapy sessions.

Phase II

In phase II speech intelligibility data were evaluated within the framework of the following questions: (1) How closely did the laryngectomized subjects maintain their intelligibility rankings during the three year period between Phase I and Phase II? (2) What was the relationship between months after surgery and speech intelligibility in Phase II? (3) Does speech improvement continue beyond a twenty-four month postoperative period?

Speech intelligibility

To ascertain how closely the laryngectomized subjects maintained their speech intelligibility rankings for both words and sentences during the three year period between Phase I and II, Spearman rank order correlations were obtained for each of the two speech indices. The correlations of 0.73 for sentence intelligibility and 0.85 for word intelligibility suggest relatively close correspondence between speech intelligibility measures over a period of time. Further tests for reliability of measures were completed by correlating word and sentence materials. In Phase I, a correlation of 0.85 was obtained, and in Phase II a correlation of 0.87. Reliability between speech indices was relatively high and tended to maintain itself over the three year period.

Speech intelligibility subgroups

The eighteen subjects in Phase II were divided into high and low groups as in Phase I. Those subjects falling above the median speech intelligibility score on both measures of intelligibility were designated as "high" intelligibility speakers, and those below the median score as "low" intelligibility speakers.

The subjects were further divided into smaller subgroups with the four most intelligible speakers designated as the "high four" and their least intelligible counterparts as the "low four".

Months after surgery

In Phase I, statistically significant correlations were obtained between months after surgery and both indices of speech intelligibility (word: 0.54, $p<0.05$, sentence: 0.46, $p<0.05$). These correlations were based on a range of 4 to 191 months, with a mean of 39.6 and a median of 28.5. For Phase II, comparable correlations of 0.43 for word intelligibility and 0.58 for sentence intelligibility were obtained. Only the second of these correlations (0.58, sentence intelligibility) reached significance at the 0.05 level. The range of months after surgery in Phase II was 37 to 229, with a mean of 80.5 and a median of 67. These correlations again suggested only a moderate relationship between speech intelligibility and months after surgery.

The *t* tests indicated that months after surgery did not differentiate between the high and low speech intelligibility groups nor the highest four and lowest four subjects on the speech indices. These results were comparable to Phase I findings.

Speech improvement and postoperative time

The question of whether speech improvement continues after a twenty-four month postoperative period was evaluated by comparing speech intelligibility scores of those subjects in Phase I twenty-four months or less postoperative with those who were postoperative twenty-five months or longer. No statistically significant difference was found for either word or sentence intelligibility.

Further information was obtained by comparing the intelligibility scores of those subjects in Phase I who were 24 months postoperative or less with their own intelligibility scores obtained in Phase II after a three year interval. The *t* test for related measures showed no statistically significant difference between mean intelligibility scores above and below two years.

Social adjustment

No essential changes were noted for marital, social and vocational adjustment during the three year intervening period between Phase I and II of this investigation. Marital status was unchanged and the adjustment between marital partners was considered adequate. The majority of subjects reported greater financial security at this time due to increased veterans benefits and higher Social Security payments. As in Phase I, it was not possible to accurately predict speech intelligibility levels on the basis of the social adjustment data.

In the course of the social service interview, each subject was asked to judge whether his speech had improved, regressed or remained essentially the same during the preceding three years. Seven of the speakers reported improvement, five regression, and six noted no essential change in their speech patterns. In general, this self-evaluation of speech proficiency tended to be inaccurate when compared with the obtained speech intelligibility scores. The closest correspondence between self-evaluation and speech intelligibility scores occurred for those laryngectomized subjects who indicated that their speech had improved.

Further examination of the speech intelligibility data revealed that deterioration of speech intelligibility had occurred with the passage of time for 7 of the 18 subjects on one or both of the speech measures employed in this study.

Discussion

On the basis of the findings in the present investigation it seems reasonable to conclude that none of the psychosocial dimensions clearly differentiated the laryngectomized subjects (Group A) from subjects who received surgery for nonlaryngeal malignancy (Group B) or from those who had no history of malignancy (Group C), nor did these variables effectively differentiate the laryngectomized subjects with respect to speech intelligibility. Although the data did indicate that one of the variables, frustration tolerance, statistically differentiated the laryngectomized subjects from the remaining two groups, the value of this positive finding is limited in view of the probability of a chance significant difference occurring more frequently as the number of analyses increases. It was also observed that the groups themselves did not differ significantly from one another as revealed by t test data. Furthermore, subjects in Group C exhibited the greatest frustration during the task with the largest mean difference in frustration scores occurring between subjects in Groups B and C.

Statistically significant correlations were obtained for the speech intelligibility of the laryngectomized subjects and the variables of achievement motive, anxiety level, months after surgery, years of education and verbal intelligence. It should be stressed, however, that no single correlation was of sufficient magnitude to be considered useful as a predictive index. In addition, the lack of consistency of these relationships between word and sentence intelligibility as well as between speech intelligibility sub-groups, further limits the predictive value of these variables.

Future investigation of the possible relationships between psychosocial variables and speech after laryngectomy should include diversified samples and a variety of psychosocial instruments. Such research should be initiated prior to surgery and continue throughout the speech rehabilitation program focusing attention on the interrelationships involved in the therapeutic process.

Analysis of the audiometric data did not reveal word or sentence intelligibility to be significantly related to hearing acuity for pure tones or speech nor was it found to be related to speech discrimination. It is important to note, however, that only 4 of the 38 subjects, two in the laryngectomized group and one in each of the two remaining groups, exhibited a substantial degree of hearing loss (30 dB or more in the better ear). For the two laryngectomized subjects evidencing such hearing loss, one placed in the high speech intelligibility group, while the other scored low with respect to speech intelligibility.

It therefore seems improbable that any real relationship between hearing loss and the indices of speech intelligibility would be demonstrable on the basis of the sample employed. Thus, the non-significant findings obtained should not necessarily be interpreted as contradictory to the reports of Berlin (1963), Shames, Font and Matthews (1963) and Diedrich and Youngstrom (1966) which indicated an apparent relationship between speech intelligibility and hearing loss.

Deterioration of speech intelligibility with the passage of time for some laryngectomized subjects noted by Diedrich and Youngstrom (1966) was also evidenced in the present study. No explanation for this finding was readily apparent. The influence of possible neurological and physiological changes, debilitating illness, and psychosocial adjustment requires further evaluation.

In reviewing the data of Phase I and II, it would appear that the variable, months after surgery, correlated only moderately with speech intelligibility, offered limited predictive value and failed to differentiate intelligibility levels for the laryngectomized speakers. These results are in agreement with Damsté (1958) but differ somewhat from the reported findings of Berlin (1965) and Diedrich and Youngstrom (1966).

A postoperative period of more than 24 months did not result in significant differences in speech intelligibility for the laryngectomized subjects in this investigation. Damsté (1958) and Diedrich and Youngstrom (1966) noted similar trends. It was not possible, on the basis of the present data, to designate a discrete maximum improvement cut-off point during or after the 24 month time interval.

The laryngectomized subjects achieved a higher level of social adjustment than might have been anticipated. This appeared to be related in part to the supportive attitudes of family members and the duration and quality of relationships with physicians and paramedical personnel following surgery.

Vocational data revealed that prior to surgery the laryngectomized group comprised 14 subjects retired because of age or disability, 2 unemployed and 4 employed. Post-surgery information (Phase I) indicated an increase in the laryngectomized group employed with 7 of the original 14 who were previously retired working part-time or full-time. Employment status remained essentially the same during the three year intervening period between Phase I and II of this investigation. Beamer (1954) reported similar findings regarding the vocational adjustment of her subjects.

The relationship between years of education and speech intelligibility found to be significant by Shames, Font and Matthews (1963) was not completely substantiated by the results of the present study. In this regard, Hudson (1965) reported that educational level did not significantly differentiate her laryngectomized speakers with respect to speech intelligibility.

Examination of questionnaire responses involving speech rehabilitation did not reveal any apparent relationship between the number of months in therapy or the number of therapy sessions and speech intelligibility. These findings are in agreement with Robe et al. (1956) but are in contrast to the results reported by Shames, Font and Matthews (1963).

Research concerned with speech rehabilitation of the laryngectomized should attempt to control such factors as the time interval between surgery and the initiation of therapy, as well as the length, frequency, and type of therapy. Clinical circumstances in the present investigation did not permit systematic evaluation of these issues.

Acknowledgement

The authors are indebted to Louis M. DiCarlo, Ph. D., of the Veterans Administration Hospital, Syracuse, New York and Ithaca College, Ithaca, New York, and Bernard Locke, Ph. D., of the John Jay College of Criminal Justice of the City University of New York, for their helpful guidance and counsel.

References

Ammons, R.B. and H.S. Ammons, 1948, Full-Range Picture Vocabulary Test. Missoula, Montana, Psychological Test Specialists.

Baker, H.K., 1948, The rehabilitation of the laryngectomized. Trans. Am. Acad. Ophthalmol. Otolaryngol., 52, 227–233.

Barrabee, P., E.L. Barrabee and J.E. Finesinger, 1955, A normative social adjustment scale. Am. J. Psychiatry, 112, 252–259.

Bartlett, M.D., 1967, The use of transformation. Biometrics, 3, 39–52.

Bayton, J.A., 1943, Aspiration, performance and past performance. J. of Exp. Psychol., 33, 1–32.

Beamer, M.W., 1954, A qualitative study of the personality adjustment of laryngectomized subjects. Unpublished Master's Thesis, Texas State College for Women.

Berlin, C.I., 1963, Clinical measurement of esophageal speech: I. Methodology and curves of skill acquisition. J. Speech Hearing Dis., 28, 42–51.

Berlin, C.I., 1965, Clinical measurement of esophageal speech: III. Performance of nonbiased groups. J. Speech Hearing Dis., 30, 174–183.

Damste, P.H., 1958, Oesophageal speech after laryngectomy. Univ. of Groningen, Netherlands.

Davis, H. and S.R. Silverman, 1960, Hearing and deafness (Rev. ed.) New York, Holt, Rhinehart & Winston, Inc.

DiCarlo, L.M., W.W. Amster and G.R. Herer, 1955, Speech after laryngectomy. Syracuse, Syracuse University Press.

Diedrich, W.M., and K.A. Youngstrom, 1966, Alaryngeal speech. Springfield, Charles C. Thomas.

Ebel, R.L., 1951, Estimation of reliability ratings. Psychometrika. 16, 407–424.

Edwards, A.L., 1950, Experimental design in psychological research. New York, Rhinehart.

Egan, J.P., 1948, Articulation testing methods. Laryngoscope, 58, 955–991.

Ellis, N.R., C.D. Barnett, and M.W. Pryer, 1957, Performance of mental defectives on the mirror drawing task. Percept. Motor Skills, 7, 271–274.

Fontaine, A., and J. Mitchell, 1960, Oesophageal voice: a factor of readiness. J. Laryng. (London), 74, 870–976.

Frank, J.D., 1941, Recent studies in level of aspiration. Psychol. Bull., 28, 218–225.

Gardner, W.H., 1951, Rehabilitation after laryngectomy. Public Health Nursing, 43, 612–615.

Greene, J.S., 1947, Laryngectomy and its psychologic implications. New York J. Med., 47, 53–56.

Heaver, L. and G.E. Arnold, 1962, Rehabilitation of alaryngeal aphonia. Postgrad. Med., 32, 11–17.

Heaver, L.W., W. White and N. Goldstein, 1955, Clinical experience restoring oral communication to 274 laryngectomized patients by esophageal voice. J. Amer. Geriat. Soc., 3, 687–690.

Hudson, A., 1965, Influences on the acquisition of esophageal voice in a group of laryngectomized veterans. Proceedings 13th International Society of Logopaedics and Phonetics, Vienna Academy of Medicine, 2, 183–185.

Levin, N.M., 1940, Teaching the laryngectomized patient to talk. Arch. Otolaryng., 32, 299–314.

Locke, B., 1966, Psychology of the laryngectomee. Milit. Med., 131, 593–599.

McCall, J.W., 1943, Preliminary voice training for laryngectomy. Arch. Otolaryng., 38, 10–16.

McClelland, D.C., J.W. Atkinson, R.A. Clark, and E.L. Lowell, 1953, The achievement motive. New York, Appleton-Century-Crofts, Inc.

Morrison, W.W., 1941, Physical rehabilitation of the laryngectomized patient. Arch. Otolaryng., 34, 1101–1112.

Moses, P.J., 1958, Rehabilitation of the post-laryngectomized patient; the vocal therapist: place and contribution to the rehabilitation program. Ann. Otol. Rhinol. Laryngol., 67, 538–543.

Murray, H.A., 1943, Thematic Apperception Test. Cambridge, Massachusetts, Harvard University Press.

Pinchek, L.E. and G.W. Rollins, 1960, A social adequacy rating scale: preliminary report. Soc. Work, 5, 71–78.

Pitkin, Y.N., 1953, Factors affecting psychologic adjustment in the laryngectomized patient. Arch. Otolaryng., 58, 38–49.

Putney, E.J., 1958, Rehabilitation of the postlaryngectomized patient; specific discussion of failures: advanced and difficult technical problems. Ann. Otol. Rhinol. Laryngol., 67, 544–549.

Robe, E.Y., P. Moore, A.H. Andrews, Jr. and P.H. Holinger, 1956, A study of the role of certain factors in development of speech after laryngectomy: 1. Type of operation, 2. Site of pseudoglottis, 3. Coordination of speech with respiration. Laryngoscope, 66, 173–186 (Part 1), 382–401 (Part 2) and 481–499 (Part 3).

Schall, L.A., 1938, Psychology of laryngectomized patients. Arch. Otolaryng., 28, 581–584.

Shames, G.H., J. Font and J. Matthews, 1963, Factors related to speech proficiency of the laryngectomized. J. Speech Hearing Dis,, 28, 273–287.

Snidecor, J.C., 1968, Speech rehabilitation of the laryngectomized. (2nd ed.) American Lecture Series, Springfield, Ill., Charles C. Thomas.

Stoll, B., 1958, Psychological factors determining the success or failure of the rehabilitation program of laryngectomized patients. Ann. Otol. Rhinol. Laryngol., 67, 550–557.

Svome-Knudsen, V., 1960, The substitute voice of the laryngectomized patient. Acta Otolaryngol. (Stockholm) 52, 85–93.

Taylor, J.W., 1953, A personality scale of manifest anxiety. J. Abnorm. Soc. Psychol., 48, 285–290.

United States Department of Labor, 1949, Dictionary of occupational titles, (2nd ed.) Washington, D.C., Superintendent of Documents.

Webb, M.W. and R.W. Irving, 1964, Psychologic and anamnestic patterns characteristic of laryngectomees; relation to speech rehabilitation. J. Amer. Geriat. Soc., 12, 303–322.

Wechsler, D., 1955, Wechsler Adult Intelligence Scale. New York: Psychological Corporation.

Winer, B.J., 1962, Statistical principles in experimental design. New York, McGraw-Hill.

SOCIAL AND VOCATIONAL ACCEPTABILITY OF ESOPHAGEAL SPEAKERS COMPARED TO NORMAL SPEAKERS

STUART I. GILMORE

Louisiana State University, Baton Rouge, Louisiana

This study explored the social and vocational acceptability of esophageal compared to normal speakers. Of specific interest was the estimation of the effect of (1) visual, auditory, and simultaneous audio-visual presentation of the speakers, and (2) simple expository introductions of the speakers. A group of 480 subjects, members of business and professional men's groups, evaluated the four speakers on one social and three vocational criteria. Statistical analysis indicated the esophageal speakers were perceived as being significantly less acceptable than the normal speakers regardless of whether the judgments were based on visual, auditory, or simultaneous visual and auditory impressions. Information about the esophageal speakers significantly raised their acceptability, with the exception of the criterion of public contact in employment. The criterion measures used in this study might serve as objective indicators of the degree to which communicative disorders handicap adults.

Increased attention is being given to the psychosocial factors involved in physical disability, including communicative disabilities. Concern has been directed toward economic and social integration of the disabled, originally because of humanitarian considerations and later because rehabilitation was found to be economically sound. As with other socially significant minority groups, recent attention has been focused on the civil rights of the physically and mentally handicapped, and legislation amending the Civil Rights Act of 1964 to prohibit discrimination against the disabled has been introduced. (Senate Bill 1780, and House Bills 2685, 10960, 11986, and 11987, of 1973.) Public Laws 92-515 (1972) and 93-112, sections 503 and 504 (1973) have been enacted to guarantee the rights of the handicapped.

Equality of opportunity for the disabled is restricted in two ways: (1) by the negative attitudes of the nondisabled, which presumably are learned and therefore changeable or preventable, and (2) by the consequent negative attitudes the disabled may develop toward themselves. Both clinical and research literature suggest that the handicapped, generally, and the communicatively handicapped, specifically, do indeed experience rejection, penalty, and consequent anxiety, frustration, and withdrawal (Ashmore, 1958; Gelman, 1959; Horowitz, 1957; Ingwell, Thoreson, and Smits, 1967; King, Lowlks, and Peirson, 1968; Kleck, Ono, and Hastorf, 1966; Kleffner, 1952; Masson, 1970; Meyerson, 1955; Perrin, 1954; Suinn, 1967).

Reprinted by permission from *Journal of Speech and Hearing Research*, 1974, *17*, 599–607.

Laryngectomized individuals are particularly interesting subjects for research regarding the psychosocial concomitants of a communicative disorder. Laryngeal cancer usually occurs in individuals who, as normal speakers, have already established themselves socially and vocationally. In general, they learn to use esophageal speech, about which literature indicates mixed reactions. The more optimistic writers envision the return of normal conversational ability, natural and fluent speech, and the absence of untoward curiosity on the part of the listener for the proficient esophageal speaker (Damste, Van Den Berg, and Moolenaar-Bijl, 1956; Gatewood, 1946; Levin, 1940, 1955; Lindsay, Morgan, and Wepman, 1944; Stetson, 1937). Many writers, however, find esophageal speech less intelligible than normal speech, uneconomical of air and effort, reduced in rate and intensity, reduced in flow rate, lower in fundamental frequency, restricted in range, possessing significant noise elements, incapable of expressing meaning beyond rational content, and requiring listeners who will take the trouble to listen (Bateman, Dornhorst, and Leathart, 1952; Bisi and Conley, 1965; Jesberg, 1954; Martin, 1963; Moses, 1958; Snidecor, 1971; Tato, 1954; Tikofsky, 1965). Stoll (1958) states that society will accept only the more intelligible esophageal speaker. Several writers acknowledge a need for public education regarding the capabilities and problems of laryngectomees, especially for employers and business associates (Greene, 1947; Heaver, White, and Goldstein, 1955; Jesberg, 1954; Masson, 1970; McCall, 1943; Schall, 1938; Waldrop, 1954).

The present study was designed to explore the social and vocational acceptability of esophageal speakers to the business and professional community, who control considerable economic and social power. Three specific questions were asked: (1) Do business and professional men rate esophageal speakers differently from normal speakers in terms of social and vocational acceptance? (2) If esophageal speakers are rated unfavorably, are the ratings due to audible, visible, or both audible and visible differences between the esophageal and normal speakers? (3) Are attitudes toward esophageal speakers, as indicated by the ratings of social and vocational acceptability used in this study, influenced by simple explanatory introductions of the speakers?

METHOD

Selection of Experimental Speakers

Two of a group of esophageal speakers were selected following evaluation by audiences consisting of both trained speech correctionists and laymen. These evaluations indicated that these esophageal speakers were easily intelligible and had no attention-attracting characteristics other than those considered normal concomitants of esophageal speech. Both held high prestige positions that required considerable public contact and were reportedly highly acceptable socially. The two normal speakers used in the study met the same requirements as the esophageal speakers and appeared to be within five years of their ages. Two pairs of speakers were used; one pair in their forties, the other in their fifties. Each pair was composed of a normal speaker and an esophageal speaker. Women speakers were not used because of possible differences in social and vocational acceptability related to sex differences.

EXPERIMENTAL FILMS AND TAPES

To insure uniformity of speaker presentation to the subjects, the speakers were filmed and a tape recording of the sound tracks was made. The two normal and two esophageal speakers were filmed while sitting behind a business desk and dictating a one-minute telegram, via telephone, to a Western Union operator. This situation permitted the subjects to see and/or hear the speakers individually, at a distance and close up, using speech that had no emotional content but that needed to be easily understood.

Subjects

The listeners were 480 members of business and professional men's groups. Business and professional men were chosen because they represent the potential employer and are important in the community power structure. Moreover, they could be obtained as captive rather than volunteer subjects, thus eliminating any effects of greater initial interest or sympathy that might typify volunteers. Fortunately, the program chairmen of the groups contacted were eager to provide time for a program they felt would be of interest to their members and would aid research.

CRITERION MEASURES

Four criteria of acceptability were used for this study. The sum of the levels of closeness of social contact at which the speaker is acceptable to the subjects is referred to as social acceptability. The three vocational acceptability criteria are (1) the sum of the prestige levels associated with the various jobs which the subjects felt the speaker could handle adequately, called "job prestige"; (2) the total number of jobs the subjects felt the speaker could adequately handle, called "number of jobs"; and (3) the public contact entailed in the jobs that the subjects felt the speaker could handle adequately, called "degree of public contact."

Social acceptability was assessed by means of an adaptation of the Bogardus Scale of Social Distance, a seven-point scale ranging from close acceptance (admission to kinship by marriage) to relative rejection (relegating the individual being judged to residence outside the judge's country) (Campbell, 1953). Each subject checked any of the seven statements with which he agreed relative to the speaker he was evaluating. Scores ranged from a maximum of 28 to a minimum of 0.

The vocational acceptability judgments were obtained by means of a scale devised by the investigator, on which subjects checked the jobs they thought the speaker capable of handling. Fourteen jobs were listed alphabetically on the form, ranging across seven levels of job prestige, with one job requiring public contact and one not requiring public contact at each prestige level. The results of the study from which the prestige ratings were obtained (National Opinion Research Center, 1947) indicated that the chief factors of job prestige are highly specialized training and a considerable degree of responsibility for the public welfare. Unskilled, low-paid, and "dirty" jobs involving little public responsibility were considered the least desirable occupations. The ranges of possible scores a subject could give a speaker were 56 to 0 for job prestige, 14 to 0 for number of jobs, and +7 to −7 for degree of public contact.

The social and vocational scales were placed on a single response form along with the directions for the subject. Each subject was given four forms, one for his reactions to each speaker. The forms were designed to obtain reactions quickly and with minimal self-criticism, to be easily and quickly completed by the subject (requiring 21 checks at most), and to give quantitative ratings that could be objectively and quickly tabulated. To minimize the pressure to respond "humanely," no subject-identifying data were requested.

EXPERIMENTAL VARIABLES STUDIED

The experimental questions listed earlier suggest the variables of interest, the type of speaker, the manner of presentation of the speaker, the information provided the subjects before their judging the speakers, and the order in which the speakers were presented.

The speaker variable involved four levels: two normal and two esophageal speakers. The use of two speakers of each type constituted a form of replication designed to establish the reliability of differences found between normal and esophageal speakers. All subjects judged each of the four speakers, alternating normal and esophageal speakers, so that ample opportunity would be available for comparing the speakers.

The presentation variable involved three levels: by tape (speech only), by silent film (appearance only), and by sound films (simultaneous speech and appearance). This permitted evaluation of subject reactions to speaker appearance alone, to speech alone, and to speech and appearance combined.

The information variable involved two levels: no information or a simple statement presented before having the subjects judge the speakers. This statement was to the effect that two of the speakers were normal and two laryngectomized and included a brief explanation of the effects of laryngectomy.

The order variable grew out of the alternate presentation of the normal and esophageal speakers to all of the subjects. By counter-balancing order over speaker in a Latin Square design, each speaker's total judgment was comprised of equal numbers of subjects having rated him first, second, third, or last of the four speakers. The main effect of order and its interactions with the other experimental variables, the significance of which proved to be inconsistent from one criterion variable to the other, are outgrowths of the intended interspeaker comparison but are of little practical importance. They were included in the analyses of variance so that they could be isolated from the error variance, thereby increasing the efficiency of the design. Each subject judged all four speakers, one order of presentation, and one manner of presentation, and was either exposed to the directions only or to the informative introduction before judging the speakers.

An extension of the Type IV analysis of variance described by Lindquist (1953, pp. 285-288) was used to analyze the data, and separate analyses were conducted for each of the four criterion variables. Analyses by individual degree of freedom (orthogonal comparisons) were subsequently employed to test the differences between the normal and esophageal speakers, the two normal speakers, and the two esophageal speakers (Snedecor, 1950, pp. 403-406).

TABLE 1. Means of the four criterion measures for normal (N) and laryngectomized (L) speakers according to manner of presentation and presence or absence of information.

Condition	Social Acceptability		Job Prestige		Number of Jobs		Degree of Public Contact	
	N	L	N	L	N	L	N	L
Tape presentation	14.20	9.47	31.99	24.39	7.20	6.35	0.39	−0.95
Silent film	14.08	10.69	28.90	22.36	6.22	5.46	0.19	−0.85
Sound film	15.47	12.10	31.58	25.56	7.05	6.06	0.35	−1.08
Mean	14.58	10.75	30.82	24.10	6.83	5.96	0.31	−0.96
No-information	13.25	8.50	26.63	20.45	5.65	5.13	0.37	−0.59
With-information	15.92	13.00	35.01	27.75	8.00	6.79	0.25	−1.34
Mean	14.58	10.75	30.82	24.10	6.83	5.96	0.31	−0.96

RESULTS

The results of this study are summarized in Table 1, which shows the means for each of the four criterion measures for two normal and two esophageal speakers for each of the three modes of presentation. In addition this table shows the means for the *no-information* and *with-information* conditions.

Speaker Comparisons

Laryngectomized speakers received significantly poorer scores than the normal speakers on all four criteria, regardless of manner of presentation or the presence or absence of information ($F = 163.69$, 128.27, 39.41, and 139.64; $df = 3,1368$; $p < 0.001$, for the social acceptability, job prestige, number of jobs, and degree of public contact criteria, respectively). For the most part, the two normal speakers received similar ratings, whereas there was usually a significant separation between the two laryngectomees.

Differences in Presentation

For the criterion of social acceptability, sound-film presentation (13.78) resulted in significantly higher scores ($F = 5.51$; $df = 2,456$; $p < 0.005$) than either tape (11.83) or silent-film presentation (12.38), which were not different from one another. Manner of presentation did not have a significant effect on the other three criterion measures (job prestige, number of jobs, and degree of public contact). In every case, however, the speaker-by-presentation interaction was statistically significant, resulting in part from the varying differences between the normal speakers and laryngectomees and in part from the varying differences between the two speakers in each category.

In the case of social acceptability, a source of the speaker-by-presentation interaction ($F = 3.89$; $df = 6,1368$; $p < 0.001$) was that the ratings for normal speakers were relatively independent of mode of presentation (14.20, 14.08, and 15.47 for tape, silent-film, and sound-film, respectively) while the ratings for esophageal speakers varied significantly (9.47, 10.69, and 12.10, respectively). For job prestige, the speaker-by-presentation interaction ($F = 2.34$; $df = 6,1368$; $p < 0.05$) was related to differences between the two speakers within each group rather than to the differences between the normal and laryngectomized groups. The speaker-by-presentation interaction for number of jobs ($F = 2.76$; $df = 6,1368$; $p < 0.025$) also reflects presentation variations within groups rather than between groups. Finally, the significant speaker-by-presentation interaction for degree of public contact ($F = 2.45$; $df = 6,1368$; $p < 0.025$) can be explained by the fact that the laryngectomized speakers received their best ratings for silent-film and their poorest ratings for presentations involving voice, whereas the normal speakers received their poorest ratings for silent-film and their best ratings for presentations involving voice.

Effect of Information

Interestingly, telling the judges that two of the speakers they would be rating were laryngectomized and describing the effects of this surgery significantly influenced their ratings of both the normal and the laryngectomized speakers ($F = 52.54$, 38.99, 36.75, and 19.65; $df = 1,456$; $p < 0.001$, for the social acceptability, job prestige, number of jobs, and public contact criteria, respectively). The changes were in the same direction for both groups, but significant speaker-by-information interactions indicate that their amounts of change were not similar for three of the criteria. For social acceptability ($F = 11.04$; $df = 3,1368$; $p < 0.001$) the ratings for esophageal speakers rose from 8.50 to 13.00, while those for the normal speakers rose only from 13.25 to 15.92. For the number of jobs ($F = 6.35$; $df = 3,1368$; $p < 0.001$) the ratings of the normal speakers rose from 5.65 to 8.00, whereas those of the laryngectomees rose only from 5.13 to 6.79. For the degree of public contact ($F = 7.52$; $df = 3,1368$; $p < 0.001$) the ratings of both groups fell, with the laryngectomees declining from -0.59 to -1.34, whereas the normal speakers declined only from 0.37 to 0.25. Job prestige demonstrated no speaker-by-information interaction, indicating that the amount of improvement due to information was similar for both groups.

DISCUSSION

The above findings indicate that business and professional men rate esophageal and normal speakers differently in terms of social and vocational acceptability. Regardless of whether or not the subjects were informed about esophageal speakers, they consistently viewed the laryngectomees as being less acceptable socially than normal speakers and capable of handling significantly fewer jobs, these jobs having significantly reduced prestige and public contact. It should be remembered that the laryngectomees used in this study were superior speakers having high-contact, prestige positions in real life.

The fact that the esophageal speakers experienced reduced social and vocational status when judged from silent films as well as from tape recordings and sound films indicates that there is a negative visible concomitant of esophageal speech. The visible difference probably results from perceptible muscular contractions of the face, neck, and mouth associated with "trapping" and releasing esophageal air. These visible characteristics would be analogous to differences in fundamental frequency, phrasing, inflection, loudness, and extraneous noises that constitute the negative auditory stimuli.

Explanations of what esophageal speech is and why it is used significantly improved the acceptability of the esophageal speakers in three of the four criteria evaluated: social closeness, the number of jobs relegated to the speaker, and the prestige associated with those jobs. Introductory information, however, decreased the degree of public contact afforded the laryngectomees.

The degree of public contact criterion appears to be an especially significant measure of acceptability. It represents the subjects' willingness to accommodate the speaker in the formal, competitive, impersonal world as distinct from the family-friend relationship or the recognition of prestigious attributes. Of the four criteria studied, it is probably the best measure of anticipated speaker effectiveness and desirability in business interaction. It is interesting to note that the normal speakers were placed primarily in positions requiring public contact, whereas the laryngectomees were relegated to a majority of positions isolating them from the public. Moreover, when information made the subjects aware of the specific nature of the disorder, rejection of the laryngectomees in public-contact positions increased, whereas acceptance increased in the other criterion measures.

The literature regarding the adjustment of the laryngectomee to his suddenly altered status deals primarily with physical, speech, and family readjustments. It appears that problems involved in gaining social and vocational acceptance may be even more insidious. Reductions in feelings of personal worth and motivation to communicate are reasonable expectations, especially since the esophageal speaker has at one time been "normal."

This study suggests that intelligible and fluent esophageal speech, although important, is not enough to insure the rehabilitation of the laryngectomee. Elimination of visible stigmas, psychological preparation and support for return to the previous level of social and vocational influence, and public education to facilitate that return, are also important.

With regard to the communicatively handicapped in general, this study suggests the need for (1) measures of speech proficiency that reflect the speaker's capacity to gain social and vocational access and influence; (2) the analysis of the effect of variables such as intelligibility, fundamental frequency, fluency, stress, voice quality, appearance, and sex, on speaker acceptability; and (3) the effect of listener attributes such as sex, age, and socioeconomic level on speaker acceptability. It is suggested that the criterion measures used in this study might serve as objective indicators of the degree to which communicative disorders handicap adults.

ACKNOWLEDGMENT

This research was supported in part by Project Grant RD 421, U. S. Department of Health, Education, and Welfare, Office of Vocational Rehabilitation. Requests for reprints should be sent to Stuart I. Gilmore, Speech and Hearing Clinic, 217 Music and Dramatic Arts Building, Louisiana State University, Baton Rouge, Louisiana 70803.

REFERENCES

ASHMORE, L. L., Effects of indoctrination on audience ratings of the personality characteristics of individuals with articulatory defects. Doctoral dissertation, Univ. of Wisconsin (1958).

BATEMAN, G., DORNHORST, A., and LEATHART, G., Oesophageal speech. Brit. med. J., 2, 133-139 (1952).

BISI, R., and CONLEY, J., Psychologic factors influencing vocal rehabilitation of the post-laryngectomy patient. Ann. Otol. Rhinol. Laryng., 74, 1073-1078 (1965).

CAMPBELL, D., The Bogardus Scale of Social Distance. In O. K. Buros (Ed.), The Fourth Mental Measurements Yearbook. Highland Park, N. J.: Gryphon (1953).

DAMSTE, P., VAN DEN BERG, J. W., and MOOLENAAR-BIJL, A., Why are some patients unable to learn esophageal speech? Ann. Otol. Rhinol. Laryng., 65, 998-1005 (1956).

GATEWOOD, E., A new and simple procedure for developing esophageal voice in the laryngectomized patient. Virginia med. mon., 73, 206-209 (1946).

GELLMAN, W., Roots of prejudice against the handicapped. J. Rehab., 25, 4-6, 25 (1959).

GREENE, J. S., Laryngectomy and its psychologic implications. N. Y. St. J. Med., 47, 53-56 (1947).

HEAVER, L., WHITE, W., and GOLDSTEIN, N., Clinical experience in restoring oral communication to 274 laryngectomized patients by esophageal voice. J. Amer. geriat. Soc., 3, 687-690 (1955).

HOROWITZ, L. S., Attitudes of speech defectives toward humor based on speech defects. Speech Monogr., 26, 46-55 (1957).

INGWELL, R., THORESON, R., and SMITS, S., Accuracy of social perception of physically handicapped and non-handicapped persons. J. soc. Psychol., 76, 107-116 (1967).

JESBERG, N., Rehabilitation after laryngectomy. Calif. Med., 70, 80-82 (1954).

KING, P., LOWLKS, E., and PEIRSON, G., Rehabilitation and adaptation of laryngectomy patients. Amer. J. phys. Med., 47, 192-203 (1968).

KLECK, R., ONO, H., and HASTORF, A., The effects of physical deviance upon face-to-face interaction. *Hum. Relat.*, 19, 425-436 (1966).

KLEFFNER, F., A comparison of the reactions of a group of fourth grade children to recorded samples of defective and non-defective articulation. Doctoral dissertation, Univ. of Wisconsin (1952).

LEVIN, N., Teaching the laryngectomized patient to talk. *Arch. Otolaryng.*, 32, 299-314 (1940).

LEVIN, N., Total laryngectomy and speech rehabilitation. *Eye, Ear, Nose Thr. Mon.*, 34, 585-592 (1955).

LINDSAY, J., MORGAN, R., and WEPMAN, J., The cricopharyngeus muscle in esophageal speech. *Laryngoscope*, 54, 55-65 (1944).

LINDQUIST, E. F., *Design and Analysis of Experiments in Psychology and Education*. Boston: Houghton Mifflin (1953).

MARTIN, H., Rehabilitation of the laryngectomee. *Cancer*, 16, 824-833 (1963).

MASSON, R. L., The laryngectomee: Obstacles to vocational rehabilitation. *J. Rehab.*, 36, 33-34, 44 (1970).

McCALL, J. W., Preliminary voice training for laryngectomy. *Arch. Otolaryng.*, 38, 10-16 (1943).

MEYERSON, L., Somatopsychology of physical disability. In W. Cruickshank (Ed.), *Psychology of Exceptional Children and Youth*. N. J.: Prentice-Hall (1955).

MOSES, P., Rehabilitation of the post-laryngectomized patient; 2. The vocal therapist: Place and contribution to the rehabilitation program. *Ann. Otol. Rhinol. Laryng.*, 67, 538-543 (1958).

NATIONAL OPINION RESEARCH CENTER, Jobs and occupations: A popular evaluation. *Opinion News*, 9, 3-13 (1947).

PERRIN, E., The social position of the speech defective. *J. Speech Hearing Dis.*, 19, 250-252 (1954).

SCHALL, L., Psychology of laryngectomized patients. *Arch. Otolaryng.*, 28, 581-584 (1938).

SNEDECOR, G. W., *Statistical Methods*. Ames, Iowa: Iowa State Univ. Press (1950).

SNEDECOR, J., Speech without a larynx. In L. E. Travis (Ed.), *Handbook of Speech Pathology and Audiology*. New York: Appleton-Century-Crofts (1971).

STETSON, R. H., Esophageal speech for any laryngectomized patient. *Arch. Otolaryng.*, 26, 132-142 (1937).

STOLL, B., Rehabilitation of the post-laryngectomized patient; 4. Psychological factors determining the success or failure of the rehabilitation program of laryngectomized patients. *Ann. Otol. Rhinol. Laryng.*, 67, 550-557 (1958).

SUINN, R. M., Psychological reactions to physical disability. *J. Ass. phys. ment. Rehab.*, 21, 13-15 (1967).

TATO, J. M., Study of the sonospectrographic characteristics of the voice in laryngectomized patients. *Acta otolaryng.*, 44, 431-438 (1954).

TIKOFSKY, R. S., A comparison of the intelligibility of esophageal and normal speakers. *Folia Phoniatr.*, 17, 19-32 (1965).

WALDROP, W., Rehabilitation of the laryngectomized patient. *Neb. St. med. J.*, 39, 419-422 (1954).

Received August 23, 1972.
Accepted December 1, 1973.

PART IV

EXTRINSIC FORMS OF ALARYNGEAL VOICE AND SPEECH: ARTIFICIAL LARYNGES

Extrinsic forms of alaryngeal speech and voice are discussed in this section of the book. The term *extrinsic* was chosen to highlight the fact that the forms of phonation and oral communication depend upon man-made voicing prostheses (artificial larynges) or surgically created structures developed specifically for the purpose of voice production (surgical-prosthetic approaches to speech and voice restoration).

The second most common form of alaryngeal speech involves the use of a prosthetic voicing source, or artificial larynx. There are two principal reasons for the widespread and increasing use of artificial larynges: 1) patient preference for the artificial larynx as a primary method of oral communication and 2) failure of large numbers of laryngectomized patients to attain functionally serviceable esophageal speech.

Although a wide variety of artificial larynges are currently available, clinical or basic research studies concerned with important aspects of artificial larynges are scarce. This situation is primarily the result of a long-standing view in which the artificial larynx was regarded as a back-up method for patients who failed to achieve esophageal speech (Lauder, 1968). This philosophy was popular until about a decade ago when Diedrich argued that a primary goal of alaryngeal speech rehabilitation was to develop functional communication, regardless of the mode of voicing. The Diedrich concept, coupled with the fact that there is no evidence that the use of an artificial larynx reduces the laryngectomized patient's ability to learn esophageal speech, gave rise to increasing interest in the use of artificial larynges as alternative and primary modes of voicing support for speech. Current clinical philosophy embodies the implementation of the artificial larynx as a compliment to esophageal voice training. This philosophy is sound for a variety of reasons. For example, the artificial larynx may 1) facilitate the development of oral communication, 2) reduce communicative frustration on the part of the patient and others, and 3) facilitate the acquisition of esophageal voicing.

Efficient use of an artificial larynx as a voicing source clearly does not depend on the integrity of the esophagus and the P-E segment. The prosthetic device itself serves as the vibratory source. The voicing source of these devices are powered either by pulmonary air or by electronic means. Stated differently, pneumatic instruments utilize pulmonary air from the stoma to activate a voicing source. Electronic artificial larynges are battery powered and generate a sound into the vocal tract on either a transcervical or intraoral basis. The characteristics of the voice produced by an artificial larynx depend on the acoustic characteristics of the source and the properties of the laryngectomized patient's altered vocal tract.

It is generally agreed that desirable attributes (Barney, 1958) of any type of artificial larynx should include:

1. Output speech intensity equal to that of normal speech
2. Output speech quality and prosody comparable to that of normal speech
3. Inconspicuousness
4. Hygienically acceptable to the user
5. Simple to operate
6. Reliability
7. Inexpensiveness

Descriptive study and clinical experience indicate that none of the artificial larynges currently available adequately meet all of these design attributes (see Bennett and Weinberg, 1973; Weinberg and Riekena, 1973). In summary, voice produced by most artificial larynges is characterized by a mechanical or electronic quality with limited variation in f_0 (pitch) or intensity (loudness) (Barney, 1958; Weinberg and Bennett, 1973).

Lauder (1968), a laryngectomee and a speech pathologist, summarizes the results of a questionnaire soliciting "opinions, observations, and experiences, if appropriate, as to the usefulness, intelligibility of, and the acceptance/rejection of the artificial larynx...." The major issues concerning the philosophical debate concerning the use of artificial voicing prostheses are raised in this important contribution.

Barney (1958) provides information about four important areas related to the development of speech aids: design objectives, acoustic factors that affect speech quality, consonant production, and speech intelligibility. Barney's discussion of these critical areas is lucid, technically sound, and clinically relevant. Barney (1959) also describes the development of the Western Electric Model 5 (A & B) artificial larynx. This electronic device is currently the most widely used artificial larynx. Hence, both the historical perspectives and the technical background surrounding its development should be understood. Both articles by Barney should be required reading for all persons involved in speech rehabilitation for laryngectomized patients.

Weinberg and Riekena (1973) describe an inexpensive, mechanically simple pneumatic artificial larynx. This Japanese-made device is now quite readily available in the United States and a large number of patients now use this voice prosthesis as a primary method of speech communication. Weinberg and Riekena conclude their article by stating "...In our opinion, speech produced with the Tokyo larynx is not characterized by an overwhelming mechanical or electronic quality.... We hope this report will stimulate consideration and study of this additional method of alaryngeal speech." This opinion, now verified by additional years of experience and shared by others, is offered as strongly now as it was at the time of original publication.

The remaining articles in this section deal with experiments conducted to compare various types of alaryngeal speech. For example, Hyman (1955) represents one of the earliest attempts to compare esophageal speech, artificial larynx speech, and normal speech. This early project is a landmark paper highlighted by the observation that speech produced by artificial larynges may, in some cases, be preferred over esophageal speech. Mc-Croskey and Mulligan (1963) sought information about the intelligibility of esophageal speech and artificial larynx speech. The results of their study revealed that differences in the intelligibility of these two forms of alaryngeal speech varied as a function of a listener sophistication and level of professional training.

Bennett and Weinberg (1973) provide comparative information about the ultimate acceptability of various types of speech (esophageal speech, pneumatic artificial larynx speech and electronic larynx, or alaryngeal, speech). The results of this work clearly show the substantial preference listeners have for normal speech over any form of alaryngeal speech produced by persons without a larynx. The findings of this project also uncovered specific speech and vocal attributes of various forms of alaryngeal speech listeners rated as abnormal.

THE LARYNGECTOMEE AND THE ARTIFICIAL LARYNX

Edmund Lauder

San Antonio, Texas

The publication of Diedrich and Youngstrom's book *Alaryngeal Speech* (1966) has, despite their proposal that "the dichotomy between esophageal speech and the artificial larynx . . . be abandoned . . . ," reawakened this interesting subject. This was particularly manifest during one part of the Sixteenth Annual Meeting of the International Association of Laryngectomees. A professional panel of three physicians, a registered nurse, and a speech pathologist was asked by a laryngectomee member of the audience whether or not they subscribed to the use of the artificial larynx as an adjunct to the teaching of esophageal voice. The majority of the panel members stated that they were in favor of the practice; however one of the physicians rejected this technique. He was applauded by the audience for his position and it was obvious that, insofar as the laryngectomees in that audience were concerned, the issue is still a controversial one.

Many speech pathologists, physicians, laryngectomees, and paramedical specialists claim that the early introduction and use of the artificial larynx following laryngectomy is a psychological as well as an economic necessity for the

Reprinted by permission from *Journal of Speech and Hearing Disorders*, 1968, *33*, 147–157.

new laryngectomee; that esophageal voice can be developed later when the patient has recovered from this traumatic experience. They assert that the instrument is much more understandable than esophageal voice and it enables the user to communicate much sooner and more effectively, particularly in situations involving emotional stress or when more volume than is normally possible with esophageal voice is required. The opponents of the artificial larynx claim that the use of this instrument is an unnecessary crutch and interferes with the development of esophageal voice; that its use, other than in an emergency situation, should be discouraged. Both the advocates and opponents agree that the artificial larynx is a vital requirement for those who cannot take advantage of esophageal voice instruction due to rural residence, old age, poor health, insufficient knowledge of the national language, or those who fail to learn esophageal phonation in spite of sufficient instruction.

An "either-or" solution is not readily apparent. In seeking the information presented in this paper, I wrote to more than 100 persons with special background in this subject. They were asked for their opinions as well as their personal observations and experiences, if appropriate, as to the usefulness, intelligibility, and the acceptance/rejection of the artificial larynx as compared with the esophageal voice in laryngectomees. Response to this inquiry was gratifying.

The replies are presented here in the form of a round-table discussion using the words of the writers. Not every letter could be used since duplication had to be avoided. The letters "SP," "MD," or "L" in parenthesis adjacent to the

contributor's name identify that person as a speech pathologist, physician, or laryngectomee.

LAUDER: The purpose of this presentation is to examine some of the advantages and disadvantages associated with the use of the artificial larynx as it applies to the person who has been laryngectomized. As far as I am able to determine, there is no objection to the use of the electrolarynx by the laryngectomee who is in poor health, suffers from weakness associated with old age, or is otherwise physically incapable of learning postlaryngectomy voice. For example, few will argue with Levin (1952), who recommends the use of an artificial larynx when: (1) stenosis of the esophagus occurs after extensive removal of a widespread malignant lesion; (2) resection of the cervical portion of the esophagus is necessary; (3) multiple handicaps are present such as laryngectomy plus deafness; (4) a suspected recurrence, metastasis, or multiple lesions occur; or (5) when senility or other feebleness is present.

In a questionnaire survey of 3366 laryngectomees conducted in 1960-61, Horn (1962) found that 64% of this number spoke with esophageal voice, and 5% used esophageal voice but also used artificial devices. Ten percent spoke entirely with artificial devices and 12% did not speak at all. The remainder did not indicate the status of their speech. Gardner and Harris (1961) reported that 40% of all laryngectomees never acquire intelligible speech and that an artificial speech aid should be recommended for them. In evaluating 302 laryngectomees, Green (1949) found that 81% acquired a serviceable esophageal voice while 19% were not successful, and 5-6% of those failures appeared to be due to a physical inability to master this technique. Putney (1958) found in a survey of 440 laryngectomized patients that 166 (38%) failed to develop a useful voice and of this group 25 (5.7%) used an artificial larynx. Of these and other surveys Martin (1963) says:

> Despite optimistic claims (some as high as 80%), I would estimate that less than half of all laryngectomees ever acquire a reasonably adequate and socially acceptable esophageal voice, that is, better than "indifferent," "poor," "offensive," or "absent."

Lueders (1956) maintains that approximately one third of all patients do not learn to speak and that in his judgment of some patients who consider themselves able esophageal speakers, the proficiency of the remaining two thirds might be questioned. He states further:

> The psychological importance of an early return to communicative ability should be considered. Speech, being a most important social function, should be restored to the patient as soon as possible. The psychological effect of enforced silence during a protracted learning period for esophageal speech is the building of resentments and frustration that tend to make the patient uncooperative. It is perhaps better to offer him the help of the electrolarynx, with which he can at least satisfy his all-important sense of speech.

In comparing esophageal speech with electrolarynx speech Martin (1963) asserted that the electrolarynx voice tends to be of uniform quality; that it is far less rasping in tone than many otherwise acceptable esophageal voices; and, furthermore, that it is always devoid of intake burps, facial grimaces, and concomitant forced expulsion of air from the stoma. Martin also has a very definite opinion as to when the electrolarynx should be introduced to the laryngectomee. He states:

> Furthermore, contrary to the pronouncement of many esophageal voice teachers, resorting to such a device promptly after operation in my experience does not preclude or discourage the patient from later efforts to the attainment of esophageal speech, nor does it lessen the chance of ultimate success in that endeavor. It can, however, serve as a stopgap in all cases and give the laryngectomee an unprejudiced, eventual choice between the two methods. Also it makes possible that use of either one as a supplement to the other, depending on the requirements of the occasion. Elimination of any unnecessary delay in achieving a practical means of audible communication transcends any and all other considerations.

BRODNITZ (MD): I am not a great friend of offering the artificial larynx at an early stage. I have done it only rarely, and only in such cases where I had strong doubt whether the patient would be able to learn esophageal speech (age, poor physical condition, difficulty hearing). The laryngectomee has the tendency to retire to his own little "island" and to use this handicap as an unconscious motive to retire from active life. It is difficult enough, in many of these cases, to induce the patient to practice constantly as a requisite to the development of esophageal voice. With the crutch of a primary introduction of the artificial larynx one diminishes the often poor motivation of the patient to learn esophageal voice.

HYMAN (SP): It has been my experience that people who start out with the artificial larynx will generally be poor esophageal speakers. Apparently the habit of using the artificial larynx, the reliance on this, the lack of real practice with esophageal speech (no doubt esophageal speech is much more difficult at first and the artificial larynx is much easier to use), help to bring about the lack of development of esophageal speech. Of course, there are always some who do develop good esophageal speech, but in my experience it has been the minority. I feel that very few people fail to learn esophageal speech.

FARR (MD): I agree with many of those who say that thrusting this machine upon the patient at an early stage tends to take away his desire to learn esophageal speech. The use of an electrolarynx immediately postoperative is difficult because the tissues of the surgical wound and the neck are stiff and will not permit a good result with the machine.

GRANT (MD): In the past undue emphasis has been placed on keeping artificial equipment from the laryngectomee. This is fallacious thinking based on the idea that once such equipment has been used the patient will not get around to learning esophageal voice. It is my understanding that experience has shown that this is not the case. However, human nature, being what it is, and the learning process being essentially one of response to irritation or discomfort or great need, it does seem that esophageal voice should be offered first with considerable backing in order to have the patient put forth maximum efforts to learn the technique.

EDELMAN (SP): I do not feel that the artificial larynx should be introduced during the immediate postoperative period. My answer assumes that the individual has been fully prepared for surgery and that he is receiving a good deal of emotional support from the surgeon, family, and speech clinician. Although economic problems are very real, I would tend to discourage early use of an artificial larynx should the individual return to work prior to the development of pseudo-voice. My rationale is based on the following observation: The use of an artificial larynx does not require the same pattern of air intake that is needed for esophageal voice production. If the greater part of a person's communication efforts is dependent upon the action of a finger on a button instead of on the coordinated movements of the oral structure, that person will be establishing habit patterns for voice production which are opposed to those needed for esophageal voice.

DIEDRICH (SP): No research as yet has shown that an artificial aid precludes or slows down the learning of esophageal speech. It might show that the aid speeds up learning esophageal speech. If the laryngectomee accepts the artificial larynx as a means of communication, the clinician should feel rewarded that he has provided a means by which this was accomplished and not feel guilty that he was unable to teach the person esophageal speech. It was a decision for the client to make, not the clinician.

Articulatory skill is an additional speech benefit which might accrue from the use of the artificial larynx during the immediate postoperative period. The user of the artificial larynx must articulate precisely or the speech will be unintelligible. He must learn, for example, to make voiceless consonant sounds with intraoral-pharyngeal air pressure and not with pulmonary air. The learner of esophageal phonation must also learn to articulate voiceless consonants in a like manner. Clinical observation indicates that persons articulate well who had successfully used the artificial larynx before acquiring esophageal speech.

Another secondary benefit of good articulation is its influence on air intake. Precision in articulatory movements aids in the injection process, especially during the syllable-pulse of plosives and sibilants. Because of these possible speech gains through the use of the artificial larynx it is suggested that the esophageal speech learning period can be shortened, not lengthened.

Another reason for believing this is the additional practice time which would now be available. If the laryngectomee practices 10 minutes an hour on esophageal speech each day and uses writing for all other communication, he achieves 100 minutes of verbal practice in a 10 hour day. Most of this practice is concerned with learning air intake, developing phonation, and acquiring new phrase patterns. He could be talking at least another 100 minutes during the day on an artificial larynx. This additional practice should have some effect on learning better articulatory performance as well as phrasing. It is agreed that not all impromptu talking necessarily results in improvement, but the odds seem better than chance that with speech training, articulation would improve. With the combination of the two types of practice, one phonation and the other articulatory, the total speech learning period should be reduced.

KALTENBORN (SP) : It has been our experience that those who learn to use the artificial larynx before learning esophageal speech do not do as well with esophageal speech because they can always fall back on the artificial larynx. They also do not practice as much as the person who must use esophageal speech if he is to be understood at all.

LANPHER (L) : Based upon my limited experience, however, and taking cognizance of some few of my students who were given artificial larynges by their surgeon in the hospital and who were using them proficiently when the surgeon referred them to me for speech work, my opinion is that the use of the artificial larynx is no deterrent to the learning of efficient esophageal speech by those who really have the desire to learn it. In fact, it may be an aid inasmuch as it permits the person to keep his communication alive, to return sooner to his job; it helps keep his morale high and tension low, and thus helps establish a favorable climate for learning esophageal speech. I would raise the question of whether those who rely upon an artificial larynx to the exclusion of attempting esophageal speech would achieve as serviceable speech through their esophageal voice as they do by artificial means—whether for physical or other reasons. In my experience most people have learned a serviceable esophageal speech and have not supplemented with artificial aids. I wonder whether they might have learned it with greater relaxation, ease, and speed if they had also been given an artificial crutch. I do not know.

McQUEEN (L) : In general I object to the use of an artificial speech aid. I do not think it is the best approach for the majority of people. Of the claims substantiating the use of an electrolarynx, I agree with only one—

old age. Although this instrument is normally easy to use I have known a number of people who have trouble learning to use it and never used it well. The instrument has its limitations also—the extent of surgery occasionally becomes a factor in its limitations. The electrolarynx is not a panacea.

HEBERT (L): My experience with the electrolarynx has been one of the most wonderful things that happened to me while I was trying to learn esophageal speech. I acquired an electrolarynx and in a day or so learned to operate it sufficiently well to carry on a good conversation, the results of which relieved that terrible frustration and anxiety. It gave me a new incentive to learn to speak. While I now speak with good esophageal voice, I do not hesitate to use the electrolarynx in situations where it is necessary to talk above the noise of the shop or to a friend who is hard of hearing.

PERSCH (L): First, I prefer the electrolarynx for myself—not because I am too lazy to use an esophageal voice; I can speak with an esophageal voice but I do it poorly and it is very exhausting for me. I still practice with our club because I don't want to be a stumbling block for others. I am told I use an electrolarynx well and am easily understood. All users do not use them well, as all esophageal speakers do not speak well. This I believe is up to the individual. I am a very busy person. If I were to spend more time practicing esophageal speech I would have to give up other activities I enjoy. Therefore, time being an element, I have had to evaluate the worth of such a voice against the value of my other interests. As long as I can speak clearly with an electrolarynx, I chose to use my time in enjoying other interests. I feel too, the moment I speak, people know I have something "different" or a "limitation." So there is no need to explain. I find it easier on my listeners for me to use an electrolarynx.

WHITNEY (MD): Since the inception of the American Telephone and Telegraph Company's interest in a method for artificial speech, it has been my understanding that our role is limited to making such a device available. The selection of cases and the principles for the use of an artificial larynx are appropriately left to the professional disciplines primarily responsible for medical care and rehabilitation. I have been aware that there is some divergence of opinion as to the most effective time for the introduction of an artificial larynx. At the time the new electronic larynx was introduced to our sales representatives in the Bell System Companies in 1960, I stressed that the patient or relative making the contact should be sure that the procurement of an artificial larynx met with the approval of the physician in charge of the case. At the same time, I also stressed to our company representatives that esophageal voice was considered by the vast majority of the experts in the field to be the method of choice, and that we have no quarrel with this viewpoint. There are cases and times in which the artificial larynx serves a useful purpose.

CORGILL (MD): I agree. I am more than ever convinced that more than half of laryngectomized patients can benefit by the use of an artificial larynx. My patients live such varied existences and great distances from Dallas that speech instruction is a matter of too of an artificial larynx. Unless there has been very radical surgery involving tongue I am convinced that all laryngectomized patients can learn esophageal speech. Of course it does require determination and practice and many patients lack motivation and also the realization that this speech cannot be acquired overnight. It is my personal feeling that in many instances the clinicians are responsible if the patient resorts to an instrument. Either they give up too early or indicate in some way that they feel the patient cannot acquire esophageal speech.

PERRY (SP): Our routine procedure with the newly laryngectomized is to introduce them to both the artificial larynx and esophageal speech. Esophageal speech is demonstrated by a range of adequate to very good laryngectomized speakers. The artificial larynx demonstration, by the clinic staff, is probably less impressive than the esophageal speech demonstration. We explain to the patients that the Veterans Administration is reluctant to provide an artificial larynx unless the patient has demonstrated that he cannot successfully use esophageal speech. A typical reaction of patients upon introduction to the artificial larynx, when esophageal speech has also been demonstrated, is to reject the artificial larynx.

FERGUSON (SP): I have always avoided mentioning the artificial larynx until it has become obvious that the patient cannot learn esophageal speech. If the patient asks about the artificial larynx before he has acquired fluent esophageal speech I explain the instrument to him and assure him that it will be given to him should that be necessary. I believe that to put too

many of those people can be understood by their relatives, close friends, and neighbors, much as the small child is understood by his parents but not by strangers. These people are severely limited in their contacts. For example when trying to ask the bus driver street directions, they are unable to make themselves heard or understood. I think this is a great handicap and I think that there has been too much downgrading of the artificial larynx.

CAMPIGLIA (L): I personally do not approve of the artificial larynx. I feel it is more difficult to learn to speak after becoming dependent upon the artificial larynx. If a patient cannot learn to speak after sufficient training, then the use of the artificial larynx is suggested. The instrument is too artificial. A patient's voice is more understandable and pitch may be accomplished with time and training. The artificial larynx should be used as a last resort.

DOEHLER (L): I must be counted among those who do not favor the use many miles, too many times. Most of them do not receive any organized speech therapy. Some of my very best speakers, using esophageal speech, are self taught. But all of them need a quiet environment to be heard and they are unable to communicate under noisy circumstances. I was very distressed at our last cancer recheck day when we examined some 36 returning patients to discover that only five could give me their names so that I could understand them. The patient very often does not attain adequate speech and now is not motivated to seek an artificial larynx since we have downgraded it. Also he does not know where or how to purchase one. Of course, much importance in the artificial larynx will in some cases undermine the patient's motivation to learn esophageal speech quickly and well. Most patients who have even poor esophageal speech seem to prefer doing the best they can to using the artificial larynx because of the flat, expressionless tone of the instrument and the obvious drawbacks to relying on mechanical equipment. The artificial larynx, like any other crutch, is to be avoided until it is clear that the patient either cannot or will not learn to speak unaided.

HUDSON (SP): We do not use an artificial larynx in teaching esophageal voice. For those veterans who cannot learn to communicate with esophageal speech we provide an artificial aid.

ZIMMERMAN (SP): No artificial larynx produces more understandable or more audible speech than even fair-to-middling esophageal speech. And some of them produce speech that is much less audible and intelligible than esophageal production. They all "squawk" too, which is distracting, and they are a nuisance to carry around. Particularly so for one who also has a severe hearing loss and has to wear a body hearing aid and wear glasses. Most of our patients don't like them and that fact has motivated their desire to develop speech without them.

DUGUAY (SP): There is no right or wrong regarding the use of the artificial larynx. Each case must be individually evaluated. Anyone who will say, "Do not let him use one," or, "Give him one to use," does not know what he is talking about. Every laryngectomee is a special individual with a particular set of circumstances and no set formula will work in every situation. It is extremely important that the person responsible for the speech rehabilitation of the laryngectomee be a person of the highest professional and ethical background and training. He must see each patient as an individual and make the decision for or against the artificial larynx on the basis of the particular need of each patient entrusted to him.

SNYDER (SP): A central principle in rehabilitation as I understand it is to train people to employ their own natural resources wherever feasible rather than to rely on artificial or prosthetic devices. Where it is possible for such individuals to learn good esophageal voice, the artificial larynx has little or no place.

MAWHINNEY (SP): For my students the artificial larynx has been a crutch, and I prefer to have nothing to do with it. I found the patients who used this device to "tide them over" never got over the tide. There was much rationalization over its use. Also, the patients who were extremely interested in learning to speak orally found the artificial larynx very distracting to the listeners and discarded it themselves.

SNIDECOR (SP): Esophageal voice should be used whenever it can become sufficiently effective to compete with the artificial larynx. The latest surveys indicate that approximately 69% of all laryngectomees learn esophageal speech. It also seems obvious that the artificial larynx is far better than no vocal communication whatsoever. There is a very critical moment at which the skilled clinician must judge whether or not esophageal speech can be learned. If it cannot be learned, it is then the clinician's obligation to lead the laryngectomee into adequate use of the artificial larynx.

EISENSON (SP): I do not think any hard and fast values in one direction or the other can be esablished without special regard for the individual laryngectomee. Some persons, laryngectomees included, must use a "crutch" so that they will know that they are not cut off from communication despite their new condition. Some will be willing to discard this instrument as soon as they are able to get along without it. Others may be unwilling to risk giving up the useful instrument and to learn to get along with their own modified organic equipment. I wish some studies could be made of criteria to indicate when and for whom an artificial larynx rather than esophageal voice training is indicated.

SHANKS (SP): Discussion about an artificial larynx to provide the laryngectomee with a pseudo-voice devolves into not "if" but "under what conditions" an instrument should be used. A distinction should be made between the use of an instrument on a permanent as opposed to a temporary basis—during the hospital or immediate postlaryngectomy period. I assume that postsurgical expressive communication will be limited, that ordinarily the laryngectomee can print or write his needs, that he can mouth, without sound, answers which are brief or readily anticipated. Thus the decision to employ the instrument temporarily should hinge on the presence of a secondary or multiple handicap such as blindness, inability to read or write, or lack of familiarity with the extant language. The decision to use an instrument on a temporary basis should take cognizance of the likelihood that its temporary use will extend into prolonged use. Implicit in this discussion is an assumption that the decision to use an artificial larynx will not be dependent upon such factors as the bias of the surgeon or the ability of the manufacturer to sell his instrument. There appear to be many benefits stemming from the professional demonstration or description of one or more instruments to the laryngectomee during his convalescence. The essence of such an explanation is that an instrument would be available as needed or desired, that its use would not be an indication of failure.

DIEDRICH (SP): The International Association of Laryngectomees through their Lost Chord Clubs can do much to help users of the artificial larynx to be more accepted. Often there is the subtle but extremely provocative indication that one with an aid is not as good as one who can speak without it. It does not take long for the laryngectomee who comes to a club meeting with an artificial larynx to feel different and guilty about being unable to achieve esophageal speech. This individual soon drops out and is no longer seen at the meetings. There are exceptions, of course, usually someone who has considerable ego strength. It would be preferable to listen to someone talk with intelligible speech with the use of an artificial larynx than to see him write or struggle along with raucous, clunking noises, facial grimaces, or interminable pauses only to have to go through it again when he is told, "I didn't understand you. Would you please repeat that?"

KALTENBORN (SP): We have also observed that in some Lost Chord Clubs the use of any artificial device is frowned upon by the members or their sponsors and as a result the person becomes discouraged. He is rejected in the very place he should be accepted. From our experience there seems to be no particular difference in the intelligibility between esophageal speech and the speech with an artificial larynx. We are aware of some studies which would indicate that the artificial larynx is easier to understand; however we have not felt this to be true.

BRODNITZ (MD): The artificial larynx is at best a poor substitute for any form of active speech. Lately many of the laryngectomies are done in combination with radical neck dissections. In these cases the shape of the neck is considerably altered and I have had difficulty to find a flat place on the neck that accommodates the head of the instrument high enough to transmit enough vibration into the mouth.

DIEDRICH (SP): One must experiment with a variety of spot placements along the neck and floor of the mouth to determine the best place. With radical neck dissection there is additional scar tissue and there may be more complaint of pain by the laryngectomee. Some laryngectomees have so much scar tissue that smooth contact of the vibrator head against the neck is impossible. Others cannot get good resonance for intelligent speech because the sound waves are dissipated before they can be amplified in the oral and pharyngeal cavities due to a thick neck, edema, or postradiation fibrosis of the tissues. A few clients complain of so much pain when the head of the vibrator is pressed firmly against the neck that they cannot use it.

CONCLUSION

The opinions expressed are so varied as to preclude any attempt to draw all-encompassing conclusions. Nevertheless, certain aspects of this controversial subject are clearly evident. For example, those who oppose the use of the electrolarynx generally assert that:

1. The instrument will interfere with the development of esophageal voice.
2. It should not be introduced to a new laryngectomee until he has tried to learn esophageal voice.
3. The instrument has too many limitations, not the least of which is the unacceptable sound it makes.
4. The user of such an instrument cannot produce speech as intelligible as esophageal speech.
5. Except for those who are physically infirm, it presents too easy an escape from the onerous task of learning esophageal voice; in short, it is a crutch.

Advocates of the electrolarynx maintain that:

1. An early return to work made possible by the electrolarynx provides rehabilitative as well as economic dividends.
2. The instrument need not interfere with the development of esophageal voice so long as the patient's teacher perseveres in teaching the proper technique of esophageal voice.
3. When properly used, the instrument enables the patient to produce intelligible speech; again the responsibility for teaching him the proper technique of using the electrolarynx rests with the teacher.
4. Too many laryngectomees speak poorly with esophageal voice; they would be better off using an instrument part of the time or even all of the time.
5. The electrolarynx should be given to the patient as soon after his operation as the physician permits. Immediate communicative ability will be maintained during

the period it takes to learn efficient esophageal speech. Such ability also provides a favorable psychological impetus to learning the new technique.

The entire subject was summarized by Diedrich and Youngstrom (1966), who stated:

The philosophy which the speech clinician should maintain does not appear to be a simple decision between esophageal speech or an artificial larynx. They are not mutually exclusive. The question is not which method is better, but which methods are best, not only for any given patient, but also for any given time within the rehabilitation period. What may be appropriate right after surgery may not be so appropriate in a year; what is adequate speech at home may not be adequate at work. Also, the clinician's choice of method may not be in harmony with the wishes of the patient. Herein lies a professional ethic which cannot be ignored—the patient must have freedom of choice after he has been provided with the best available information about his problem.

Editor's Note: Edmund Lauder is a laryngectomee, a retired lieutenant colonel, United States Air Force, a member of ASHA, and a member of the Board of Directors, International Association of Laryngectomees. This article is based primarily on correspondence received from many otolaryngologists, speech pathologists, and lay laryngectomized voice instructors.

ACKNOWLEDGMENT

The author would like to thank the following people, whose personal communications were of great assistance in the preparation of this article: F. S. Brodnitz, P. Campiglia, Donald A. Corgill, William M. Diedrich, Mary Doehler, Marshall S. Duguay, F. Edelman, J. Eisenson, H. W. Farr, Jack D. Ferguson, Roald Grant, A. J. Hebert, A. Hudson, M. Hyman, A. L. Kaltenborn, Jr., Anne G. Lanpher, Clara K. Mawhinney, Elsie McQueen, Peter S. Perry, Mabel R. Persch, James C. Shanks, J. C. Snidecor, Murray A. Snyder, J. M. Wepman, L. H. Whitney, and J. D. Zimmerman.

REFERENCES

DIEDRICH, W. M., and YOUNGSTROM, K. A., *Alaryngeal Speech.* Springfield, Illinois: Charles C Thomas (1966), pp. 138, 148.

GARDNER, W. H., and HARRIS, H. E., Aids and devices for laryngectomees. *Arch. Otolaryngol.,* **73,** 145 (1961).

GREEN, J. S., Statistical study of 300 patients. *N. Y. St. J. Med.,* **49,** 272 (1949).

HORN, D., Laryngectomee Survey Report presented at the 11th annual meeting of the International Association of Laryngetomees, August 21, 1962.

LEVIN, N. M., Speech rehabilitation after total removal of larynx. *J. Amer. Med. Ass.,* **149,** 1285 (1952).

LUEDERS, O. W., Use of the Electrolarynx in speech rehabilitation. *Arch. Otolaryngol.,* **63,** 134 (1956).

MARTIN, H., Rehabilitation of the laryngectomee. *Cancer,* **16,** 824, 835 (1963).

PUTNEY, F. J., Rehabilitation of the postlaryngectomized patient, *Transactions Amer. Laryngolog. Ass.,* **79,** 91 (1958).

A Discussion of Some Technical Aspects of Speech Aids for Postlaryngectomized Patients

Harold L. Barney (by invitation)

Murray Hill, N.J.

Since the development of the Western Electric Models 2A and 2B artificial larynges about thirty years ago,[1] there have been a number of developments in the general fields of acoustics and electronic circuitry which would be applicable to the design of an improved artificial larynx. A major development in electronic circuitry has been the invention and perfection of the transistor; this, coupled with miniaturization of circuit components such as acoustic transducers and batteries, has made possible radical improvements in hearing aids and other similar types of devices. Also improved acoustic and electronic circuit measurement techniques are now available using new instruments such as the sound spectrograph, for example. It would certainly be of interest to examine the possibilities afforded by these new techniques in the design of an artificial larynx. But before a choice can be made of a particular method of operation of an artificial larynx, there are a number of acoustic and electronic circuit aspects of the problem to be considered. It will be the purpose of this paper to examine some of these aspects in detail.

DESIGN OBJECTIVES FROM THE VIEWPOINT OF THE PATIENT

An exhaustive survey of opinions of postlaryngectomized patients has not been made to determine what would be an ideal type of artificial larynx, but the consensus of those patients and doctors who have been consulted is that an ideal device should have the following attributes:

1. Output speech volume equal to that of a normal speaker.
2. Output speech quality and pitch inflection like that of normal speech.
3. Unobtrusive; without visible wires, tubes, or other appurtenances, and small in size.
4. Reliable; with trouble-free operation for long periods of time.
5. Hygienically acceptable to the user.
6. Inexpensive price and low operating cost.

In addition, the device should be simple to operate so that a minimum of training is required. A design which attempts to satisfy all the above objectives must necessarily involve some compromises, if for no other reason than that an uncompromising compliance

Reprinted by permission from *Annals of Otology, Rhinology, and Laryngology*, 1958, 67, 558–570. Copyright 1958, Annals Publishing Company.

with the first four objectives would certainly require a design that would not be inexpensive.

In cases where good proficiency with esophageal speech can be acquired by the patient, this provides a solution to the problem that is generally acceptable, although the speech volume is usually weaker and the speech quality is considerably inferior to that of normal speech. However, there is a sizeable fraction, about a third, of all laryngectomized patients who cannot master esophageal speech for one reason or another, according to O. W. Lueders.[2] For this group an improved design of artificial larynx is needed.

The first design objective listed above, namely, that of a normal speech output volume, is a relatively easy one to meet. Normal conversational speech requires a total acoustic output of only about 20 microwatts when integrated over an interval of several seconds or more. The short term peak factors are such that on the peaks of strong syllables in conversational speech, the acoustic power output may be as much as 1,000 microwatts. Acoustic powers of this magnitude are quite easily radiated with small transducers, and various types of artificial larynges could be designed which would meet this requirement.

The second objective, of obtaining speech quality like that of normal speech, will be somewhat more difficult of attainment. To sound natural, speech should have pitch inflection, should have both voiced and unvoiced types of output, and should have spectra of energy distributions versus frequency that are rather carefully controlled according to the various speech sounds that are intended. These aspects will be discussed in more detail later in this paper.

The third objective, of making the device unobtrusive, is considered by all to be highly desirable. It is in this respect that the Western Electric Model 2 device is felt to be seriously deficient. Many postlaryngectomized patients express the view that the insertion of the tube into the mouth and the connection at the throat constitute sources of embarrassment. Judging from the efforts of hearing aid manufacturers to produce unobtrusive hearing aids, this desire to avoid the appearance of anything that would call attention to an infirmity is one to which serious attention should be given.

The fourth, fifth and sixth objectives of reliability, acceptability from a hygienic standpoint, and low cost are also obviously desirable. For an electronic device, the battery power consumption should be kept to a minimum in order to reduce costs of battery replacement. The manufacturing cost can be minimized by the use of commercially available transducers, transistors, and other component parts. In this respect, the Western Electric Model 2 device has been an expensive one to manufacture because of the special reed mechanism that has to be machined to close tolerances especially for it.

ACOUSTIC FACTORS WHICH AFFECT SPEECH QUALITY OF AN ARTIFICIAL LARYNX

In the normal production of voiced speech sounds, the initial source of sound is provided by the vocal cords. This source produces a complex sound which is rich in harmonic content. The quality of this sound is modified by the resonating action of the cavities of the pharynx, mouth and nose, and by constrictions at the back of the tongue and at the lips and teeth. The different combinations of the shapes of these cavities and constrictions give rise to the various voiced sounds of speech. The upper part of Figure 1 shows a sagit-

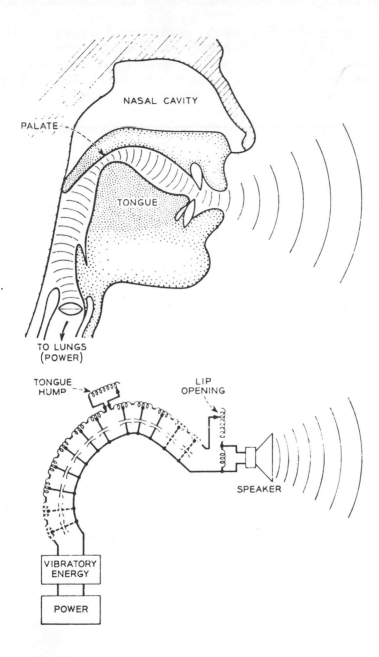

FIG. 1.—Sagittal section of the head showing vocal tract cavities and points of constriction. Lower part of the figure shows an electrical circuit analogue of the vocal tract.

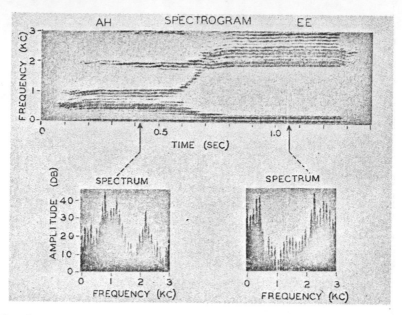

FIG. 2.—Sound spectrogram and spectra of the vowel sounds, "ah" and "ee," as spoken by a normal male talker.

tal section of the head and illustrates these cavities and constrictions. The lower part of Figure 1 shows an electrical circuit analogue of the vocal tract developed by H. K. Dunn, which has been found useful in studies of speech processes.[3]

As an illustration of the way in which the harmonic content of the speech wave is modified by a simple change in the vocal tract, consider the sound spectrogram of the sounds "ah" and "ee" shown in Figure 2. In going from "ah" to "ee," the only change in the vocal tract is the movement of the tongue hump from a back to a front position in the mouth. The patterns of Figure 2 present an analysis of the sounds by visible speech techniques developed at Bell Telephone Laboratories by Potter, Kopp, and Green.[4] In this spectrogram, time is portrayed on the horizontal scale from left to right, frequency on the vertical scale, and the intensity of a component of the sound at any time and frequency position is indicated by the darkness of the marking on the pattern at that time and frequency. This is a narrow band spectrogram, and the individual harmonics of the speech sound appear as closely spaced horizontal lines whose changing intensities determine the over-all pattern. Individual spectra may be portrayed at any particular time in the sound; for instance, spectra taken in the middle of the "ah" and "ee" sounds are also shown on Figure 2. In these spectra, frequency is indicated by the horizontal scale, and amplitude by the vertical scale. The individual spikes in the spectra are the fundamental and the harmonics of the sound, and the regions in which the cavity resonances of the vocal tract result in groups of harmonics being enhanced in amplitude are called formants. These formant positions along the frequency scale are distinguishing characteristics of the various voiced sounds, and one requirement of any artificial larynx which pro-

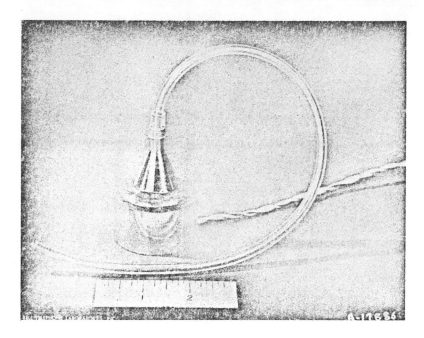

FIG. 3.—Special transducer for producing buzz tones, and a plastic tube for insertion of sound in pharynx or mouth.

duces natural sounding speech is that it be capable of producing formant patterns resembling those of normal speech sounds.

When the source of sound is introduced into the mouth cavity, as it is with the Western Electric Model 2 artificial larynx, the pharynx and nasal cavities do not have the same resonating effect to shape the spectrum of the output speech as they would if the sound were introduced at the glottis; consequently the formant patterns of some sounds cannot be made satisfactorily. This causes a loss of naturalness and intelligibility.

In order to study the effect of inserting the sound source at different points in the vocal tract, a standard ring armature receiver unit such as is used in telephone handsets, was equipped with a conical throat and a small flexible tube, as shown in Figure 3. With the tube as shown, the sound generated by the receiver could be inserted in the mouth. With the same tube, having the end inserted through the nasal cavity, down through the pharynx to a point just above the glottis, the sound could be inserted in a location to simulate the normal production of speech.

In order to simulate normal speech quality as closely as possible, considerable attention was given to getting a satisfactory sound source spectrum. For this purpose, a spectrum was desired which had the harmonic amplitudes approximately inversely proportional to the 1.5 power of the harmonic number. Although the spectrum of the volume velocity for normal vocal cords varies somewhat with the intensity of the cord tone produced, and also varies to some extent from one individual to another, the 1.5 power law is representative of an average condition. The acoustic properties of transducers and the tubes used to convey the sound to the mouth or to the throat ordinarily cause pronounced

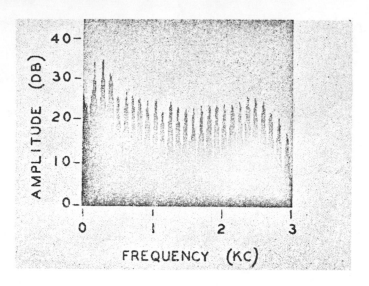

FIG. 4.—Sound spectrum of output of special transducer.

peaks or valleys in the spectrum of the sound source, unless careful attention is given to these factors in the design. A representative spectrum of the sound source with plastic tube is shown in Figure 4. This departs somewhat from the 1.5 power law, but is of the right general slope, and is free enough from pronounced peaks or valleys to be quite satisfactory.

With the sound source inserted near the vocal cords, brief listening tests showed that speech had a more natural quality than when the source was inserted in the mouth. This result confirmed the thesis that the most natural sounding speech would be that in which all of the vocal tract would be effective in shaping the output spectrum. Examples of sound spectra for a vowel sound spoken normally by a male speaker, then with the sound source in the pharynx and finally with the source in the mouth of the same male talker, are shown in Figure 5. This shows the spectra of the "oo" sound as in "book" for the three conditions. Inspection of these patterns shows that for the normal and artificial speech with the source in the throat, the four principal formants have nearly identical frequency positions. Their relative amplitudes, while different, are not so far out of line as to appreciably change the phonetic value of the sound. With the source in the mouth, however, the second formant is considerably more prominent than any of the others, the third formant is at a higher frequency than in the other two conditions, and the fourth formant is completely missing. The presence of the tube in the mouth, preventing the tongue from assuming the appropriate position to form the vowel, plus the difference in effect of the vocal tract cavities in shaping the resonances which control the formant frequency positions and amplitudes, combine to give the result shown in Figure 5.

The effect of introducing the sound source in the mouth rather than at the glottis was also studied with the aid of the electrical analogue vocal tract which was shown on the

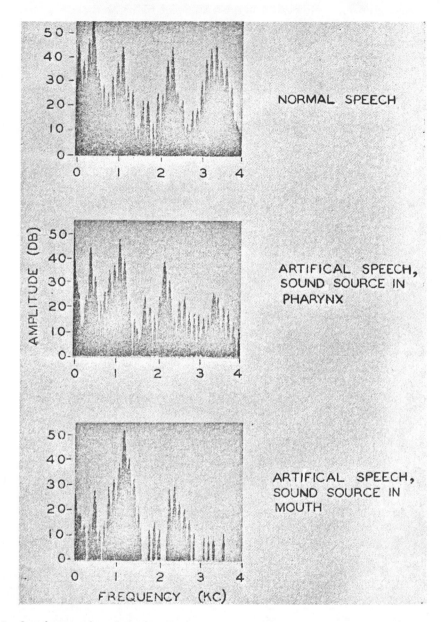

FIG. 5.—Sound spectra of vowel sound "oo" (as in "book") as spoken by a normal talker, and as produced artificially with the sound source in the pharynx, and in the mouth.

lower part of Figure 1. In this circuit, the buzz tone was inserted in the line between the inductance simulating the tongue hump, and the output. This corresponded to insertion of the acoustic signal in the mouth, and the results were similar in that the vowel quality was appreciably inferior as judged by listening tests and by spectrographic analyses.

Since it appears that the preferred position for the sound source is in the pharynx, it is appropriate to consider the advantages and disadvantages of introducing the sound from the outside of the throat by means of a buzzer-like transducer. This has the advantage that has just been discussed, of using the entire vocal tract to modulate the source sound. However, it poses two obstacles to the attainment of satisfactory artificial speech. One of these is the large amount of power output required of the buzzer in order to get an acoustic signal through the flesh and cartilage into the pharynx. This is particularly true if a natural sounding speech output is desired, which requires a source spectrum having strong low frequency components. It is not too difficult to transmit acoustic energy into the flesh from a small transducer, if one is concerned only with components lying in the upper part of the audible frequency range. Such a source, having principally the higher frequencies in its output, would give a buzzy kind of quality rather than a normal sounding one. The acoustic problems attendant to radiating into the flesh, a broad band of frequencies extending from about 100 to several thousand cycles with a small transducer having a high efficiency, are too involved to be considered here, but they are formidable.

A second difficulty with an external transducer is the direct radiation of sound into the air, which, of course, is unmodulated by the vocal tract, and therefore appears as a steady buzz accompanying the speech.

Inflection of the voiced sounds was mentioned previously as a factor in the naturalness of artificial speech. The degree of inflection need not be great, to obtain a considerable improvement in naturalness, as compared with monotone speech. Normal conversational speech contains inflections which correspond to a range of about an octave in the fundamental pitch frequency. A half octave range is quite sufficient for very acceptable inflections of speech. The inflection can be easily provided by a small rheostat in the appropriate part of an electronic driver circuit which actuates the transducer. For optimum effect, it should be operable in conjunction with the off-on button which starts the circuit buzzing. An arrangement of this sort for an electrical artificial larynx was developed by R. R. Riesz of Bell Telephone Laboratories at the time the original development work was being done on the Western Electric Model 2 artificial larynx.

PRODUCTION OF CONSONANT SOUNDS WITH ARTIFICIAL LARYNGES

Most of what has been discussed so far has dealt with the production of vowel sounds. The unvoiced sounds which are produced normally by turbulent air flow at some point in the vocal tract, can still be produced to some degree by the laryngectomized patient, even though there is no connection between the breath stream and the vocal tract. This is particularly so for plosive consonant sounds like "p," "t," and "k," which require only a small amount of air under pressure in the mouth to be released suddenly. Some of the fricative consonant sounds like "s," "f," and "th" (as in "thin") can be produced for short durations by forcing some of the air out of the mouth by tongue, jaw or cheek movements.

The Western Electric artificial larynx is well adapted to the production of these unvoiced sounds, particularly when they follow vowels in a word, since it provides a flow of air into the mouth cavity. Other types of artificial larynges, operated from electrical circuits, would not have this advantage and would have to depend on the method of forcing out impounded air from the mouth cavity, as described above.

The intelligibility of consonant sounds is an important aspect of an artificial larynx, and various expedients have been considered for improving it. One idea that might be effective would be to provide two sources of sound energy, one the buzz for vowel sounds, and the other a hiss for sibilant or fricative consonants. If these were applied to the transducer alternatively under control of the talker, by a simple switch arrangement, improved naturalness and articulation might be obtained.

INTELLIGIBILITY OF ARTIFICIAL LARYNX SPEECH

In a study of artificial larynx and esophageal speech made at Ohio State University, Melvin Hyman[5] measured the word articulation of a group of users of the Western Electric Model 2 artificial larynx, and found the average score to be about 48 per cent. In this study a multiple-choice intelligibility test list of phonetically balanced words was used. Corresponding scores on normal speech would be in the order of 98 per cent. Although the figure of 48 per cent may appear to be quite low, it is a characteristic of speech intelligibility that with a word articulation score of this value, discrete sentence intelligibility will be in the order of 96 per cent. Hyman also found that the articulation scores with his group of esophageal speakers were not significantly different from the scores obtained with the Western Electric larynx, and that the quality of speech obtained with the artificial larynx was definitely preferred to that of esophageal speech by a large group of observers.

Some preliminary tests of word articulation with various types of artificial speech have been made at Bell Telephone Laboratories recently, in which it has been found that somewhat higher scores are made by expert users of the Western Electric device, and also by well-trained esophageal speakers. A very skilled user of the Western Electric larynx may have articulation scores as high as 70 per cent on multiple-choice phonetically balanced word lists. This would correspond to a discrete sentence intelligibility of about 99 per cent. It would seem that a desirable objective for a new artificial larynx design would be to obtain articulation scores of this order with a reasonably short period of training for the average user.

SUMMARY

To summarize, a number of aspects of the speech process have been considered, with the objective of shedding some light on the artificial larynx problem. It has been shown that the most suitable point to introduce the sound from a transducer is into the pharynx. Ideally, the best solution from an acoustic standpoint would be to use surgical means to place a small transducer so that its output could be applied to the pharyngeal cavity directly. If this is not advisable because of danger of possible infections or for other medical considerations, two possible alternatives are to conduct the sound into the mouth through a tube, as is done with the Western Electric Model 2 device, or by means of a vibrating driver applied to the outside of the throat. It is anticipated that both of these would fall somewhat short of the tentative design objectives enumerated at the beginning of this paper, in one or more respects. However, with proper acoustic and electronic circuit design, either should be capable of giving adequate intelligibility in the hands of the average user, and the addition of a conveniently operated pitch inflection control will provide a much more natural sounding speech.

REFERENCES

1. Riesz, R. R.: Description and Demonstration of an Artificial Larynx. J. Acoust. Soc. Am. 1:273–289, 1930.
2. Lueders, Oscar W.: Use of the Electrolarynx in Speech Rehabilitation. A.M.A. Arch. of Otolaryng. 63:133–134, 1956.
3. Dunn, H. K.: The Calculation of Vowel Resonances and an Electrical Vocal Tract. J. Acoust. Soc. Am. 22:740–750, 1950.
4. Potter, R. K., Kopp, G. A., and Green, H. C.: Visible Speech. D. Van Nostrand, New York, 1947.
5. Hyman, Melvin: An Experimental Study of Artificial Larynx and Esophageal Speech. J. Speech and Hearing Disorders 20:291–299, 1955.

AN EXPERIMENTAL TRANSISTORIZED ARTIFICIAL LARYNX

By H. L. Barney, F. E. Haworth and H. K. Dunn

(Manuscript received July 23, 1959)

A new experimental artificial larynx, which makes use of transistors and miniaturized components to provide a voice for those who have lost the use of their vocal cords by surgical removal or paralysis, is described. The larynx operates by introducing a substitute for the sound of the vocal cords into the pharyngeal cavity by means of a vibrating driver held against the throat. The acoustic principles of normal and artificial speech production that were followed in arriving at the new design are presented, along with descriptions of the transistor circuit and its operating characteristics.

I. INTRODUCTION

It is sometimes necessary, for the health of an individual, to remove his entire larynx by surgery. His trachea is then terminated at an opening (stoma) in the throat, and no connection between the lungs and the vocal tract remains. Since the normal source of energy for the speech process is provided by the lungs, such an individual loses his natural means of speaking.

These persons are usually advised by their surgeons and speech therapists to learn esophageal speech, and classes for this purpose are set up in various centers. In producing esophageal speech, the upper end of the esophagus serves as the substitute larynx and provides the necessary complex tone at an appropriate point in the vocal tract—the bottom of the pharynx. The esophageal speaker must learn to swallow air, or force air into the esophagus and then control its escape, in such a manner as to cause sustained vibrations of tissues at the upper end of the esophagus. Not all patients can do this successfully. In fact, surveys have shown that about a third of all laryngectomized patients are unable to master esophageal speech for one reason or another.[1] In addition, the quality of speech produced by this method is generally rather unpleasant—to such a degree that, in a comprehensive comparison test, listeners were unanimous in their preference for speech produced by a reed-type artificial larynx rather than esophageal speech.[2]

The use of an artificial larynx is therefore frequently desirable, and is often a necessity if the laryngectomized patient is to communicate by speaking. At the present time, there are several different artificial larynges available, including the Western Electric reed-type which has been distributed by the Bell System since 1930. However, both doctors and users are generally agreed that there are various deficiencies in the performances of all the available models, and that none are really efficient in their function. In the past few years, suggestions for the improvement of the Western Electric reed-type larynx have been received with increasing frequency, along with suggestions that a totally different design making use of transistors could provide improved performance. Accordingly, it was decided to investigate the problem further to see how modern components and techniques might be used to make an improved artificial larynx.

The experimental artificial larynx to be described here is a result of these studies. Its characteristics are such that it provides an efficient means of communication for laryngectomized patients, while being more convenient and less conspicuous in use than the Western Electric Model 2 or other available larynges. It includes, in one small hand-held unit, a modified telephone receiver used as a vibrating driver that is held against the throat, a transistorized pulse-generating circuit and a battery power supply. When the pulse generator is switched on, vibrations are transmitted through the throat wall into the pharynx cavity and transformed into speech by the normal use of the articulatory mechanisms of the vocal tract. The loudness of the speech obtained with this unit is comparable with that of a normal person speaking conversationally. The artificial speech so produced sounds somewhat mechanical, but it is quite intelligible. By the use of an easily operated inflection control, a degree of naturalness heretofore unobtainable in artificial larynges may be achieved.

II. HISTORY OF BELL SYSTEM ARTIFICIAL LARYNX WORK

There is substantial evidence that artificial larynges were used as early as 1874, but it was not until 1925 that the Bell System became concerned with this area of communications. F. B. Jewett, who was president of Bell Telephone Laboratories at that time, suggested the development of an artificial larynx. His suggestion was prompted by discussions with a friend who had been laryngectomized and had impressed him with the need for a device that was more satisfactory than any then obtainable.

The Laboratories' initial efforts resulted in an instrument that employed rubber bands stretched in a manner to simulate the vocal cords, and was designated type 1A. These rubber bands deteriorated rapidly and were a source of considerable dissatisfaction. Consequently, during 1929 a new larynx, designated type 2A, was developed that incorporated several refinements,[3] including the substitution of a vibrating metallic reed for the elastic bands. It is this model, with a few minor changes, that is currently being manufactured by the Western Electric Company and distributed by the Bell System operating companies. The method of operation of the 2A artificial larynx is illustrated by the sagittal section view of the head in Fig. 1. The metallic reed is connected by tubing to the stoma in the throat, so that the user's breath can actuate the reed. The sound of the vibrating reed is conducted through another tube into the mouth, and this sound is used in the production of artificial speech sounds with normal tongue, lip and jaw movements.

In all, about 200 of the Model 1A larynges were made between 1926 and 1930, and about 5500 of the Model 2A larynges have been made to date. Since about 1950, the de-

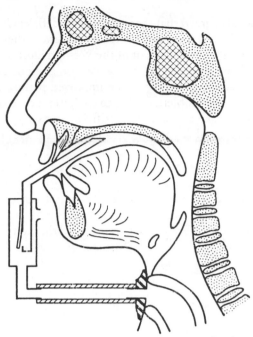

FIG. 1—Sagittal section showing method of operation of reed-type larynx.

mand has remained constant at approximately 300 per year, although the number of laryngectomies performed annually has increased steadily. This leveling-off has occurred partly because there has been a marked increase during the last ten years in the use of esophageal speech, with the establishment of many speech clinics for the purpose of training laryngectomized patients in this method of speaking.

However, as noted previously, about a third of the total number of laryngectomized patients are unable to use esophageal speech, and consequently the need for an improved artificial larynx has become more urgent. In response to this need an advisory committee on artificial larynges was set up in 1956 by the National Hospital for Speech Disorders in New York, and its recommendations have provided helpful stimulation and guidance in the development of the new experimental model.

III. DESIGN OBJECTIVES FOR AN IMPROVED ARTIFICIAL LARYNX

In determining objectives toward which artificial larynx experimentation should be directed, preliminary discussions were held with the committee mentioned above, whose members include several surgeons, speech therapists and postlaryngectomized patients. To supplement the information obtained from them, all of the artificial larynges that were commercially available were studied and analyzed to ascertain their individual advantages and deficiencies.

The primary requirements, of course, were that the artificial speech be loud enough and natural enough so that the speaker could be easily understood. For the speech to sound natural, it should have pitch inflection, and, like the natural voice, should have a suitable fundamental pitch accompanied by harmonics that can be used to produce the various vowel sounds. These objectives were discussed in some detail in a recent paper.[4]

Secondary to the above, but still of great importance to the user, were the objectives that the device be inconspicuous and hygienic. It is in these respects that most of the presently available devices are deficient. If the user has to insert a tube into his mouth, it not only calls attention to his disability, but is also hygienically undesirable. Any connection at the opening in the throat, such as that required for the Western Electric Model 2, leaves much to be desired from the hygienic standpoint. In electrical devices, dangling wires leading to battery cases are also embarrassing and are liable to become entangled with other objects. The importance of making prosthetic devices inconspicuous may be inferred from the great efforts that hearing aid manufacturers have expended to make their product less noticeable in use.

Other desirable characteristics were simplicity of operation, reliability and low cost. Simplicity of operation is very desirable so that the patient will require only a minimum of training and, as soon as possible, gain the psychological benefits of vocal communication with his family and friends. Reliability and low cost can probably be attained most easily by the use of components that are already available commercially.

The design objectives, therefore, can be listed as follows:

1. having output speech volume equal to that of a normal speaker,
2. having output speech quality and pitch inflection like that of normal speech,
3. inconspicuous,
4. hygienically acceptable to the user,
5. simple to operate,
6. reliable,
7. inexpensive.

IV. ACOUSTIC FACTORS IN PRODUCTION OF ARTIFICIAL SPEECH

4.1 Types of Sound Source Needed

In the production of normal speech, two types of sound energy are involved. One is a periodic tone produced by the vocal cords. It is variable in frequency and rich in harmonics, and is introduced into the pharyngeal cavity of the vocal tract. Except in whispered speech, this tone is always used in vowels and semivowels, including the nasal consonants, and is present in some other "voiced" consonants.

This normal vocal cord tone is completely lost when the larynx is removed. The esophageal speaker has learned to substitute the vibration of membranes at the mouth of the esophagus. But, if this sound cannot be produced and controlled adequately, another tone source must be supplied, and this is the chief function of the artificial larynx. For intelligibility of the speech produced, it is essential that the tone contain a wide range of harmonics, and, for naturalness, the harmonic amplitudes should fall off toward higher frequencies at the same rate that the real vocal cord tone does. Also, the tone should match that of the normal larynx in fundamental frequency and in frequency variability.

The second type of sound energy in speech is random noise, which is produced when the breath stream passes through a constriction formed by tongue or lips. It is present in stop and sibilant consonants, sometimes alone and sometimes in combination with the vocal-cord tone. These sounds are vital for the intelligibility of speech.

The normal means of generating random noise by the breath stream is also lost in the usual laryngectomy. However, it is not necessary to supply a substitute in an artificial larynx. Air trapped in throat and mouth can be forced out in such a way as to take the place of the normal breath stream in forming most of these sounds. Some deficiencies occur, such as a shortening of continuants like "s" and "sh," due to an insufficient volume of the trapped air; and the sound "h" is usually completely lost. The Western Electric reed-type artificial larynx improves the ability to make some of these sounds, by allowing some breath stream to pass through the reed chamber into the mouth.

4.2 Point of Application of Substitute Tone

To match as nearly as possible the natural speech process, the artificial tone should be applied in the pharyngeal cavity. This requirement is not met in the Western Electric reed-type artificial larynx, yet understandable speech is produced. It is of interest to see just what changes in the quality of speech sounds result from a change of source application from pharynx to mouth.

It may be shown theoretically that a change from throat to mouth application, keeping the vocal tract configuration constant for a given vowel, does not change the resonant frequencies characteristic of that vowel. It does, however, change the relative amplitudes of the different resonances. The extent of the change depends upon the degree of constriction imposed by the tongue, which is different for different vowels. Another manifestation of the change is the appearance of antiresonances, which are not present when the source is in the throat.

To confirm these conclusions, two experiments were performed. In the first, an artificial tone was introduced into the pharynx of a human subject. A tube was attached to a transducer that produced the tone, and passed through the nose of the subject and into his pharynx until the opening of the tube was not far from his vocal cords.

Fig. 2 shows spectra taken as the subject made the vowel sound of "book." The first was made with his own vocal cords. The same vowel made with the artificial source yields the second spectrum. Although some pains were taken to make the spectrum at the output of the tube approach that of the real cord tone, some differences can be seen. The third spectrum was produced with the artificial source withdrawn from the pharynx and placed in the mouth of the subject. Particularly to be noticed are the change in relative amplitudes of the first two resonances and the "holes" in the mouth spectrum due to the antiresonances.

The second experiment made use of the Electrical Vocal Tract,[5, 6] an analog of the vocal tract in which cavities are represented by lengths of transmission line and constrictions by inductances placed in series with the line (the tongue), or at its termination (the lips). An electrical complex tone can be applied easily to either throat or mouth cavity. Settings of such a device can be held constant more easily than a human subject can maintain a particular vocal tract configuration. On listening to the output of the artificial

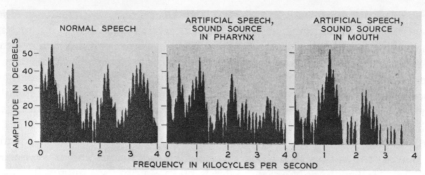

FIG. 2—Sound spectra of vowel sound "oo" (as in "book") spoken normally and as produced artificially with sound source in pharynx, and in mouth.

tract, it was found that vowel sounds changed considerably in character when the source was moved to the mouth. However, some but not all of their original naturalness could be restored by manipulation of the settings. It seems likely that the reed-type larynx user makes these readjustments naturally under the guidance of his own hearing, and that this accounts for the fact that his speech is still very intelligible.

Fig. 3 shows transmission measurements made with a sine-wave input on the Electrical Vocal Tract, in the three settings determined by previous listening tests: (1) the vowel

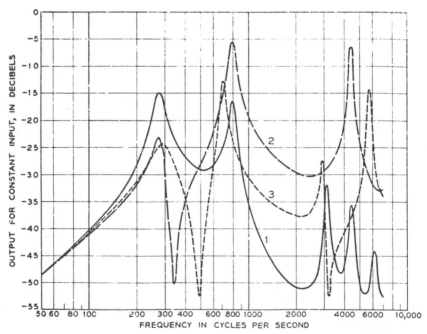

FIG. 3—Transmission vs. frequency characteristic of electrical vocal tract: (1) adjusted for vowel "oo" (as in "fool") with source in throat position; (2) same settings, but with source in mouth position; (3) with source in mouth, but with controls readjusted to restore the "oo" sound as nearly as possible.

"oo" (as in "fool") with a source in throat, (2) the same settings with source in mouth and (3) with controls readjusted to restore "oo" as nearly as possible.

Although it would seem that excitation in the mouth is not as disadvantageous as it at first appears, pharynx excitation is still preferable. It is, of course, not practicable to introduce the sound through the nasal cavities as was done for the subject in the experiment described. In fact, insertion of any outside bodies into throat and mouth tends to be unhygienic. However, sound can be introduced into the throat from outside by transmission through the throat wall. This principle was used in an artificial larynx designed by Wright.[7] In the present development, it has been found possible to produce an adequate spectrum in the pharynx by this method, while at the same time limiting to a reasonable level the sound radiated directly from the device.

4.3 The Use of a Throat Vibrator to Provide Substitute Vocal-Cord Tone

The experiments just described indicate that the preferred position for the sound source is in the pharynx. Some thought was given to the use of a transducer surgically embedded in the throat. However, this would require a second operation for those who already had been laryngectomized, and the opinions of doctors consulted on the subject were divided as to its advisability. Accordingly, it was considered to be outside the scope of the present artificial larynx project. The problem then became one of transmitting through the flesh and cartilage around the pharynx a complex signal with a broad frequency spectrum. In order to obtain natural-sounding speech, the source spectrum must have strong low-frequency components. The total frequency range required extends from about 100 to several thousand cycles per second.

Experiments were conducted using a variety of vibrating devices held against the outside of the throat. Some of these were constructed especially for these tests and the rest were devices obtainable commercially. Of all these, the HA-1 telephone receiver used in the type 300 telephone sets proved the most promising.[8] However, when pressed against the throat, the loading on the diaphragm was far different from what it is when working into air, since the characteristic mechanical impedance of flesh is some 4000 times that of air. This heavy loading made desirable a number of modifications in the receiver to enable it to give a greater amplitude of vibration into the throat. These modifications are described in Section 5.4.

V.   CIRCUIT AND MECHANICAL CONSTRUCTION

The circuit of the new experimental artificial larynx uses a highly efficient arrangement of transistors powered by mercury batteries to provide a compact, self-contained unit. In its design, an objective was to use commonly available, inexpensive components wherever possible. Fig. 4 illustrates the cylindrical configuration of the unit, with the combined on-off switch and pitch-inflection control knob arranged for operation by thumb or forefinger.

5.1   Transistor Circuit

A schematic diagram of the circuit is shown in Fig. 5. It is essentially a two-stage relaxation oscillator followed by a power stage that works into a transducer. The relaxation os-

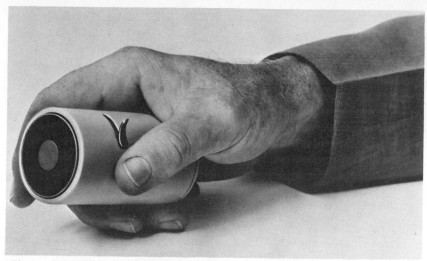

FIG. 4—Picture of artificial larynx showing thumb-operated on-off switch and inflection control.

cillator uses a p-n-p transistor, Q_1, and an n-p-n transistor, Q_2, coupled together with regenerative feedback. The frequency of oscillation is determined by the pitch-control resistance, R_1, in combination with capacitance C_1. The output of the relaxation oscillator appears across resistance R_5 as a series of short periodic pulses. The width of these pulses is determined by resistance R_2 and capacitance C_1. The values shown in Fig. 5 give a pulse width of 0.0005 second.

The periodic pulses generated in the relaxation oscillator are transmitted through the semiconductor diode, CR_1, to the base of power transistor Q_3. The HA-1 receiver is connected in the collector circuit of Q_3, and receives short periodic current pulses of about 0.45 ampere peak value at the oscillation frequency.

The range of oscillating frequency may be adjusted by changing the range of resistance R_1 available in the pitch-control rheostat, to simulate either a man's or a woman's

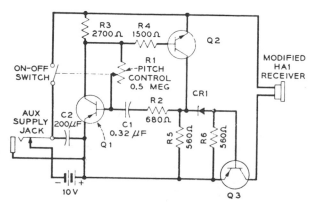

FIG. 5—Schematic of artificial larynx circuit.

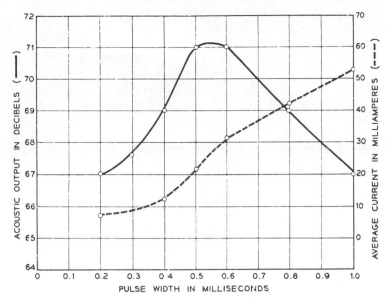

FIG. 6—Characteristics of acoustic output vs. pulse width, and average battery supply current vs. pulse width.

pitch range. For men, the range is from 100 to 200 cycles and, for women, it is from 200 to 400 cycles. This is an octave range in either case, and is sufficient to duplicate the pitch inflection used in normal speech. The on-off switch and pitch-control rheostat are arranged so that the switch is closed at the lowest oscillating frequency, and further movement of the control causes the frequency to increase. The control knob is spring-loaded so as to return it to the off position when released.

Two 5.2-volt mercury batteries in series provide the necessary power to operate the circuit. Although the peak is 0.45 ampere, the pulse duty factor is so small that the average current drain from the batteries is only about 22 milliamperes. The rating of the batteries is 250 milliampere hours.

As an alternative to the self-contained mercury batteries, a small rectifier operated from 115-volt, 60-cycle line voltage may be substituted. This arrangement may be useful at an office desk or other fixed location. When the rectifier power supply is plugged into the auxiliary power jack shown in Fig. 5, the batteries are disconnected from the circuit.

5.2 Selection of Pulse Duty Cycle

The average current drain on the batteries, the spectrum of the acoustic output of the artificial larynx and the loudness of the output, are all functions of the pulse width, assuming a fixed supply voltage. For widths of a few tenths of a millisecond, the average current drain would be low, and the spectrum would have a wide frequency band with strong harmonics running up to several thousand cycles per second, but the acoustic output would be weak. Fig. 6 shows the relation between acoustic output and pulse width, and also the relation between current drain and pulse width. The acoustic outputs displayed were obtained by measuring the output from a single subject saying "ah" at a distance of

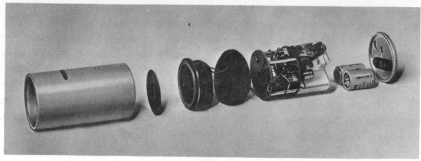

FIG. 7—Exploded view of artificial larynx, showing modular construction.

3 feet from the sound level meter. Pulse widths of 0.5 to 0.6 millisecond gave near-maximum output. For wider pulses, the acoustic output decreased, and the speech became somewhat muffled and nasal in quality. A pulse width of 0.5 millisecond was adopted. Correspondingly, the average current drain was 22 milliamperes at a frequency of 100 pulses per second. Sound spectrograms of speech using the 0.5-millisecond pulse width indicated a satisfactory spectrum.

5.3 Mechanical Construction

For simplicity of construction, a cylindrical container was chosen to house the artificial larynx. The dimensions of the experimental model are 1¾ inches in diameter and 3¼ inches long. The weight, including batteries, is 8 ounces. To package all the components in this volume, a modular type of construction was used, as shown in the exploded view in Fig. 7.

The HA-1 receiver is at the front end of the unit, with the diaphragm flush with the end of the cylinder. The back of the receiver is wrapped with sponge rubber, and two discs of sponge rubber and one of thin brass sheet are placed between it and the adjacent components to attenuate the backward radiation of sound. Were it not suppressed, this direct radiation back through the shell and into the surrounding air would tend to mask the speech sounds and contribute a buzzy, mechanical quality to the over-all effect.

The next two modules back of the receiver contain the pitch-control rheostat, the transistors and associated circuit elements. The last module contains the two mercury batteries in a plastic shell and the jack for the external power supply. The back plate may be removed by unscrewing a single machine screw which has a slot large enough so that a thin coin may be used in place of a screwdriver. This permits convenient access to the mercury batteries for changing them without disturbing the rest of the circuit.

While the experimental model is a compact unit, some further miniaturization could be achieved by the use of printed circuit techniques and closer component spacing.

5.4 HA-1 Receiver Modifications

The HA-1 receiver as normally used in a telephone set has a protective metal grid and cloth cover over the diaphragm. For use in the artificial larynx these are removed. And, in order to achieve greater efficiency in terms of output volume of artificial speech for a given battery supply power, several additional modifications were made.

The permanent magnets were magnetized to full strength, instead of being only partially magnetized. The diaphragm was correspondingly shimmed out from the pole pieces, so that it would not be pulled into contact with them. The spacing between diaphragm and pole pieces in this condition measures between 0.002 and 0.003 inch, and a slight push on the diaphragm is sufficient to make it adhere to the pole pieces. The electrical pulses from the transistor circuit are so poled as to oppose the permanent magnet field and release the diaphragm to spring outward. This driving polarity gives higher speech volumes than the opposite one.

In order to obtain sufficient current from the 10.4-volt supply to counteract the permanent magnetization, it was necessary to decrease the impedance of the receiver winding by connecting its two coils in parallel instead of in the usual series arrangement. In order to improve the match of mechanical impedances between the receiver and the throat, a diaphragm of 0.0083-inch permendur was used in place of the standard 0.011-inch thickness provided in the HA-1. A series of tests was made with a range of thicknesses from 0.0065 to 0.011 inch, and it was found that the highest speech volumes were obtained with a thickness in the order of 0.0083 inch.

In order to reduce the magnetic saturation of that area of the diaphragm between the pole pieces, a small center patch of permendur, 0.54 inch in diameter and 0.011 inch thick, was spot-welded to the diaphragm before heat treatment. This addition improves the magnetic circuit and does not materially affect the stiffness of the diaphragm.

The HA-1 receiver normally has a small resonance damper provided by a cloth-covered hole in the plastic back under the diaphragm. This damps the natural diaphragm resonance, which in air falls at about 3000 cycles. The cloth covering this hole is removed in the artificial larynx, and diaphragm damping is obtained by contact with the flesh of the throat. Removal of the cloth damping patch slightly increases the output of high-frequency harmonics in the artificial speech.

5.5   On-Off Switch and Inflection Control

The arrangement of the on-off switch and inflection control was designed for ease of manipulation. With practice on the present arrangement, either rising or falling inflection can be achieved at the beginning or ending of voicing.

Several other methods of control were tried. One made use of a rack and pinion gear arrangement, in which a button was pushed straight into the shell of the unit. Precise control of frequency was not easily obtained with that method. It was found more satisfactory to push the control sideways over a distance of a half-inch or more. Another early version depended for control on application of pressure along the longitudinal axis of the artificial larynx. This seemed satisfactory from the functional standpoint, but was more difficult to implement mechanically than the arrangement finally adopted.

VI.   ACOUSTIC PERFORMANCE

Tests of the acoustic performance of the new artificial larynx have been made to find how nearly it meets the original design objectives with respect to output volume and speech quality.

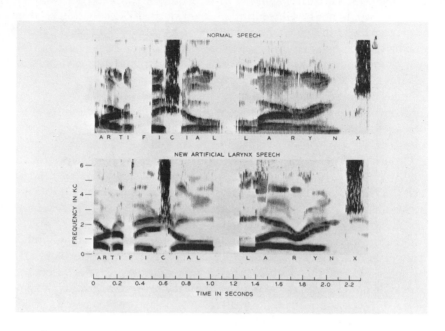

FIG. 8—Sound spectrograms of the words "artificial larynx" as spoken normally and with the new experimental artificial larynx.

6.1 Loudness

A little practice is required to find the proper pressure and placement on the throat that yield the best results. Output volume measurements on subjects who have acquired a moderate amount of proficiency show sound pressure levels on the vowel peaks of 70–75 db above 0.0002 microbars at a distance of three feet from the speaker's mouth. This is approximately a normal conversational level. However, in an environment so noisy as to require a speaker to raise his voice appreciably above the normal level, this volume would limit the separation between talker and listener to shorter distances than those possible for a normal speaker.

6.2 Frequency Spectra

Speech quality has been checked by comparisons of frequency spectra, and by measurement of the ratio of speech signal to directly radiated buzz. Spectrograms[9, 10] of the words "artificial larynx" and amplitude sections of ten vowel sounds were made from the speech of one subject, using both the new artificial larynx and his natural voice. These are reproduced in Figs. 8 and 9 respectively. In Fig. 8, it may be seen that the "f" and "sh" sounds in the word "artificial" are shorter in duration for the artificial larynx speech than for the normal speech. With the artificial larynx, the speaker must make such sounds by means of the air trapped in his mouth and pharynx since his normal air supply is cut off.

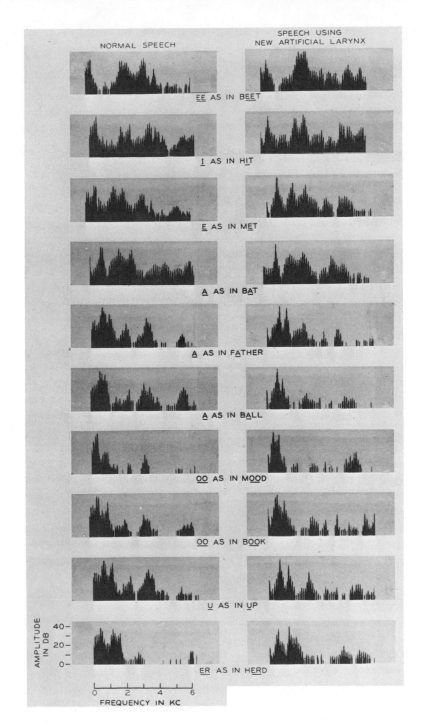

FIG. 9—Sound spectra of ten sustained vowel sounds as spoken normally and with the new experimental artificial larynx.

This small air supply thus tends to shorten fricatives and sibilants, but the spectrogram indicates that they can be made satisfactorily. Some practice was required to make the "sh" sound in "artificial" as long as that which is shown.

In using the artificial larynx it is more convenient to leave it turned on through several syllables or words than to turn it on and off as one does in natural voicing. That this does not make the speech as unnatural as one might expect is indicated also in Fig. 8. The instrument was turned off between the two words, but it can be seen that, for the "t," "f," "sh" and "x" sounds, very little of the voicing comes through, although the device was operating while those sounds were being produced. For the unvoiced fricatives and stop consonants, the sound transmission path from the pharynx is evidently nearly closed off.

In the comparison of the vowel spectra shown in Fig. 9, it is apparent that the new artificial larynx is able to transmit sufficient power into the pharynx throughout the spectrum to permit satisfactory development of the high-amplitude regions (formants) of the vowel sounds. It has been indicated[4] that the harmonics in the source spectrum of the natural voice are strongest at the low frequencies, dropping in amplitude toward the high frequencies at about the inverse 1.5 power of the harmonic number. A cross comparison in Fig. 9 shows that, for some vowels, the difference in the high- and low-frequency amplitudes is greater for the natural source, and, for others, it is greater for the artificial source. This observation leads to the conclusion that, on the average, the artificial source has approximately the right spectrum.

6.3 Externally Radiated Interference

Some of the sound produced by the vibrating diaphragm does not pass through the speaker's throat but is radiated directly by the instrument itself or from areas of the throat around the place where the unit is pressed. This external radiation, of course, would interfere with the intelligibility of the speech if it were not well suppressed. Measurements taken in an anechoic chamber with the unit pressed against the throat but with the mouth closed showed an intensity level for this interference 20–25 db below the level when the vowel "ah" was being voiced. When the unit is operated with the vibrating end working into a sound-absorbing cavity, the level is about 6 db lower still, indicating that most of the interfering sound is from the throat areas immediately adjacent to the artificial larynx rather than from the instrument itself. If it should be desirable to reduce this noise still further, the end held against the throat might be specially shaped to reduce the external vibration of the throat tissues.

6.4 Reactions of Laryngectomized Users

In collaboration with the Advisory Committee on Artificial Larynges of the National Hospital for Speech Disorders, a limited field test was conducted with several laryngectomized patients to obtain their reactions. Four units of the new design were used in the field test; two were assigned to two laryngectomized patients for the entire period of four weeks, and the other two units were used for shorter periods by several other patients. In all cases, favorable comments were made on the speech quality and the lack of externally radiated buzz. Comments of friends and relatives of the patients using the new model

Table I—Percentages of PB words heard correctly, from natural and substitute-larynx speech

Natural voices	97.3
	96.6
Esophageal speech	79.0
	64.1
Reed-type artificial larynx	63.4
	40.3
Throat-type artificial larynx	58.1
	40.3

generally indicated that they liked the intelligibility and speech quality of the artificial speech produced by it.

One comment was made to the effect that, for optimum comfort in use, the diameter of the unit should be somewhat less. Adoption of this suggestion would preclude the use of the HA-1 receiver. The Advisory Committee on Artificial Larynges of the National Hospital for Speech Disorders felt that, for nearly all patients, the present diameter of 1 ¾ inches would be satisfactory, and did not recommend such a change.

Battery life was indicated to be satisfactory in these tests. The new units were used alternately with other models by the two patients who had them for the entire test period, and it is not known just what their cumulated operating times were. One of the two patients estimated that he had used the new unit for about half of his talking. None of the four units in the limited field test required a change of batteries during the four-week period.

VII. ARTICULATION TESTS

Articulation tests using speech produced by practiced talkers with previously available artificial larynges have been carried out. These tests were intended as a guide in the development of the new instrument. A second set of tests was made after the new experimental model was available, comparing it with previous types.

7.1 Tests with Previous Types

For the first test, it was possible to obtain two experienced users of esophageal speech, of the reed-type artificial larynx, and of an available type using throat application. These individuals were asked to read five of the Harvard PB (phonetically balanced) lists of 50 monosyllabic words.[11] Their utterances were recorded on tape and presented later, in a suitably mixed order, to a crew of seven listeners who recorded their responses. Two speakers with normal voices were included for comparison. The percentages of words heard correctly are given in Table I.

To understand the significance of these scores, it has been found that a 60 per cent articulation from such isolated words corresponds to a sentence intelligibility of more than 95 per cent, and that even 40 percent in the word score means that more than 90 per cent of sentences would be understood.

In a test supplementary to the above, it was found that the articulation score with the throat type tested could be improved to about 70 per cent if the directly radiated sound were reduced about 20 db.

The number of individuals in the tests was too small to indicate an over-all ranking for the different types. It can be concluded, however, that either the reed type (with mouth application) or the external throat type could be sufficiently intelligible to give good conversational ability. The choice between these types could therefore be made by other criteria.

7.2 Comparison of New with Best of Older Types

The second set of tests was abbreviated, and was intended to provide a comparison between the new larynx and the previous types. Thus, only the higher-scoring individuals using the reed and throat types in the previous tests, with two PB lists (100 words) each, were incorporated. These utterances were compared with 100 words from the new experimental model. Because of changed conditions (principally the use of a crew of listeners who were less familiar with laryngectomized speech) the results shown in Table II are not directly comparable with the previous tests. They are comparable with each other, however.

With regard to population averages, these figures cannot be considered indicative. The differences, however, are favorable for the new model.

VIII. CONCLUSIONS

An artificial larynx has been developed that is hygienic, convenient and inconspicuous. It has a fundamental tone that is similar in pitch range and variability to the real voice, and near enough in spectrum to produce natural-sounding speech. The loudness of the speech produced with it is comparable to that used in normal conversation, and the speech is generally free of masking effects of directly radiated noise. The essential characteristics and performance of this experimental model will be incorporated into a commercial design to be manufactured by the Western Electric Company. Distribution of the new model, beginning some months hence, will be through the Bell System operating companies, following procedures similar to those used with the Model 2 reed-type larynx for the past 30 years.

IX. ACKNOWLEDGMENTS

We wish to thank Dr. L. H. Whitney, medical director of the American Telephone & Telegraph Company, and L. C. Withers of the Western Electric Company for their continued interest and encouragement, and Dr. Hayes Martin of New York and Dr. Lynwood Heaver, medical director of the National Hospital for Speech Disorders, for assisting us in finding expert laryngectomized talkers. Some ten of the latter were very cooperative and generous of their time in recording our test sentences and lists of words with esophageal speech and various models of artificial larynges. Our thanks are also due to D. J. MacLean for his valuable aid in many technical phases of the work, to Miss E. A.

Table II—Articulation scores from new experimental artificial larynx and from the more successful users of older types

Older throat type	43 per cent
Reed type	52 per cent
New experimental model	59 per cent

Klarmann for assistance in preparation and scoring of the articulation test and to J. H. Kronmeyer for aid in mechanical design and construction of the new model.

REFERENCES

1. Heaver, L., White, W. and Goldstein, N., Clinical Experience in Restoring Oral Communication to 274 Laryngectomized Patients by Esophageal Voice, J. Am. Geriatrics Soc., 3, September 1955, p. 678.
2. Hyman, M., An Experimental Study of Artificial-Larynx and Esophageal Speech, J. Speech and Hearing Disorders, 20, September 1955, p. 291.
3. Riesz, R. R., Description and Demonstration of an Artificial Larynx, J. Acoust. Soc. Amer., 1, January, 1930, p. 273.
4. Barney, H. L., A Discussion of Some Technical Aspects of Speech Aids for Postlaryngectomized Patients, Ann. Otology, Rhinology and Laryngology, 67, June 1958, p. 558.
5. Dunn, H. K., The Calculation of Vowel Resonances and an Electrical Vocal Tract, J. Acoust. Soc. Amer., 22, November 1950, p. 740.
6. Schott, L. O., An Electrical Vocal System, Bell Lab. Record, 28, December 1950, p. 549.
7. Wright, G. M., U.S. Patent No. 2,273,077, February 17, 1942.
8. Jones, W. C., Instruments for the New Telephone Sets, B.S.T.J., 17, July 1938, p. 338.
9. Koenig, W., Dunn, H. K. and Lacy, L. Y., The Sound Spectrograph, J. Acoust. Soc. Amer., 18, July 1946, p. 19.
10. Kersta, L. G., Amplitude Cross-Section Representation with the Sound Spectrograph, J. Acoust. Soc. Amer., 20, November 1948, p. 796.
11. Egan, J. P., Articulation Testing Methods, Laryngoscope, 58, September 1948, p. 955.

SPEECH PRODUCED WITH THE TOKYO ARTIFICIAL LARYNX

Bernd Weinberg

Speech Research Laboratory, Indiana University Medical Center,
Indianapolis, Indiana

Ann Riekena

Veterans Administration Hospital, Indianapolis, Indiana

This report provides basic information about a relatively unknown pneumatic artificial larynx called the Tokyo artificial larynx. Part of the report describes a clinical study of a highly skilled American user of the Tokyo larynx. Descriptive information is provided about important acoustic and perceptual characteristics of speech produced with this Japanese-made device.

A paramount objective of postlaryngectomy rehabilitation is the restoration of speech. One essential feature of a comprehensive alaryngeal speech program is the early presentation of information about the various methods of speech available to laryngectomized patients. This discussion must include the exchange of information about esophageal speech and artificial speaking devices. A variety of artificial larynges are now available, and the more widely used instruments have been described in the literature (Snidecor, 1969; Diedrich and Youngstrom, 1966; Shanks, 1971). This report provides basic information about a relatively unknown pneumatic artificial larynx now available to speech specialists and laryngectomized patients. The instrument, called the Tokyo artificial larynx, was developed in Japan and is not widely used in the United States. This report also describes a clinical study of a highly skilled American user of the Tokyo larynx. Important acoustic and perceptual characteristics of the speech he produced with this device were measured and are presented here.

THE TOKYO ARTIFICIAL LARYNX

The Tokyo artificial larynx is an inexpensive ($15), mechanically simple pneumatic artificial larynx. Like other pneumatic artificial larynges, this instrument (Figure 1) consists of a stoma cover (A), a vibratory mechanism (B),

Reprinted by permission from *Journal of Speech and Hearing Disorders*, 1973, 38, 383–389.

and a sound-conduction tube (C). A patient uses the Tokyo larynx by placing the cover against his stoma, directing pulmonary air through a vibrator to produce voice, and transmitting the psuedoglottal sound to the vocal tract through a sound-conduction tube placed in his mouth.

The vibratory mechanism consists of a strip of rubber placed over a stainless steel base and fastened to the base with a rubber band. The stoma cover and the base of the vibratory mechanism are made of stainless steel, while the sound-conduction tube is plastic. These materials permit easy cleaning and sterilization. Moreover, repair, adjustment, and cleaning are easy because the components can be taken apart by hand (Figure 1).

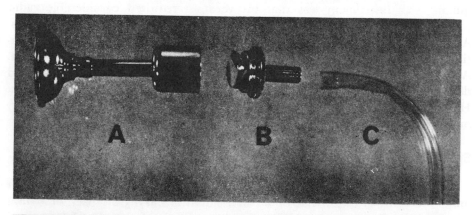

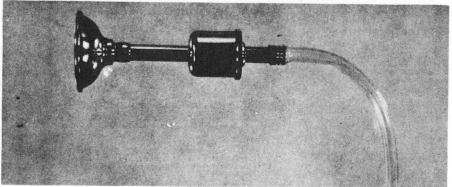

Figure 1. The Tokyo artificial larynx. The components of this instrument are a stomal cover (A), a vibratory mechanism (B), and a sound-conduction tube (C).

CLINICAL STUDY

Recently we had the opportunity to meet and study a laryngectomized patient who taught himself to speak with the Tokyo artificial larynx. We were impressed with his speaking proficiency. In our opinion, his Tokyo artificial speech was far superior to speech produced with other more widely used artificial larynges. In an attempt to provide information about this relatively unknown form of alaryngeal speech, we measured selected acoustic and perceptual attributes of the speech of this patient.

The Subject

The subject (ASG) is a 64-year-old laryngectomee who taught himself to speak with the Tokyo artificial larynx. He was laryngectomized in June 1967 and used esophageal speech as a primary method of communication before acquiring this instrument. ASG was a ship's navigator who purchased his first instrument in Japan around December 1967. His chief motivation for acquiring this instrument was that his vocation required considerable radio communication in shipboard environments with high ambient noise levels. Although his esophageal speech was serviceable under relatively quiet conditions, he could not fulfill his job responsibilities using esophageal speech. Accordingly, he taught himself to speak with the Tokyo artificial larynx and developed socially and vocationally serviceable speech in about three months. He has used both esophageal and Tokyo artificial larynx speech as primary methods of communication since 1968.

Speech Materials and Procedures

The materials used in this clinical study were collected during the eleventh annual meeting of the International Association of Laryngectomees, in Kansas City in 1971. By this time, ASG had been using the Tokyo larynx for three and a half years and, in our opinion, was a highly proficient alaryngeal speaker.

A high-quality recording of ASG reading a standard passage (Fairbanks, 1960) was used to measure fundamental frequency (f_0), rate, and phonation time characteristics. This recording was duplicated and the second sentence was extracted for analysis. The recording was played at half-speed by a high-quality tape recorder to one channel of a Honeywell Visicorder Model 1508. For calibration purposes, a counter-monitored 1000-Hz signal was simultaneously played into the second channel of the Visicorder. Visicorder chart speed of 1000 mm/sec and mirror galvanometers M-5000 were used. The Visicorder record of the sentence material was segmented into categories of periodicity, aperiodicity, and silence. The individual periods of each periodic wave form and the segment lengths of aperiodicity and silence were measured. Fundamental frequency mean, standard deviation, range, duration, and phonation time characteristics were obtained from these measurements.

To evaluate the intelligibility of Tokyo artificial larynx speech, ASG recorded the six 50-item word lists of the consonant rhyme-test described by House et al. (1965) and the six 24-item vowel rhyme-test word lists described by Horii (1969). The recorded words were played into a Bruel and Kjaer graphic-level recorder (Model 2305) and the level of the vocalic maxima of each word was measured relative to a 1000-Hz reference signal. The range in average level of the six consonant test lists was 1.8 dB, while the range in average level among the six vowel lists was 1.6 dB. Consequently, the recordings were not adjusted for level variations. The word lists were presented to 16 listeners under earphones through high-quality listening equipment. The average level of speech was 75 dB SPL measured under the headphones.

RESULTS AND DISCUSSION

Acoustic Characteristics

The average fundamental frequency of speech with the Tokyo artificial larynx was 71 Hz, f_0 standard deviation was 2.1 semitones, and f_0 full range was 10.3 semitones. The 71-Hz average fundamental frequency was comparable to the 65-Hz average reported for excellent male esophageal speakers (Curry and Snidecor, 1961; Weinberg and Bennett, 1972), but considerably lower than expected for normal men of this subject's age (Hollien and Shipp, 1972). The f_0 standard deviation of 2 semitones and full range of 10 semitones were much smaller than the 4 semitone SD and 12 to 14 semitone 90%-range values reported for excellent esophageal speakers (Shipp, 1967; Curry and Snidecor, 1961; Weinberg and Bennett, 1972).

The phonation time characteristics of this speaker using the Tokyo artificial larynx compared favorably with those reported for normal speakers (Hanley, 1951). For example, 60% of his total speaking time was spent producing periodicity, 17% was aperiodicity, and 23% was silence. These data show that, in comparison with esophageal speakers, this speaker using the Tokyo artificial larynx spent a significantly greater percentage of time producing periodicity and significantly less time in silence (Curry and Snidecor, 1961; Shipp, 1967; Weinberg and Bennett, 1972). Such observations were not unexpected, since the phonation time characteristics of speech with the Tokyo larynx are largely regulated by the patient's preoperative respiratory speech patterns.

ASG's total duration for reading the 12-word sentence was 5.14 sec or 138 words per minute. These values were smaller than the 5.5–6.0-sec averages reported for excellent esophageal speakers (Curry and Snidecor, 1961; Shipp, 1967; Weinberg and Bennett, 1972) and support the widely held belief that alaryngeal speech is characterized by lower-than-average (166 wpm) speaking rates (Darley, 1940; Curry and Snidecor, 1961).

Speech Intelligibility Characteristics

The subject's average speech intelligibility for monosyllabic consonant rhyme-test words was 95% correct. Average intelligibility scores for individual consonants under test are shown in Table 1. The mean intelligibility scores for word-initial and word-final consonants were 91 and 95% correct, while for voiced and voiceless consonants they were 97 and 90% correct. With respect

TABLE 1. Average intelligibility (percentage correct) of consonants. Initial (I), final (F), and initial + final word position (I + F) are tabulated.

Consonant	I	F	IF		I	F	IF			I	F	IF
p	63	85	74	m	98	88	93	f		97	86*	94
b	99	100	99	n	100†	99	99	v		100†	84*	86
t	89	95	92	ŋ	–	95*	95	θ		100†	80*	84
d	90	100	96					ð		100†	100†	100
k	76	98	91					s		99	98	99
g	98	100*	99	w	88	–	88	z		–	95	95
				r	94	100	95	ʃ		100†	–	100
‡	88*	100*	95	l	96	100*	98	ʒ		–	98*	98
								dʒ		100†	100*	100
								h		84	–	84

* Sound is in at least two but less than six test forms.
† Sound occurs in only one test form.
‡ Consonant is not present.

to consonant type, the order of correct identification, from most to least intelligible, was affricates, nasals, fricatives, plosives, and glides. For vowel rhyme-test words, average intelligibility was 95% correct. The mean scores for individual vowels under test are as follows:

Vowel	Percentage Correct	Vowel	Percentage Correct
ɝ	93	ʌ	93
o	99	ɔ	97
e	99	ɪ	97
ɛ	99	i	99
æ	97	ɑ	80
ʊ	97	u	94

The high intelligibility scores for both consonant and vowel rhyme-test words show that the speech produced by this man using the Tokyo larynx was characterized by near-perfect intelligibility of monosyllabic rhyme-test materials. Under the optimal signal-to-noise conditions used in this experiment, both normal and excellent esophageal speakers also exhibit near-perfect intelligibility for these same materials (House et al., 1965; Horii, 1969; Weinberg and Horii, 1972[1]).

CLINICAL PERSPECTIVES

This study was based on the performance of a single talker, and we caution the reader not to overgeneralize. ASG taught himself to speak with the Tokyo

[1] B. Weinberg and Y. Horii, unpublished work on the effects of noise on the intelligibility of excellent esophageal speech (1972).

artificial larynx and was able to achieve a superior level of speech proficiency. This may not be the case for others learning to speak with this instrument.

For example, some patients may have difficulty effecting proper placement of the stomal cover and the sound-conduction tube. The stomal cover must fit tightly against the tracheal opening to prevent loss of respiratory power and to prevent audible air loss between the cover and the stoma. Improper placement of the sound-conduction tube may interfere with articulatory maneuvers of the tongue. To prevent interference, the patient should be instructed to place the sound-conduction tube in the side, rather than the front, of the mouth. The subject of our clinical study placed the tube between his upper and lower molars and stated that he "chewed on the tube as he talked." ASG used a very stiff plastic sound-conduction tube to prevent tubal collapse and aphonia.

Like other artificial speaking devices, the Tokyo artificial larynx is highly visible. The visibility factor calls attention to the speech differences occasioned by the patient's surgery and may affect his willingness to use the device. As with other instruments, speakers must hold the Tokyo larynx in place and, therefore, do not have full use of both hands when they talk. Thus, the Tokyo artificial larynx is not unlike available artificial instruments in its practicality and visual appeal. We believe that the Tokyo larynx is unlike available instruments in the pleasantness of tone it produces. In our opinion, speech produced with the Tokyo larynx is not characterized by an overwhelming mechanical or electronic quality so often associated with speech produced by artificial devices. We hope that this report will stimulate consideration and study of this additional method of alaryngeal speech.

ACKNOWLEDGMENT

This work was supported in part by a grant from the Delaware County Cancer Society, Muncie, Indiana. We acknowledge the assistance and cooperation of Alfred St. Germaine, the subject of our clinical study. Harry Brittian provided biostatistical and programing consultation. Suzanne Bennett provided many helpful suggestions. In the United States, Tokyo artificial larynges may be purchased through Red Woodward, 3132 Waits Street, Fort Worth, Texas 76109. Requests for reprints may be directed to Bernd Weinberg, Speech Research Laboratory, Rotary Building, Indiana University Medical Center, Indianapolis, Indiana 46202.

REFERENCES

CURRY, E. T., and SNIDECOR, J. C., Physical measurement and pitch perception in esophageal speech. *Laryngoscope,* **71,** 415-424 (1961).

DARLEY, F., *A Normative Study of Oral Reading Rate.* Master's Thesis, State Univ. of Iowa (1940).

DIEDRICH, W., and YOUNGSTROM, K., *Alaryngeal Speech.* Springfield, Ill.: Charles C Thomas (1966).

FAIRBANKS, G., *Voice and Articulation Drillbook.* New York: Harper (1960).

HANLEY, T. D., An analysis of vocal frequency and duration characteristics of selected samples of speech from three American dialects. *Speech Monogr.* **18,** 78-93 (1951).

HOLLIEN, H., and SHIPP, T., Speaking fundamental frequency and chronologic age in males. *J. Speech Hearing Res.,* **15,** 155-159 (1972).

HORII, Y., *Specifying the Speech-to-Noise Ratio: Development and Evaluation of a Noise with Speech Envelope Characteristics.* Doctoral dissertation, Purdue Univ. (1969).

HOUSE, A. S., WILLIAMS, C. E., HECKER, M. H. L., and KRYTER, K. D., Articulation testing methods: Consonantal differentiation with a closed response set. *J. acoust. Soc. Amer.,* **37,** 158-166 (1965).

SHANKS, J. C., The use of the manufactured larynx for alaryngeal speech training. Ch. V in *Therapy for the Laryngectomized Patient.* New York: Teacher's College Press (1971).

SHIPP, T., Frequency, duration, and perceptual measures in relation to judgments of esophageal speech acceptability. *J. Speech Hearing Res.,* **10,** 417-427 (1967).

SNIDECOR, J. C., *Speech Rehabilitation of the Laryngectomized.* Springfield, Ill.: Charles C Thomas (1969).

WEINBERG, B., and BENNETT, S., Selected acoustic characteristics of esophageal speech produced by female laryngectomees. *J. Speech Hearing Res.,* **15,** 211-216 (1972).

Received December 13, 1972.
Accepted March 27, 1973.

An Experimental Study of Artificial-Larynx And Esophageal Speech

Melvin Hyman

Laryngectomized patients may be trained to develop esophageal speech or advised to use an artificial larynx. In the absence of experimental evidence, the choice of method has necessarily been determined by previous experience or personal preference of the physician or speech pathologist in charge of the case.

Several writers advocate esophageal speech, with little evidence to support their views; others write in Aristotilean terms of employing either the artificial larynx or the esophageal method of speech production.

The purpose of this experiment was to compare selected aspects of esophageal speech, artificial-larynx speech, and normal speech.

Procedure

Twenty-four persons participated as experimental subjects in the investigation. They included equal numbers of (a) artificial-larynx speakers,[1] (b) esophageal speakers, and (c) normal speakers. The age

[1]The artificial larynges employed by the subjects were of a reed type, number two, produced by the Western Electric Company.

Melvin Hyman (Ph.D., Ohio State University, 1953) is Assistant Professor of Speech and Director of the Speech and Hearing Clinic, Bowling Green State University. This article is based on a Ph.D. dissertation completed under the direction of Professor John W. Black and adapted from a paper presented at the 1953 Convention of ASHA in New York.

range for the three groups was from 40 to 65 years. All of the subjects except two were men; there was one woman in the esophageal group and one woman in the normal group. The investigator and two trained assistants established the following criteria for the selection of laryngectomized cases: (a) the respective type of speech had been used for at least six months, and (b) individuals selected were considered to be 'good' or 'effective' speakers. The laryngectomized speakers were matched with normal speakers in occupational and educational backgrounds.

Each subject spoke into an Altec Lansing microphone, model 200B, located six inches directly in front of his lips. The speech was recorded on a Magnecorder tape recorder, model PT6-A at a speed of 7.5 inches per second.

Preferences. This phase of the study was concerned with the preferences of college students for the voices of artificial-larynx or esophageal speakers.

Each speaker read a standard prose selection of 132 words entitled, 'My Grandfather.' (Henceforth this will be referred to as the 'standard passage.') The informal directions given to each speaker were: 'Read this paragraph as though you were reading it aloud to your wife (husband) or a friend. Read it naturally.' Each speaker was given one practice read-

Reprinted by permission from *Journal of Speech and Hearing Disorders*, 1955, 20, 291–299.

TABLE 1. Order of presentation of recordings of subjects (S) to listeners in a modified paired comparison technique. Only one half of the order of presentation is represented in this table.

Subject (S)	Compared With	Subject (S)	Subject (S)	Compared With	Subject (S)
1		2	12		13
1		3	12		14
2		3	13		14
2		4	13		15
3		4	14		15
3		5	14		16
			15		16

ing in which he demonstrated that he could recognize and say the words in the selection.

The first sentence of the passage, 'You wish to know all about my grandfather,' was removed from the selection recorded by each artificial-larynx and esophageal speaker and was employed in a paired-comparison technique to determine preferences of voices by college students. To compare 16 sentences with each other in two orders would involve $N(N-1)$ or $16 (16-1)$ comparisons, and would require an hour and 15 minutes. In order to reduce the time required of the judges, a special technique suggested by Guilford (3) was employed. The sentences were ranked 1 to 16—most preferred to the least preferred voice—by three students of speech correction. Recordings of the 16 were then rearranged on the magnetic tape. The reading that was ranked highest became the first recording on the tape and was designated *Subject One* (S_1). This reading was succeeded by *Subject Two* (S_2), etc.

Each subject was compared with the two subjects immediately preceding and following in rank according to the scheme in Table 1. This scheme

illustrates only one half of the presentation of stimuli, or one order. A counterbalanced or two-order system was employed to negate an order effect in the presentation. For example, subject rank one was both the first and second member of pairs in the comparison with subject rank two (*ab* and *ba*). These recordings of the subjects were rearranged (by editing and splicing the tape) in the indicated order, and copied onto 12-inch discs to facilitate the presentation of the pairs to the listeners. The disc recordings of the subjects were then played in random order to 100 college students in elementary speech and English courses. The following directions were given to the listeners:

> You will hear two speakers reading the same materials. After the second speaker has finished, write the number *1* or *2* according to the speaker whose *voice you would prefer to listen to*. Do the same for the other pairs of speakers. Do not leave any space blank—guess if you have to—but write only one number for each space. Remember, write only after the second speaker of a pair has finished.

The recordings were heard in classroom quiet. Two subjects had a sound level that equalled the average sound level of all the subjects as measured with a VU meter. The recordings of these two subjects were played to the listeners at an approximate level of 60 db. The distance from the loudspeaker to the middle of a row of 12 listeners was approximately three feet. The level was determined with the sound level meter[2] placed three feet from the loudspeaker, along the axis of the cone of the loudspeaker. The attenuator on the phonograph was fixed throughout the entire testing procedure. For each aspect studied, the listeners gave a total of 200 judgments regarding each pair of speakers. The number of judgments in which one subject was preferred over the second subject of a pair was tabulated. These figures were tested by chi-square to determine whether the results could have occurred by chance alone.

The procedures for determining the preferences among college students of loudness levels and duration of reading of artificial-larynx and esophageal speakers were similar to those described for determining preferences of voices. Ranks of the same subjects' recordings of the sentence, 'You wish to know all about my grandfather' were determined by the therapists for each attribute of voice investigated. The recordings of these subjects were rearranged on the magnetic tape according to the scheme described previously and copied on the 12-inch discs. Three groups of 100 college students participated as listeners, one group for each aspect of voice studied. Chi-square tests were employed for both loudness levels and duration of reading.

Physical Measurements. This phase of the study was concerned with the physical measurements of sound pressure and duration of reading of artificial-larynx, esophageal, and normal speakers.

While magnetic tape recordings were being made of the first reading of the standard passage, the attenuator dial on the recorder was fixed. Thus, variations in relative sound pressure from subject to subject were included on the records. The magnetic tape recorder fed a level recorder (Sound Apparatus Company; 50 db potentiometer), and graphic records of the duration and pressure characteristics of the readings were obtained. The three highest amplitudes or peak deflections of the stylus within each second of reading time were measured and the mean of the three was computed. The level for the entire selection was computed, in turn, from these means as an arbitrary indication of each speaker's sound pressure level. These mean values were treated as basic measures in a three by eight array, three columns (type of speech) with eight (subject) values in each column and subjected to analysis of variance.

According to Fletcher (2), the average speech power is the 'total speech energy radiated over any period, divided by the length of the period.' Somewhat in keeping with Fletcher, the graphic tracings enclosed an area in which horizontal dimensions represented time and vertical dimensions represented relative sound pressure levels. A planimeter was employed to integrate the graphic records. These measurements were of two kinds: (a) integrated sound pressure levels for the first five seconds of graphic level recordings of speech and (b) integrated sound pressure levels for the first five seconds of speech omitting pauses. In each case,

---

[2]General Radio Sound Level Meter, type 759-B, scale C, setting slow.

measurements of two five-second periods of recording were obtained. Since the second measurement never differed by more than 1/20 from the first, the first measurement was taken as representative of integrated sound pressure level for each speaker. Analysis of variance was employed to test for significant differences among the means of the three groups of speakers.

Another aspect considered was the range of sound pressure of the speakers. Each speaker produced three vowel [ɑ] sounds as 'loud' as possible and as 'soft' as possible. The mean value of the 'loud' vowel sounds was obtained by averaging the three highest peak deflections (one peak from each sound) recorded by the stylus on the power level recorder. The same procedure was employed in obtaining the mean of the 'soft' productions of the vowel. The difference between the two means represented the range of sound pressure for each speaker.

Values of the duration of the readings were computed from the horizontal dimensions of the graphic recordings of the spoken materials. The original measurements were transferred into time units (seconds).

Intelligibility. This phase of the study was concerned with the identification by listeners of words and sounds produced by artificial-larynx, esophageal, and normal speakers. Lists of words from a multiple-choice intelligibility test (*1, 4*), recorded by the speakers on magnetic tape were played to a total of 120 listeners in five sound-level conditions. There were 24 listeners for each condition; 12 listeners were located approximately nine feet from the loudspeaker and 12, thirty-six feet from the loudspeaker. The five conditions were:

(1) the speaker with the 'softest' sound level was heard at 68 db as measured by a sound level meter placed midway between the two rows of listeners; the remaining speakers were relatively 'louder'; (2) the esophageal speakers with the modal sound level for their group were heard at 68 db and the remaining speakers were heard relatively louder; (3) artificial-larynx speakers with the modal sound level for their group were heard at 68 db and the remaining speakers were heard relatively 'softer'; (4) each speaker was heard at a sound level of 78 db; (5) each speaker was heard at a sound level of 78 db with a background of 73 db of white noise. The intelligibility score for each speaker was the percentage of words correctly identified by the listeners. Analyses of variance were employed to test for significant differences among the mean intelligibility scores of the three groups of speakers.

In another measurement of intelligibility, each speaker read aloud a total of 58 monosyllables; these were composed of 21 consonants in the initial position followed by [ɑ], 21 consonants in the final position preceded by [ɑ], and 16 vowels and diphthongs. These were recorded and presented to seven college students who transcribed the monosyllables into phonetic symbols. The number of sounds correctly identified for each speaker was tabulated and converted into percentage values. The differences in intelligibility among the 24 speakers were tested by means of analysis of variance.

Results

Preferences. In comparing the voices of the artificial-larynx and eso-

phageal speakers, *the artificial-larynx speakers were always preferred.* Twelve out of the thirteen comparisons were significant at the one per cent level of confidence and one comparison was significant at the five per cent level of confidence. There were individual differences among the speakers with artificial larynx and among the esophogeal speakers. The results of the chi-square anaylses revealed that 28 out of 29 comparisons (artificial-larynx *vs.* artificial-larynx as well as *vs.* esophageal speakers) were significantly different from chance at the one per cent level of confidence. One of the 29 comparisons did not show significance at the five per cent level of confidence or above. This comparison was between two speakers with artificial larynx, both considered by the original judges to be in the top quartile of preferred voices. Since 13 out of 13 comparisons of esophageal *vs.* artificial-larynx speakers were in favor of speakers with artificial larynx, it appears that college students believed the voices of the artificial-larynx speakers to be more pleasant than the voice of the esophageal speakers.

When the judges were asked to indicate which loudness level was preferred, the loudness levels of the speakers with artificial larynx were preferred over the esophageal speakers in 10 out of 12 comparisons at the one per cent level of confidence. In the two remaining comparisons, the esophageal speakers were preferred over the artificial-larynx speakers at the one per cent level of confidence. There were individual differences among the speakers in each group. Of the 29 comparisons, 27 were significant at the one per cent level of confidence and one comparison was significant at the five per cent level of confidence.

With respect to duration of reading, the speakers with artificial larynx were preferred over the esophageal speakers in four out of eight comparisons at the one per cent level of confidence. In one comparison, the esophageal speaker was preferred over the artificial-larynx speaker at the one per cent level of confidence. Thus, the artificial-larynx speakers were preferred more than 50 per cent of the time in judgments of duration of reading. Results of the chi-square tests also revealed individual differences in each group of speakers. Twenty-five

TABLE 2. Summary of means and (t) values.

	Artificial Larynx	Esophageal	Normal	t
Sound Pressure	33	23	29	A and N $t=3.86$* E and N $t=4.01$* A and E $t=7.01$*
Range of Sound Pressure	7	11		A and E $t=2.12$†
Duration	350.2	384.8	311.5	A and N $t=4.04$* E and N $t=3.64$* A and E $t=2.21$‡

* Significant at the one per cent level.
† Approximates significance at the five per cent level.
‡ Significant at the five per cent level.

out of twenty-nine comparisons were significant at the five per cent level of confidence.

Physical Measurements. Using the highest amplitudes or peak deflections of the stylus on the power level recorder as an indication of sound pressure levels, the relative means[3] for the the three groups of speakers were found to be 33, 23, and 29 db for artificial-larynx, esophageal, and normal speakers, respectively. The *F*-ratio was significant at the one per cent level of confidence and each group was significantly different from every other. These results are summarized in Table 2.

The values of the *F*-ratios were significant at the one per cent level of confidence when the planimeter was employed in measuring sound pressure for speech with pauses and without pauses. In considering the integrated sound pressure for speech (including pauses), the esophageal group was 4 db lower than the artificial-larynx and normal speakers; the artificial-larynx and normal speakers were approximately the same. The mean values for the three groups of speakers for integrated sound pressure levels of their speech (omitting pauses) were computed and the esophageal group was 3 db lower than the artificial-larynx and normal speakers. The normal speakers were approximately 0.3 db less intense than the artificial-larynx speakers. In each case the mean of the normal and artificial-larynx speakers was significantly different from the esophageal speakers at the one per cent level of confidence. The normal and esophageal speakers were significantly different from one another at the one per cent level of confidence. The artificial-larynx and normal speakers were not significantly different from each other with either set of measurements (speech including pauses and speech omitting pauses).

The mean range of sound pressure for artificial-larynx speakers and esophageal speakers was 7 db and 11 db respectively. The difference between the two groups approximated the five per cent level of confidence. The esophageal speakers had a wider range of sound pressure than did the artificial-larynx speakers.

The mean values of the groups in duration of reading of the standard passage were 350.2, 384.8 and 311.5 seconds for artificial-larynx, esophageal, and normal speakers respectively. The *t* values between the means of normal and artificial-larynx speakers, and between normal and esophageal speakers respectively were significant at the one per cent level of confidence. The means of esophageal and artificial-larynx speakers were significantly different at the five per cent level of confidence. Differences in duration of reading were significant among the three groups of speakers. The normal speakers were the fastest talkers and esophageal speakers the slowest talkers.

Intelligibility. In the first four conditions tested, the normal speakers were significantly more intelligible than artificial-larynx and esophageal speakers at the one per cent level of confidence with either row of listeners. The artificial-larynx and esophageal speakers were significantly different at the five per cent level of confidence in *Condition One* when listeners were located nine feet from the loudspeaker; in the other condi-

---

[3]These figures are above a reference level of 50 db relative to .0002 dynes/cm².

TABLE 3. Summary of analyses of variance of the means for intelligibility conditions one to five.

Location of Listeners from Loudspeaker	Conditions	Source of Variation	df	Variance	F
9 Feet	One	Between Groups	2	1301.40	13.86*
		Within Groups	21	93.88	
		Total	23		
36 Feet	One	Between Groups	2	806.14	11.42*
		Within Groups	21	70.62	
		Total	23		
9 Feet	Two	Between Groups	2	900.16	17.47*
		Within Groups	21	51.53	
		Total	23		
36 Feet	Two	Between Groups	2	798.10	18.33*
		Within Groups	21	43.53	
		Total	23		
9 Feet	Three	Between Groups	2	593.20	12.17*
		Within Groups	21	48.75	
		Total	23		
36 Feet	Three	Between Groups	2	449.42	13.09*
		Within Groups	21	34.33	
		Total	23		
9 Feet	Four	Between Groups	2	703.40	13.13*
		Within Groups	21	53.58	
		Total	23		
36 Feet	Four	Between Groups	2	570.37	10.45*
		Within Groups	21	54.58	
		Total	23		
9 Feet	Five	Between Groups	2	61.47	2.15†
		Within Groups	21	28.56	
		Total	23		
36 Feet	Five	Between Groups	2	16.32	0.81†
		Within Groups	21	20.08	
		Total	23		

* Significant at the one percent level of confidence.
† Not significant at the five percent level of confidence.

tions they were not significantly different from each other at the five per cent level of confidence. There were no significant differences among the groups in *Condition Five*. These results are summarized in Tables 3 and 4.

The mean gross scores for sounds that were correctly identified were 160, 188, and 288 for artificial-larynx, esophageal, and normal speakers, respectively. The F-ratio was significant at the one per cent level of confidence. The normal and artificial-larynx speakers, and the normal and esophageal speakers were significantly different from each other at the one per cent level of confidence. The artificial-larynx and esophageal speakers were not significantly different at the

TABLE 4. Summary of means and t values of eight artificial-larynx (A), eight esophageal (E) and eight normal (N) speakers when reading lists from the multiple-choice intelligibility test.

Location of Listeners from Loudspeaker	Condition	Groups	Means	t
9 Feet	One	A	48.0	A and N t=5.72*
		E	56.4	E and N t=3.34*
		N	73.0	A and E t=2.83†
36 Feet	One	A	44.6	A and N t=4.14*
		E	50.4	E and N t=3.33*
		N	64.5	A and E t=1.68‡
9 Feet	Two	A	44.0	A and N t=5.55*
		E	50.9	E and N t=4.46*
		N	64.9	A and E t=1.81‡
36 Feet	Two	A	40.3	A and N t=5.97*
		E	46.2	E and N t=4.22*
		N	59.5	A and E t=1.67‡
9 Feet	Three	A	43.4	A and N t=4.37*
		E	50.2	E and N t=3.49*
		N	60.8	A and E t=2.01‡
36 Feet	Three	A	41.8	A and N t=4.42*
		E	45.8	E and N t=4.17*
		N	56.1	A and E t=1.32‡
9 Feet	Four	A	48.2	A and N t=4.91*
		E	51.8	E and N t=3.90*
		N	66.1	A and E t=0.98‡
36 Feet	Four	A	43.1	A and N t=4.24*
		E	46.2	E and N t=3.71*
		N	58.9	A and E t=0.79‡
9 Feet	Five	A	34.6	
		E	35.8	
		N	38.9	
36 Feet	Five	A	33.2	
		E	35.1	
		N	36.4	

* Significant at the one per cent level of confidence.
† Significant at the five per cent level of confidence.
‡ Not significant at five per cent level of confidence.

five per cent level of confidence. The rank order correlations between the five intelligibility conditions and the monosyllabic test for esophageal and artificial-larynx speakers were .80, .69, .62, .66, and .36 respectively. The ranks in the first four intelligibility conditions appeared to be related to the ranks in the monosyllabic test at the one per cent level of confidence.

The English speech sounds of the monosyllabic test given to the three groups of speakers were categorized into consonants and vowels. The vowel sounds for all three groups were identified more times than con-

TABLE 5. Summary of percentages of the four consonant phonemes most rarely identified and most frequently identified.

	Most Rarely Identified		Most Frequently Identified	
Artificial	[θ]	1.8	[s]	58.9
Larynx	[ð]	2.7	[w]	57.1
	[ŋ]	7.1	[ʃ]	54.5
	[h w]	8.9	[n]	50.0
Esophageal	[h]	0	[r]	73.2
	[h w]	5.4	[d ʒ]	69.6
	[ð]	9.8	[d]	62.5
	[θ]	12.5	[w]	60.7
Normal	[θ]	17.0	[w]	91.1
	[ð]	22.3	[t]	91.1
	[ŋ]	37.5	[n]	89.3
	[h w]	44.6	[s]	88.4

sonants at the one per cent level of confidence. The consonants were further subdivided: (a) The voiced consonants were identified more times than voiceless consonants for the esophageal speakers whereas the opposite effect took place for the artificial-larynx and normal speakers; (b) The initial consonants for all three groups of speakers were identified more times than final consonants. In a further division of consonants, the following types of consonants are placed in order from most to least frequently correctly identified: affricates, glides, nasals, plosives, and fricatives for the esophageal group; affricates, nasals, fricatives, glides, and plosives for the artifical-larynx speakers; and affricates, plosives, nasals,

glides, and fricatives for the normal group of speakers.

Table 5 summarizes for each speaker four consonant phonemes most rarely identified and most frequently identified by the listeners.

Summary and Conclusion

The results of the study indicate that *acoustically*, speech production by means of the artificial-larynx was preferred over esophageal speech. There is probably no significant difference in intelligibility between good speakers who employ the artificial-larynx and the esophageal methods. Further research is needed in testing the *visual* aspects of these two types of speech, to determine whether or not listeners object to seeing the artificial-larynx, and how detrimental this is to the effectiveness of the speaker. Motion picture films with sound could be employed for testing the visual aspects of the speech of the artificial-larynx and esophageal speakers.

References

1. BLACK, J. W. Final report and summary of work on voice communication. *OSRD Report No. 5568.* Psychological Corporation, September 11, 1945.

2. FLETCHER, H. *Speech and Hearing in Communication.* New York: Van Nostrand Co., 1953.

3. GUILFORD, J. P. *Psychometric Methods.* New York: McGraw-Hill Book Co., 1936.

4. HAAGEN, C. H. Intelligibility measurement techniques and procedures used by the voice communication laboratory. *OSRD Report No. 3748.* The Psychological Corporation, May 1944.

The Relative Intelligibility of Esophageal Speech and Artificial-Larynx Speech

ROBERT L. McCROSKEY

MARIGENE MULLIGAN

Research concerned with the speech of the laryngectomee has been focused on various acoustic properties of speech and voice production (*4, 12, 8*) or judgments by listeners of their preferences for various voice types (7). There is a dearth of objective information regarding the intelligibility of the laryngectomized individuals who use esophageal speech as compared with that of those who employ an artificial larynx.

Several writers have discussed the relative merits of speech resulting from the use of artificial-larynx and esophageal speech (*11, 1, 10*). According to Gardner and Harris (*6*) approximately 40 per cent of successfully laryngectomized patients never acquire intelligible esophageal speech. Nevertheless, those who are concerned with speech rehabilitation frequently introduce psychological bias against the use of the artificial larynx (*11*), a bias apparently based in part upon the opinion that esophageal speech is preferred by listeners. Hyman's findings (7), for example, appeared to show that esophageal speech is preferred when judgments are based on auditory cues alone. It has also been demonstrated that esophageal speech is preferred by sophisticated and naive listeners when judgments are based on combined auditory and visual stimuli (*3*). Listener preference is a valuable means of determining the better system of speech production, but another dimension, intelligibility, remains relatively unexplored.

Speech pathologists have generally agreed that esophageal or pharyngeal speech is to be preferred over the artificial-larynx method (*1, 4, 5, 6*) there has seemed to be a general consensus that this mode of speech production was more convenient for the speaker, more sanitary, and more easily understood. While the opinion of the speech specialist is of importance, it is also of interest to know the judgment of the naive listener since he certainly constitutes the typical audience of the laryngectomee.

It was the purpose of the present investigation to study the intelligibility of two methods of producing speech by laryngectomees, esophageal and artificial-larynx, as determined by both sophisticated and naive listeners.

Robert L. McCroskey (Ph.D., Ohio State University, 1956) is Associate Professor of Teacher Education, Emory University, and Director of Speech at the Atlanta Speech School, Inc. Marigene Mulligan (M.A., Ohio State University, 1954) is Lecturer, Emory University, and Speech Pathologist at the Atlanta Speech School, Inc.

Reprinted by permission from *Journal of Speech and Hearing Disorders*, 1963, *28*, 37–41.

445

Procedure

Speakers. Ten laryngectomized individuals, five of whom used esophageal speech and five of whom employed an artificial larynx, served as speakers. All had employed their method of speaking for more than one year. The average number of years' experience among users of the artificial larynx was 13.8; the average duration of experience for the esophageal speakers was 6.1 years. Three of the artificial larynx speakers employed electrically produced sound sources while the remaining two speakers used mechanical devices involving the insertion of a sound-conducting rubber tube to the side of the mouth. All speakers were obtained through the cooperation of the Georgia Association of Laryngectomees. It should be noted that all laryngectomees employed in this experiment were considered to be proficient speakers, based on self-ratings and judgments of the experimenters.

Stimulus Material. Each speaker read different multiple-choice intelligibility lists (2) composed of nine groups of three words each. All speakers were given cards on which was printed identifying information and stimulus words. For example the first speaker read:

I am speaker one. I say again I am speaker one.

Number 1 (5 second pause)	grew	modest	vicc
Number 2 (5 second pause)	stay	purveyed	chink
. . . .	. . . . . .	. . . .	. . . .
Number 9	craft	bowled	polo

Equipment. All speech samples were recorded on an Ampex 960 using an Altec 661-B microphone in a sound-

isolated room. Visual monitoring of the recorder's VU meter was the method for equating SPL between groups of speakers. The recorded stimuli were played back through the same system coupled with a Pilot 240 amplifier and two Altec 1-755-A speakers.

Listeners and Listening Conditions. Three panels of 10 listeners each were required to make judgments in accordance with the procedures described by Black (2). The listeners were given multiple-choice forms which provided four alternatives for each stimulus word. It is felt that this procedure reduces the role of various levels of linguistic sophistication among listeners in the testing of intelligibility. It was the listener's task to cross out the word he heard. For example, using the first set of three stimulus words shown above, the listener would mark his paper in the following manner, provided he had understood the stimulus:

SPEAKER 1

1	groove	modern	~~vice~~
	drew	moderate	fight
	crew	modesty	mice
	~~grew~~	~~modest~~	bite

One panel of listeners was composed of experienced speech therapists, another panel was made up of graduate students with some prior exposure to speech of the laryngectomee, and the third panel was composed of naive listeners, i.e., those who had never heard or been exposed to either of the modes of speech under investigation.

Prior to the experiment, each listener's auditory acuity was determined by administering a pure-tone audiometric test using a sweep-check technique at 10 db. Only those with normal bilateral hearing in the speech range were used in the actual experiment.

TABLE 1. Summary of analysis of variance for testing differences in intelligibility of esophageal and artificial-larynx speech according to professional, student, and naive listeners.

Source	df	ss	ms	F	$F_{(.01)}$	$F_{(.05)}$
Between panels	2	117	58.50	3.578		3.17
Between groups	1	304	304.00	18.593	7.12	
Between cells	5	759	151.80	9.183	3.37	
Interaction	2	338	169.00	10.336	5.01	
Within cells	54	883	16.35			

The listeners' responses on the first two groups of three words each in each list were not included in the final analysis of the data. This allowed each listener equal time to adjust to the speakers' manner of talking.

All stimuli were presented free-field to the panels of listeners at 74 db SPL (Scott sound level meter C-scale, fast), as measured at the ear of a listener seated directly in front of the sound source at a distance of nine feet.

Analysis of Data. The data were analyzed by an analysis of variance by double entry table according to Lindquist (9, pp. 108-120). The criterion measure was the number of correct responses by listeners for all speakers in each group.

Results and Discussion

Analysis of the data revealed differences between the judged intelligibility of the two groups of speakers which were statistically significant beyond the .01 level of confidence (F = 18.543; 1 and 54 df). The differences among the three panels of listeners were also statistically significant as was the interaction. Table 1 is a summary of the analysis of variance by double entry table.

A summary of the distribution of mean intelligibility for the two groups of speakers, according to listeners, is shown in Table 2. An inspection of the means reveals agreement among speech pathologists and graduate students in speech therapy with the higher mean intelligibility in the direction of the esophageal speakers; however this direction was reversed where intelligibility was determined using naive listeners. This fact would appear to account for the significant interaction which makes it impossible to generalize the between-groups findings to all listeners. The differences found among listeners seems to indicate that the listener who has never been exposed to the laryngectomee, or has never heard

TABLE 2. Summary of means and standard deviations for esophageal and artificial-larynx speakers with respect to intelligibility.

Speakers	Listeners					
	Professional		Student		Naive	
	M	SD	M	SD	M	SD
Esophageal	66.8	4.0	62.9	3.5	58.2	3.8
Artificial-larynx	57.9	3.6	56.2	3.2	60.3	4.7

the laryngectomee speak in any manner, finds speech more intelligible when produced by means of an artificial larynx.

The fact that intelligibility is determined by listeners implies that it is a joint function of the speaker and the receiver. The unanticipated, contradictory intelligibility scores obtained from the naive listeners as compared with the sophisticated ones suggests that professional preferences or training may have had an effect on the way in which the sophisticated listeners understood the stimuli.

Those speakers who used an artificial larynx were generally apologetic for their speech. The comments made during the recording reflected a feeling that they were less easily understood and that the device was not pleasant to hear. There was a tone which suggested that their having had to resort to a mechanical aid, either because of difficulty with learning esophageal speech or because it was necessary following additional surgery in the laryngeal area, meant that communication by means of artificial larynx was inferior. It was inferred from statements made to the experimenters that the artificial larynx was a symbol of failure for most of the speakers.

It is unfair to create bias against mechanical speech when many laryngectomees do not have a reasonable chance of achieving satisfactory skill otherwise. Speech pathologists should continue to urge these clients to strive for functional nonmechanical speech, but guard against creating a mental set toward the artificial larynx which may influence the user's security in social and business situations.

Summary

It was the purpose of this investigation to study the intelligibility of two methods of producing speech by laryngectomees, esophageal and artificial-larynx. The speakers were 10 laryngectomees, five of whom used esophageal speech and five of whom employed an artificial larynx. Each speaker read a different multiple-choice intelligibility list. Three panels of 10 listeners each responded independently to the spoken stimuli in a standard multiple-choice setting. One panel was composed of speech therapists, one of graduate students and one of naive listeners. All stimuli were presented free-field at a sound pressure level of 74 db at the listener's ear.

Statistical analysis of the data indicated that both speech therapists and graduate students found esophageal speakers to be significantly more intelligible than the artificial-larynx speakers; however, higher intelligibility was obtained for the artificial-larynx user when the stimuli were heard by naive listeners. These results suggest that intelligibility scores may be influenced by professional training or bias.

References

1. ARNOLD, G. E., Alleviation of alaryngeal aphonia with the modern artificial larynx: I. Evolution of artificial speech aids and their value for rehabilitation. *Logos*, 3, 1960, 55-67.
2. BLACK, J. W., Multiple-choice intelligibility tests. *J. Speech Hearing Dis.*, 22, 1957, 213-235.
3. CROUSE, G., An experimental study of listener preferences for artificial larynx or esophageal speech by comparison of audio with audio-visual presentation. Master's project in progress, Emory Univ., 1962.

4. CURRY, E. T., and SNIDECOR, J. C., Physical measurement and pitch perception in esophageal speech. *Laryngoscope*, 71, 1961, 415-424.

5. DI CARLO, L. M., AMSTER, W. W., and HERER, G. R., *Speech after Laryngectomy*. Syracuse: Syracuse Univ. Press, 1956.

6. GARDNER, W. H., and HARRIS, H. E., Aids and devices for laryngectomees. *Arch. Otolaryng.*, 73, 1961, 145-152.

7. HYMAN, M., An experimental study of artificial-larynx and esophageal speech. *J. Speech Hearing Dis.*, 20, 1955, 291-299.

8. LAFON, J. C., and CORNUT, G., Etude de la formation impulsionnelle de la voix et de la parole. *Folio Phoniat.*, 12, 1960, 176-188.

9. LINDQUIST, E. F., *Design and Analysis of Experiments in Psychology and Education*. Boston: Houghton Mifflin Co., 1953.

10. LUEDERS, O. W., Evaluation of postlaryngectomy rehabilitation programs. *Arch. Otolaryng.*, 65, 1957, 572-574.

11. REED, G. F., The long-term follow-up care of laryngectomized patients. *J. Amer. Med. Assn.*, 175, 1961, 980-985.

12. SNIDECOR, J. C., and CURRY, E. T., How effectively can the laryngectomee expect to speak? Norms for effective esophageal speech. *Laryngoscope*, 70, 1960, 62-67.

ACCEPTABILITY RATINGS OF NORMAL, ESOPHAGEAL, AND ARTIFICIAL LARYNX SPEECH

SUZANNE BENNETT *and* BERND WEINBERG

Indiana University Medical Center, Indianapolis, Indiana

To provide information about the ultimate acceptability of various types of alaryngeal speech, 37 listeners rated nine speakers with normal phonation in relation to two groups of superior alaryngeal speakers: five who used esophageal speech and four who used artificial larynges. Normal speech was rated significantly more acceptable than any form of alaryngeal speech studied. Speech produced with a Tokyo artificial larynx was rated significantly more acceptable than all other types of alaryngeal speech. Superior esophageal speech was significantly preferred over Western Electric reed and Bell electrolarynx speech. Listeners also categorized each of the 18 speakers as a normal speaker or not a normal speaker. The nine alaryngeal speakers were all classified as nonnormal, while eight of the nine normal subjects were classified as normal.

Information about the ultimate acceptability of various types of alaryngeal speech is important both to laryngectomized patients and to professionals providing rehabilitative services. Experiments have been performed to specify vocal attributes which differentiate good and poor esophageal speakers (Snidecor and Curry, 1959; Shipp, 1967; Hoops and Noll, 1969), and to compare listener preferences of esophageal and artificial larynx speech (Hyman, 1955; Crouse, 1962; Snidecor, 1968). To our knowledge, there has been no research comparing listeners' acceptability ratings of superior alaryngeal speech with ratings of normal speech.

The present work compared listeners' acceptability ratings of esophageal, artificial larynx, and normal speech. Since the principal aim was to obtain information about the ultimate acceptability of alaryngeal speech, only highly proficient laryngectomized speakers were studied.

METHODS

Subjects and Recordings

The subjects were 18 men between the ages of 50 and 82. Included in this group were five superior esophageal speakers, four superior artificial larynx speakers, and nine normal speakers matched to the laryngectomized subjects on the basis of age. Of the four subjects who spoke with artificial larynges,

Reprinted by permission from *Journal of Speech and Hearing Research*, 1973, *16*, 608–615.

one used the Bell 5A electrolarynx, while three used pneumatic devices powered by air from the tracheal stoma. Two subjects used the Western Electric 2A reed larynx, and the third used the newly developed Tokyo artificial larynx. Pictures and descriptions of each of these instruments are available (Diedrich and Youngstrom, 1966; Snidecor, 1968; Shanks, 1971; Lauder, 1972; Weinberg and Riekena, 1973).

The principal factors governing selection of the laryngectomized subjects were that they exhibit clearly superior speech and that among this group of speakers there be represented a variety of methods of alaryngeal speech which could be equated on the basis of their superiority. The laryngectomized subjects were selected from recordings of a large group of alaryngeal talkers ($N = 70$) representing various types of alaryngeal speech and the full continuum of speech proficiency. The two investigators independently rated the speech proficiency of each of these subjects on the basis of four broad categories: superior, above average, average, or below average. The category *superior* was used only when the sample was representative of the best alaryngeal speech the authors had ever heard. On the basis of this criterion, nine laryngectomized speakers were given superior ratings by both investigators; five were esophageal speakers and four were artificial larynx users. Hence, the number of subjects ($N = 9$) and their distribution within each alaryngeal subgroup was not predetermined. The small size of this group occurred as a result of the very strict speech proficiency requirements adopted by the investigators.

The characteristics common to all the esophageal and artifical larynx speakers selected for study were that they spoke fluently and with continuity. Their speech was easily understood and naturally produced without apparent thought or effort. The esophageal speakers evidenced minimal respiratory and air intake noise and had short latencies between air intake and esophageal phonation. The speaker using the Bell electrolarynx had minimal neck sound radiation, while the three speakers using pneumatic instruments had no perceptually identifiable stomal air loss. All the esophageal and artificial larynx speakers studied were able to effect perceptually identifiable variations in pitch and stress, thereby minimizing the monotonous quality often present in less proficient alaryngeal speakers.

High-quality tape recordings of the 18 speakers reading the second sentence of a standard passage (Fairbanks, 1960) were randomized to provide a tape for perceptual study.

Listeners and Listening Tasks

The listeners were 37 young adults who had little or no experience judging speech or familiarity with alaryngeal voice. The listening experiment was conducted in a college classroom, and the recordings were presented over a high-quality tape loud-speaker system.

Two listening sessions were conducted. In the first session, judges rated the acceptability of each subject's speech using a seven-point equal-appearing-interval scale, where 1 represented speech which was least acceptable and 7 speech which was highly acceptable. Listeners were told only that they would hear recordings of men between the ages of 50 and 82. The nature of the voices to be rated was not discussed with them. Listeners were given the following specific information concerning speech acceptability:

> In making your judgments about the speakers you are about to hear, give careful consideration to the attributes of pitch rate, understandability, and voice quality. In other words, is the voice pleasing to listen to, or does it cause you some discomfort as a listener?

Before the actual rating session, a tape of the 18 recordings was presented to acquaint the listeners with the voices to be rated.

In the second listening session, the recordings were rerandomized and again presented for evaluation. The listeners' task was to decide whether each recording was produced by a normal speaker or not a normal speaker. If the response was "not a normal speaker," listeners were instructed to indicate their reasons for this choice by checking one or more of the following categories: (1) voice pitch too high, (2) voice pitch too low, (3) voice quality does not sound normal, (4) speech is too slow, (5) speech is too fast, (6) voice is monotonous, (7) speech sounds mechanical, and (8) other comments.

Statistical Analyses

Ebel's (1951) intraclass correlation technique was used to evaluate the reliability of the average speech acceptability ratings made by the 37 listeners and to provide an estimate of the average reliability of individual raters. An analysis-of-variance procedure was used to test the significance of the differences between average acceptability ratings for esophageal, artificial larynx, and normal speakers. A Bartlett test was used initially to evaluate homogeneity of variance. In cases where heterogeneity of variance was found, the Welch F' test was used (Welch, 1951). When F tests were significant ($p < 0.05$), individual comparisons of the average scale values between speaker groups were evaluated using t-test procedures. When there was heterogeneity of variance, t' tests were used (Welch, 1951).

RESULTS

Reliability of Ratings

The intraclass correlation coefficient estimating average reliability of individual listeners was $r = 0.77$, showing that about 59% of the variance in ratings by one listener was predicted by the ratings of another listener. This coefficient is essentially the same as an average Pearson r computed for the ratings from each possible pair of judges. The intraclass correlation coefficient estimating the reliability of mean scale values of speech acceptability was $r = 0.99$, showing that the 37 listeners provided highly reliable average ratings of these 18 voice samples.

Speech Acceptability Judgments

. The mean scale values of speech acceptability for each of the 18 speakers and the average ratings for speaker groups are shown in Figure 1. The average acceptability rating was 5.48 for the normal speakers, 2.54 for the esophageal speakers, 1.59 for the Western Electric reed and Bell electrolarynx speakers, and 3.62 for the Tokyo artificial larynx speaker. In order to compare the alaryngeal speakers with normal speakers, it was necessary to remove one of the normal speakers from the analysis because 20 of the 37 listeners classified him as not a normal speaker in the second listening session. Consequently, the mean for normal speakers in Figure 1 is based upon eight rather than nine subjects. The data in Figure 1 also show that the average rating for the Tokyo artificial larynx speaker was markedly higher than the ratings for the five

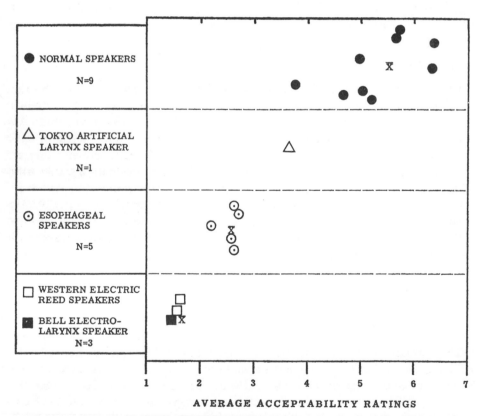

FIGURE 1. Mean scale values of speech acceptability for nine alaryngeal and nine normal speakers. The mean rating for each speaker group is noted by X.

esophageal speakers and the remaining three artificial larynx users. This subject was treated as a separate speaker group in the statistical analysis.

The results of the analysis of variance indicated that there was a significant difference in the average acceptability ratings among the types of speech studied ($F' = 184.3$, $df = 2$ and approximately 8, $p < 0.05$). The Tokyo artificial larynx group contained only a single case. Consequently, this group had a variance of 0 and could not be included in the F' test. Comparisons between the Tokyo artificial larynx speaker and the other three speaker groups were made with t tests, where the variance of the comparison group was used in the denominator (Sokol and Rohlf, 1969).

The multiple comparisons of the four speaker groups are summarized in Table 1. Listeners rated normal speech significantly more acceptable than all forms of alaryngeal speech. Comparisons between esophageal and artificial larynx speech were especially interesting, since they provided information about the relative acceptability of various types of alaryngeal speech. Superior esophageal speech was significantly ($p < 0.01$) preferred over speech produced with the Western Electric reed larynx and the Bell electrolarynx. Tokyo artificial larynx speech was judged significantly more acceptable than esophageal, Western Electric reed, and Bell electrolarynx speech.

Normal and Not Normal Speaker Categorizations

The listeners' categorizations of these 18 voices as normal or not normal were subjected to sign-test analyses (Sokol and Rohlf, 1969). Every alaryngeal speaker was consistently judged to be not a normal speaker, while eight of the nine normal speakers were consistently judged to be normal speakers. This finding emphasizes the fact that naive listeners perceived significant differences in the speech of superior alaryngeal and normal talkers.

A Pearson product-moment correlation coefficient was computed to assess the relationship between listeners' "normal" and "not normal" categorizations and ratings of speech acceptability. The correlation of +0.97 between these variables shows that as speech became more acceptable, the number of listeners responding "normal speaker" increased. This finding emphasizes the marked similarity of the listeners' behavior on the two perceptual tasks used here and suggests that judgments of speech acceptability may be based on a perceptual model of normalcy.

The reasons listeners gave for classifying alaryngeal speakers as nonnormal speakers are summarized in the Appendix and provide a basis for identifying the specific vocal attributes listeners perceived as abnormal. The most frequent complaint in response to esophageal speech was that its quality did not sound normal. Not surprisingly, disturbances in speaking rate and vocal pitch were the next most frequent reasons given for perceiving esophageal speech as abnormal. The almost unanimous complaint in response to the Bell electrolarynx speaker was that his speech sounded mechanical. In addition, his voice quality was not normal and his voice was monotonous. Nonnormal voice quality was

TABLE 1. Comparisons between speech acceptability ratings of normal, esophageal, and artificial larynx speech.

Speaker Groups	Mean Values	Mean Difference	Approx. df	Multiple Comparisons
Normals vs Esophageal	5.48 vs 2.54	2.94	9	$t' = 13.435$*
Normals vs W. E. Reed and Bell Electrolarynx	5.48 vs 1.59	3.89	8	$t' = 18.850$*
Normals vs Tokyo Artificial Larynx	5.48 vs 3.62	1.86	7	$t = 3.109$**
Esophageal vs W. E. Reed and Bell Electrolarynx	2.54 vs 1.59	0.95	6	$t' = 9.029$*
Tokyo Artificial Larynx vs Esophageal	3.62 vs 2.54	1.08	4	$t = 4.879$*
Tokyo Artificial Larynx vs W. E. Reed and Bell Electrolarynx	3.62 vs 1.59	2.03	2	$t = 18.579$*

*$p < 0.01$.
**$p < 0.05$.

also identified as the chief disturbance of speech produced with the Western Electric reed larynx. In addition, listeners indicated that speech produced with this reed larynx was too slow and sounded mechanical. The most frequent reasons given for Tokyo artificial larynx speech not sounding normal were that vocal pitch was too low, speaking rate was too slow, and the speech sounded mechanical.

DISCUSSION

The listener preferences described here provide useful information about the ultimate acceptability of various forms of alaryngeal speech. Superior esophageal speech was significantly more acceptable than speech produced by highly competent users of the Western Electric reed larynx and the Bell electrolarynx. This finding is in agreement with the work of Crouse (1962) and Snidecor (1968) which showed that esophageal speech was preferred over speech produced with an electrolarynx, but is in conflict with Hyman's (1955) conclusion that speech produced with a reed-type artificial larynx is more acceptable than esophageal speech. It is difficult to resolve this discrepancy, since the speaking proficiency of Hyman's (1955) subjects (good or effective) differed from the superior proficiency of the subjects used in the present experiment. These differing results point strongly to the need to define and equate the speaking proficiency of subjects to be compared.

The listeners' responses to Tokyo artificial larynx speech were particularly interesting. Speech produced with this instrument was judged significantly more acceptable than all other forms of alaryngeal speech studied. Unlike other forms of alaryngeal speech, a disturbance in voice quality did not emerge as the chief reason listeners cited to indicate that Tokyo artificial larynx speech did not sound normal (see Appendix). In our opinion, the more normal voice quality produced with this device was, in large part, responsible for Tokyo artificial larynx speech being judged more acceptable than other forms of alaryngeal speech.

ACKNOWLEDGMENT

This research was supported by the Delaware County Cancer Society, Muncie, Indiana. James Norton and Harry Brittain provided biostatistical consultation. Recordings of normal speakers were made available to us by William Ryan, University of New Mexico. Reprint requests should be directed to the authors at their current address, Department of Audiology and Speech Sciences, Purdue University, West Lafayette, Indiana 47906.

REFERENCES

CROUSE, G. P., An experimental study of esophageal and artificial larynx speech. Master's thesis, Emory Univ. (1962).

DIEDRICH, W. M., and YOUNGSTROM, K. A., *Alaryngeal Speech*. Springfield, Ill.: Charles C Thomas (1966).

EBEL, R. L., Estimation of the reliability of ratings. *Psychometrika*, 16, 407-424 (1951).

FAIRBANKS, G., *Voice and Articulation Drillbook.* New York: Harper and Row (1960).

HOOPS, H. R., and NOLL, J. D., Relationship of selected acoustic variables to judgments of esophageal speech. *J. Comm. Dis.,* 2, 1-13 (1969).

HYMAN, M., An experimental study of artificial larynx and esophageal speech. *J. Speech Hearing Dis.,* 20, 291-299 (1955).

LAUDER, E., *Self Help for the Laryngectomee.* San Antonio, Texas (1972).

SHANKS, J. C., The use of the manufactured larynx for alaryngeal speech training. In S. Rigrodsky and J. Lerman (Eds.), *Therapy for the Laryngectomized Patient.* New York: Columbia Univ., Teachers College Press, 53-66 (1971).

SHIPP, T., Frequency, duration, and perceptual measures in relation to judgments of alaryngeal speech acceptability. *J. Speech Hearing Res.,* 10, 417-427 (1967).

SNIDECOR, J. C., *Speech Rehabilitation of the Laryngectomized.* Springfield, Ill.: Charles C Thomas (1968).

SNIDECOR, J. C., and CURRY, E. T., Temporal and pitch aspects of superior esophageal speech. *Ann. Otol.,* 68, 623-636 (1959).

SOKOL, R. R., and ROHLF, F. J., *Biometry.* San Francisco: W. H. Freeman (1969).

WELCH, B. L., On the comparison of several mean values: An alternative approach. *Biometrika,* 38, 330-336 (1951).

WEINBERG, B., and RIEKENA, A., Speech Produced with the Tokyo Artificial Larynx. *J. Speech Hearing Dis.,* 38, 383-390 (1973).

Received January 3, 1973.
Accepted August 13, 1973.

APPENDIX

Reasons Listeners Cited for Classifying Alaryngeal Speakers as Nonnormal Speakers*

Esophageal Speech

Quality does not sound normal (53%)
Speech too slow (32%)
Pitch too low (24%)
Speech sounds mechanical (21%)
Voice is monotonous (19%)
Pitch is too high (3%)
Speech is too fast (3%)
Other: breathing sounds funny (1%)
    jagged, hesitant (3%)
    sounds harsh (1%)

Bell Electrolarynx Speech

Speech sounds mechanical (95%)
Quality does not sound normal (50%)
Voice is monotonous (47%)
Speech is too slow (28%)
Pitch is too low (11%)
Speech is too fast (6%)
Pitch is too high (3%)
Other: produced by machine (3%)
    robot (3%)

Western Electric Reed Speech

Quality does not sound normal (68%)
Speech is too slow (32%)
Speech sounds mechanical (31%)
Voice is monotonous (25%)
Pitch is too high (13%)
Pitch is too low (4%)
Speech is too fast (0%)
Other: nasal (3%)
    intoxicated (3%)

Tokyo Artificial Larynx Speech

Pitch is too low (48%)
Speech is too slow (41%)
Speech sounds mechanical (41%)
Voice is monotonous (27%)
Quality does not sound normal (20%)
Pitch is too high (4%)
Speech is too fast (0%)
Other: too dramatic (4%)

*Values reflect the percentage of listeners citing a given category to explain their response of "not a normal speaker."

PART V

EXTRINSIC FORMS OF ALARYNGEAL VOICE AND SPEECH: SURGICAL-PROSTHETIC METHODS OF SPEECH RESTORATION

An obvious primary postsurgical rehabilitation objective for laryngectomized patients involves the restoration of oral communication. To date, speech rehabilitation of laryngectomized patients has been accomplished chiefly with the time-honored methods of esophageal speech or through the use of artificial larynges. Study of the articles in Parts I–IV of this readings text reveals that each of these time-honored methods is characterized by some functional liabilities.

In this final section, information is provided about a field of alaryngeal speech rehabilitation that is undergoing a renewed period of resurgence and the more recent history of surgical-prosthetic approaches to voice and speech restoration is reviewed. In these approaches, the laryngectomized patient produces voice and speech by relying upon surgically created structures developed specifically for the purpose of voice production. All methods discussed in this section are also characterized by functional liabilities and all have one common feature—the surgical reconnection between the pulmonary airway and the laryngectomized patient's vocal tract or new phonatory apparatus. For example, some of these methods seek to develop an air shunt, or connection, between the trachea and the esophagus or between the trachea and the pharynx (Conley, DeAmesti, and Pierce, 1958; Miller, 1967; Calcaterra and Jaffek, 1973; Taub and Bergner, 1973; Komorn, 1974; Sisson, McConnel, Longemann, and Yeh; 1975). Others seek to interpose both an air shunt and a mechanical voicing source between the trachea and pharynx (Weinberg, Shedd, and Horii, 1978). Finally, there is a method known as the Staffieri technique, in which a new mucosal-muscular neolarynx is created at the superior end of the trachea.

The originator of this technique is Professor Staffieri, an Italian surgeon, who has not published in English texts. However, Griffiths and Love (1978) and Vega (1975) provide adequate coverage of this topic.

Conley, DeAmesti, and Pierce (1958) describe the creation of a mucosal, or vein, tract developed to connect the posterior wall of the trachea with the esophagus. This tract serves as an air shunt and is used to power esophageal voice with pulmonary air. The more recent work of Calcaterra and Jafek (1971) and of Komorn (1974) delineates a revision of the Conley procedure. Basically, a full-thickness, cervical esophageal wall flap is used to form a tracheo-esophageal air shunt.

Taub and Bergner (1973) describe a combined surgical-prosthetic approach to the problem of connecting the trachea and the esophagus. The surgical portion of this method involves completing a modified cervical esophagostomy, a procedure leading to the development of an opening between the esophagus and the outer neck. The prosthetic portion involves incorporating an air bypass device to connect the patient's pulmonary airway (stoma) and the surgically created opening. This combined approach enables laryngectomized individuals to use pulmonary air to power esophageal speech and voice. The second major form of combined surgical prosthetic form of speech restoration is described by Sisson, McConnel, Logemann, and Yeh (1975). In this case, a prosthetic air bypass device (the Northwestern prosthesis) is used to connect the laryngectomized patient's tracheostoma with a surgically created fistula in the upper neck.

Miller (1967) describes early experiences with a surgical approach to speech and voice restoration developed by the Japanese surgeon, Dr. Ryozo Asai. The basis of this technique is the construction of a dermal tube connecting the upper end of the trachea with the hypopharynx. Some speech characteristics of Asai speakers are described by Curry, Snidecor, and Isshiki (1973). Readers of these articles will readily discover that the source of voicing associated with the production of Asai speech is unknown.

By way of summary, all methods of surgical-prosthetic speech restoration discussed involve the surgical creation of a connection between the trachea and esophagus or hypopharynx (Conley, DeAmesti, and Pierce, 1958; Calcaterra and Jafek, 1973; Miller, 1973; Taub and Bergner, 1973; Komorn, 1974; Sisson et al., 1975). This connection serves as an air shunt that enables laryngectomized patients to power esophageal phonation with pulmonary air (Conley, DeAmesti, and Pierce, 1958; Calcaterra and Jafek, 1973; Taub and Bergner, 1973; Komorn, 1974) or to power an unspecified vibratory source with pulmonary air (Miller, 1973; Sisson et al., 1975). In view of this situation, speech produced by the methods should not be expected to exceed levels obtained by highly proficient esophageal speakers. These methods may enable patients to acquire voice and speech more rapidly, since the need to learn esophageal insufflation techniques is eliminated by virtue of their reliance upon pulmonary air.

In contrast to air-shunt methods, the surgical-prosthetic approaches to speech and voice restoration discussed by Vega (1975), by Griffiths and Love (1978), and by Weinberg, Shedd, and Horii (1978) enable laryngectomized patients to power newly formed vibratory sources with pulmonary air. Vega (1975) and Griffiths and Love (1978) highlight the techniques described by Staffieri. The Staffieri technique has attracted the attention of a number of American surgeons who are currently adopting this method of voice restoration. Basically, this method involves reconstruction of what Staffieri calls a "phonatory neoglottis" as part of total laryngectomy. Although this method has attracted world-wide attention in recent years, readers will soon realize that the belief that the surgically created "neoglottis" serves as a vibratory or voicing source remains undocumented.

Weinberg, Shedd, and Horii (1978) describe the reed-fistula method of speech, a surgical-prosthetic approach to speech rehabilitation for patients who have undergone extensive resection of the pharynx in association with total laryngectomy. The reed-fistula approach consists of interposing an external air bypass and pseudolaryngeal mechanism between the laryngectomized patient's tracheal stoma and a surgically created pharyngeal fistula. The pseudolarynx is a modified Tokyo artificial larynx mechanism (Weinberg and Riekena, 1973). This method differs from other approaches in that it is modeled on principles of normal speech production. Simply stated, the reed-fistula approach consists of developing an external larynx (voicing source) and incorporating this new mechanism into the patient's highly integrated speech production system.

Simpson, Smith, and Gordon (1972) describe four types of surgical reconstructions of the pharyngoesophageal segment. Speech and surgical specialists have often expressed the view that improvement in the rate and efficiency of voice reacquisition with esophageal phonation might be increased if consideration were given to surgically altering the morphology of the P-E segment following laryngectomy. Simpson, Smith, and Gordon (1972) describe just this and the results of their work should provide thought-provoking information to all readers.

The articles in Part V of the text provide information about a variety of surgical-prosthetic approaches to speech and voice restoration. The majority of these reports highlight the surgical-prosthetic techniques used to implement these methods, while the information about the speech characteristics effected is scanty. The observations support the hypothesis that functionally serviceable speech has been provided to some laryngectomized patients by each of these methods. Although this is true, each of the methods is characterized by some relative liabilities. Thus, as was the case for esophageal speech and speech powered by artificial larynges, surgical-prosthetic forms of speech are also not characterized by functional universality.

Although the articles in this section of the text indicate that it is possible, in some instances, to restore speech following laryngectomy on a surgical-prosthetic basis, the process of accomplishing this task involves attempting to find solutions to a number of difficult biomedical and speech-related problems. It is hoped that, in addition to providing information, the material covered in this section will serve to interest others in the problem of surgical-prosthetic voice restoration, to stimulate participation in this area of basic and clinical research and rehabilitation, and to highlight the need for continued interdisciplinary cooperation so essential to the improved ultimate quality of future rehabilitation of laryngectomized persons.

A New Surgical Technique for the Vocal Rehabilitation of the Laryngectomized Patient

John J. Conley, M.D.

New York, N.Y.

Felix DeAmesti, M.D.

(By Invitation)
Santiago, Chile

Max K. Pierce, M.D.

(By Invitation)
Los Angeles, Cal.

One of the most distressing aspects of the total laryngectomy operation is the loss of the ability to produce sound. The threat of the denial of this projectory capacity causes the patient confusion and depression. In his efforts to avoid this unhappy situation he has often delayed or even substituted an inferior method of treatment for his disease, and in some instances forfeited his life.

It is true that there are rehabilitative measures available in the use of the esophageal voice or mechanical appliances. The latter are cumbersome, and their substitution for the human voice is so inferior that few patients accept them. Technical improvements in these mechanical aids are badly needed and long overdue. The use of esophageal speech has been very effective in many instances, yet it requires considerable discipline and effort for months postoperatively, under the leadership of a vocal rehabilitationist. Some patients attain a high degree of proficiency in this method but many more are left with inadequate voice, and some are simply not rehabilitated. Forty per cent discontinue training against the advice of the therapist. The reasons for these failures are associated with the size and character of the wound relating to the excisional operation and the psychological determinations of the patient.

It was hoped that a new operation to supply adequate air easily for phonatory purposes would eliminate the "gulping" technique, and permit the patient to talk with ease. It is likely that this technique will prove to be more of a help in accomplishing a

From the Head and Neck Department, Pack Medical Group and the Surgical Service, St. Vincent's Hospital, New York, N.Y.

Prosthesis made by Joseph A. Salviolo, D.D.S., New York City, N.Y.

speech technique that a permanent part of the particular activity of speaking. It was recognized that this new voice would never attain the capacity of the natural vocal organ, yet the ease of speaking postoperatively might partially remove one of the serious disadvantages to the operation which has proved most effective against cancer of the larynx.

INDICATIONS

The vast majority of patients on whom vocal rehabilitation operations can be considered fall into the group where extirpation of the larynx and associated organs have been carried out for the treatment of cancer. This includes laryngectomies alone, or as part of the composite operations incorporating the lateral neck, pharynx, tongue and mandible. The new technique can be carried out at the time of the primary excision, or as a separate, secondary procedure. Individuals who have had the larynx destroyed by irradiation comprise a smaller group who can usually not be benefited by vocal rehabilitation operations.

Individuals who have been subjected to extirpation of the larynx and have not mastered esophageal speech, or adjusted to an artificial mechanism, and who desire speech development, may be considered for the rehabilitation operation.

THE PROBLEM

The technical problem to overcome consisted of creating a passageway that would permit the free flow of air from the trachea into the esophagus without the passage of food or saliva from the gullet into the trachea. The great inconvenience caused by an inadvertent small pharyngeal or esophageal fistula would unquestionably condemn any such uncontrolled communication. It was therefore conceived that the communication should provide the following principles:

1. It should be tubed, as a tunnel or flap.
2. The act of swallowing should close the tunnel automatically.
3. The tracheal air inlet should be 3 to 5 cm higher than the internal esophageal opening.
4. A muscle should be used to suspend the superior portion of the tunnel.
5. The main portion of the tunnel should be positioned in the narrowed area of the esophagus so that the passage of food or fluid through this area would enhance the collapse of the tunnel and prevent the ''fistula'' phenomenon.
6. The external opening should be easily adapted to the airway system so that exhaled pulmonary air could be directed into the gullet for phonatory purposes, without a complicated apparatus.

THE OPERATION

It is essential that adequate preparation for this operation be carried out in the experimental laboratory on dogs and cadavers. When the procedure is incorporated as part of the primary excisional operation of the larynx and associated tissues, a mucosal flap is

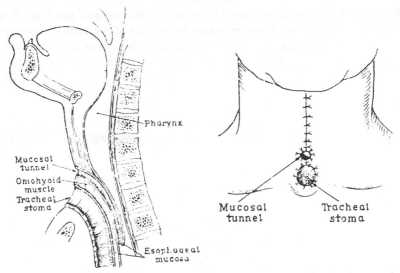

FIG. 1.   Mucosal tunnel opens just above tracheostome and extends inferiorly along esophagus.

FIG. 2.   One position for tunnel opening.

created along the anterior portion of the cervical esophagus. The dimensions of the flap are 1½ cm wide by 5 cm long. Its position may begin at the borders of the external wound of the cricopharyngeus or several centimeters lower in the esophagus, to accommodate the remaining mucosal pattern and also the tracheostome. The muscular element of the esophagus is not included in this flap. The flap is then tubed with No. 5-0 atraumatic chromic catgut over a No. 9 rubber catheter, with the mucosa forming the inside lining of the new tube. The lateral walls of the esophagus are approximated over this tube, thus forming a mucosal tunnel emerging from the lower anterior wall of the esophagus. The catheter remains as a stent in the tunnel for six weeks. It communicates with the esophagus below and with the external portion of the neck above. This catheter is tied off so that it will not leak. The superior portion of the tunnel is then fixed to a buttonholed aperture in the posterior part of the trachea, or sutured just above the tracheostome, according to the relative positions of these structures. A muscle sling or loop may be positioned under the upper segment of the tunnel in an attempt to assist in its compression upon swallowing. The omohyoid or scalene muscles were used for this maneuver. Three cases did not have the muscle sling and worked satisfactorily. The pharyngeal and neck wounds are closed in the routine manner following laryngectomy and excision of associated tissues.

The use of an autogenous anterior jugular vein has been used upon two occasions to create the communication of the tracheal air with the esophagus. This free graft is inserted in a tunnel in the adventitia of the anterior esophageal wall 5 cm long. At the inferior aspect of the tract the vein threaded over a No. 8 catheter perforates into the lumen of the esophagus. The superior segment of the vein graft is attached at the opening of the trachea or in the skin just above it. This vein graft is not in direct contact with the mucosal pharyngeal repair but approximately 2 to 3 cm below this critical area. The technical fea-

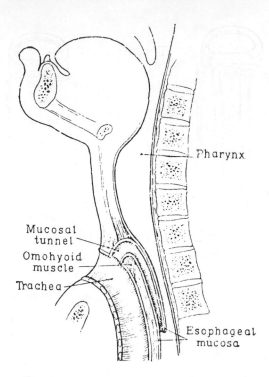

FIG. 3. Mucosal tunnel opens in trachea, extends upward then inferiorly. It is suspended on a neck muscle (omohyoid).

tures of the vein graft operation in this instance are much easier to carry out than the creation of the mucosal tunnel.

In individuals who have been given the opportunity to study hypopharyngeal or esophageal speech and have failed to rehabilitate their voices, and individuals who have had not only laryngectomy but unilateral or bilateral neck dissection, where normal vocal rehabilitation is considerably more difficult, a modification of the tunnel technique is applied. A free mucous membrane tubular graft approximately 5 cm in length is procured from the inferior buccal aspect of the oral cavity and tubed over an appropriate catheter. Full thickness supraclavicular skin has been used for the same purpose. By means of a puncture wound and stylet this free mucous membrane graft, or skin graft, is inserted into the space between the trachea and the cervical esophagus. It is threaded through this space inferiorly for a distance of approximately 5 cm. Under direct laryngoscopy it is perforated through the anterior wall of the cervical esophagus. The catheter is maintained in position for six weeks or longer if there is a tendency toward stenosis. The patient is fed with a nasogastric tube for the first four postoperative days.

After an interval of two weeks postoperatively, the patient can use the new esophageal tunnel to facilitate his speech rehabilitation. This is accomplished by the use of a specially adapted plastic tracheostomy tube with a superior connecting outlet over which a soft rubber tube can be fixed in order to fit into the new mucosal tunnel. The air stream

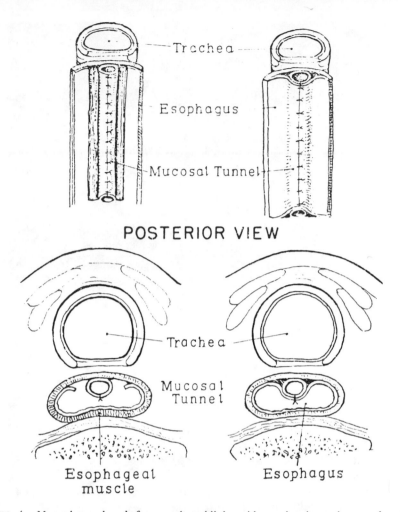

POSTERIOR VIEW

FIG. 4. Mucosal tunnel made from esophageal lining with openings in esophagus and trachea.

is directed by placing the finger over the external opening of the tracheostomy tube. This might be improved by the use of a flutter valve.

RESULTS

The technique has been carried out on fifteen patients, twelve primary procedures and three delayed procedures. Of the twelve primary procedures there were three technical failures, two stenosis of the tube and one fistual formation. It is believed that the stenosis resulted from removing the catheter stent after seven to ten days, thus permitting scar to close the tunnel. This caused no added inconvenience to the patient. The patient with fistula formation had been treated with irradiation prior to his laryngectomy. The fistula leaks intermittently when the patient takes liquids by mouth, but has not caused him enough inconvenience for him to request it to be closed, as a minor office surgical pro-

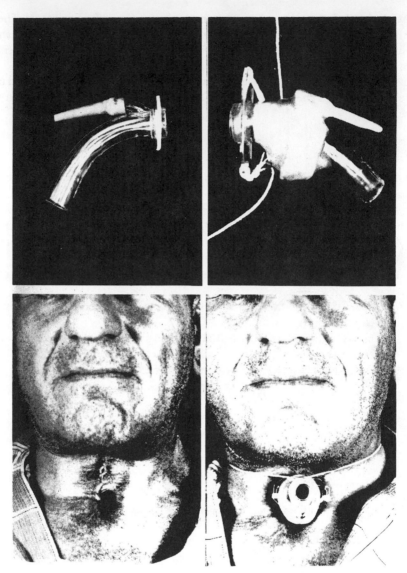

FIG. 5. Original plastic tracheostomy tube with tunnel adapter. This adapter is custom fitted to the size and angle of the mucosal tunnel.

FIG. 6. A. Airway adapter. B. Patient, showing controlled tunnel. C. Patient, showing adapter in position in trachea and tunnel.

cedure, for a period of over eighteen months. Two of the successful patients leaked a few drops as a result of pressure from a poorly adapted air tube connection. This improved when the curve and length of the tube was corrected. It is conceivable, however, that the delicate plastic tunnel could be destroyed by pressure and abuse from the adapter.

With simple instructions, patients can usually speak on the first effort. The quality of the voice is essentially that of pharyngeal or esophageal speech, with better air control and supply, and greater ease of production. It has assisted all in understanding esophageal speech techniques and in using the two methods in combination.

Four patients rarely use the tube now that they have become accomplished in esophageal speech through their own training. The presence of this tunnel is not an inconvenience.

CONCLUSIONS

1. A new surgical technique for the vocal improvement of the laryngectomized patient has been presented.
2. It consists of creating a mucosal tunnel through the wall of the cervical esophagus, causing a controlled communication between the trachea and gullet. The tube is constructed in such a manner that air can pass into the esophagus without the disadvantage of food and saliva passing onto the neck or into the trachea.
3. It is not a dangerous procedure and can be carried out with an acceptable margin of success.
4. There is an obvious and immediate improvement in the patient's adaptive capacity to the laryngectomized status.
5. It is hoped that this will stimulate thought in this neglected field with advancements in speech rehabilitation instruction and technical aids for these patients.
6. Results from the operative technique warrant further investigation.

Tracheo-Esophageal Shunt for Speech Rehabilitation After Total Laryngectomy

Thomas C. Calcaterra, MD, and Bruce W. Jafek, MD

Los Angeles

It is well established that if a vibrating column of air is introduced into the esophagus or pharynx, understandable speech can be formed by the oral cavity. Several methods of creating a tracheo-esophageal fistula have been attempted in the laryngectomized patient; however all have been beset by stenosis, aspiration, or both. An esophageal tube anastomosed to an opening in the trachea has been constructed in dogs to provide an air shunt. Stenosis is avoided by using a full-thickness esophageal flap, and aspiration is prevented by using a narrow lumen tube which runs upward from the esophageal opening. There has been no evidence of aspiration or shunt closure for one year.

For almost 100 years, surgeons have been confronted with the problem of providing a method of speech for the patient who has undergone laryngectomy. It was known as early as 1874 that if a communication could be established between the trachea and pharynx, intelligible speech could be restored.[1] Two major complications have beset all attempts to establish a tracheo-pharyngeal communication for speech production: aspiration of saliva and food and eventual stenosis of the communication.

Early attempts to maintain a tracheopharyngeal fistula employed mechanical devices. Gussenbauer[1] and Park[2] both designed a type of metallic tube extension that was inserted into a fistula to the pharynx and connected to the tracheostomy tube. During swallowing an obturator was placed into the pharyngeal extension to prevent aspiration. As with most exposed prosthetic implants, the problems of poor tissue tolerance, leakage around the prosthesis, and stenosis upon removal were never overcome.

In 1958, Conley et al[3] described a tunnel fashioned from esophageal mucosa which received a special air outlet device attached to the tracheostomy tube. He later modified this mucosal tunnel and inserted an autogenous vein graft.[4] He found that placing the trachea inlet above the esophageal outlet almost prevented aspiration, and attempts to fashion a muscular sling which would close the tunnel during deglutition were unnecessary. The voice produced, while essentially the quality of esophageal speech, was much better controlled and provided more words per phrase, since the vibrating air stream

Accepted for publication Feb 19, 1971.

From the Department of Surgery (Head and Neck), University of California School of Medicine, Los Angeles.

Reprint requests to Department of Surgery (Head and Neck), University of California School of Medicine, Los Angeles 90024 (Dr. Calcaterra).

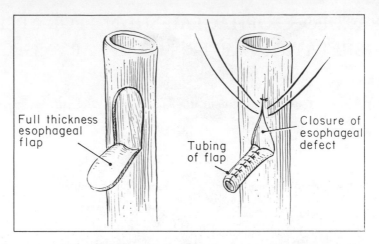

FIG 1.—Construction of the tracheo-esophageal air shunt using a full-thickness esophageal flap.

came during pulmonary exhalation as in normal speech rather than the air-gulping method of esophageal speech. In addition, the new voice technique could be learned almost immediately and thus did not require prolonged training with a speech therapist necessary for most candidates learning esophageal speech. The most distressing complication of this operation was a predisposition to stenosis. Even with placement of a small plastic catheter to preserve patency, many patients had closure of the lumen.

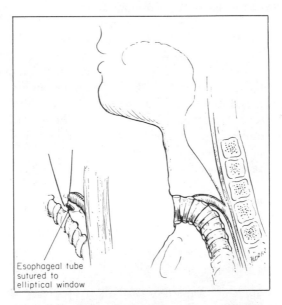

FIG 2.—**Left,** Anastomosis of the esophageal tube to a window in the membranous portion of the trachea. **Right,** Schematic sagittal view demonstrating relationship of shunt to esophagus and trachea following total laryngectomy.

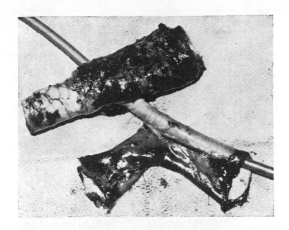

FIG 3.—Excised segments of trachea and esophagus demonstrating shunt with indwelling catheter.

Ogura et al,[5] in 1962, performed a direct mucosa-to-mucosa anastomosis of the trachea and pharynx in ten dogs. Although no scarring or stenosis of the anastomosis occurred, all dogs eventually died of aspiration pneumonia. They also attempted to create a laryngeal substitute with an artificial prosthesis, but regardless of the material used, every prosthesis was rejected by at most three months.

Asai[6] developed a subcutaneous skin-lined tube from the trachea to the oral cavity, a technique popularized in this country by Miller,[7] who found the voice production early

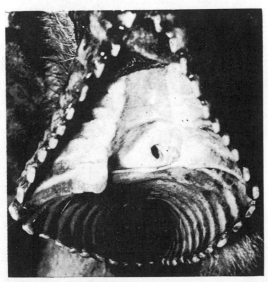

FIG 4.—View of trachea from above demonstrating upper orifice of shunt.

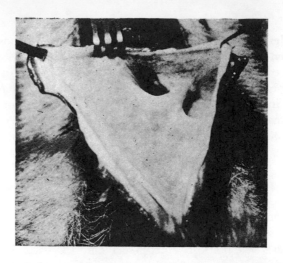

FIG 5.—View of esophagus demonstrating lower orifice of shunt.

in the postoperative period remarkably good. However, many patients were troubled by aspiration, and most of the tubes became obstructed by either hair growth or scarring. This operation was not advised in patients who had received preoperative irradiation because of the decreased healing capacity of the irradiated neck skin.

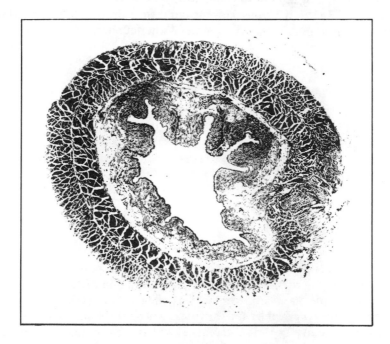

FIG 6.—Cross-section histomicrograph of tracheo-esophageal shunt demonstrating intact mucous membrane with no evidence of scarring or necrosis.

EXPERIMENT

An air shunt was designed specifically to avoid the problems of stenosis and aspiration. Stenosis was avoided by using a 4½ cm × 2½ cm full-thickness cervical esophageal wall flap which was tubed and sutured end-to-side to a fenestra excised in the membranous portion of the trachea (Fig 1 and 2). A two-layer mucosa-to-mucosa anastomosis was accomplished using fine chromic and silk suture, and the resultant esophageal defect was closed in a similar manner. Aspiration was prevented by running the tube upward about 4 cm from the esophageal opening and constructing a narrow lumen tube which would remain collapsed and perhaps close by esophageal muscular contraction during peristalsis.

This procedure was carried out in ten dogs who have been followed for as long as one year. One animal died from a massive wound infection, leaving nine available for study. The surgical technique presented no problems in execution and was completed in about 45 minutes without special instruments. Only local tissues were used, and no prosthetic or transplanted tissues were necessary other than a temporary indwelling silicone rubber (Silastic) stent which was used in the first five animals. The larynx was preserved because laryngectomy is so poorly tolerated in dogs.

RESULTS

The dogs were fed orally on the fifth postoperative day, and all tolerated feedings without apparent aspiration. The shunt was evaluated during the fourth postoperative week by esophagoscopy and bronchoscopy, and several dogs were killed at periodic intervals to determine patency of the shunt and to observe the lungs for evidence of aspiration. In all dogs the shunts were found to be patent (Fig 3 to 5) and no evidence of aspiration pneumonia was seen on gross or microscopic examination of the lungs. Serial sections of the shunt showed a healthy mucous membrane lining the shunt and no evidence of tissue necrosis or scarring (Fig 6).

Several special studies were carried out to determine the functional status of the shunt. A cine-esophagram was performed, and although a small amount of barium was seen to enter the esophageal end of the shunt, no barium reached the respiratory tract. Since these studies were performed with the dog in the usual horizontal stance, it is assumed that humans in a vertical stance will show even less tendency for spill into the trachea.

COMMENT

This tracheo-esophageal shunt affords at least two sources for potential vibration of the air stream—the vibrating characteristics of the shunt itself and the cricopharyngeal inlet of the esophagus. Conley et al[3] assumed that with their air tunnel the primary vibrating source was the cricopharyngeal inlet and thus the character of the voice produced was similar to esophageal speech. Asai[6] and Kitamura et al[8] have shown that their dermal tubes have inherent vibratory characteristics which depend upon the length, lumen diameter, and tension on the tube. Although the vocal frequency range was considerably narrower than normal, loudness and pitch could be controlled by variation of the expiratory air pressure. In general, the voice was loud and low with a wide fistula, and soft and high for a narrower one. The mechanism of phonation was considered to be the vibration at the edges of the pharyngeal opening; this was confirmed by roentgenographic studies and indirect laryngoscopy. Kitamura and associates found that the best internal diameter of the dermal tube was 5 mm, and the optimal configuration of the pharyngeal opening was ellipsoidal.

Studies of the vibratory characteristics of the tracheo-esophageal shunt have been carried out, and results will be presented in a subsequent report. Using air-flow rates of 2 to 10 liters/minute, a direct correlation was found between increased flow rate and increased pitch; similarly, increased tension on the shunt also raised the pitch. The average fundamental frequency was 300 cps at 6 liters/second air-flow rate, the usual flow rate for human speech.

In an attempt to improve the vibratory or reed characteristics of the shunt, a bivalving technique was used (Fig 7). Before the esophageal flap was tubed, two narrow strips of mucosa were shaved longitudinally along the flap. These were approximated with fine chromic suture and the shunt completed in the usual manner. On postmortem examination, the double lumen shunt was found to be patent, as demonstrated in the histomicrograph (Fig 8).

We have limited our study to research animals to allow full experience for technical problems that might be encountered in humans. The operation also has been carried out on fresh cadavers and found to be technically feasible. The human esophagus is somewhat smaller in circumference than the esophagus of a large dog, but this operation has

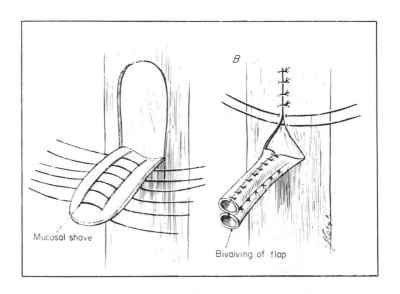

FIG 7.—Construction of bivalve shunt utilizing linear shaves of esophageal flap mucous membrane.

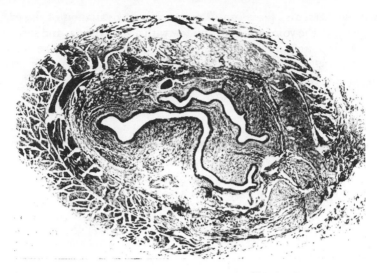

FIG 8.—Cross-section histomicrograph of bivalve shunt.

been performed in small dogs with no evidence of esophageal stenosis. The proposed shunt will be outside the primary field of preoperative irradiation.

When the patient with the tracheo-esophageal shunt desires to speak, he will simply place his finger over the tracheostoma and exhale. A controlled stream of air will pass via the shunt and esophagus to the oral cavity where words can be formed.

REFERENCES

1. Gussenbauer C: Über die erste durch Th. Billroth an Menschen ausgeführte Kehlkopf-Exstirpation, und die Anwendung eines künstlichen Kehlkopfes. *Verh Deutsch Ges Chir,* 1874, p 250.
2. Park R: A case of total extirpation of the larynx. *Ann Surg* 3:28–38, 1886.
3. Conley JJ, De Amesti F, Pierce MK: A new surgical technique for the vocal rehabilitation of the laryngectomized patient. *Ann Otol* 67:655–664, 1958.
4. Conley JJ: Vocal rehabilitation by autogenous vein graft. *Ann Otol* 68:990–995, 1959.
5. Ogura JH, Shumric DA, Lapidot A: Some observations on experimental laryngeal substitutions in laryngectomized dogs. *Ann Otol* 71:532–550, 1962.
6. Asai R: A new voice production method: A substitution for human speech. Read before the eighth International Congress for Otolaryngology, Tokyo, 1965.
7. Miller AH: First experiences with the Asai technique for vocal rehabilitation after total laryngectomy. *Ann Otol* 76:829–835, 1967.
8. Kitamura T, Toshio K, Kiyoshi T, et al: Supracricoid laryngectomy. *Laryngoscope* 80:300–308, 1970.

VOCAL REHABILITATION IN THE LARYNGECTOMIZED PATIENT WITH A TRACHEOESOPHAGEAL SHUNT

ROBERT M. KOMORN, M.D.

HOUSTON, TEXAS

SUMMARY — A tracheoesophageal shunt was used for vocal rehabilitation in 29 laryngectomized patients. Twenty-three patients had the shunt constructed at the time of laryngectomy. Radiation therapy or radical neck dissection did not limit the usefulness of the shunt. Twenty of the 29 patients acquired useful speech (69%). T-E shunt speech equals or exceeds other forms of alaryngeal speech when measured against the parameters of rate, duration, and intelligence. Failure to acquire useful speech occurred in nine patients because of either stenosis of the shunt (10%), aspiration (7%), or wound problems (14%). Stenosis of the shunt was primarily a problem in patients who received postoperative radiation therapy without a stent in the shunt. Wound problems were related to either our previous use of a lateral based flap or diabetes mellitus. Since January 1973 there has only been one failure in fourteen shunts constructed. The technique as now used is simple, applicable in a wide variety of clinical situations and associated with a low incidence of complications.

Any surgeon who has had to remove a larynx in a vigorous, energetic patient and then sees that patient become depressed, despondent, and withdrawn because of lack of speech, understands the need for rapid vocal rehabilitation. Providing this vocal rehabilitation by a surgical procedure which reconnects the pulmonary air supply to the hypopharynx in a manner that duplicates the vocal function of the larynx has intrigued and tantalized generations of surgeons.[1-7] In order for any surgical vocal rehabilitation technique to be considered successful, it must satisfy several important requirements. Technically, the connection must be easy to construct, preferably in one stage, applicable in a wide variety of clinical conditions, not contraindicated by radiation therapy, and relatively permanent in that stenosis or plugging of the connection by keratin debris is not a major problem. Physiologically, aspiration of any clinical significance should not occur, and the speech produced should equal or exceed the speech produced by nonsurgical methods. The procedure, obviously, must also work in the majority of patients and it must also be relatively safe in that if it does fail or complications develop, there is no significant increase in morbidity or mortality.

After almost three years' experience with a tracheoesophageal shunt, we feel that this technique meets most of these requirements. The tracheoesophageal shunt is a modern day improvement on the diathermy needle tracheo-hypopharyngeal fistula technique described by Guttman in 1935.[2] It was reintroduced in its present form by Calcaterra and Jafek.[6]

SURGICAL TECHNIQUE

The shunt is constructed from a full thickness, inferiorly based, esophageal mucosal flap that is developed either at the time of laryngectomy or as a one-staged procedure subsequent to laryngectomy if nonsurgical vocal rehabilitation has not been achieved. There have

From the Department of Otorhinolaryngology and Communicative Sciences, Baylor College of Medicine and the Veterans Administration Hospital, Houston, Texas.

Presented as part of a panel on Vocal Rehabilitation Following Laryngectomy at the meeting of the American Laryngological Association, Palm Beach, Florida, April 26-27, 1974.

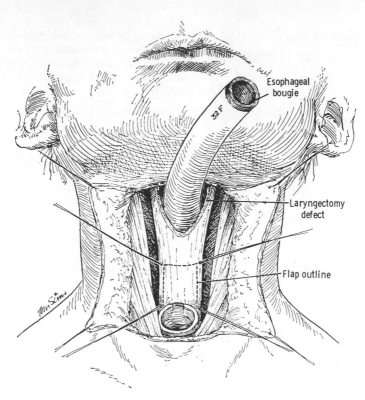

Fig. 1. Methylene blue and silk stay sutures outlining a 2½ x 5 cm full thickness inferior based esophageal flap. A bougie inserted either through the mouth or through the hypopharyngeal defect present at the time of laryngectomy stabilizes the esophagus.

been several minor changes in the technique since our previous reports.[7,8]

We now begin construction of the shunt by outlining and stabilizing the esophagus with a 32 or 34 F esophageal bougie. A flap, measuring 2½ x 5 cm, based inferiorly and placed in the center of the anterior wall of the esophagus, is outlined with stay sutures and methylene blue dye (Fig. 1). This flap design was used in 26 of the patients. An oblique flap was used in three patients but is no longer recommended. Placing the flap high in the cervical esophagus but not compromising the final inferior position of the shunt in respect to the trachea, appears to result in better speech. When the shunt is constructed as part of the laryngectomy procedure, a 2 cm margin is maintained between the superior edge of the flap and the hypopharyngeal defect.

After the flap is cut, a tracheal meatus for the shunt is formed from a 1½ cm horizontal incision in the middle of the posterior wall of the trachea. The incision is placed 2 cm below the distal end of the trachea. A single layer of submucosal interrupted 3-0 dexon sutures is used to accurately approximate the mucosa of the flap to the tracheal mucosa (Fig. 2). Before completing this end-to-side anastomosis, a 12 or 14 F catheter is inserted through the tracheal meatus and directed into the esophagus. The flap is then tubed around this catheter by using a continuous 3-0 dexon suture that begins at the superior end of the esophageal defect and runs up to the flap-trachea anastomosis (Fig. 3). The bougie is left in the esophagus during closure to help maintain the esophageal lumen and permit more precise mucosal approximation. A second layer of 4-0 silk is used to re-

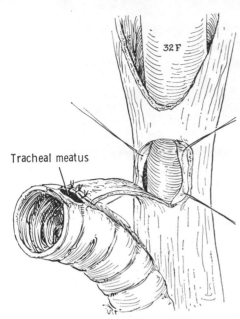

Fig. 2. Approximation of the flap to the posterior wall of the trachea with a single layer of interrupted sutures. The incision for the tracheal meatus of the shunt is horizontal, measures 1½ cm and is placed approximately 2 cm below the distal end of the trachea.

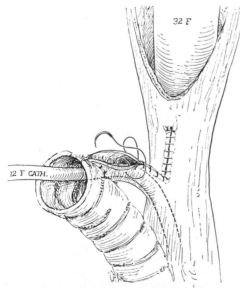

Fig. 3. After the flap to trachea anastomosis is completed, a catheter is placed through the meatus into the esophagus and the flap tubed around this catheter. A continuous Connell suture is used to close both the esophageal defect and tube the flap.

inforce this closure (Fig. 4). After 10-18 days, or when healing is complete and there is no crusting or raw surface around the shunt meatus, the indwelling stent is removed and speech training is begun.

CLINICAL MATERIAL AND INDICATIONS

Since 1971, this technique has been used 30 times in 29 male patients between the ages of 42 and 69. One patient had a second shunt constructed 28 months after the first shunt stenosed while he was receiving planned postoperative radiation therapy. The main indication for the procedure was that the patient either required a total laryngectomy, with or without a radical neck dissection, or was not vocally rehabilitated after a previous laryngectomy. Twenty-three shunts were constructed at the time of laryngectomy, and seven were constructed 4 to 77 months after laryngectomy. Four patients had a widefield laryngectomy and 25 patients had an ipsilateral radical neck dissection with the laryngectomy. There were no bilateral radical neck dissections in this group. Radiation therapy with a minimum dose of 5000 rads was used in four patients preoperatively and in nine patients postoperatively. Postoperative radiation was begun 2-4 weeks after surgery and is part of our approach to the management of advanced laryngeal cancer. The fields included the area of the shunt in one preoperative and all nine of the postoperative patients. We did not construct a shunt in any patient where a laryngectomy was done solely for palliation of advanced disease. We also had a firm requirement that the patients understood and accepted the risk of this new procedure. Diabetes, cardiovascular or pulmonary disease, if controlled medically, were not initially considered to be limitations.

RESULTS

Twenty-four of twenty-nine patients (83%) spoke 8-44 days after the shunt was constructed, but only 20 patients (69%) have retained shunt speech. The patient who had the second shunt constructed after the first one stenosed is

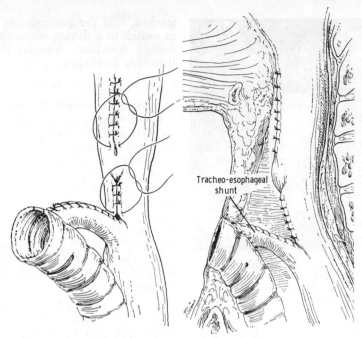

Fig. 4. A second layer of interrupted silk sutures reinforces the continuous suture closure. The hypopharyngeal defect is closed after the shunt is completed (left). Appearance of the completed shunt showing its inferior position in relation to the meatus in the trachea (right).

only counted once in these results because it is too soon postsurgery to analyze the outcome of the second procedure. Speech is produced by having the patient cover the tracheal stoma while exhaling.[†]

Speech quality depends on many variables including education levels, previous dialectic patterns, and the proficiency of coordinating stoma coverage with expiration. All our patients benefited from instruction and practice sessions with a speech pathologist. When measured against the parameters of duration, rate and intelligibility, T-E shunt speech equals or surpasses other forms of vocal rehabilitation (Table I).[9] Mean duration of sustained /a/ and counting with one breath surpasses asai[10] and

TABLE I

COMPARISON OF T-E SHUNT SPEECH

	T-E Shunt	Asai[*]	Esophageal	Air Bypass
Mean Sustained /a/	7.20 sec (N = 8)	7.34 sec (N = 5)	2.37 sec + (N = 30)	—
Mean Counting/Breath	34 (N = 8)	17 (N = 5)	8 [*] (N = 7)	—
Mean Rate (WPM)	133 (N = 8)	133 (N = 5)	117 ++ (N = 5)	141 [**] (N = 6)

　 [*] Adapted from Snidecor (1969)
　 + Adapted from Berlin (1969)
　 ++ Adapted from Snidecor (1955)
　 [**] Adapted from Blom (1972)

[†] Brief movie illustrating T-E shunt speech was presented at this point.

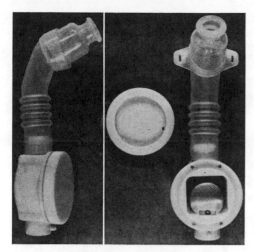

Fig. 5. Modified air bypass device wih a silastic tracheal connector (left). Adjustable valve mechanism that closes with rapid or forced expiration permitting the air to enter the hypopharynx via the T-E shunt.

esophageal speech.[11] The rate is essentially equal for T-E shunt, asai[11] and air bypass (voicebak) speech.[12] All these methods have a better rate than esophageal speech.[13]

The median score for intelligibility as tested by the Black and Haagen Multiple Choice Intelligibility Test was 82% in eight shunt speakers.[9] Six of the eight scored above 75% and three of these six were above 90%.[9] Blom[12] has reported intelligibility scores of 90% for air bypass (voicebak) speakers. Excellent esophageal speakers usually score between 60-80%.[14]

Recently we have tried to overcome the disadvantage of the patient's having to use one hand to talk by modifying the air bypass* device for T-E shunt use. Theoretically, the valve mechanism would be activated by rapid expiration and the air forced back into the shunt in the same manner that occurs when the trachea is covered with a thumb or forefinger (Fig. 5). It has not received wide acceptance by our patients. The main drawbacks are that it causes tracheal irritation, is difficult to seal in the

trachea, and the patients are reluctant to switch to a device when they can so readily produce speech with their thumb or forefinger.

DISCUSSION

Stenosis or aspiration have not been major problems in our experience with the T-E shunt. Stenosis, where the shunt becomes completely occluded and nonfunctional, occurred in one of 17 patients who received no radiation, none of four patients who received preoperative radiation, and in the first two of eight patients who received postoperative radiation. Since we began using an indwelling catheter during postoperative radiation two years ago, the remaining six patients in this group have not had stenosis.

Relative stenosis has occasionally occurred in our patients. By this, we mean either difficulty in initiating speech if the shunt has not been used for several hours, or the necessity to strain or use excessive force to initiate speech. This problem was frequently overcome by having the patients occasionally dilate the shunt with a catheter or sleep with the catheter in place for several additional weeks or until the shunt stabilized. Two patients appeared to be developing a stricture at the tracheal meatus of the shunt, but surgical revision of the meatus corrected this problem. It is important to be aware of this problem of relative stenosis in the immediate postoperative period. Close follow-up of the patients and aggressive use of dilatation or revision of the meatus will prevent permanent stenosis and results in better speech.

Aspiration does not occur with solid foods, but did appear with liquids in 14 patients. In six patients it was asymptomatic and only presented as a small drop of moisture at the meatus of the shunt. In eight patients, five of whom had a documented hiatus hernia, it was symptomatic in that it either was esthetically annoying or caused coughing. Cinefluoroscopic studies suggest that

* La Barge, Inc., St. Louis, Mo.

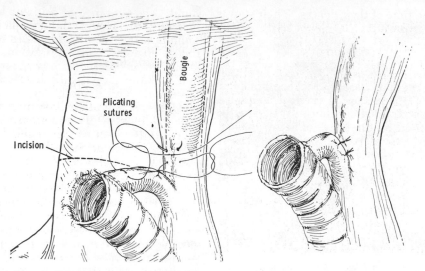

Fig. 6. Plicating nylon sutures (2-3) used to narrow the lumen of the shunt and shift the shunt upward and backward. The esophageal bougie is reinserted during the revision (left). Completed revision showing the changed angle of the now narrowed T-E shunt (right).

this is a reflex phenomenon and not direct entrance of fluid into the shunt.[7] All eight of the symptomatic patients had the shunt revised. The revision is accomplished under local anesthesia. The shunt is tightened with several plicating sutures of interrupted 3-0 nylon and shifted upward and backward by anchoring these sutures in fibrous tissue near the esophagus (Fig. 6). Six of the eight patients had elimination of the aspiration by this technique. In the two patients that had persistent symptomatic aspiration after revision, the shunt was closed at their request by simply oversewing the meatus under local anesthesia in the office. Useful speech was present for several weeks in one of these patients and for over a year in the other. In no instance, even in the two patients who had their shunt closed, has the asymptomatic or symptomatic aspiration caused weight loss, tracheitis, pneumonia or pulmonary complications. It is also interesting to note that aspiration tends to decrease with time. Careful observation in the immediate postsurgical period will help determine which shunts should be revised.

Wound infection, cicatrix formation, and stenosis of both the trachea stoma and shunt meatus occurred in two of 26 patients who had the shunt constructed from a medial based flap. Both patients had diabetes mellitus. One also had significant arteriosclerosis and required a carotid endarterectomy and bilateral aorto-femoral bypasses two months after the shunt was constructed. Both of these patients had beginning speech but lost it when the scarring became significant enough that dilatation or revision surgery was not practical.

The only major complications or wound problems occurred in the three patients with a shunt constructed from the lateral based flap. One patient was free of problems but the other two had wound breakdown and fistula formation. Even though the shunt stenosed and the fistula closed spontaneously in both of these latter two patients, one of them had a severe esophageal stricture and died one year later of bronchopneumonia and rupture of a right lower lobe abcess. The other patient healed without an esophageal stricture and now uses excellent esophageal speech.

Two other patients in our series have died. Both had myocardial infarctions and no evidence of cancer or aspiration at the time of their deaths. Their shunts were working.

CONCLUSIONS

Our results have convinced us that the medial based tracheoesophageal shunt is a successful surgical technique for vocal rehabilitation. It satisfies the technical requirements of being an easy, one-stage procedure that can be used in a wide variety of clinical situations. Radiation therapy or radical neck dissections are not contraindications to its use. Stenosis only occurred in three of the patients, and since we began stenting the shunt during radiation therapy, have eliminated the cause for stenosis in two of the three patients.

The laterally based flap was originally conceived as a means of preventing reflux aspiration. It has failed, causing major wound problems in two of three patients. Aspiration, if it occurs in a symptomatic fashion, can best be corrected by revising the medially based

7800 FANNIN ST., HOUSTON, TEXAS 77025.

shunt. The presence of a hiatus hernia increases the change for symptomatic aspiration but we are unwilling to call this a definite contraindication. Our major wound problems have been limited to either the laterally based flap or in patients with diabetes and/or arteriosclerosis. We no longer recommend or use the laterally based flap and even though only two of our patients had diabetes, the occurrence of wound problems in both of these two patients make us feel that diabetes may be a contraindication. Again, it must be stressed that careful and close follow-up in the immediate postopetrative period must be done. Relative stenosis or aspiration can be effectively managed, and both problems usually resolve as the shunt matures or after revision surgery if revision is necessary. Overall, twenty patients (69%) have been successfully rehabilitated, and we have had only one stenosis and no major wound problems in the fourteen patients who had a shunt constructed since January 1973.

REFERENCES

1. Gussenbauer C: Uber die uste durch. Th. Billroth an menschen ausgefuhrte kehlkopf-erstirpation, und die anwendung eines kunstlichen kehlkopfes. Verh dtsch Ges Chir p. 250, 1874

2. Guttman MR: Tracheo-hypopharyngeal fistulization. Trans Am Laryngol Rhinol and Otol Society 41:219-226, 1935

3. Conley JJ, DeArnesti F, Pierce MK: A new surgical technique for the vocal rehabilitation of the laryngectomized patient. Ann Otol Rhinol Laryngol 67:644-655, 1958

4. Assai R: Laryngoplasty. J Japan Broncho-Esophagological Soc 12:1-3, 1960

5. Montgomery WW, Toohill RJ: Voice rehabilitation after laryngectomy. Arch Otolaryngol 88:499-505, 1968

6. Calcaterra TC, Jafek BW: Tracheoesophageal shunt for speech rehabilitation after total laryngectomy. Arch Otolaryngol 94:124-128, 1971

7. Komorn RM, Weycer JS, Sessions RB, et al: Vocal rehabilitation with a tracheoesophageal shunt. Arch Otolaryngol 97:303-305, 1973

8. Komorn RM: Surgical technique for vocal rehabilitation. Neoplasia of Head and Neck, Chicago, Illinois, Year Book Medical Publishers, Inc. (in press)

9. Malone P, Komorn RM: Speech rehabilitation following laryngectomy and construction of a T-E shunt. Presented at the American Speech and Hearing Association Annual Convention, Detroit, Michigan, 1973

10. Snidecor JC: Speech Rehabilitation of the Laryngectomy. Springfield, Illinois, Charles C Thomas, 1969

11. Berlin CI: Cinical measurement of esophageal speech III. J Speech Hear Disord 30:174-183, 1965

12. Blom ED, Baker OJ: A preliminary investigation of speech with an air bypass voice prosthesis. J Speech Hear Disord (in press)

13. Snidecor JC, Isshiki N: Air volume and air flow relationships of six male esophageal speakers. J Speech Hear Disord 30:205-216, 1965

14. Creech HP: Evaluating esophageal speech. J Speech Hear Assoc Virginia 2:13-19, 1966

AIR BYPASS VOICE PROSTHESIS FOR VOCAL REHABILITATION OF LARYNGECTOMEES

Stanley Taub, MD

New York, New York

Lloyd H. Bergner, MD

New York, New York

The loss of speech after a laryngectomy procedure constitutes a severe functional and social impairment that is not easily overcome. Existing electronic speech appliances have not achieved the desired goal of providing a natural, trouble-free source of speech [1]. Recent surgical technics for vocal rehabilitation as described by McGrail and Oldfield [2], Asai [3], and Montgomery and Toohill [4,5] have not eliminated the distressing problem of aspiration and fistula tract stenosis. The results of our efforts after five years of basic and clinical research have led to the development of a voice prosthesis and surgical technic that have four uniquely important features: (1) the surgical procedure is single stage; (2) in most cases the need for finger control of speech is eliminated; (3) the problem of aspiration is eliminated because there is no direct internal passage from the esophagus to the trachea; and, most importantly, (4) the procedure restores effortless speech without any training. This work was first described in a preliminary study relating our experiences with eight patients [6]. Two of these patients, who have been using the devices for more than two years, are followed up in this report.

Since then the device has been installed in twelve other patients whose case studies will be presented. The voice prosthesis herein described requires no external power supply other than the patient's own respiratory system. Incorporating a unique bypass valve arrangement, it frees the user's hands during phonation, thereby eliminating a cumbersome problem that has always existed with a manual devices. The successful use of our prosthesis is dependent upon the creation of a cervical esophageal fistula placed above the clavicle anterolaterally in the lower third of the neck. The skin fistula is directed retrograde and enters the esophagus approximately 2 cm above the level of the tracheostome in a downward direction, thereby minimizing reflux salivary secretions into the neck area. The voice prosthesis is connected between the tracheostome and the fistula in a manner

From the Department of Surgery, New York Medical College, Flower and Fifth Avenue Hospital, New York, New York.

Reprint requests should be addressed to Dr Taub, 4 East 78th Street, New York, New York 10021.

Reprinted by permission from *American Journal of Surgery*, 1973, *125*, 748–756.

which will be described in the section *Clinical Methods*. During phonation, air flows from the lungs through the device into a tube that is inserted into the fistula, thereby gaining access to the upper esophagus. The flow of air over the esophageal mucosa in the area of the cricopharyngeus muscle provides a sound source that is articulated as speech. Once the device is properly installed, the patient begins to speak immediately.

In our preliminary report [6] emphasis was placed on the use of an external reed mechanism as a source of sound. Since then, we have learned that 95 per cent of laryngectomees do not require an external reed mechanism, but merely a source of pulmonary air to vibrate their own esophageal tissues. Indeed, patients were able to speak with a closed tube attachment from the tracheostome to the fistula. However, they soon experienced shortness of breath because there was no free flow of air during the aphonatory phase of respiration. The esophageal sphincter does not open involuntarily during respiration. To solve this problem it became mandatory to recognize that there are fundamental physiologic differences between breathing and speaking. Breathing occurs at relatively low resistance levels (from 7 to 15 cm of water pressure) whereas speaking occurs at higher resistance levels (from 22 to 40 cm of water pressure). Recognition of these variations in pressure led to the development of the air bypass valve. By automatically separating these functions, the air bypass valve was successful in permitting patients to breathe and speak without difficulty.

Laryngectomees were selected for this procedure on the basis of the following criteria: (1) no evidence of recurrent laryngeal cancer; (2) no evidence of pharyngeal or esophageal stricture on clinical and barium swallow examinations; and (3) positive psychologic motivation. They were rejected if they had previous bilateral radical neck surgery because of inadequate protection to the carotid vessels. Surgery was deferred if the skin in the proposed area of the fistula was indurated, inflamed, or markedly injected, or if there was evidence of radiation skin damage.

SURGICAL TECHNIC

The technic of the modified cervical esophagostomy is shown in Figure 1. A longitudinal incision paralleling the lower anterior border of the sternocleidomastoid muscle is carried deeply between the sternal and clavicular heads of the anterior sheath into the retroesophageal space. This incision is preferably made in the left side of the neck unless a radical neck dissection had been performed on that side. By means of a previously inserted Foley catheter the esophagus is exposed posteriorly and laterally. By maintaining pressure against the medial wall of the esophagus with the tip of a Kelly clamp, the esophagus can be immobilized. Stay sutures of number 3–0 chromic catgut are placed in the margins of an opening made into the lumen of the esophagus, wide enough to admit the tip of the fifth finger. This opening should be made approximately 2 to 3 cm above the level of the tracheostome. If the opening is made below this point, there is a chance that air will not flow freely upwards into the oral cavity but be forced into the stomach. The sternal head of the sternocleidomastoid muscle is severed and rotated over the carotid vessels for added bulk and protection, and sutured with number 3–0 chromic cat-

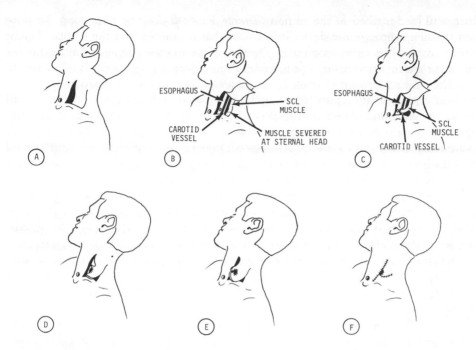

FIGURE 1.   A, a vertical incision is made, paralleling the anterior border of the sternocleidomastoid muscle. Adjacent skin flap is outlined, measuring approximately 7 cm in width and 9 cm in length. B, the esophagus is exposed and a small opening is made into the lumen as low as feasible. The superiorly based skin and platysma flap is raised from the lateral portion of the vertical incision. C, the sternal head of the sternocleidomastoid muscle is severed and rotated over the carotid vessels for added bulk and protection. It is sutured to the prevertebral fascia and to the esophagus, posterior to the margins of the fistula. D, suturing of the skin fistula to the posterior margins of esophagostoma is begun. E, with skin turned inwards, the skin flap is tubulated for approximately 4 to 5 cm. F, suture line shows appearance of wound at closure.

gut to the prevertebral fascia and to periesophageal tissue, posterior to the margins of the fistula.

A superiorly based skin flap (including platysma) is then raised from the lateral side of the original incision and sutured to the circumference of the esophageal opening with the skin surface inwards. The flap is approximately 9 cm in length and 7 cm in width. The tubulation of the skin flap is facilitated by inserting the bevelled tip of a number 26 Bardex nasopharyngeal airway into the esophagus in the downward direction. The tubing of the flap is carried for a distance of 4 to 5 cm, after which the skin of the medial edge of the longitudinal neck incision is drawn over the raw surface of the tubed flap and sutured to the skin edge of the inverted flap. The donor flap defect in the lower part of the neck is closed by local approximation of tissues, and it is facilitated by flexing the neck at the time of skin closure. Small dog ears may have to be excised from the upper and lower poles of the skin incision. Number 4–0 Dexon® is used to close the subcutaneous layer and interrupted number 4–0 nylon sutures are used to close the skin and number 3–0 chromic catgut sutures are used to perform the esophagocutaneous anastomosis. A

Hemovac is used postoperatively to minimize fluid and blood collection and is removed on the third postoperative day.

The Bardex tube is secured in the fistula by placing a neck band made out of 1/2 inch gauze attached to a rubber plug inserted into the flanged opening of the rubber tube. This tube is removed after ten days and is replaced with a new number 26 Bardex tube. The new tube, if it is well lubricated, should pass easily into the esophagus. If it does not, it may be necessary to reverse the angle of the bevel at the tip of the tube by cutting it and smoothing the edges with a medium grain emery. During the first three postoperative days the patient is fed a pureed diet by gravity drainage through a number 18 gauge Levin tube inserted through the fistula tube into the stomach. There may be some reflux leakage around the Bardex tube, but this is not cause for concern. On the fourth postoperative day, oral feeding may be started. If subcutaneous leakage of salivary secretions and oral feedings occurs through the suture line inferior to the external opening of the skin fistula, then nasogastric tube feedings should be resumed through the fistula tube until the leakage subsides. Antibiotics should be administered throughout the entire postoperative period. Sutures are removed from the eighth to the tenth postoperative day.

CLINICAL METHODS

An air bypass mechanism was designed by one of us (ST) for the purpose of allowing the laryngectomee to breathe, talk, and eat without having to remove or adjust the device. Made out of light plastic materials the air bypass mechanism is supported on the upper part of the chest by rubber connections to laryngectomy and fistula tubes. Inhalation and exhalation occur through the air bypass valve from a breathing port on its undersurface. (Figure 2.) During phonation a natural increase in breath pressure activates the bypass valve, allowing air to flow into the esophagus via the fistula valve and fistula tube. Breathing and speaking do not require finger control. However, an initial adjustment of the manual turn valve is necessary to achieve proper balance between the two functions during routine use. The bypass valve can be opened for greater air exchange as may be required during increased physical activity.

Installation of the Device

Installation of the device should not be attempted until after the third postoperative week, when wound healing is complete. With practice the patient can install the voice prosthesis in less than five minutes and it can be worn continuously for twelve to eighteen hours daily. The individual parts are assembled prior to insertion of laryngectomy and fistula tubes.

Installation at Tracheostomy Site

The sizes of the tracheostomal openings in laryngectomees usually vary from 10 to 16 mm (inner diameter). Standard stainless steel or silver-plated tracheotomy tubes are individually cut to proper length and fitted to a plastic angled connecting tube to which the prosthesis is attached. (Figure 2.) The inner tube is not recommended because it narrows

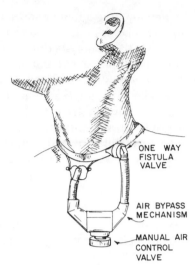

FIGURE 2. Inhalation and exhalation occur through the air bypass valve from a breathing port on its undersurface. During phonation a natural increase in breath pressure activates the bypass valve allowing air to flow into the esophagus via the fistula valve and fistula tube. Breathing and speaking do not require finger control. However, an initial adjustment of the manual turn valve is necessary to achieve proper balance between the two functions during routine use. Manual use of the device is optional.

down the inside diameter and contributes to the accumulation of mucus. Once installed, the laryngectomy tube is rarely changed during daily use. If the laryngectomy tube does not provide an airtight seal, an inflatable endotracheal cuff may be slipped over the tube with its distal portion overhanging the end of the metal tube. This also provides a shield for the tracheal mucosa against trauma during coughing. The endotracheal cuff may be inflated with 1 to 2 cc of water to provide an airtight seal.

For laryngectomees who cannot tolerate the insertion and maintenance of a laryngectomy tube, an overlying Silastic® rubber mold can be formed with an attachment for

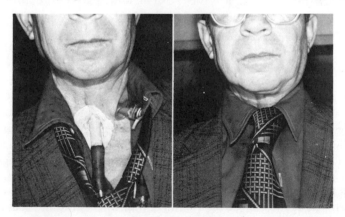

FIGURE 3. A, for laryngectomees who cannot tolerate the insertion and maintenance of a laryngectomy tube, an overlying Silastic plug can be molded with an attachment for the air bypass mechanism. B, satisfactory cosmetic appearance of patient wearing device covered by shirt and tie

the air bypass mechanism. (Figure 3.) Using a room temperature curing silicone rubber with an added catalyst, the liquid rubber is poured around a 1/2 inch right-angled hollow plastic tube that fits directly over the stoma. As the Silastic begins to cure, its shape conforms exactly to the skin contour peripheral to the stoma. When curing is complete, the rubber plug with its enclosed airway is removed and the edges trimmed. This plug can be sprayed with a Dow Corning medical grade adhesive ("B") and recemented over the stomal opening with the voice prosthesis attached. The cement remains tacky over a twenty-four hour period. If there is any hissing due to air escape beneath the rubber plug, gentle manual pressure over the Silastic will prevent this during phonation. The plug can be removed with the aid of an adhesive solvent before sleep and reapplied after cleansing in the morning.

Installation of Fistula Tube

It is important to maintain fluid-tight systems in the fistula; otherwise leakage will occur that can be a source of great annoyance to the laryngectomee, particularly during swallowing.

Two types of fistula tubes have been developed. The type I tube is a Bardex rubber nasopharyngeal airway number 26 to 28, approximately 1.5 inches in length with a 3/8 by 1 inch endotracheal cuff positioned over its proximal end (near the flange). The length of this tube can vary from patient to patient and is critical for adequate sound production. With the tip bevelled smoothly, a hinged rubber flap is cemented to the top end of the bevel to act as a flap valve. With this arrangement the external fistula valve can be completely eliminated. The flap prevents secretions from entering the tube lumen during swallowing. Leakage around the tube is controlled by inflating the endotracheal cuff with 1 to 3 cc of water to provide a snug fit within the fistula. The flanged tube is secured around the neck by means of a band. At night the cuff is deflated and the fistula tube is replaced by a narrower diameter tube (size 26) without an endotracheal cuff. This allows the fistula walls to contract in diameter.

The type II fistula tube employs the use of an inner flange worn inside the esophagus. The tube is not to be inserted until after the third postoperative week after satisfactory wound healing. The diameter of the flange is 2.5 cm and is sufficiently thin to allow easy insertion into the fistula. As the flanged portion of the fistula tube enters the esophagus, it opens. The high intraesophageal pressures exerted during swallowing force the rubber flange against the mucosa, thereby preventing leakage around the tube into the neck area. To maintain a good contact seal against the inner esophageal walls, the internal flange is pulled against the opening by slipping an outer flanged tube over the proximal end of the shaft of the fistula tube. This outer flange is snugged up against the external opening of the fistula, thereby sandwiching the fistula tract between both flanges. No neck band is required to support this tube. The arrangement is advantageous because it eliminates the need for an endotracheal cuff and prevents distention of the fistula tract. Its length is not critical as with the type I tube for optimal sound production. In fact, the use of such a tube has facilitated voice production in a patient who was unable to speak with the type I tube. The reason for success was that the inner flange acted as a bolster or support for patulous esophageal mucosa that caused obstruction to the flow of air near the source of vibration.

All but one of the patients currently using the device have been successfully fitted with an inner flanged tube; however, the cuffed fistula tube had been used for more than two years without causing any irritation to fistula and esophageal tissues. However, caution is recommended with the use of a cuffed fistula tube because of its tendency to cause dilatation of the fistula tract. In any case, periodic examination of the fistula walls is recommended to insure against irritation or erosion. At the present time an external fistula valve must be used with the inner flanged tube in order to prevent reflux of secretion from entering the tube lumen and contaminating the prosthesis. An internal valve mechanism is now being investigated for this purpose.*

Maintenance of the Air Bypass Voice Prosthesis

The air bypass valve and component parts may be disassembled and rinsed with warm water and peroxide to loosen accumulated mucus. The laryngectomy tubes with plastic and rubber connections are easily cleansed with a baby bottle brush. The plastic fistula valve can be opened and the rubber stem valve cleansed or replaced if the edges are frayed. Fistula tubes and endotracheal cuffs should be replaced when they show signs of deterioration. To prevent halitosis the entire prosthesis should be rinsed with a mouthwash solution prior to use. Before the laryngectomee is discharged he is instructed in the use of his device, its maintenance, and in the care of his fistula. If the air bypass mechanism should become defective, it can easily be replaced or it can be used manually by digitally occluding the breathing port during phonation. The air bypass valve, which functions twelve to eighteen hours a day during speech, has lasted for as long as six months without requiring any major repair.

Speech Production

There is no training required for speech production. Once the voice prosthesis is properly installed, the laryngectomee can begin to speak immediately. However, there is usually a short adjustment period required for accommodation to the device, its installation, and its use.

In one of our earlier cases, after the fitting of a voice prosthesis, speech could not be produced above a whisper. This was attributed to an unusually dilated esophageal sphincter at the level of the cricopharyngeus muscle or a paralyzed cricopharyngeus muscle. This was also demonstrated in patients who underwent laryngopharyngectomy with reconstruction of the upper esophagus and pharynx. For these patients, a mechanical reed of varying pitch can be incorporated into the air bypass mechanism as a source of sound.

CASE REPORTS

Case I

The patient (CG), a fifty-six year old businessman, underwent laryngectomy in October 1969. He was unable to learn any esophageal voice and used a writing pad for communi-

*Under a grant ("Clinical Investigation and Refinements in the Development of a Prosthetic Larynx") sponsored by the American Cancer Society.

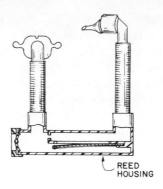

REED
HOUSING

FIGURE 4. Earlier reed-type device found to be impractical in patients with low cervical esophagostomy, who have a vibrating sound source at the level of the cricopharyngeus muscle.

cation. A right cervical esophagostomy was performed in May 1970. After an uneventful postoperative course, the patient was discharged on the fifth postoperative day. He was fitted with a reed type device (Figure 4) and was unable to produce speech. In spite of all attempts to improve the reed apparatus, phonation was impossible because intraesophageal resistance was too great to permit vibration of the reed. However, by merely blowing air into the fistula at a higher gradient of pressure than that required for normal respiration, the patient could speak easily. He could whisper at a pressure of 15 cm of water and speak with normal volume at 24 cm of water. Shortly thereafter, an air bypass valve was developed that allowed him to phonate without any manual finger control and permitted normal breathing between 5 to 14 cm of water. The patient has a normal speaking rate, can whistle, sing, shout, and count to 50 in one breath. After taking only two to three minutes to install the device, he wears it from twelve to fourteen hours a day and removes it only at night before sleeping. He has excellent control of fistula secretions and uses a cuffed fistula tube with an external fistula valve. He has spoken before the International

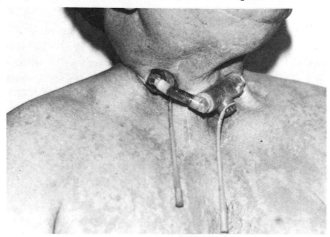

FIGURE 5. Case I. Patient using a custom-fitted air bypass mechanism. Note the two rubber tubes used to inflate the fistula tube cuff and the cuff of the laryngectomy tube to provide an air-tight seal.

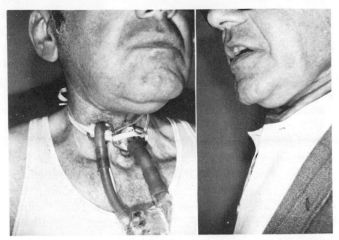

FIGURE 6.   Case III. A, patient has air bypass mechanism installed using a type I fistula tube. B, natural appearance after installation of prosthesis.

Association of Laryngectomees in 1970, where he received a standing ovation, and has been invited to speak publicly on many occasions since. The patient (Figure 5) is pleased with his new voice and has been using the air bypass valve over two and a half years.

Case II

The patient (DL), a fifty-seven year old steelworker, underwent laryngectomy in 1968, but was unable to learn esophageal speech. In May 1970, left cervical esophagostomy was performed. The patient's postoperative course was uneventful, and he was discharged on the fifth postoperative day. After installation of the newly developed air bypass valve, he spoke immediately. Because of a sensitive tracheostome, he could not tolerate the continual use of a laryngectomy tube. A molded Silastic plug with an airway and a connection for the air bypass valve was then tried. The patient found that the Silastic plug was very satisfactory, but he preferred a manual control device. By occluding the inhalation port digitally, the patient could direct air through a rubber side tube into the fistula. In addition to directing air flow for speech, finger pressure prevented leakage of air from beneath the Silastic plug into the neck area. Cementing the plug and inserting the fistula tube required only a few moments. This patient prevents leakage from the fistula by means of a short number 34 fistula tube with a rubber flap cemented over the distal end of the tube. The fistula tube is secured around the neck with a Velcroix band and is angled downwardly in the retrograde esophagostomy opening. The patient has been using the device successfully for more than two years and is quite independent, being able to make his own repairs. He communicates well on the job, where there is a great deal of noise, and his wife complains that he talks too much!

Case III

The patient (DR), a fifty-five year old salesman (Figure 6), underwent laryngectomy and left radical neck dissection in July 1970. Shortly thereafter he became acutely depressed over the disintegration of his family, business, and social life. Because of his progressive psychologic deterioration, it was decided to perform right cervical esophagostomy in November 1970. After installation of the bypass mechanism, the patient spoke without any difficulty. He was able to return to work and carry on his business activities in usual fashion. His speech was exceptional, very expressive, and with a normal range of inflection. He was able to sing and to modulate his speech for whispering or shouting, and he could count to 45 in one breath. In May 1971 he appeared on a local television program demonstrating his success with the device and told how it had dramatically improved his psychologic outlook. He had no problems with fistula leakage and managed secretions by means of a 1.5 inch fistula tube and a 3/8 inch endotracheal cuff inflated with 2.5 cc of water. The tube was deflated at night and replaced with a number 30 Bardex nasopharyngeal airway. Within four months of using the device he incidentally developed a very effective esophageal voice. However, in October 1971 symptoms of hemoptysis developed. A chest roentgenogram revealed a lesion in the apex of the right lung. His attending physician in Oklahoma performed lobectomy and the pathology report was positive for carcinoma with spread to mediastinal nodes. The patient died in the hospital during the second postoperative week.

Case IV

The patient (PC) is a fifty-four year old lumberman who performs daily strenuous physical activity outdoors. His larynx was removed in June 1970, after which he was unable to develop an esophageal voice. Right cervical esophagostomy was performed in January 1971, after which the patient was discharged on the fifth postoperative day. During the procedure, a solitary lymph node was removed for biopsy. The pathology report was squamous cell carcinoma. The family refused radical neck surgery and insisted that cervical esophagostomy be performed. Since then there has been no evidence of recurrent disease. It is interesting to note that this lymph node might never have been discovered or perhaps discovered too late had cervical esophagostomy not been performed. After installation of the air bypass mechanism, the patient immediately spoke with his usual Southern drawl. He now uses the device for sixteen hours a day, and although he has one arm, he can install it in less than five minutes.

Case V

The patient (GC) was a fifty-two year old autobody repairman, in whom carcinoma of the larynx developed in June 1967. A full course of radiotherapy was completed in August 1967. Recurrence was discovered in January 1968, necessitating laryngectomy and left radical neck dissection. A small fistula developed postoperatively that was closed in March 1969. After two years of unsuccessful esophageal voice training, the patient volunteered for right cervical esophagostomy, which was performed in December 1970. He was discharged on the seventh postoperative day and subsequently had the air bypass mechanism installed. Speech returned within moments. The quality of the speech was excellent. In addition to achieving normal volume, inflection, and speaking rate, he was able to sing a full octave. He was able to count to 40 in one breath. The patient works outdoors and uses the air bypass mechanism under strenuous physical and environmental conditions. For secretion control he uses an inner flanged tube and an external fistula valve. He is extremely pleased with the device.

Case VI

The patient (AJ), a moderately obese sixty-four year old man, underwent total laryngectomy and left radical neck dissection in 1963. He developed an esophageal voice that was low in volume and difficult to produce. Right cervical esophagostomy was performed in December 1970, and the patient was subsequently discharged on the fifth postoperative day. After installation of the device the patient was able to speak with much less effort and with greater volume. Subsequent to surgery, he had difficulty managing secretions. The cuffed fistula tube could not be retained because the fistula tract was extremely short and too medially placed. At that time, an inner flanged tube was unavailable for trial. Because of the progressive annoyance to the patient, we elected to close the fistula three months later.

Case VII

The patient (BW), a thirty year old man, underwent laryngectomy in October 1969. He achieved very good esophageal speech and was able to count to 6 on one air charge. However, he desired greater volume and complained of fatigue and indigestion with daily esophageal voice production. Left cervical esophagostomy was performed in October 1970 and he was discharged on the fourth postoperative day. After the air bypass mechanism was installed, an improvement in his voice was noted immediately. He could count to 40 in one breath, was speaking with greater volume, and experienced no fatigue. After several weeks, the patient began to complain of stomal irritation and objected to wearing anything around his neck. After several months, he rarely used the voice prosthesis and spoke with his own esophageal voice, using a plugged fistula tube with a cuff to control secretions. Seven months later the cervical esophagostomy was closed.

Case VIII

The patient (MA) had a severe cardiac condition. He underwent laryngectomy in September 1969. He was unsuccessful at learning esophageal speech and strongly desired to undergo esophagostomy. His cardiac status had stabilized over the previous six months and upon recommendation of his personal physician, cervical esophagostomy was performed in March 1971. After successful installation of an air bypass mechanism, the patient was able to speak, whistle, and count up to 20 in one breath. Shortly thereafter he began to experience tracheal irritation on insertion of the laryngectomy tube. He was gradually becoming more debilitated because of his poor cardiac status. Ultimately, it became too great an effort for him to install the prosthesis. For these reasons, the fistula was closed. While the fistula was open, secretions were managed successfully with the use of a number 28 nasopharyngeal airway replaced at night by a narrower tube to allow for contraction of the fistula.

Case IX

The patient (FM) was a salesman (Figure 7) who had had his larynx removed twenty-two years ago. He was unable to learn esophageal speech but developed expertise in the use of the Bell Electrolarynx. Right cervical esophagostomy was performed in April 1971. Postoperatively, an abscess developed beneath the skin-lined tube adjacent to the lateral skin

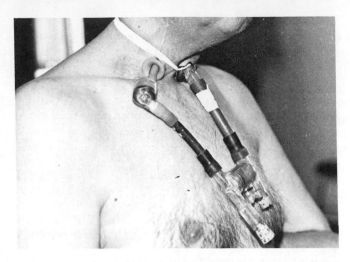

FIGURE 7. Case IX. Patient using the air bypass mechanism with an inner flanged fistula tube and external fistula valve.

flap from an infected hematoma. Wound healing was delayed by oral secretions into this area. Nasogastric tube feedings through the esophagostomy opening were instituted and continued for ten days, after which the abscess cavity healed. Subsequently the patient was fitted with an air bypass mechanism. His voice was immediately impressive. He could count to 50 in one breath and wear the device for sixteen hours. The patient thoroughly enjoys his new means of communication. Because of the previous infection, the skin-lined tube was more horizontal than retrograde. The patient had difficulty managing secretions with a cuffed fistula tube. This was greatly reduced with the use of an inner flanged tube and an external fistula valve.

Case X

The patient (HS) was treated by radiotherapy for carcinoma of the larynx and he subsequently underwent laryngectomy in July 1970. Having been unable to develop understandable esophageal speech, he underwent left cervical esophagostomy in March 1971. Postoperatively an abscess developed in the base of the skin flap, but it spontaneously drained. The cavity was packed with iodoform gauze, and the patient received esophagostomy feedings for approximately one week. Leakage under the flap stopped and the abscess cavity closed. Shortly thereafter he was fitted with an air bypass mechanism and spoke with great clarity within minutes. He wears the device for fourteen hours during the day and can install it in one minute. He counts to 50 in one breath and can sing anything. He is pleased with his new voice and has had excellent comments from co-workers and friends. He has successfully managed secretions from the fistula with a cuffed fistula tube and is able to use the voice prosthesis when working or engaged in any physical activity. (Addendum: It was recently learned that the patient developed recurrent cancer on the right side of the neck for which he was treated elsewhere. He subsequently died.)

Case XI

The patient (AP) is an accountant who had undergone laryngectomy in October 1970. He had no desire to learn esophageal voice and became proficient in the use of the Electrolarynx. He became dissatisfied with the mechanical quality of his speech and the fact that he could not speak in a whisper. In September 1971 he volunteered for left cervical esophagostomy and installation of the voice prosthesis. He is elated with his present voice, which he feels is equal to that of a highly trained esophageal speaker. He wears the voice prosthesis for eighteen hours daily and requires only two minutes to install it. Because of a cough-sensitive tracheostome he prefers the use of an overlying Silastic plug to support the air bypass valve. (Figure 3.) By exerting manual pressure over the cemented plug, he can effect an air-tight seal. He is able to count to 45 in one breath, and he can whistle and communicate normally. Fistula secretions are completely controlled by the use of an inner flanged tube and an external fistula valve.

Case XII

The patient (IP) is a retired Air Force Colonel who is presently self-employed as a salesman. He underwent laryngectomy in June 1971 for carcinoma of the larynx. Unable to learn esophageal speech, he managed to communicate with an Electrolarynx. Desiring a more natural means of communication, he volunteered to undergo cervical esophagostomy, which was performed in October 1971. Upon installation of the voice prosthesis, he began speaking; however, his speech was somewhat strained and he required more effort to produce a smooth flow of speech. Tensing of the cricopharyngeus muscle was noted upon direct observation with the Taub oral panendoscope [7]. After 5 mg of Valium® was given intramuscularly, the patient relaxed and his flow of speech improved. After a short period of adjustment, he was able to overcome this difficulty without medication. When he plays golf, he adjusts the air bypass valve for manual control. When speaking before groups or business meetings, he uses the automatic adjustment. Leakage is controlled by means of an inner flanged tube and an external fistula valve. He is very pleased with the voice prosthesis and rarely uses the Electrolarynx.

Case XIII

The patient (HH) is an employee of the Federal Aviation Agency as a flight service engineer. His job requires air to ground radio communication. After undergoing laryngectomy in February 1970, he developed poor esophageal speech. Fearing imminent loss of his job, he volunteered for right cervical esophagostomy, which was performed in October 1971. After an uneventful postoperative course, the air bypass mechanism was installed. At the present time, the patient is continuing in his job, having regained a highly acceptable means of communication. Secretions are controlled by a cuffed fistula tube with an internal flap valve and now recently with an inner flanged tube.

Case XIV

The patient (HL), a fifty-eight year old woman, underwent laryngectomy in July 1970. One year later recurrence developed in the left side of the neck and radical neck dissection was carried out. In April 1972 the patient underwent right cervical esophagostomy and she was discharged from the hospital after six days. After installation of the air bypass device, she immediately spoke with an excellent voice. Her speech had a completely normal range of inflection; she could shout, whisper, and sing. Her Southern accent was quite apparent (she had been born in Atlanta, Georgia). She does a great deal of laughing, talking, and counts to 45 in one breath. The patient wears the device for eighteen hours a day and has been promoted to a supervisory position as an instructor. Before the operation she was without oral communication and was forced to take a job that demeaned her intelligence. Her outlook on life is extremely bright and she states that no one takes notice of her new voice. Secretions are controlled by means of an inner flanged tube and an external fistula valve.

COMMENTS

Of the fourteen cases reported, three laryngectomees had their fistulas closed for the following reasons: (1) leakage related to a short, medially placed fistula (case VI); (2) a previous dependency on a very good esophageal voice and lack of motivation in the use of an external apparatus (case VII); and (3) progressive physical weakness and chronic tracheal irritation (case VIII). Two patients died (case III and X) due to recurrence of disease unrelated to the use of the prosthesis. Nine patients are currently using the device regularly.

We do not recommend this technic for patients who have achieved superior esophageal speech. Our most successful results were in patients who had no satisfactory means of vocal communication and who were psychologically well motivated. As described in the case reports, the speech produced is quite acceptable and is capable of a variety of modifications from extreme volume changes to fine modulations in frequency. These observations remain to be scientifically evaluated. In those instances in which patients are severely depressed because of social "excommunication" and loss of income, we recommend the use of this technic at the earliest opportunity.

Management of salivary leakage from the fistula was a problem in some patients; however, leakage has been practically eliminated by the use of the inner flanged tube.

SPEECH RESULTS

A recent research study [8] was designed to compare acoustical and perceptual features of six superior esophageal speakers with six untrained patients using the air bypass voice prosthesis. The speech of both groups was judged as to intelligibility and listener acceptibility. Loudness, ease of voice production, and pitch variability were not studied. The following conclusions were drawn: the data failed to show any significant difference between untrained speakers using the air bypass mechanism and highly trained superior esophageal speakers. The investigator believed that this information was highly significant since none of the speakers using an air bypass mechanism was able to learn esophageal speech. The obvious conclusion is that speakers using the air bypass voice prosthesis are as intelligible as highly trained esophageal speakers, although no training is required.

CONCLUSIONS

The results of efforts after five years of basic and clinical research have led to the development of an air bypass voice prosthesis and the refinement of a surgical technic that has several uniquely important features: (1) a single stage surgical procedure, low retrograde cervical esophagostomy, that is functionally and cosmetically feasible, since it permits hidden use of the device; (2) elimination of need for finger control of speech in most cases; (3) elimination of the problem of aspiration because there is no direct internal passage from the esophagus to the trachea; and, most importantly, (4) a natural speech mechanism without any training period.

Patients who are subjected to laryngectomy procedures suffer severe psychic trauma since they are deprived of a major line of communication with the world around them. We believe that the work accomplished here is valid and offers an opportunity in carefully selected patients to help restore the lost cord.

Acknowledgment

We would like to thank Dr Ronald Spiro for his initial contributions in the development of the surgical technic, Mr Elliot Eckhaus for his technical assistance during the earlier (HEW) phase of research, and Dr Walter L. Mersheimer and the Department of Surgery of the New York Medical College for their continued support. The senior author would like to express his gratitude to Dr Arnold Davidson for his helpful suggestions over the past years and Eric Blum, PhD, for his investigative analysis of the speech quality of laryngectomees using the air bypass voice prosthesis.

ADDENDUM

Since this paper was written, we have performed six additional cervical esophagostomies for vocal rehabilitation, bringing our total to twenty-six. Eight cases were reported in an earlier paper [6], and twelve new cases are reported herein along with two follow-up cases from the first group of eight.

In the first eight patients, one patient (now deceased) spoke with a reed device and the other with a reed in combination with an air bypass prosthesis to facilitate breathing (fistula closed because of salivary leakage). All the remaining patients in this group spoke with an air bypass mechanism. Four patients had the fistula closed for the following reasons: salivary leakage (two patients), lack of interest and poor articulation (one), difficulty in sound production and loss of interest (one). Two patients are currently and successfully using the device. (One uses an air bypass, the other a manual prosthesis.)

The second group of twelve patients are discussed in the paper.

Of the six additional cases, two have been successfully fitted with the air bypass prosthesis. Of the remaining four, one had the fistula closed before installation of the prosthesis because of a carotid hemorrhage that occurred ten days postoperatively. One has a valvelike stricture at the cricopharyngeus that allows food and fluid to pass into the stomach but permits no regurgitation. This has been visualized by a fiberoptic esophagoscope, but was not visible on a routine barium swallow. In retrospect, this stricture could have been detected by passing a #18 rubber Foley catheter transnasally into the upper esophagus to a point approximately 2 to 3 cm above the level of the tracheostome. By blowing air through the tube, one should be able to hear air passing into the pharynx. If there is a tight cricopharyngeus or a stricture present, no air will pass around the tube and the normal reflux of air necessary for sound production would not occur. This particular patient never experienced eructation. The air-blowing test can be used to determine the exact site of the inner esophagostomal opening. As the sound is produced, the patient can be asked to articulate. If a whisper type speech is heard, most likely the catheter has been pulled above the cricopharyngeus into the hypopharynx. It is essential that the opening be made below the cricopharyngeus. In one patient, the fistula was placed low in the esophagus at a level of the tracheostomal opening. Air only intermittently flows into the oral cavity and mostly passes into the stomach. The third patient has had a simple cervical esophagostomy performed without exposure of the carotid vessels and without the rotation of a skin flap. This operative procedure is being evaluated. We are considering using this type of fistula because it eliminates carotid exposure and minimizes postoperative wound healing difficulties such as early subcutaneous salivary leakage in the area of the skin fistula tube. At present, there are a total of eleven patients who are currently using the air bypass voice prosthesis successfully.

A detailed tabulation of all cases to date is available from the senior author on request.

REFERENCES

1. Gardner WH, Harris HE: Aids and devices for laryngectomees. *Arch Otolaryngol* 73: 145, 1961.
2. McGrail JS, Oldfield DL: One-stage operation for vocal rehabilitation at laryngectomy. *Trans Amer Acad Ophthalmol Otolaryngol* 75: 510, 1971.
3. Asai R: Laryngoplasty after total laryngectomy. *Arch Otolaryngol* 95: 114, 1972.
4. Montgomery WW, Toohill RJ: Voice rehabilitation after laryngectomy. *Arch Otolaryngol* 88: 499, 1968.
5. Montgomery WW: Postlaryngectomy vocal rehabilitation. *Arch Otolaryngol* 95: 76, 1972.
6. Taub S, Spiro RH: Vocal rehabilitation of laryngectomees: preliminary report of a new technic. *Amer J Surg* 124: 87, 19/2.
7. Taub S: The Taub oral panendoscope: a new technique. *Cleft Palate J* 3: 328, 1966.
8. Blom ED: A comparative investigation of acoustical and perceptual features of esophageal speech and speech with the Taub voice prosthesis. (Unpublished PhD dissertation, University of Maryland, 1972.)

VOICE REHABILITATION AFTER LARYNGECTOMY
Results With the Use of a Hypopharyngeal Prosthesis

George A. Sisson, MD; Fred M. S. McConnel, MD;
Jerilyn A. Logemann, PhD; Stephen Yeh, Jr., MD

The Northwestern voice prosthesis for laryngectomees is described. The prosthesis contains no vibrator but activates vibration of the patient's pharyngeal or upper esophageal tissue by transporting air from the tracheostoma to a fistula in the upper neck, well away from major blood vessels. The prosthesis fits directly onto the laryngectomy tube and allows the patient to breathe, speak, and cough without any manual adjustments.

The important advantage of this prosthesis is the fistula location. It can be placed at the time of original surgery and is also workable in patient who have had radiation and extensive radical surgery with total reconstruction of their gullet. The prosthesis can be used by primary total laryngectomees while learning esophageal speech or installed in those who are unable to use the electronic larynx or to learn esophageal speech. Four case studies are presented.

One hundred years ago, Gussenbauer[1] designed an artificial larynx that was used by Billroth's first laryngectomy patient. The device was a modified tracheostomy tube with a series of one-way valves that allowed air to be transferred from the trachea to the hypopharynx through a pharyngostoma. The apparatus reportedly produced a loud, clear voice with only air injection into the hypopharynx and contained no mechanical vibrator.

During the last century, a number of artificial larynges have been developed, the majority of which have been discarded.[2] Presently, in this country, the only widely used artificial larynges are the hand-held electronic transcervical type. Many patients object to the mechanical-sounding, monotonous voice produced by this device.[3] Esophageal speech is the most popular means of vocal rehabilitation for laryngectomees today. Unfortunately, not all patients can develop this type of speech. Goode[4] cites studies in which 17% to 50% of laryngectomees fail to develop esophageal speech despite the duration and quality of speech therapy. Of the esophageal speech failures, Putney[5] and MacComb and Fletcher[6] found that only approximately 20% of their patients learned to use the electronic transcervical artificial larynx, the remainder being aphonic.

This study was supported in part by the American Cancer Society, Illinois Division, March 1, 1974–March 1, 1975 (Northwestern University Grant No. 4269–250). The pressure sensitive flapper valve in the prosthesis was designed by the ARO Corporation in conjunction with the Sparta Instrument Corporation.

Accepted for publication Sept 20, 1974.

Read before the Tenth Annual Meeting of the American Academy of Facial Plastic and Reconstructive Surgery, Inc., Palm Beach, Fla, April 20, 1974.

From the Department of Otolaryngology & Maxillofacial Surgery (Drs. Sisson, McConnel, Logemann and Yeh), and the Department of Neurology (Dr. Logemann), Northwestern University-McGaw Medical Center, Chicago.

Reprint requests to the Department of Otolaryngology & Maxillofacial Surgery, Northwestern University-McGaw Medical Center, 303 E Chicago Ave, Chicago, IL 60611 (Dr. Sisson).

During the last 15 years, a number of surgical procedures have been proposed to form a pseudoglottis for total laryngectomees. The Asai procedure[7] and its variations[8-11] have received much attention. These procedures have been used satisfactorily by some surgeons in nonirradiated patients. The failure rate of the Asai-type procedure increases significantly when attempted in irradiated patients. The difficulties encountered with the Asai procedure are dehiscence of the tissue tube constructed for air transfer from the tracheostoma to the hypopharynx and stenosis of the hypopharyngeal fistula. With the current emphasis being placed on the combined therapy of radiation and surgery for laryngeal carcinoma, there are few candidates for the Asai-type reconstruction. With the wound dehiscence problems that are encountered with irradiated tissue, the most logical alternative is the use of prosthetic tubes for air transfer from the trachea to the esophagus or hypopharynx to produce speech. After 100 years, therefore, we find ourselves again evaluating the originally proposed solution to the problem of replacing the cancerous larynx.

Currently, Taub et al[12,13] have produced an artificial larynx called the LaBarge Voice-Bak Prosthesis. This apparatus fits on the laryngectomy tube, hangs down onto the chest, and conducts air into the esophagus through an esophagostoma low in the neck. An air bypass mechanism allows the patient to breathe and speak without any manual adjustments. A very similar device was described by Briani,[14] in 1952, that also had an air bypass valve. Both devices depend on vibration of the esophagus in the area of the cricopharyngeus sphincter to produce speech. With the low placement of the fistula, the LaBarge VoiceBak can be concealed under clothing. In a series of 26 patients using the LaBarge device, the major problems have been salivary leakage from the esophagostoma, two deaths from carotid hemorrhage, and tracheostoma irritation. Reportedly, 14 of the 26 patients have been rehabilitated successfully with an excellent voice. The major disadvantage of this prosthesis is the location of the esophagostoma in the immediate proximity of the carotid artery. Due to the dangers of carotid rupture, the esophagostoma should not be placed in necks violated previously by surgery or irradiation. These contraindications, as with the Asai procedure, reduce the number of total laryngectomees who are potential candidates for the prosthesis.

Of utmost importance with any surgical rehabilitative procedure is that it have no associated mortality. A safe fistula is one located in the neck away from major vessels that lead into the hypopharynx. Shedd et al[15] reported on a series of patients in whom they tried a hypopharyngeal fistula prosthesis that contained a reed as a vibrator. The major disadvantages to this attempt are the mechanical quality of the voice and salivary leakage from the pharyngostoma.

In our experience, most patients selected for total laryngectomy have 5,500 rads of preoperative radiation or have been radiation failures. In patients in whom radiation has failed, the recurrences may require extensive esophageal resection a mediastinal dissection, or both. None of the surgical or prosthetic methods presently proposed for vocal rehabilitation are utilized easily in these patients. Therefore, we have been interested in developing a means of vocal rehabilitation applicable to this problem. During the last year, we have developed a voice prosthesis that utilizes a hypopharyngeal pseudoglottis for voice. A hypopharyngeal pseudoglottis is also the basis for voice production in the Asai-type laryngoplasty patients and can produce an excellent voice.

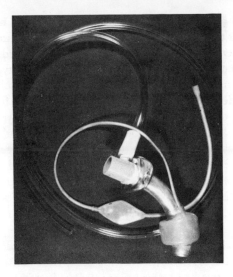

FIG. 1.—Test device for locating critical vibratory area in hypopharynx.

The vibrator utilized in the Northwestern voice prosthesis varies in each patient depending on the type of previous surgery and the anatomy of his residual neck structures. Fluoroscopic studies of our patients have proven the vibrator to consist of the internal aspect of the pharyngostoma, a portion of the walls of the hypopharynx, or the base of the tongue, or both. The location of the fistula in the hypopharynx is a critical factor in determining the quality of voice obtained. The fistula must be in an area where air, which is introduced into the hypopharynx, sets the mucosal walls into vibration. In postlaryngectomy patients, fluoroscopy has been helpful in determining the best location for the internal os of the fistula. With a small amount of barium to coat the hypopharyngeal walls, the level at which the mucosal walls most closely approximate may be observed.

The vibrator potential of this area can be tested in the following manner. A No. 16 nasogastric tube is attached to the patient's laryngectomy tube by a side arm (Fig 1). The tubing is introduced into the hypopharynx through the nose. When the patient wants to speak, he closes the laryngectomy tube lumen and air is diverted through the nasogastric tube into the hypopharynx. The level of the nasogastric tube in the hypopharynx may be changed until the best voice is obtained. The quality of the voice appears to correlate to the magnitude of the vibratory motion in the hypopharynx as observed on fluoroscopy. It is at this point at which the internal os of the fistula should be located. If the fistula is located above this point, a breathy voice or whisper will be obtained and if the fistula is located more than 3 cm below this point, the voice will sound similar to esophageal voice with lower frequency and increased roughness. No single anatomical point may be said to be correct for all patients, but each patient should be studied to locate the critical vibratory area.

The prosthesis fits onto the laryngectomy tube and allows the patient to breathe, speak, and cough without making any manual adjustments (Fig 2). A single pressure-sensitive flapper valve remains open during respiration and closes on exhalation for speech. On coughing, the valve disengages to allow an unobstructed airway and is reset

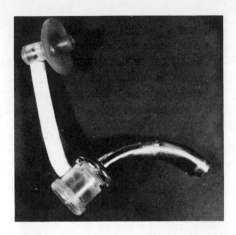

FIG. 2.—Northwestern voice prosthesis.

on inspiration. There is also a duckbill valve mounted in the top of the pharyngostomy tube that prevents salivary leakage and allows the patient to eat without removing the device.

Since the fistula is 0.25 to 0.50 cm in diameter, it may be sealed easily with a plug to allow the patient to practice esophageal speech. Thus, the voice prosthesis not only can aid those unable to develop esophageal speech, but can make possible the rapid vocal rehabilitation after the initial laryngectomy.

There are three types of patients who can use this voice prosthesis: (1) the total laryngectomy patient who fails to learn esophageal speech; (2) the irradiated total laryngectomy patient who has also had extensive neck and reconstructive esophageal surgery; and (3) the total laryngectomy patient who must return to his occupation promptly with a quality voice after the initial surgery.

Case 1 is an example of the latter type of patient.

REPORT OF CASES

Case 1

A 39-year-old football coach had a subglottic reoccurrence of his T_1 glottic cancer after 6,500 rads irradiation that required a total laryngectomy and neck dissection. Since he had unplanned preoperative irradiation, a controlled fistula or small pharyngostoma was fashioned to aid in healing. The fistula was formed at the level of the valleculae with the internal os in the closure line of the pharynx and the external opening located in the lateral aspect of the neck 2 cm anterior to the carotid artery and 6 cm superior to the tracheostoma. The mucosa of the pharynx was sutured to the skin. The postoperative period was uncomplicated and during this time the controlled fistula was used for feeding. The patient was discharged on June 15 and was anxious to resume his coaching responsibilities the first of August. Therefore, three weeks after surgery, he was fitted with the speaking

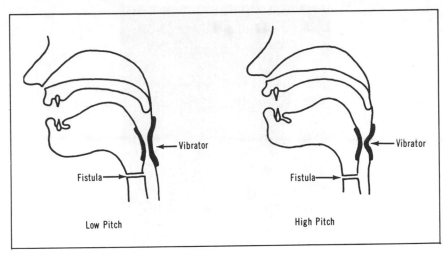

FIG. 3.—Location of vibrator in hypopharynx with pitch change.

device that immediately produced an intelligible voice. At the same time, he began esophageal speech instruction. With the artificial larynx, he was able to resume his full teaching and coaching responsibilities, which require him to talk 8 to 12 hours a day. It is necessary to replace the pharyngostoma seal every 24 hours. With the pharyngostoma located in the hypopharynx, there are minor problems with salivary leakage.

It is important that the external opening of the fistula is horizontal or above the location of the pharyngeal opening to prevent salivary leakage.

On fluoroscopy, the patient's vibrator consisted of the base of the tongue and pharyngeal walls (Fig 3). The location of the vibrator remained the same when the patient used his alaryngeal voice, his prosthesis, or when he had air injected into his hypopharynx by a nasogastric tube. The patient can sing simple tunes with change in pitch. When singing with the prosthesis, one can see on fluoroscopy, the mass of his hypopharyngeal vibrator change as he changes pitch, reducing mass as pitch is elevated (Fig 3).

This case is an example of a highly motivated individual whose livelihood depended on his ability to communicate. The voice prosthesis allowed rapid vocal rehabilitation. His esophageal speech development has been progressing but he still uses the prosthesis for teaching and coaching.

It is too early to report whether this patient will be able to develop his esophageal speech skills to the point where he will no longer need a voice prosthesis for teaching. Will the prosthesis or the presence of the fistula deter the development of esophageal speech if this method is used immediately after laryngectomy? This is a question we are currently studying.

Another category of patients, who are candidates for the voice prosthesis method, are those who have undergone extensive neck and esophageal reconstructive surgery and who find it more difficult to develop esophageal speech. The following patients are examples of this type.

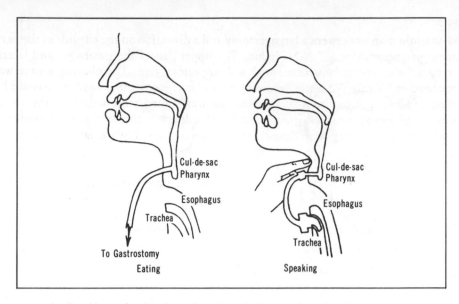

FIG. 4.—Speaking and eating device for patient during staged esophageal reconstruction.

Case 2

Two and one-half years ago, a 52-year old man had à $T_3N_0M_0$ glottic lesion with subglottic extension. A total laryngectomy with neck dissection was performed. He learned esophageal speech and returned to his former occupation as a truck driver. One year ago, he developed a stomal recurrence and was referred to Northwestern University for treatment. A mediastinal dissection with partial esophagectomy was performed. Postoperatively he developed a fistula that resulted in a 6 × 4 cm esophageal defect. Since anterior chest flaps were used to stabilize his mediastinum, a bipedicled abdominal tube was developed and migrated in stages to close the esophageal fistula. After surgery the patient's hypopharynx formed a cul-de-sac at the base of which a No. 22 Foley catheter was used to divert saliva from the esophageal reconstruction area. A valve mechanism was mounted on the tracheostomy tube and the Foley catheter from the hypopharynx was attached to the valve. With this arrangement (Fig 4) the patient was able to speak in a whisper by means of air injected into his hypopharynx. Since there was no tissue pseudoglottis to act as a vibrator, as with the lateral pharyngostoma, a foam rubber external dressing was used to compress the walls of the hypopharynx above the level of air injection. With this compression, the patient had a very intelligible voice. He reported that it was less tiring to speak with the prosthesis than it had been with his former esophageal voice. When the patient ate, he disconnected the Foley from the prosthetic valve mechanism and attached it to his gastrostoma, which allowed him to eat by mouth. The patient ate a soft diet. Before this arrangement, he had not been able to eat by mouth for a four-month period. After completion of the esophageal reconstruction, a lateral pharyngostoma was developed and the voice prosthesis was used successfully.

Case 3

A 68-year-old man underwent a laryngectomy and a dissection on the left side of the neck with esophagectomy for a $T_3N_1M_0$ lesion. The upper part of the esophagus and lateral pharyngeal wall were reconstructed with a deltopectoral flap. The pharyngostoma was surrounded by very flaccid tissue devoid of muscular support, but a good voice could be obtained. When the patient's pharyngostoma was stinted with a tube or the tissue around the pharyngostoma was immobilized with a dressing, the voice would be reduced to a whisper. Fluoroscopy shows the vibrator to be composed of the lateral pharyngeal walls.

Patients who have had esophageal reconstruction, as in the last case, are the most difficult to rehabilitate vocally. They are frequently unable to learn esophageal speech because of structural incompetence and may use the electronic larynx poorly.

The third category of patients who are candidates for the voice prosthesis are the esophageal speech failures. The following case history illustrates the importance of preoperative fluoroscopic evaluation.

Case 4

A 69-year-old woman had a total laryngectomy and radical neck dissection and could not develop esophageal speech despite two years of speech therapy. A pharyngostoma was placed at the base of her tongue in the lateral pharyngeal wall. Her voice with the prosthesis was only a whisper. On fluoroscopy, the patient was noted to have a large osteophyte projecting into the hypopharynx. Her best vibratory area was on the inferior aspect of the osteophyte and the fistula was above this area.

Of our eight patients, this patient was the only one in whom a voice was not produced with a hypopharyngeal fistula.

REFERENCES

1. Gussenbauer C: Uber die erste durch Th. Billroth am Menschen ausgefuhrte Kehlkopf-Exstirpation und die Anwendung eines Kunstlichen Kehlkopfes. *Arch Clin Chir* 17:343–356, 1874.
2. Hanson WL: A new artificial larynx with a historical review. *Ill Med J* 78:483–486, 1940.
3. Martin H: Rehabilitation of the laryngectomee. *Cancer* 16:823–841, 1963.
4. Goode RL: The development of an improved artificial larynx. *Trans Am Acad Ophthalmol Otolaryngol* 73:279–287, 1969.
5. Putney FJ: Rehabilitation of the post-laryngectomized patient. *Ann Otol Rhinol Laryngol* 67:544–549, 1958.
6. MacComb WS, Fletcher GH: *Larynx: Cancer of the Head and Neck*. Baltimore, Williams & Wilkins Co, 1967.
7. Asai R: Laryngoplasty after total laryngectomy. *Arch Otolaryngol* 95:114–119, 1972.
8. Conley J: Surgical techniques for the vocal rehabilitation of the post-laryngectomized patient. *Trans Am Acad Ophthalmol Otolaryngol* 73:288–299, 1969.
9. Miller AH: Further experience with the Asai technique for vocal rehabilitation after laryngectomy. *Trans Am Acad Ophthalmol Otolaryngol* 72:779–781, 1968.
10. Montgomery WW, Toohil RJ: Vocal rehabilitation after laryngectomy. *Arch Otolaryngol* 88:499–506, 1968.

11. Karlan MS: Two-stage Asai laryngectomy utilizing a modified Tucker valve. *Am J Surg* 116:597–599, 1968.
12. Taub S, Spiro RH: Vocal rehabilitation of laryngectomees. *Am J Surg* 124:87–90, 1972.
13. Taub S, Bergner LH: Air bypass voice prosthesis for vocal rehabilitation of laryngectomees. *Am J Surg* 125:748–752, 1973.
14. Briani AA: Il ricupero sociale dei laringectomizzati attraverso un metido personale operatirio. *Med Sociol* 8:265–269, 1958.
15. Shedd D, Bakamjian V, Sako K, et al: Reed:-fistula method of speech rehabilitation after laryngectomy. *Am J Surg* 124:510–514, 1972.

FIRST EXPERIENCES WITH THE ASAI TECHNIQUE
FOR VOCAL REHABILITATION
AFTER TOTAL LARYNGECTOMY

ALDEN H. MILLER, M.D.

LOS ANGELES, CALIF.

Late in 1965, it was my privilege and pleasure to see and hear a sound movie by Dr. Ryozo Asai, in which he demonstrated a method of providing laryngectomized patients with an almost normal voice. The basis of his technique was the construction of a dermal tube from the upper end of the trachea into the hypopharynx. When the lower tracheal fistula, which had been placed for breathing, was closed with the patient's finger, air could then be expired up the dermal tube and into the pharyngeal cavity with sound produced there and transformed into speech. The voices of these patients had an excellent quality and a wide range of pitch. They could sing; whistle with ease; and speak sentences of average length with normal pauses for inspiration.

In January of 1966, I used Dr. Asai's technique for the first time, performing the first stage at the conclusion of a wide field laryngectomy. I have now completed the final stage in four such patients and have completed the first or second stage in another three patients. The four have excellent voices, far superior, in my opinion, to the average esophageal voice after laryngectomy. There are two slight inconveniences for these patients. First, one has to use a hand to close the tracheal opening when he talks and second, he has to manually press the skin over the upper end of the dermal tube sometimes when swallowing saliva or liquid foods.

TECHNIQUE

The technique consists of three stages or operations. The first stage is employed at the end of an ordinary wide-field laryngectomy. After removal of the larynx, the open end of the trachea is sutured to the skin opening of the mid-line of the neck in the usual fashion. I continue to use a posterior triangular tongue of tracheal mucosa in making this stoma. When using the usual mid-line vertical skin incision for the laryngectomy, I place the open end of the trachea a centimeter or two higher than that usually done. This necessitates some closure of the lower end of the incision below the tracheal stoma thus being formed. A permanent tracheal stoma is then made through the fourth or fifth tracheal ring with 2 cm of skin between it and the upper opening. This will be the

Read before the eighty-eighth annual meeting of the American Laryngological Association, Seigniory Club, Province of Quebec, Canada, May 15-16, 1967.

Reprinted by permission from *Annals of Otology, Rhinology, and Laryngology*, 1967, 76, 829–833. Copyright 1967, Annals Publishing Company.

patient's permanent opening for breathing the remainder of his life. The stoma made above it will become the lower opening of the final dermal tube into the pharynx. This completes the first stage of the technique.

The second stage consists in making, a month or so later, a fistula into the pharynx, suturing mucosal edges to skin edges. This fistula should enter the pharynx just under the overhang of the bulge posteriorly of the base of the tongue. The patient now has three stomae in a vertical line.

The third and final stage, another month or so later, forms a tube of skin with its lower opening being the upper tracheal stoma and its upper opening being the fistula into the pharynx. This tube is formed by making a vertical skin incision one centimeter on each side of the mid-line of the neck and curving these incisions around and above the pharyngeal stoma by one centimeter, and below and around the upper tracheal stoma by the same centimeter. The cut edges of this island of skin are then approximated and sutured vertically in the mid-line. Thus is formed a tube of skin connecting the uppermost end of the trachea and the pharynx. The remaining cut skin edges are now closed vertically in the mid-line over the dermal tube, burying it.

The first six patients have taught me certain rules and measurements to follow during the surgery of each stage and in postoperative management. In the first stage, I prefer to insure that the lowermost opening, the permanent tracheal stoma, be a little smaller than usual. A diameter of about 12 mm is probably the best. This may mean the use of a number seven or eight laryngectomy tube instead of a number nine. I would like the middle stoma, the uppermost end of the trachea, to end up being about six millimeters in diameter. This may necessitate the wearing of a small plastic tube or plug in this opening during the month intervening between the first and second stage and even that month between the second and third stages of the technique.

In the second stage I attempt to place the pharyngeal stoma in such a way that it runs downhill from its skin opening to its pharyngeal opening. I place the pharyngeal opening just under the ledge formed by the remaining floor of the valleculae left at the conclusion of the laryngectomy. This, of course, necessitates leaving some of this anterior floor when the larynx is severed from the base of the tongue. I use a direct laryngoscope during this second stage to direct the insertion to this spot of a large needle through the skin of the mid-line of the neck at just about where the skin of the neck angulates with that of the underside of the floor of the mouth. This is about the level of the removed hyoid bone. When the needle is angulated properly, an incision then follows it into the pharynx. The skin opening is kept high when mucosal edges are sutured to skin edges. This pharyngeal stoma is made vertically with a vertical diameter of one centimeter. The pharyngeal stoma will narrow in the postoperative course of this second stage. Ideally, it should end up remaining with a diameter of about four millimeters. This may necessitate the wearing of a plastic tube or plug in this stoma or in daily dilations for a few weeks.

During the third operation, I form the dermal tube over a section of plastic tubing having an outside diameter of six millimeters. This tubing is left in

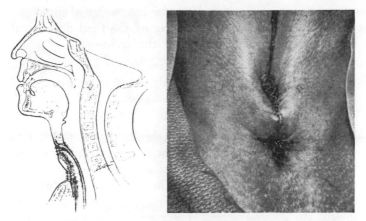

Fig. 1.—End of first stage.

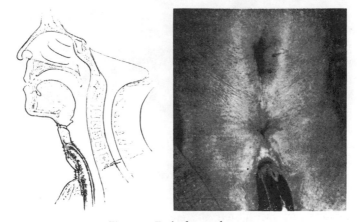

Fig. 2.—End of second stage.

place for two or three weeks from just where it can be seen through the permanent tracheal stoma, up the dermal tube, into the pharynx and standing with its upper end at the level of the top surface of the tongue. Suture is tied into both ends of it to form an endless circle in order to replace it if it moves upwards or downwards. At the conclusion of the third stage, the patient will immediately be able to talk in a hoarse whisper even with the plastic tube in place.

RESULTS

The first two patients, the two who have had their final operation completed the longest, have excellent voices. They can talk with inflection and a wide range of pitch and tonal quality and can even sing. The oldest patient has been

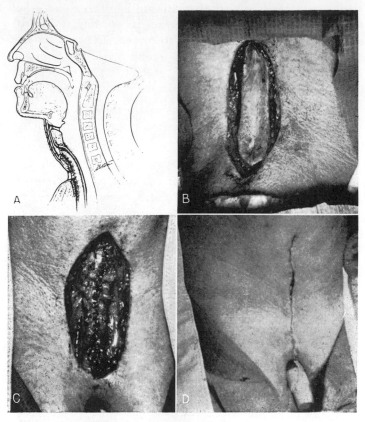

Fig. 3A.—End of third stage.
Fig. 3B.—First step of third stage.
Fig. 3C.—Second step of third stage.
Fig. 3D.—Third step of third stage.

completed nine months and his voice continues to improve. The second patient has had her procedures completed four months and she, too, has continued to have a voice that steadily improves in loudness, range and singing ability and she has retained her Southern accent. The third and fourth patients' voices are still rather soft after just the month following their final surgery but are steadily improving.

The first patient has no difficulty with swallowing solids, but sometimes must use digital pressure over the skin over the upper end of the dermal tube with drinking some liquids. The second patient must use the digital pressure with the swallowing of all liquids. The third patient, in whom for the first time the pharyngeal stoma was deliberately slanted downwards from the skin, has absolutely no leak of either liquids swallowed or of his saliva. None of the patients report any cough resulting from the trickling down of saliva and none have had any infections of their respiratoy tract. All report that talking seems to keep the dermal tube clear of saliva.

The first two patients report that talking is much easier when they leave their laryngectomy tubes in place and occlude its opening rather than occluding the tracheal stoma when the tube is not in place. The first patient obtains his loudest and clearest voice when he uses a second finger for digital pressure over the lowermost end of the dermal tube in order to narrow its lumen. Interestingly, the greatest vibration of the dermal tube is felt where it is narrowed.

Only the first patient has had hair grow up through the pharyngeal stoma from the dermal tube. This has given him no symptoms and the hairs are being evulsed at direct or indirect laryngoscopy.

Hinged trap-door tracheotomy tubes or tubes with diaphragms have been used so as to allow the patient to close off the tube on expiration and thus talk without having to use one hand to close the opening of the tracheotomy tube. Their voices have remained almost the same as with digital closure of the stoma but both patients report an uncomfortable, suffocating-like feeling after a minute or so of talking as if they could not expire enough air. They have insisted that these hinged tubes are too uncomfortable. It seems sure that soon a trap-door can be fashioned that will allow the patient to flip it open to relieve this sensation.

CONVERSION

Can this technique be used to convert the patient who has had the usual laryngectomy with just the formation of one rather low-lying stoma? A few weeks ago, I assisted Dr. Fred Turnbull of Los Angeles in completing the technique on such a patient. Dr. Turnbull had placed a pharyngeal fistula as a second stage. At the time of the third and final stage, the stoma was freed in its anterior 180° of circumference and the trachea was elevated 2 to 2½ cm. A new lower permanent tracheal fistula was formed and the upper two openings connected in forming a dermal tube in the usual manner. This patient had an uncomplicated postoperative course and has a good voice. The actual steps of this technique will be reported later.

SUMMARY

My first experience with the usage of the Asai technique for vocal rehabilitation of the laryngectomized patient have been recounted. I am convinced that these patients will continue to have excellent voices far superior to those with esophageal voices. However, they must put up with some discomforts in order to have these voices. Instead of one, there will be three operations and convalescent periods. They must use one hand to close the tracheal stoma when talking and some patients will experience slight annoyance in having to close the dermal tube with digital pressure when swallowing liquids. These drawbacks must be pointed out to the patient contemplating such surgery. The patients who have an excellent esophageal voice will probably not choose to be converted to the Asai technique, nor would I encourage them to have the conversion, although I think we will be able to convert almost any laryngectomized patient.

FUNDAMENTAL FREQUENCY CHARACTERISTICS OF JAPANESE ASAI SPEAKERS.*

E. Thayer Curry, Ph.D.,

University, Ala.,

John C. Snidecor, Ph.D.,

Santa Barbara, Calif.,

and

Nobuhiko Isshiki, M.D.,

Kyoto, Japan.

ABSTRACT.

The purpose of this study is to evaluate the Asai procedure in terms of the postoperative fundamental vocal frequency of a group of native Japanese Asai speakers and to ascertain if auditory impressions are related in fact to acoustical impressions of higher fundamental vocal frequency. Study results indicate a postoperative vocal frequency of 97 Hz, which is significantly higher than the previous frequencies reported near 65 Hz. Of special note is the much higher percentage of aperiodicity among the Asai speakers when compared with a group of United States superior esophageal speakers.

—— O ——

INTRODUCTION.

One of the voice characteristics of the individual speaker who has had his larynx surgically removed is the relatively low frequency of the typical esophageal speech. The present authors[1] have reported this usual postoperative fundamental frequency to be about 63.3 Hz. Various clinical techniques have been used to attempt to raise this fundamental vocal frequency, in an effort to make the voice more acceptable.

Ryozo Asai, a Japanese laryngologist, has developed a new surgical technique for removal of the larynx. The general principles of this procedure are described in Snidecor by Miller.[2] Basically, the Asai operation provides an airway for utilization of pulmonary air introduced into the lower pharynx for vocalization efforts. Asai speech sounds higher pitched than esophageal speech, and it also seems to be more rapid and more

---

*Some portions of this study were presented as part of a paper at the American Speech and Hearing Association in San Francisco, November 18, 1972.

Reprinted by permission from *The Laryngoscope*, 1973, *83*, 1759–1763.

breathy. As an aside, Asai speech is learned almost instantly as compared with much longer training periods for csophageal speech. Snidecor has observed a Japanese patient phonating while still on the operating table. The purpose of this present study is to evaluate the Asai procedure in terms of the postoperative fundamental vocal frequency of a selected group of native Japanese Asai speakers and to ascertain whether or not auditory impressions are related in fact to acoustical measurements.

PROCEDURE.

At the time of his recent stay in Japan, Snidecor obtained recordings of Asai speakers reading the Japanese version of the "Rainbow Passage." The laryngeal surgery had been performed by Ryozo Asai or Teru Kimura, a student of Ryozo Asai, of Kobe University Medical Institute. The fundamental vocal frequency of these Asai speakers was obtained by use of a Visicorder Oscillograph (Honeywell Model 906C). Visual measurements of the Visicorder periodic phonations, recurring in 1/10 second segments, were made. The selected group of five Japanese Asai speakers was compared with three other speaking groups:

1. Normal (laryngeal) native Japanese male speakers, (five subjects).

2. Normal (laryngeal) United States male speakers, (10 subjects).

3. Laryngectomized (esophageal) United States male speakers, (six subjects).

These latter two speaker groups were analyzed by use of the conventional photophonellographic technique described by Cowan.[3] Fundamental frequency for the first group was determined with the Visicorder.

RESULTS.

Since two unlike languages are being compared in this study, it seemed essential to make phonemic comparisons between Colloquial Japanese and General American dialects. Table I provides a "Phonemic Analysis of the 'Rainbow Passage' " for these two dialects. The following aspects of this table are noteworthy. For this reading passage the total number of phonemes is very similar, 177 in General American (GA), 170 in Colloquial Japanese (CJ). The passage contains a considerably higher percentage of back vowels in Japanese, 20.6 percent compared with 3.8 in General American; also, there are more central vowels (largely the Schwa) in General American. The total of vowels and diphthongs is somewhat greater in Japanese, 51.6 percent, than in General American, 38.3 percent.

Despite these vowel/diphthong differences, the total percentage of voiced elements in the two dialects is very similar: 78.4 percent in GA and 82.7 percent in CJ. For the dialects the percentages of voiceless elements are 21.4 percent in GA and 17.0 percent in CJ; thus, for the read-

TABLE I.

Phonemic Analysis of "Rainbow Passage."

	"General American"		Colloquial Japanese	
Total Words	51		37	
Total Syllables	66		86	
Total Phonemes	177		170	
	Number	Percent	Number	Percent
Front Vowels	21	11.8	27	15.8
Back Vowels	7	3.9	35	20.6
Central Vowels	24	13.6	5	2.9
Diphthongs	16	9.0	21	12.3
Total Vowels and Diphthongs	68	38.3	88	51.6
Voiced Consonants and Combinations	71	40.1	53	31.1
Voiceless Consonants and Combinations	38	21.4	29	17.0
Total Consonants and Combinations	109	61.5	82	48.1
Total Phonemes	177	99.8	170	99.7
Total Voiced Elements:				
Vowels		29.3		39.3
Diphthongs		9.0		12.3
Consonants and Combinations		40.1		31.1
		78.4		82.7
Total Voiceless Consonants and Combinations		21.4		17.0

TABLE II.

Analysis of Phonation During Speaking Performances.

Percentage of Overall Duration	Japanese Asai Speakers					Asai Group	Superior U. S. Esophageal Group
	Orita	Momota	Hicki	Enuma	Kuroda		
Periodic Intervals (%)	31.9	40.3	4.5	53.9	22.1	30.3	59.5
Aperiodic Intervals (%)	33.9	8.7	66.3	19.0	32.2	30.7	1.9
Total Phonation (%)	65.8	49.0	70.8	72.9	54.3	61.0	61.4
Silence (%)	34.2	50.9	29.0	26.9	45.7	38.9	38.5
Overall Duration (in Seconds)	30.4	31.0	22.0	21.5	37.0	28.38	27.73

ing passage of this study, the overall language structure of the American and Japanese dialects is remarkably similar as far as the voiced/voiceless element concept is concerned. It, therefore, seems reasonable to compare the phonation characteristics of these two dialects, at least for the purposes of this study.

Table II present the results of an "Analysis of Phonation During Speaking Performances." The following values from Table II should be commented upon: the overall reading duration for the speaker groups for the two dialects was very similar, 28.4 seconds for CJ and 27.7 seconds for GA. The two speaker groups spent essentially the same amount of time in pauses, 28.9 percent for CJ and 38.5 percent for GA. Similarly, the total phonation time was very much alike. The greatest difference between the two speaker groups is seen with 30 percent of the Asai phonation being aperiodic; in contrast, only 1.9 percent of the GA esophageal phonation was aperiodic. Why the Asai airway should result in this greater aperiodicity is a matter for further investigation. Perhaps this unusual amount of phonational aperiodicity is simply the nature of a simple tubular vibrator supplied with an ample supply of pulmonary air. The idea that this attribute is characteristic of this specific group of Japanese Asai speakers can be discarded, for American Asai speakers perceptually have comparable aperiodicity. Nichols, reporting in Snidecor[2] describes this as follows: "The growth of the breathiness ratings for the male Asai speaker, over the months in which he was acquiring control over his voice, and the female speaker's breathiness are striking." It may be inferred that less complete closure of the pseudoglottis was made as the voice developed, producing the turbulent airflow which results in broad-band noise acoustically. Yanigahara[4] has discussed at length such effects in the pathological larynx.

Three distinct factors which may be responsible for the large amount of aperiodicity may be set forth briefly as follows:

1. The first factor may relate to the looseness or mobility of the mucosa from the underlying tissue. The neoglottis in the Asai speaker is usually formed high at the roof of the tongue or the vallecula, where the mucosa is not so movable from the underlying tissue as that of the esophagus. If the covering mucous membrane were not movable, the closure of the glottis by the Bernoulli effect would be disturbed, as in the pathological larynx such as a cicatrical vocal fold after irradiation.[5] The vocalizations from scarred vocal folds are also very breathy (aperiodic).

2. The narrow cavity below the neoglottis in the Asai speaker is also assumed to be related to the breathy vocal quality in these speakers. Since the tube below the neoglottis is very narrow, the neoglottis is not so convex in a relative sense, thus making the vibration of the neoglottis difficult.

3. In addition, a large amount of air supply from the lung produces turbulent air flow of high velocity at the neoglottis, thus making the noise level of the aperiodic breathiness very high.

Table III presents "Measures of Fundamental Vocal Frequency Usage." The median value of 97.08 Hz found for the Asai speakers of the present study should be contrasted with the previous median results from esophageal studies of Damste (1958), 67.5 Hz, Snidecor and Curry (1961), 63.3

TABLE III.

Measures of Fundamental Vocal Frequency Usage.

	Damste (1958)	Snidecor and Curry (1961)	Shipp (1967)	Rollin (1967)	Present Data (1972)	Normal Laryngeal Group
Fundamental Frequency						
Mean (in Hz)			94.38	65.6		
Median (in Hz)	67.5	63.3	86.1			132.1
SD (in Tones)		2.30	2.56			
90 Percent Range (in Tones)		6.5	8.25			
Highest Frequency (in Hz)	(185*)	135.5			149.0	262.0
Lowest Frequency (in Hz)		17.2			40.8	42.0

*Estimate.

Hz, Shipp (1967), 86.1 Hz, and a mean value for Rollin (1967), of 65.6 Hz. This median value for the present group of Asai speakers, 97.08 Hz, is thus perceptually and significantly higher than the previous results obtained with any of the cited study groups of esophageal speakers.

If this significantly higher fundamental frequency is substantiated in other study groups — then seemingly the Asai procedure has a very important positive feature in achieving this more desirable higher fundamental frequency, a feature especially important to the female speaker whose esophageal voice will have likely dropped nearly two octaves. The aperiodicity reported in this study will be further investigated in additional Asai speakers.

BIBLIOGRAPHY.

1. SNIDECOR, J. D., and CURRY, E. T.: Temporal and Pitch Aspects of Superior Esophageal Speech. Ann. Otol., 68:623-636, 1959.

2. SNIDECOR, J. C.: Speech Rehabilitation of the Laryngectomized. Second Edition. Charles C. Thomas, Springfield, Ill., 1968.

3. COWAN, M.: Pitch and Intensity Characteristics of Stage Speech. Arch. Sp., Suppl., 1936.

4. YANIGAHARA, N.: Significance of Harmonic Changes and Noise Components in Hoarseness. Jour. Speech and Hearing Res., 10:531-541, 1967.

5. ISSHIKI, N., ET AL.: Differential Diagnosis of Hoarseness. Folia phoniat., 21:9-19, 1969.

LARYNX RECONSTRUCTIVE SURGERY — A STUDY OF THREE-YEAR FINDINGS — A MODIFIED SURGICAL TECHNIQUE.*

MANUEL F. VEGA, M.D.,

Madrid, Spain.

We were highly impressed in the larynx surgical reconstruction technique. The thought of a surgery capable of preserving the mechanism of oral communication of man, was most interesting to all of us. For many years, specialists have made every possible effort to discover a surgical means to remedy this problem; however, it must be considered that one should not expose patients to a risk greater than that existing when a conventional laryngectomy is performed. In other words, the technique must always be judged in correct measure. Attempts must also be made to improve the technique without letting past or future sacrifice involved therein, prevent us from attaining the desired target of oral preservation, together with a simultaneous elimination, from a surgical standpoint, of the risk of disease developing.

In Italy, in July, 1970, we observed some operations performed on patients with cancer in the vocal cords, using Dr. Serafini's (University of Padova) technique. In this technique the epiglottis was spared and the operation performed by a vertical central incision, raising the trachea in order to link it to the epiglottis and thus preserving the voice and, in some cases, even decannulating the patient.

We felt attracted by Dr. Serafini's technique from the beginning, nevertheless, and taking into account the fact that surgical success is limited principally by local or regional metastases and by local relapses, we believe that this technique could be performed in a similar way through removal of the whole larynx and a neck dissection on the affected area. This is the procedure aimed at in our work.

The cases involved in the development of the clinical and surgical study are from the Oncology Provintial Hospital of Madrid, directed by Professor Perez Modrego. They were larynx epidermoidal carcinoma-diagnosed patients and also included were previous laryngectomized patients, whom we have treated in collaboration with Drs. Sacristán, Scola and Bachiller.

SURVEY OF LITERATURE.

For many years specialists throughout the world have been working to

*Presented at the Centennial Conference on Laryngeal Cancer, Toronto, Ontario, Canada, May 26, 1974.

Reprinted by permission from *The Laryngoscope*, 1975, *85*, 866–881.

solve the difficult problem of conserving the voice whenever a radical larynx technique is necessary.

Many devices have been used in larynx reconstruction: artificial prosthesis, grafting, transplantation, etc., though, unfortunately, the results were not as satisfactory as desired. Numerous attempts have been made without great success: Czerny (1870), *Billroth (December 31, 1873)*, Casselli (1879), Roseell Park (1886), all using artificial laryngeal prosthesis. Föderl, in 1898, proposed the reconstruction technique described in Lauren's book in 1906. The Spaniard, Botey, in 1902, published in the Rhinology-Laryngology Latin Files (September-October, 1902, Barcelona), his reconstructive technique. Horfmann Saguez, in 1947, attempted the surgical reconstruction of the larynx. In 1952, Briani, based on an observation from Scuri (1928), attempted, through canalization of a pharyngo-precervical fistula, to improve the function of the voice. Later several authors modified and improved it: Conley (1958), Miller (1967), Montgomery (1968), and Asai (1965). Larynx transplantation has also been attempted in dogs, but difficulties of innervation and of vascular irrigation caused it to fail: Work and Boles (1965), Mounier Kuhn (1968), Ogura (1966), and Silver (1966). In 1969, Kluyskens, *et al.*, for the first time transplanted a larynx in a human being with disastrous results (massive cancer dissemination). Majer and Rieder applied the "Crico-Hyoid" technique, which, requiring the preservation of cricoid and epiglottis, reduces its application to the minimum.

Clinical Study. We are aware of the difficulties, doubts and problems that our technique may pose; however, it is through discussion of, and concern for such doubts and problems pertaining to medicine, that one can hope to reach useful conclusions.

Larynx reconstructive surgery has limited applications and reduced the number of candidates for conventional total laryngectomy.

Our contribution is intended to present a surgical technique which does not pretend to be complete and still involves many problems and disadvantages.

This technique has been used by us for three years and a study is to be carried out of all those cases wherein operations have been performed, together with a description of the surgical procedure, which is more clearly illustrated in the accompanying film.

The material used and our own experiences are based at present on the contribution of 48 operated cases at the Oncology Hospital of Madrid.

From September, 1970, to December, 1973, 187 cases involving laryngeal epidermoid carcinoma were dealt with: 18 laryngofissures (9.6 percent), 57 horizontal supraglottic and amplified laryngectomies (30.5 percent), 59 conventional total laryngectomies (31.6 percent), five pharyngo-

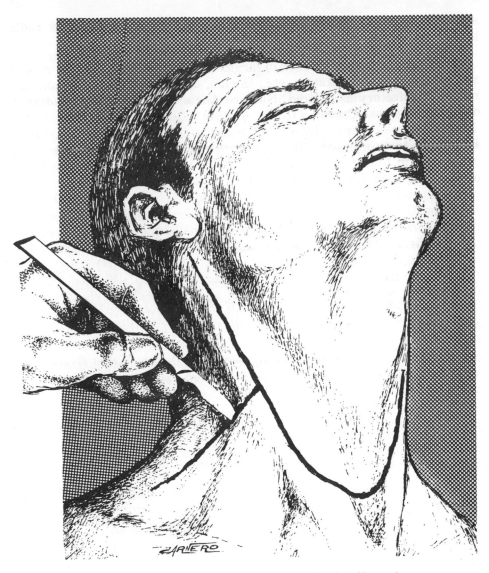

Fig. 1. Customary incision and tracheotomy in cricothyroid membrane.

glosso-laryngectomies (2.6 percent), and 48 cases reconstructive laryngectomies (25.7 percent) (Figs. 1 and 2).

Laryngofissures	18 cases	9.6 percent
Horizontal supraglottic and amplified	57 cases	30.5 percent
Conventional laryngectomy	59 cases	31.6 percent
Pharyngo-Glosso-laryngectomy	5 cases	2.6 percent
Reconstructive laryngectomy	48 cases	25.7 percent

Of the 48 cases of reconstructive laryngectomy, the techniques used were Serafini-Arslan, Labayle, Staffieri, our own personal technique, including reconstruction with epiglottis and tracheoplastic, these latter only being used in exceptional cases.

The 48 cases broken down in the reconstructive laryngectomy used and number of cases of each:

Serafini	12 cases
Personal technique	17 cases
Tracheoplastic	2 cases
Reconstructive with epiglottis	4 cases
Staffieri	9 cases
Labayle	4 cases

Of the 48 cases of reconstructive laryngectomies, all the patients were males, with an average age of 55 years. The youngest was 38 and the oldest 70. The disease treated was epidermoid carcinoma, except for one patient who had undergone a previous operation of conventional total laryngectomy and on whom a tracheoplastia was performed.

It should be stressed that the indications must be carefully studied as there are factors which play a most important role (these to be explained shortly).

From a macroscopic point of view, the patients with the following lesions have been selected:

Endolaryngeal lesions of the true and false cords and ventricle.

Vestibular-epiglottic carcinoma not permitting an amplified horizontal supraglottic.

Patients previously laryngectomized. Regarding adult papillomatosis, we have no experience in this field, but do not discount the possibility of the technique being used.

The contra-indications, from an oncological point of view, are classified as follows: patients with lymph nodes N-2 and N-3; infiltration of laryngeal cartilage; lesion in prelaryngeal muscles; invasion of thyroid gland, or extension of cancer of the thyroid gland to larynx; exteriorization of tumor to skin; invasion of tumor to hypopharyngeal mucus to valleculas, or base of the tongue, or to hyoid bone.

Of the 48 cases treated, 17 were operated with total removal of the larynx.

Location. Without cricoid 15 cases. Lesions in base of epiglottis, preepiglottic space, ventricle, false cords, true cords and beneath cords not

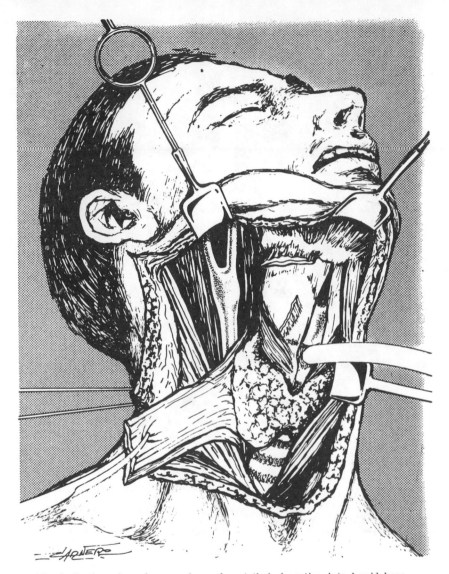

Fig. 2. Section of pre-laryngeal muscles at their insertion into hyoid bone.

exceeding 5 mm. Of the 15, conservative neck dissection was carried out on 11.

With cricoid two cases, lesions in base of epiglottis, pre-epiglottic space, false cords and ventricle. Both with conservative neck dissection.

In our opinion, we have introduced some very important modifications in a series of cases which permit the reconstructive technique to be employed in a greater number of patients affected by laryngeal epidermoidal

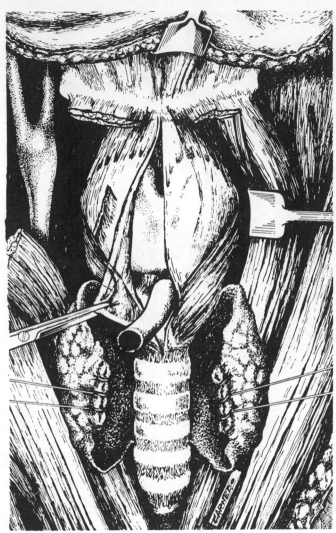

Fig. 3. Dissection of external pericondrium of thyroid cartilage and of pharyngeal constricting muscles.

carcinoma, since they offer optimal oncologic conditions, as a total larynx removal is performed together with a simultaneous neck dissection.

Such modifications consist of:

a. Larynx removal, without preservation of epiglottis and pre-epiglottic space, and maintaining a triangular posterior segment of the cricoid cartilage of the first tracheal ring, which would act as a "posterior neo-epiglottis."

b. Horizontal section of trachea, at level of first tracheal ring, with total removal of cricoid cartilage.

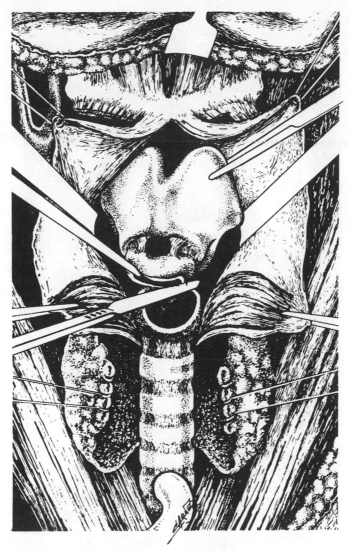

Fig. 4. Displacement of tracheotomy to fourth or fifth tracheal ring and removal of larynx from below upward.

c. Section of hyoid bone horns, and in other cases, section of hyoid body, in order to permit a greater downward displacement of the said body, thus helping the "tracheo-hyoid" linking.

d. Reconstruction purse string suture of pyriform sinus at the expense of the hypopharyngeal mucus, preserving as far as possible the original anatomical conditions, in order to ensure phonation and deglutition, as a defense mechanism.

e. Finally an intercrossing is sometimes performed with the prelaryn-

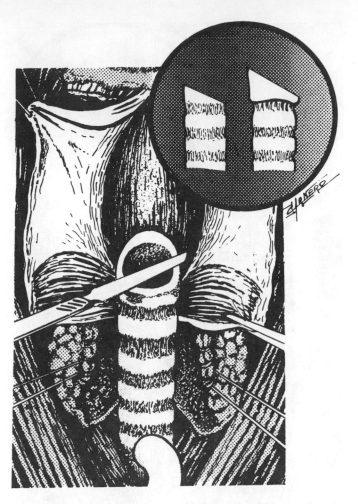

Fig. 5. Bevelling of first tracheal ring or of cricoid cartilage, when the latter has been retained in order to act as a "neo-epiglottis."

geal muscles, for a better protection of the trachea after raising it and loose suture stitches of front edge of E.C.M. whenever a functional dissection of the neck is made (Suarez type).

When it can be avoided we do not perform dissection of the thyroid gland, nor do we separate the tracheal walls too much, so that the vascularization can be made under better conditions.

Our present surgical technique is as follows:

Surgical Technique.

1. Preliminary tracheotomy with local anesthesia in the cricoid membrane, if possible, to be followed with total anesthesia. The surgeon's customary incision.

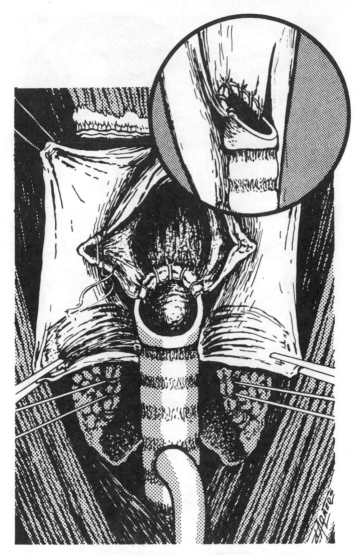

Fig. 6-A. Reconstruction of pyriform sinus at the expense of the hypopharyngeal mucous membrane. Suture of hypopharyngeal mucous membrane to rear wall of "stoma-tracheal" with 3-0 or 4-0 dexon stitches.

2. We use either the H. Martin or Hautant incision, amplifying the latter at both sides of the neck, in order to effect neck dissection, according to Martin or Suarez techniques.

3. Incision of pre-laryngeal muscles at their insertion point into the hyoid bone, dissecting them as far as their lower insertion point and preserving them.

4. The larynx is dissected and the external pericondrium detached from

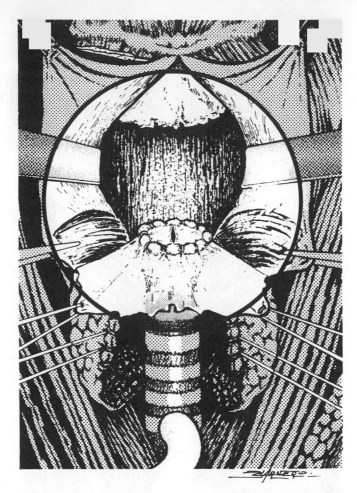

Fig. 6-B. In some cases the hypopharyngeal mucous membrane is placed in the "stoma-tra-cheal," performing at its center a "tailor's buttonhole." Staffieri's variant.

thyroid and cricoid cartilages with pharyngeal constricting muscles, for later reconstruction of "tracheal neo-larynx."

5. Section of the isthmus of the thyroid; detachment of the latter from the trachea, and dissection of front and side walls of the trachea as far as the fourth or fifth tracheal rings. In this way we have the larynx and trachea exteriorized in a single block.

6. A lengthwise opening (laryngotomy) is made in the larynx in order to determine the size of the lesion. Tracheostomy is displaced to the fourth or fifth tracheal ring. Subsequent removal is carried out from below upward, trying to preserve the maximum amount possible of retrocricoid hypopharyngeal mucosa.

7. Reconstruction of the pyriform sinus at the expense of the hypo-

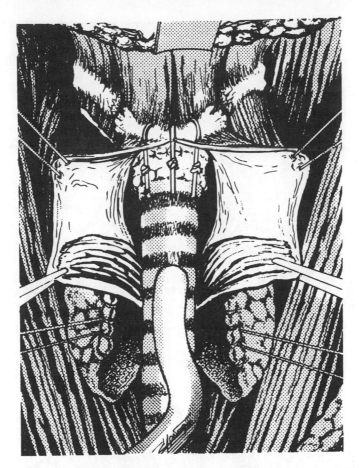

Fig. 7. Elevation of trachea passing three stitches with thick 2 or 3 chromated catgut from trachea to hyoid bone. Sometimes, section or fracture of horns of hyoid bone is made in order to facilitate tracheo-hyoid linking.

pharyngeal mucosa. Since recently, and in some cases, the hypopharyngeal mucosa has been placed over the tracheal-stoma, making "a tailor's buttonhole" in the center for oral reproduction and using the Staffieri technique.

8. When the cricoid cartilage is conserved, it is cut obliquely, in order to make a "neo-epiglottis" with a portion of the cricoid cartilage or with the first tracheal ring.

9. Reconstruction. The stoma-hypopharyngeal wall is sutured to the tracheal posterior wall by means of 3-0 dexon stitches, viz. to first tracheal ring, or to the cricoid cartilage if it has been conserved. Slight elevation of the trachea, after tilting the patient's head forward, using hooks fastened to the lateral walls of the trachea, then three stitches are made with No. 2 or 3 dexon, through the front edge of the trachea and the hyoid bone, in order to raise the trachea. When the distance was too great, we

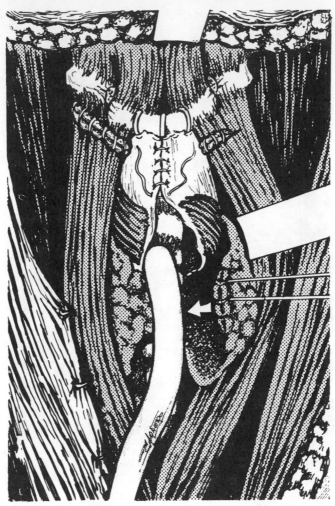

Fig. 8. The trachea raised, it is protected by the pericondrium, pharyngeal constricting muscles, thyroid gland and pre-laryngeal muscles.

performed, without any problems, the section of fracture of both horns of hyoid bone, in order to tilt its body and permit tracheo-hyoid linkage. All this is protected by the perichondrium of the thyroid cartilage which has been conserved and with the constricting muscles of the pharynx and the gland beneath the tracheostoma, if possible reinforced by stitching it with a No. 3-0 Ethicon stitch. Sometimes the prelaryngeal muscles are inter-crossed when they are restitched to hyoid bone or to front edge of E.C.M. for greater reinforcement of the trachea, in those cases in which an O. Suarez-type neck dissection emptying has been done.

10. Closing of skin with cutaneous muscle and subcutaneous tissue, plac-ing two drains.

The complications we have experienced in the immediate long term post-operative stages, are as follows.

Local complications we have encountered at the immediate postoperative stage have been:

Cartilage necrosis	4 cases
Pharyngostoma	1 case
Hemorrhage	1 case
Internal edemas	12 cases
Seromas	4 cases

The general complications encountered in the immediate postoperative stage in our techniques were: in the modified technique: one case of broncopneumonia, and in the reconstruction with epiglottis and tracheoplastia: none at all.

Among the local or regional complications encountered in our technique are:

Total laryngectomy by tracheal obliteration	1 case
Relapse base of tongue at eight months	1 case
Lymph nodes at 24 months	2 cases
Pharyngostome	1 case
Relapse in tracheostoma at 18 months	1 case
Exitus	4 cases

These four cases had relapse in the base of the tongue, tracheostoma and two cervical metastasis cases.

In the technique with epiglottis, of the four cases, there was one with endolaryngeal relapse making it necessary to perform a classic total laryngectomy.

In the immediate postoperative stage there are patients who have swallowed with relative ease during the second week. Others have encountered more difficulties and liquids posed serious problems; however, with patience and training, such difficulties have been overcome in the majority of cases.

As for phonation, it is useful from the first days and, practically in every case, the use of the voice can be considered very satisfactory. This fact was of great importance to us from the very beginning. The reconstructive technique introduces a new situation in the future of these patients: the preservation of the mechanism of communication with their fellowmen, as we mentioned earlier. In other surgical techniques of total resection this is attained only after a long arduous period of time and most often in a very restricted way.

Obviously, not all are advantages, even when preservation of the voice may represent a lot. The compromise of the respiratory function and of swallowing are problems that have yet to be satisfactorily resolved. The elimination of the larynx and the profound anatomical and functional transformations of the aero-digestive confluent, as a result of surgery, suppress in a form we may call "brutal" the protection mechanism of the respiratory system.

The respiratory phonemona are fundamentally affected in the "inhalation phase," while the "exhalation phase" is fairly well maintained; consequently, in most cases the patient cannot always be "decannulated."

In our series, for instance, we could "decannulate" only two cases, and in four other cases, the patients were able to keep the cannula closed during the daytime.

These results show that in the 17 cases operated with our technique, there were 12 in which swallowing of solids was good and one bad. Swallowing of liquids, 10 good and three bad.

The respiratory phenomena are fundamentally affected in the "inhalation phase," while the "exhalation phase" is fairly well maintained.

Swallowing	Solids	Good	12 cases	
		Bad	1 case	
	Liquids	Good	10 cases	
		Bad	3 cases	
Phonation			12 cases	
Respiration	Inhalation	Good	4 cases	
		Bad	8 cases	
	Exhalation	Good	12 cases	
		Bad	1 case	(trachea obliter.)
	Cannulated		12 cases	
	Without cannula		1 case	
	Cannula closed during daytime		3 cases	

Re-operated: one case. The trachea is closed by using hypopharyngeal mucus to form a buttonhole.

This demonstrates the functional results with reconstruction with epiglottic technique on four cases:

Swallowing good	4 cases	
Phonation good	3 cases	
Phonation nil	1 case	(Total L. for relapse)
Respiration decannulated	2 cases	
Respiration cannulated	2 cases	
Tracheoplastic two cases:		
Swallowing good	2 cases	
Phonation good	1 case	
Phonation fair	1 case	
Respiration without cannula	0 cases	
Respiration with cannula	2 cases	

Two patients who had been previously laryngectomized and had total loss of speech, were operated upon by the reconstructive technique, elevating the trachea, and linking it to the hyoid bone. Phonation was good in one and fair in the other. Deglutition was good in both. These two patients use a cannula but beforehand neither was capable of any speech whatsoever even by artificial means or esophageal speech.

To study this functional aspect we asked for the cooperation of Dr. Gálvez Galán, Chief of the Radiodiagnosis Department, since the radiological techniques, mainly the radiocinematography, proved particularly efficient in this sense.

We could verify both in the serialized images and in the radiocinematography that, during phonation and deglutition of liquids or solids, the "neo-larynx" — let's call it — shifts *en bloc* with an ascending motion, basically due to the elevation of the posterior wall of the pharynx by contraction of the pharyngeal muscles. This ascent produces a slight forward projection of the upper sector of the trachea but; above all, the forward displacement of the fold surgically created by the stitching of the hypopharyngeal anterior wall to trachea dorsal edge. With patients who still retain a portion of the cricoid cartilage, this conservation could be the fundamental element in the protection of deglutition. For this reason and because of the backward projection of the tongue base, and considering that the epiglottis plays a less important role than that supposedly conferred upon it as an occluding mechanism, we have called the artificial posterior fold the "neo-epiglottis." With patients in whom this mechanism has not been reconstructed in the same conditions, the projection mechanism is far less efficient and the inhalation of liquids rapidly sets in and becomes a very persistent phenomenon. In the radiographic images it is possible to study closely the occluding mechanism and how the pre-vertebral cavity expands, by contraction of the hypopharyngeal muscles.

The radiographs obtained during the emission of fundamental sounds show how the pharyngo-tracheal edge moves forward and upward. The space of this "neo-epiglottis" is different for the emission of open vowels than for closed vowels. The respiratory phenomena show a distinct situation.

During inhalation the hypopharynx also moves upward, with the result that the caliber of the hypopharyngeal mouth of the trachea becomes smaller. This explains in part why inhalation in these operated patients is more difficult and insufficient than exhalation. In the air-expelling phase the diameter of the air canal remains approximately two-thirds the size of the trachea.

Alterations in the trachea and in the tracheo-bronchial angle of such patients as a forced result of the elevation of the trachea, were also studied radiographically. This will be the object of another paper.

Finally, we believe that one of the most important contributions of this technique may be the functional recovery of former laryngectomized patients. This problem often appears in our clinic, with patients who have undergone a conventional total laryngectomy and who, despite a long recuperation period, could not recover the oral function by any means whatsoever; nevertheless, to make this possible, it is necessary to conserve the hyoid bone totally and conserve the cricoid or the first tracheal ring partially.

We believe that laryngeal reconstructive surgery is a step forward in the surgical treatment of laryngeal cancer. A new chapter has been opened within conventional surgery; and no doubt, with everyone collaborating, besides eliminating the cancer, we shall avoid mutilated persons and reconstruct a new larynx for them so they may be able to speak and, in the not too distant future, to breathe through their natural channels without having a cannula or using a phonatory device.

NEOGLOTTIC RECONSTRUCTION AFTER TOTAL LARYNGECTOMY

A PRELIMINARY REPORT

CERI M. GRIFFITHS, MD

J. THOM LOVE, JR., MD

GALVESTON, TEXAS

SUMMARY — This paper is a preliminary report on neoglottic reconstruction of the larynx after total laryngectomy following the techniques described by Staffieri. Also included are general observations on the criteria for selecting candidates for this procedure. At the University of Texas Medical Branch in Galveston, this procedure has been attempted on eight candidates. Reconstruction was accomplished in six, of whom five achieved satisfactory speech, providing an 80% success rate. One of the five did not like the quality of his voice and refused to use it. The sixth produced speech with difficulty and is still undergoing speech therapy. One patient died from recurrence before a second stage could be carried out, and another patient did not have sufficient tissue for neoglottic reconstruction after total laryngectomy. Three patients developed salivary fistulas at the drain site, but all closed spontaneously with the application of pressure. From this data, one may conclude that this technique offers much potential and warrants further study.

This paper is a preliminary report on neoglottic reconstruction of the larynx after total laryngectomy. This technique, developed by Staffieri,[1] has been utilized in more than 200 patients who have achieved successful voice reproduction postoperatively.

At the University of Texas Medical Branch in Galveston, this procedure has been attempted on eight occasions. One patient did not have sufficient tissue remaining after laryngectomy to perform the reconstruction. A second patient, who had preoperative radiotherapy, had only the first stage of the procedure. Before the second phase could be completed, the patient developed skin metastases and died.

Of the six patients in whom the reconstruction was completed, four developed good speech, one developed speech with difficulty, and the last, while able to phonate, did not like the quality of his neoglottic voice and refused to use it.

TECHNIQUE

A standard total wide field laryngectomy, using the modification described by Staffieri,[1] was attempted in all cases. After mobilizing the larynx in the standard manner, a permanent tracheostomy is created by excising a circle of cartilage at the level of the third and fourth tracheal rings. A similar, but slightly larger area of skin is excised over the tracheal stoma, and the skin epithelium is sutured in apposition to the tracheal mucosa. The trachea is transected at the subcricoid level, with care being taken not to enter the postcricoid esophagus. The dissection is then carried cranially, developing a flap of the postcricoid mucosa (Fig. 1). After this dissection, the larynx is entered at the point furthest from the tumor, and a standard resection is carried out. The lower margin of the resection is connected to the previously described inferior dissection at the level of the aryepiglottic folds and arytenoids. At completion of the resection, bleeding is controlled, using standard techniques.

Attention is then directed to the posterior cricoid mucosal flap. At a point in the midline that is approximately at the center of the top of the trachea, 4/0

From the Department of Otolaryngology, The University of Texas Medical Branch, Galveston, Texas.

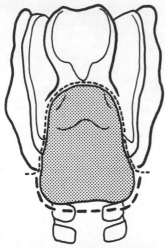

Fig. 1. The shaded area indicates the region from which the postcricoid flap is developed. The heavy dotted line indicates the standard mucosal cuts, and the light dotted line indicates the mucosal cuts used in the neoglottic procedure.

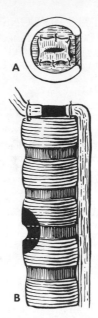

Fig. 3. A) View of neoglottis after it has been sewn in place (viewed from below). B) Side view of neoglottis sewn in position.

silk holding sutures are placed. A cutting cautery is used to incise through the muscle and submucosa to the pharyngeal mucosa (Fig. 2A). At this point, two more sutures are placed in the mucosa, which is pulled through the incision in the muscle (Fig. 2B). Using a cutting cautery, the mucosa is incised for approximately 8 mm (Fig. 2C). The mucosal edges are then sewn to the submucosal and muscle layers with 4/0 silk. One suture is placed in

each corner, as shown (Fig. 2D). The pharyngeal flap is placed over the open top of the trachea and sewn into position in two layers, using absorbable sutures (Fig. 3).

The hyoid was left intact in all of our patients. In the original reports, Staffieri[1] describes a horizontal closure with this flap. Although this method

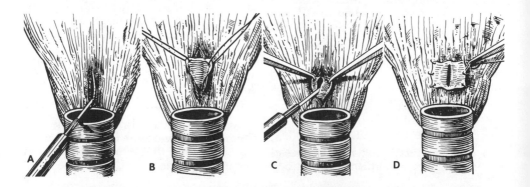

Fig. 2. A) A cutting cautery is used to make an incision through the pharyngeal muscle and submucosa. B) Holding sutures are placed in the pharyngeal mucosa, which is pulled through the opening previously created in the muscle. C) The mucosa is incised for approximately 8 mm with a cutting cautery. D) The pharyngeal mucosa is sewn back with 4/0 silk sutures.

has been attempted on several occasions, it has been abandoned due to the excessive tension produced on the flap. Hemovac® drains are placed in the gutters on each side of the pharynx, and the skin is closed in layers.

SURGICAL INDICATIONS

Neoglottic reconstruction appears to be possible in most lesions requiring a total laryngectomy. However, this procedure is contraindicated in those patients who have postcricoid or postarytenoid involvement and in those patients whose subglottic extension requires a low tracheal resection.

In patients who have had prior radiotherapy, Staffieri[1] recommends the formation of the flap and tracheostoma in the method outlined, with reconstruction delayed until healing is complete. At that time, the neoglottis is created under local anesthesia via the tracheostoma.

To date, all but two of our patients had either T_3 or T_4 endolaryngeal epidermoid carcinomas. In Case 2, the lesion was so extensive that the mucosal flap could not be developed without compromising the resection. In Case 4, the lesion, which involved the pyriform sinus, compromised the formation of the mucosal flap. In this case, a standard resection was performed, and the flap was created by mobilizing the esophagus and performing a slightly lower resection of the trachea. The neoglottis was formed in the mobilized esophageal mucosa.

CASE REPORTS

Case 1. A 56-year-old Negro male presented with a two month history of hoarseness. A squamous cell carcinoma involving the right true and false cords with minimal subglottic extension was found. The vocal cord was fixed, and no nodes were present.

A total laryngectomy with neoglottic reconstruction was performed. Postoperatively the patient healed primarily and was able to phonate on the seventh day. Subsequently, he was discharged; but when seen two weeks postoperatively, he was aspirating on water only. He was instructed to insert a cuffed tracheostomy tube when drinking water and was able to prevent aspiration satisfactorily in this way.

Case 2. A 75-year-old Negro male was transferred from another institution with a tracheostomy tube in place. The tracheostomy had been performed 24 hours previously for airway obstruction. Upon evaluation, the patient was found to have a lesion involving the entire pyriform sinus.

He underwent a total laryngectomy and right radical neck dissection. After excision of the tumor, the remaining tissue was insufficient for neoglottic reconstruction. Therefore, a normal closure was carried out, and postoperative radiotherapy was given.

Case 3. A 64-year-old Caucasian male presented with a seven month history of hoarseness. He was found to have a squamous cell carcinoma of the left true cord, left false cord and aryepiglottic fold. The cord was fixed, and no nodes were present.

He underwent a total laryngectomy with neoglottic reconstruction. Postoperatively he developed a salivary fistula from his Hemovac® drain site, which closed spontaneously with pressure in four days after removal of the drain. Although this patient phonated in 15 days, he had considerable difficulty with aspiration of liquids. The neoglottis was examined from the tracheostomy site, and it was found that the neoglottis had migrated from its original central position to the posterior lip of the tracheostomy remnant. Since the patient had good voice and was able to control aspiration of fluids with a cuffed tracheostomy tube, he declined revision.

Two months later he was still aspirating on all fluids, and it was decided to revise the neoglottis. The length of the neoglottis was reduced by approximately 50% via the tracheostoma. The procedure produced a dramatic reduction in the amount of aspiration, which was easily controlled with a cuffed tracheostomy tube. He maintained an excellent voice. Postoperatively he underwent radiotherapy.

Case 4. A 67-year-old Caucasian male presented with an eight week history of hoarseness. A lesion involving the left vocal process, true cord, the anterior commissure and one third of the opposite cord was found. A subglottic extension of 2-3 mm was noted.

A vertical hemilaryngectomy was attempted. At surgery, the subglottic extension was found to be greater than anticipated, and a complete resection could not be achieved by a partial procedure. Therefore, a total laryngectomy with neoglottic reconstruction was performed without complication.

Postoperatively there was a salivary leak in the left Hemovac® drain. The drain was removed, and the fistula healed spontaneously in four days with the application of pressure. The patient produced good speech with no aspiration 20 days postoperatively and underwent postoperative radiotherapy.

Case 5. A 63-year-old Caucasian male presented with a two week history of painful swelling in the right neck. The patient had a lesion of the aryepiglottic fold, false cord, vallecula and pharyngeal wall that involved only the right side. He also had a 1 cm node in the right jugulodigastric area.

A preoperative course of 4500 rads was given. Six weeks later he underwent a total laryngectomy and right radical neck dissection. A "neoglottic-type" flap was created and sewn in place; but due to prior irradiation, the neoglottic opening was not created at that time. Primary healing occurred, but three weeks postoperatively the patient developed skin metastases and quickly succumbed to his disease. The neoglottic aperture was never created.

Case 6. A 60-year-old Caucasian female, presented with a six month history of a sore throat. A lesion involving the entire right pyriform sinus, including the aryepiglottic fold, was found. A 2 x 2 cm node was present in the right neck.

A standard total laryngectomy was performed. Due to the size of the lesion, it was impossible to make a standard "neoglottic-type" flap. Therefore, a dissection was performed between the trachea and the esophagus, which allowed the esophagus to be mobilized cranially and utilized as the neoglottic flap. The first tracheal ring was also resected to facilitate this maneuver, and the neoglottis was then created in the esophageal flap.

Seven days postoperatively the patient appeared to be healing well, and feeding was begun. At this point, she was able to produce speech. However, on the tenth day, she developed a salivary fistula from one of the Hemovac® drain sites. The nasogastric tube was replaced, the Hemovac® drain was removed, and a pressure dressing was applied. The fistula closed in 72 hours. On the 11th day postoperatively, a course of chemotherapy using bleomycin and methotrexate was begun. On the 21st day postoperatively, another smaller fistula developed in the midline at the site of the incision. Once again, the nasogastric tube was placed, and a pressure dressing was applied. This fistula closed spontaneously in eight days.

Since that time, the patient has produced speech with difficulty. She lives many miles from the center, so she was not able to continue speech therapy. However, she will be returning for postoperative radiotherapy, and speech therapy will be resumed at that time.

Case 7. A 65-year-old Caucasian male presented with a 10 day history of hoarseness, a sore throat and a 12-pound weight loss in the past three months. On direct laryngoscopy, he was found to have a right true vocal cord lesion that extended onto the false cord subglottically for 5 mm. The cord was fixed. The patient underwent a total laryngectomy with neoglottic reconstruction.

The postoperative course was complicated by a small fistula that developed on the eighth day. This was successfully treated by reinstituting nasogastric tube feedings and applying pressure to the neck. The patient was able to phonate but did not like the quality of his voice and refused to use it. No aspiration occurred. He completed postoperative radiotherapy without sequelae.

Case 8. A 64-year-old Negro male presented with a four month history of hoarseness. A lesion of the left false cord and the left true cord with 2-3 mm subglottic extension was found. The cord was fixed.

The patient underwent a total laryngectomy with neoglottic reconstruction. Postoperatively he healed primarily, talked after three weeks and could swallow without aspiration. The patient completed postoperative radiotherapy without complications.

DISCUSSION

An 80% success rate was achieved in those patients who actually received the neoglottic reconstruction. Of the six patients in whom reconstruction was completed, one refused to use his voice, and a second had extreme difficulty with phonation. The latter case can probably be corrected by increasing the size of the neoglottis. Aspiration occurred only in the first two cases. In one of these cases, the neoglottis was found to be on the posterior lip of the trachea. The location of the neoglottis is probably important, since prevention of aspiration may depend partially upon the shielding effect of the base of the tongue. In all cases, a subsequent attempt was made to situate the neoglottis anteriorly to utilize the normal action of the tongue maximally. None of these cases had any aspiration problems. We believe, as does Staffieri,[1] that it is important to maintain the glossal musculature intact by leaving the hyoid in place so that the tongue may act in a coordinated manner during deglutition.

Three patients developed fistulas. In our experience, this is a high rate of fistula formation. Since all but one of the patients were nonirradiated, this complication was unexpected. At present, we are unable to explain this high rate of fistula formation.

All patients, except the patient discussed in Case 5 who died of his disease, have disease-free intervals of three to six months. There have been no recurrences to date.

Using Staffieri's[1] technique, vocal rehabilitation was achieved in 80% of our cases. In the authors' opinion, this technique offers great potential for the following reasons:

1) No compromise is required in the surgical resection. 2) It is a simple procedure. 3) In nonirradiated patients, it is a one-step procedure. 4) No mechanical parts are required. 5) Rehabilitation time is short. 6) Long phonation time produces much greater intelligibility of speech.

It has the following disadvantages: 1) Voice is hoarse. 2) Tracheostomy is necessary. 3) One hand is needed to block the stoma when phonating. 4) Minor aspiration problems may develop.

REFERENCES

1. Staffieri M, Serafini I, Capretti C, et al: *La Riabilitazione Chirurgica della Voce e della Respirazione Dopo Laringectomia Totale. Official Proceedings of the 19th National Congress of the Associazione Otologi Ospedalieri Italiana*. Bologna, Associazione Otologi Ospedalieri Italiani, 1976, pp 1-222

REPRINTS — Ceri M. Griffiths, MD, Deputy Chairman and Assistant Professor, Department of Otolaryngology, The University of Texas Medical Branch, Galveston, TX 77550.

REED-FISTULA SPEECH FOLLOWING PHARYNGOLARYNGECTOMY

Bernd Weinberg

Purdue University, West Lafayette, Indiana

Donald P. Shedd

Roswell Park Memorial Institute, Buffalo, New York

Yoshiyuki Horii

Purdue University, West Lafayette, Indiana

This report describes reed-fistula speech, a surgical-prosthetic approach to speech rehabilitation for patients who have undergone extensive resection of the pharynx in association with total laryngectomy and highlights some characteristics of speech produced by four subjects who use reed-fistula speech as their primary method of oral communication. Observations supported the view that the reed-fistula approach provides functionally serviceable speech to patients who have undergone pharyngolaryngectomy. A number of speech and biomedical liabilities associated with this method of speech restoration are delineated. In recognition of these liabilities, reed-fistula speech does not currently merit consideration as a routine approach to speech restoration for all laryngectomized patients. Rather, it is regarded as a potentially promising, experimental approach to speech restoration following laryngeal amputation.

A primary postsurgical rehabilitation objective for laryngectomized patients is the restoration of oral communication. To date, speech rehabilitation of laryngectomized patients has been accomplished chiefly with esophageal speech or through the use of artificial larynges. Recently, there has been much interest in surgical reconstruction (with or without incorporation of a prosthesis) as an approach to postlaryngectomy vocal rehabilitation (Asai, 1972; Conley, 1969; Komorn, 1974; Montgomery and Toohil, 1968; Taub and Spiro, 1972; Sisson et al., 1975; Vega, 1975).

For several years we have been developing and evaluating an experimental reed-fistula speech mechanism for patients who have undergone laryngectomy. In a recent paper (Shedd, Schaaf, and Weinberg, 1976), important biomedical problems incurred in the process of introducing sound into the pharynx by means of this speech mechanism were discussed. This report describes the

Reprinted by permission from *Journal of Speech and Hearing Disorders*, 1978, *43*, 401–403.

reed-fistula approach to speech rehabilitation for patients who have undergone extensive resection of the pharynx in association with total laryngectomy and highlights important characteristics of speech produced with this combined surgical-prosthetic approach under collaborative study at Roswell Park Memorial Institute (Department of Head and Neck Surgery) and Purdue University (Department of Audiology and Speech Sciences).

What is Reed-Fistula Speech?

The reed-fistula approach to speech restoration consists of interposing an external air-bypass and pseudolaryngeal mechanism between the laryngectomized patient's tracheal stoma and a surgically created pharyngeal fistula. The pseudolarynx is a modified Tokyo artificial laryngeal mechanism (Weinberg and Riekena, 1973). A diagram of a prototype reed-fistula speech appliance is shown in Figure 1. As illustrated in this figure, the vibratory mechanism (F) of the appliance is enclosed in a suitable housing and rests on the patient's

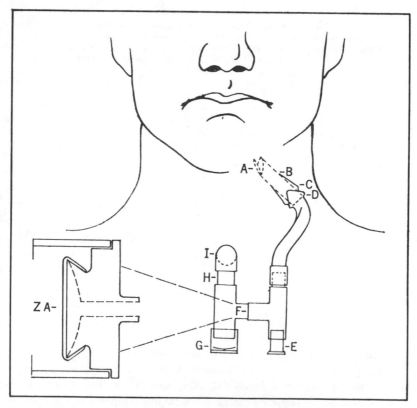

Figure 1. Diagram of reed-fistula speech appliance: (A) secretory valve (B) fistula tube; (C) secretory collar; (D) fistula opening; (E) secretory collector; (F) voicing (reed) mechanism; (G) respiratory valve; (H) tracheal connector; and (I) stomal opening. Insert (F) portrays voicing mechanism: (Z) Reed membrane.

chest wall. Pulmonary air is directed from the tracheal stoma (I) to the vibratory mechanism through a tracheal connector system (H). Sound produced by the vibratory mechanism is transmitted to the vocal tract through a fistula tube (B). The pseudovoice enters the vocal tract through a surgically created fistula (D).

Patients can place and remove the appliance into or from both the neck fistula and the tracheal stoma as needed. Moreover, the appliance is simply constructed using materials that permit easy cleaning and sterilization. Repair, adjustment, and cleaning are accomplished because the component parts of the appliance can simply be taken apart by hand. Appliances have been constructed with a minimum of monetary expense—a feature we expect to maintain in later, more biomedically finished prototypes.

An important feature of this method of speech rehabilitation is that it is modeled on principles of normal speech production. For example, the primary driving forces used to excite and regulate the pseudovoice in reed-fistula speech are those of the respiratory system. The reed larynx is viewed as a resonant device—as is the human larynx—which is set into vibration by subneoglottic forces. Simply stated, the reed-fistula approach consists of developing an external larynx and incorporating this new mechanism into the patient's highly integrated, existing speech production system.

Subjects

The speech data to be presented are based on a rather intensive study of four talkers who use reed-fistula speech as their primary method of oral communication. A brief description of each patient follows.

Patient 1. A male, born in 1927, was admitted to Roswell Park Memorial Institute in November 1971, with a large squamous cell carcinoma involving most of the right, supraglottic larynx together with a neck mass. Airway embarrassment was sufficiently severe to necessitate emergency tracheotomy. Patient underwent total laryngectomy, partial pharyngectomy, and right radical neck dissection in November 1971. Following surgery, only a thin strip of posterior pharynx remained. The pharynx was reconstructed with a delto-pectoral flap (Bakamjian, 1965), and a deliberately planned temporary fistula remained after reconstruction. Initial testing consisting of manually inserting the oral end of a Tokyo artificial larynx into the patient's fistula, and powering this voicing source externally indicated that satisfactory voice and speech could probably be attained. Accordingly, in Januray 1972, this patient's residual fistula was surgically narrowed for speech purposes and a reed-fistula appliance was fabricated for him.

The patient spent several days in the Department of Audiology and Speech Sciences, Purdue University, in March 1974, to undergo speech analysis. Hence, data for this subject reflect speech produced following more than two years of using reed-fistula speech as the sole method of oral communication.

Patient 2. A male, born in 1922, was admitted to Roswell Park Memorial

Institute with a large, transglottic squamous cell carcinoma. Patient underwent total laryngectomy, partial pharyngectomy, left radical neck dissection, and pharyngeal reconstruction with deltopectoral flap, in October 1971. Initial testing for feasibility of reed-fistula speech was conducted in November 1971, and fistula revised for long-term speech purposes in December 1971.

Patient underwent speech studies at Purdue University in October 1974. Hence, information about this patient reflects performance following about three years of using reed-fistula speech.

Patient 3. A male, born in 1929, was admitted to Roswell Park Memorial Institute with a five-month history of right neck mass. A large squamous cell carcinoma was found involving the right pyriform sinus with extension into the epiglottis and base of the tongue. Patient underwent laryngopharyngectomy and right radical neck dissection in January 1975. The pharynx was reconstructed with a deltopectoral flap deliberately leaving a temporary surgical fistula. Initial testing for feasibility of reed-fistula restoration was conducted in March 1975, and fistula was revised for speech prothesis purpose later that month. In August 1976, a small area of invasive carcinoma on the left posterior part of the tongue was excised.

Patient came to Purdue University for speech studies in May 1976, following about one year of using reed-fistula speech.

Patient 4. A female, born in 1907, was admitted to Roswell Park Memorial Institute in November 1972, with dysphagia dating back to May 1972. Diagnostic studies revealed carcinoma of the cervical esophagus and hypopharynx with involvement of the right pyriform sinus and the larynx. Patient underwent laryngopharyngectomy with deltopectoral flap reconstruction in November 1972. A deliberate fistula remained following reconstruction. Tumor involvement of mediastinal and paratracheal nodes was found. Patient had intermittent problem with stenosis of the lower end of the reconstructed pharynx. Following initial testing, fistula revision for speech purposes was performed in February 1973. In June 1973, patient required surgical revision of esophageal anastomosis, a problem unrelated to speech rehabilitation.

Patient came to Purdue University in November 1975. Hence, data for this subject reflect speech produced following about two years and six months of reed-fistula speech usage.

Speech Intelligibility Studies

The objective of one phase of this clinical project was to measure the intelligibility of speech produced by reed-fistula talkers. To accomplish this task, each of the four talkers recorded six lists of a consonant rhyme test (House et al., 1965) and six lists of a vowel rhyme test (Horii and Weinberg, 1975). Each of the consonant lists consisted of 50 monosyllabic words in which half had test consonants in the word-initial position, while the remaining half had test consonants in the word-final position. In this rhyme test, consonants appeared with frequencies approximately equal to those observed in actual English texts. On the other hand, each vowel list consisted of 24 monosyllabic words. In this rhyme test, 12 different vowels appeared twice in each list.

The recorded word lists were delivered binaurally using a high-quality tape system and matched ear phones (Grason-Stadler, Model TDH-39 with Zwislocki-type cushions). The entire perceptual experiment was conducted over a period of five, 50-min daily sessions and all listening was done in a quiet room furnished with individual listening stations. Ten young adult listeners evaluated the rhyme test recordings. Listeners were unfamiliar with alaryngeal speech and were not experienced or trained in psychoacoustic listening procedures.

The signal levels of each test list were determined by playing the test recordings into a Bruel and Kjaer graphic level recorder (Model 2305) and measuring the level of the vocalic maxima of each word relative to a 1000-Hz reference signal. The speech level of each word list was defined operationally as the mean level of the vocalic nuclei of the words in each list. Test tapes were prepared and delivered so that the average speech level of the word lists was 70-dB SPL under the ear phones.

A closed-set response strategy was used in the listening experiment (House et al., 1965). Specifically, listeners were provided answer sheets containing 50 six-word preset ensembles for each consonant list and 24 six-word preset ensembles for each vowel list. The listener's task was to identify each stimulus word from a six-word response set appearing on his answer sheet. The specific type of speech materials and response format was selected because it permitted the use of untrained listeners, provided stable scores after repeated exposure, reduced the effect of familiarity of test words, and substantially minimized the problems associated with an indeterminate response set (House et al., 1965).

TABLE 1. Average intelligibility (% correct) of vowel elements produced by reed-fistula speakers.

Subjects	S1	S2	S3	S4	Subjects Pooled
ɝ	100.0	91.7	41.2	88.3	81.0
o	97.5	82.5	89.2	96.7	91.5
e	96.7	94.2	71.7	95.0	89.4
ɛ	91.7	90.8	54.2	97.5	83.5
æ	85.0	95.8	66.7	80.8	82.1
ʊ	88.3	79.2	79.2	95.0	85.4
ʌ	85.0	73.3	52.5	93.3	76.0
ɔ	85.0	84.2	71.7	84.2	81.3
ɪ	100.0	98.3	51.7	91.7	85.4
i	97.5	97.5	91.7	97.5	96.0
ɑ	82.5	53.3	58.3	41.6	58.9
u	95.0	91.7	70.8	95.0	88.1
Overall	92.0	86.0	66.8	88.1	83.2

Intelligibility Characteristics of Reed-Fistula Talkers

The general results of vowel intelligibility testing are summarized in Table 1. Mean intelligibility for vowel materials ranged from about 67 to 92% correct for the four talkers. Overall mean intelligibility for the four subjects was 83.2% correct. Overall articulation scores for the 12 vowels ranged from about 60 to 90% correct. These data have also been analyzed in confusion matrix form and interested readers may request such data from the authors.

A summary of the mean intelligibility of consonant elements produced by the four talkers is provided in Table 2. Mean intelligibility of consonant ma-

TABLE 2. Average intelligibility (% correct) of consonant elements produced by reed-fistula speakers.

Elements	S1	S2	S3	S4	Subjects Pooled
p	90.9	70.9	79.3	94.3	83.9
b	92.5	64.0	78.5	80.5	78.9
t	82.0	88.3	79.7	93.4	85.9
d	96.3	93.7	86.8	90.0	91.7
k	93.7	90.7	91.1	97.0	93.2
g	95.0	90.7	78.2	86.4	87.7
f	94.4	65.6	74.4	99.4	83.4
v	91.7	80.0	85.0	100.0	82.2
θ	72.0	28.0	34.0	86.0	55.0
ð	95.0	00.0	65.0	95.0	63.8
s	99.6	89.6	98.5	100.0	96.9
z	100.0	100.0	100.0	100.0	100.0
ʃ	100.0	100.0	86.7	100.0	96.7
tʃ	93.3	100.0	100.0	100.0	98.3
dʒ	100.0	100.0	96.7	100.0	99.2
h	95.8	67.5	94.2	95.0	88.1
m	96.3	94.4	88.8	89.4	92.2
n	94.2	92.9	77.5	90.0	88.7
ŋ	70.0	92.0	48.0	62.0	68.0
w	96.7	98.9	93.3	100.0	97.2
r	97.5	95.8	70.3	98.3	90.4
l	100.0	100.0	83.5	94.7	94.6
#	80.0	82.0	74.0	80.0	79.0
Overall	93.1	84.8	82.8	92.9	88.4

terials ranged from about 83 to 93% correct. Overall mean average intelligibility for the four subjects was 88.4% correct. Overall articulation scores for the consonant elements ranged from about 55 for /θ/ to 100% correct for /z/. The consonant data have also been analyzed in confusion matrix form and are also available on request.

Taken together, these results indicate that reed-fistula speech restoration is capable of providing patients who have undergone pharyngolaryngectomy with speech characterized by moderate-to-high intelligible quality. Under the optimal S/N conditions used in our evaluation, normal and excellent esophageal speakers demonstrate near-perfect intelligibility for consonant and vowel rhyme test words (House et al., 1965; Horii and Weinberg, 1973). Hence, on the average, reed-fistula speakers exhibited about a 15% decrease in intelligibility for vowel elements and a 6% reduction for consonant elements when compared to normal and excellent esophageal speakers. On other comparative bases, these data support the view that the intelligibility of the four reed-fistula speakers was, in the majority of cases, superior to that reported for average esophageal and artificial larynx talkers (Hyman, 1955; Creech, 1966).

Acoustic Measurements

In a second phase of this project, high-quality recordings of each speaker reading a standard passage (Fairbanks, 1960) were subjected to various types of acoustic analyses. To obtain phonation time and fundamental frequency (f_0) measurements, the recordings were played by a Nagra IV-D tape recorder into one channel of a Visicorder Model 1508 operating at a chart speed of 500 mm/sec.

The oscillograph record of each subject's paragraph utterance was initially segmented into three basic categories: (1) periodicity, (2) aperiodicity, and (3) silence. The periodic segments of each record were divided into segments of about 50 msec and the average period of completed cycles within each segment was calculated. Fundamental frequency mean, standard deviation, and range and phonation time measures were computed for each subject. The fundamental frequency characteristics of the four talkers are summarized in Table 3. Mean f_0 values for the four talkers were 160, 121, 107, and 204 Hz

TABLE 3. Fundamental frequency and phonation time characteristics of reed-fistula speakers.

Variable	S1	S2	S3	S4
Mean f_0 (Hz)	159.90	121.50	107.50	204.50
f_0 SD (ST)	2.30	2.30	1.10	1.20
% periodicity	56.25	59.46	43.72	37.13
% aperiodicity	14.18	8.49	4.66	20.12
% silence	29.57	32.05	51.62	42.75

(S_4 is a female subject for which this pitch was appropriate). Fundamental frequency standard deviations ranged from about 1 to 2.3 semitones. These observations indicate that the average fundamental frequency of speech produced by reed-fistula speakers was (1) considerably higher than that typically found for esophageal speakers, and (2) within the frequency ranges typically used by normal speakers. Unfortunately, the reduced f_0 standard deviations observed for reed-fistula speakers highlight a relative liability. Namely, f_0 SDs of one to two semitones are smaller than observed for normal and esophageal speakers (two to four semitones) and reflect the perceptual impression of reduced pitch variation (monotonicity) that characterized the speech of this group of speakers.

The phonation time characteristics of the four talkers are also tabulated in Table 3. As can be seen, S's exhibited considerable variation in such speech parameters. For example, the range in percentages of time talkers spent producing periodicity ranged from about 37 to 60%. For aperiodicity, the percentages ranged from about 4.5 to 20%; while for silence, values ranged from about 30 to 50%. Excellent esophageal talkers spend about 50% of their speaking time in periodicity and less than 20% of the time producing noise. (Weinberg and Bennett, 1972.) A relative liability of reed-fistula speech is reflected by the rather large amount of time (40-50%) talkers (3 and 4) spent in silence.

Aerodynamic Characteristics of Reed-Fistula Speech

In this portion of the paper, some results of airflow and volume analysis of speech produced by reed-fistula speakers are delineated. Airflow and volume characteristics were measured for steady-state phonations and connected speech produced by two reed-fistula talkers (S_2, S_4). In particular, measurements were made of (1) the minimal and maximal airflow rates associated with activation and sustainment of voicing during the production of a vowel /a/, and (2) the airflow and volume characteristics associated with oral reading of a 98-word passage (Fairbanks, 1960).

Airflow and volume data were obtained through a pneumotachograph-pressure-transducer system. Oronasal air was channeled through a facemask into a pneumotachograph. Voltage change generated by a pressure transducer, corresponding to the pressure drop in the pneumotach, was amplified and recorded on one channel of an FM tape recorder. Voice signals picked up by a microphone were recorded on the second channel. The recorded signals (both airflow and voice signals) were quantitized using an analog-to-digital converter and stored on computer magnetic tape. A sampling rate of 1000 cps was used for each channel. A computer program (Horii and Cooke, 1975) was used subsequently to analyze the digital data in terms of peak and average flow rate, distribution, duration, and volume characteristics.

Some results of airflow analysis associated with sustained phonation of a vowel /a/ are shown in Table 4. Subjects were asked to sustain phonation of

TABLE 4. Mean airflow rates (cc/sec) associated with prolonged phonation of a vowel /a/.

Speech Effort Level	S2	S4
At a comfortable intensity level	211	196
Lowest flow rate	106	147
Highest flow rate	251	248

/a/ under three different conditions. (1) at a comfortable level of intensity, (2) at the lowest effort level necessary to activate and maintain sustained vibration of the reed mechanism, and (3) at the highest possible effort level permissible to maintain sustained 'voicing. The data in Table 4 indicate that at comfortable levels of speech intensity or effort, average airflow rate was about 200 cc/sec. On the other hand, flow rates associated with minimal activation and sustained voicing were about 100 cc/sec for Subject 2 and about 150 cc/sec for Subject 4. Flow rate associated with maximal effort and sustained voicing was about 250 cc/sec. These observations suggest that reed-fistula talkers are, from an aerodynamic point of view, rather limited to the higher end of the airflow continuum. For example, normal talkers sustain voicing with airflow rate at low as about 50 cc/sec at low intensity and use about 150 cc/sec airflow at a comfortable level of intensity (Isshiki, 1964). At relatively high intensity, normal talkers typically use about 250 cc/sec airflow, although rates as high as 350 cc/sec have been reported for extremely high-intensity phonations (Shipp and McGlone 1971; Faaborg-Anderson, 1957). Snidecor and Isshiki (1965) reported airflow rates of 27 to 72 cc/sec during prolonged esophageal phonation of /a/ at comfortable levels of production.

Airflow and volume characteristics associated with the oral reading of a standard passage are summarized in Table 5. For comparative purposes, data

TABLE 5. Airflow and volume characteristics associated with oral reading of a passage.

Variable	S2	S4	Normal (M)	Esophageal*
Mean airflow rate	266 cc/sec	197 cc/sec	187 cc/sec	25-100 cc/sec
Total volume out	8154 cc	9360 cc	5351 cc	871-1115 cc
Total speaking time	44 sec	75 sec	35 sec	–
Volume/syllable	67 cc/syll.	76 cc/syll.	43 cc/syll.	5-16 cc/syll.

*Isshiki and Snidecor, 1964, 1965.

for a normal male and esophageal talkers are also provided. Reed-fistula speakers were clearly characterized by higher mean airflow rates and, consequently, higher total and syllabic volume air consumption. As expected, comparable aerodynamic characteristics for esophageal talkers are considerably smaller than observed for normal and reed-fistula talkers.

The distributional properties of sampled airflow rates associated with paragraph reading are shown in Figure 2. In this figure, the relative number of occurrences is plotted against the airflow rates in cc/sec to form a frequency distribution curve. Comparable data obtained from a normal male talker are also shown. Since one of the talkers (Speaker 4) was also an effective electrolarynx user, airflow distributional properties measured for speech produced with an artificial larynx (Servox) are also plotted. Clearly, reed-fistula talkers also used high airflow rates in oral reading. Normal talkers would have to speak at production levels three times greater than normal to produce airflow distributions comparable to reed-fistula talkers. The airflow distributions of normal and reed-fistula speakers are comparable when normal talkers read the passage in a whisper (Horii and Cooke, 1975).

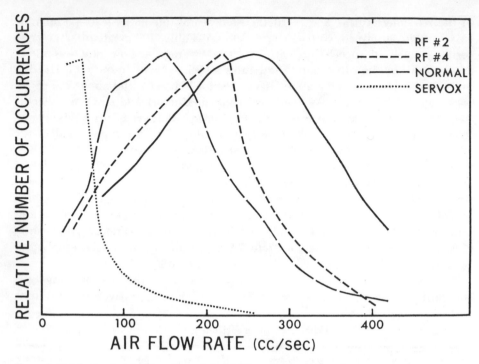

Figure 2. Distributional properties of sampled airflow rates associated with paragraph reading.

These observations emphasize the contributions aerodynamic studies may make to the design and evaluation of prosthetic speech devices. In this regard, the finding that reed-fistula mechanisms required higher airflow rates to initiate and sustain voicing was not unexpected. For example, normal talkers vary laryngeal impedance over a large magnitude. That is, impedance may range from essentially zero (glottis completely open) to relatively high levels (glottis closed and oscillating). By contrast, the voicing source in reed-fistula speech is ever present. Hence, to avoid sound generation during tidal breathing, a rather high threshold to voicing activation is required. Thus, the observed increase in airflow rate and volume consumption, coupled with the rather limited range of aerodynamic response of reed-fistula voice prostheses, specify important properties meriting future modification.

Clinical Impressions

In the preceding sections, important characteristics of speech produced by four talkers using a reed-fistula method of oral communication were described. Although such data are essential to systematic evaluation of speech restoration procedures of the type being discussed, they may not totally reflect the complete clinical picture. Some general impression of our perceptual evaluation of these speakers' effectiveness might be helpful.

For example, Subject 1 is the most experienced user of reed-fistula speech. In our opinion, he is a highly effective communicator. His speech would compare favorably with any excellent esophageal speaker, would be preferred over that produced by highly proficient users of electronic artificial larynges, and would compare favorably with that used by highly proficient users of pneumatic speech aids such as the Tokyo artificial larynx. The remaining three speakers also use reed-fistula speech as their primary method of oral communication. From their perspective, this method of speech enables them to execute activities related to daily living effectively. Our impression is that these speakers are able to communicate on a satisfactory level. Their speech would compare favorably with esophageal speakers characterized by average proficiency and with proficient users of pneumatic or electronic speech aids.

DISCUSSION

In this report, some observations about the nature of speech characteristics produced by a series of patients using an experimental, surgical-prosthetic method of speech restoration were delineated. These observations support the view that functionally serviceable speech has been provided to patients who have undergone extensive resection of the phaynx in association with total laryngectomy by use of a surgical prosthetic method called reed-fistula speech. Although this is true, reed-fistula speech is characterized by some relative speech liabilities (for example, restricted f_o variability and increased respiratory flows and volumes) that merit continued modification and study. Additional biomedical liabilities have been discussed in an earlier publication (Shedd et al., 1976).

In recognition of these liabilities, it is our belief that reed-fistula speech does not currently merit consideration as a routine method of speech restoration for all laryngectomized patients. We do not find this current situation disconcerting, since alternative forms of alaryngeal speech are also not characterized by functional universality. In this regard, it is important to emphasize that to date the reed-fistula approach has been implemented on patients who have undergone extensive pharyngeal resection in conjunction with laryngectomy. Such patients are generally unable to learn esophageal speech and must, therefore, rely on artificial speaking devices. Patients of this type clearly provide a severe test of the efficacy of the reed-fistula approach.

As is the case for other forms of artifically generated voice restoration approaches, patients are not simply fitted with an appliance. The reed-fistula approach requires considerable prosthetic fabrication time, both in terms of making the reed device itself and fitting the device to the individual patient. In general, some interval of time, including professional help from a speech-language pathologist, is required following prosthetic insertion before patients become proficient.

Among this series of patients using reed-fistula speech, we often dealt with less than optimal surgical preparations. For example, in one patient (S_3) the point of entry of the fistula orifice had to be made at the level of the tonsillar fossa. This was necessary because the patient had a moderate stenosis in the lower pharynx following laryngectomy. Among the remaining patients, all have their fistula opening into the vocal tract located slightly below the lower margin of the tongue. This lower fistula location is preferred primarily because it provides the opportunity to conceal the appliance completely with suitable attire. In the group of patients discussed here, the fistulae used to receive the reed devices were created by modifying existing deltopectral flaps created in previous pharyngeal reconstructive procedures (Bakamjian, 1965), rather than being primary fistulae created specifically for the purpose of subserving speech.

It is important to emphasize that, to date, all reed-fistula voice prostheses have been homemade. Consequently, these voice prostheses are not finished in a bioengineering sense. These limitations lead us to regard reed-fistula speech as an experimental approach to speech rehabilitation worthy of continued study and development.

Although the present clinical studies indicate that it is possible to restore speech following pharyngolaryngectomy on a surgical-prosthetic basis, the process of accomplishing this task involves attempting to find solutions to a number of biomedical (Shedd et al., 1976) and speech-related problems. It is hoped that in addition to providing information, this report will serve to interest others in the problem of surgical prosthetic voice restoration, to stimulate participation in this area of basic and clinical research, and to highlight the need for continual interdisciplinary cooperation so essential to the improved ultimate quality of future results. Finally, it is intended that this paper will highlight the belief that aerodynamic, acoustic, and perceptual analyses of alaryngeal speech can make important contributions not only to practical rehabilitative problems but also to theoretic advancement of the speech sciences.

ACKNOWLEDGMENT

This study was supported, in part, by Grant 5R01-NS10941 from the National Institutes of Health. We acknowledge the assistance provided by Peter Alfonso, Lori Ramig, Frank Vacek, and Donald Schoendorfer. Requests for reprints should be directed either to Bernd Weinberg, Purdue University, Department of Audiology and Speech Sciences, West Lafayette, Indiana 47907 or Donald P. Shedd, Roswell Park Memorial Institute, Department of Health, 666 Elm Street, Buffalo, New York 14623.

REFERENCES

ASAI, R., Laryngoplasty after total laryngectomy. *Archs Otolar.*, **95**, 76–83 (1972).
BAKAMJIAN, V. J., A two-stage method for pharyngoesophageal reconstruction with a primary pectoral skin flap. *Plast. reconst. Surg.*, **35**, 173–184 (1965).
CONLEY, J., Surgical techniques for the vocal rehabilitation of the postlaryngectomized patient. *Trans. Amer. Acad. Ophth. Otolaryng.*, **13**, 288–299 (1969).

CREECH, H. P., Evaluating esophageal speech. *J. Speech Hear. Ass. Virginia*, 2, 13–19 (1966).
FAABORG-ANDERSEN, K., Electromyographic investigations of intrinsic laryngeal muscles in humans, *Acta physiol. scand. Supp. 140*, 41, 1–148 (1957).
FAIRBANKS, G., *Voice and articulation drillbook*. New York: Harper (1960).
HORII, Y., and COOKE, P. A., Analysis of airflow and air volume during continuous speech. *Behav. res. Meth. Instr.*, 7, 477 (1975).
HORII, Y., and WEINBERG, B., Intelligibility characteristics of superior esophageal speech presented under various levels of masking noise. *J. Speech Hearing Res.*, 18, 413–419 (1975).
HOUSE, A. S., WILLIAMS, C. E., HECKER, M. H. L., and KRYTER, K., Articulation testing methods: Consonantal differentiation with a closed-response set. *J. acoust. Soc. Am.*, 37, 158–166 (1965).
HYMAN, M., An experimental study of artificial larynx and esophageal speech. *J. Speech Hearing Dis.*, 20, 291–299 (1955).
ISSHIKI, N., Regulatory mechanism of voice intensity variation. *J. Speech Hearing Res.*, 7, 17–29 (1964).
KOMORN, R. M., Vocal rehabilitation in the laryngectomized patient with a tracheoesophageal shunt. *Ann. Otol. Rhinol. Lar.*, 83, 4–7 (1974).
MONTGOMERY, W. W., and TOOHIL, R. J., Vocal rehabilitation after laryngectomy. *Archs Otolar.*, 88, 499–506 (1968).
SHEDD, D., SCHAAF, N., and WEINBERG, B., Technical aspects of reed fistula speech following pharyngolaryngectomy. *J. Surg. Oncol.*, 8, 305–310 (1976).
SHIPP, T., and McGLONE, R. L., Laryngeal dynamics associated with voice frequency change. *J. Speech Hearing Res.*, 14, 761–768 (1971).
SISSON, G. A., McCONNEL, F., LOGEMANN, J. A., and YEH, S., Voice rehabilitation after laryngectomy. *Archs Otolar.*, 101, 178–181 (1975).
SNIDECOR, J. C., and ISSHIKI, N., Air volume and air flow relationships of six male esophageal speakers. *J. Speech Hearing Dis.*, 30, 206–216 (1965).
TAUB, S., and SPIRO, R. H., Vocal rehabilitation of laryngectomees: Preliminary report on a new technique. *Am. J. Surg.*, 124, 87–90 (1972).
VEGA, M. F., Larynx reconstructive surgery. *Laryngoscope*, 5, 866–881 (1975).
WEINBERG, B., and BENNETT, S., Selected acoustic characteristics of esophageal speech produced by female laryngectomees. *J. Speech Hearing Res.*, 15, 211–216 (1972).
WEINBERG, B., and RIEKENA, A., Speech produced with a Tokyo artificial larynx. *J. Speech Hearing Dis.*, 38, 383–389 (1973).

Received June 20, 1977.
Accepted December 15, 1977.

Laryngectomy: The influence of muscle reconstruction on the mechanism of oesophageal voice production

By I. C. SIMPSON, J. C. S. SMITH, and MARGARET T. GORDON
(Glasgow)

Introduction

SINCE the first report of an oesophageal voice following glottal atresia by Reprand (1828) much has been written on the rehabilitation of the patient after laryngectomy.

Watson operated in Edinburgh in 1865, but his patient lived for only a few weeks and the first longer surviving laryngectomies were carried out by Billroth in 1874 and Kocher in 1881. During these two decades most of the patients were supplied with a primitive artificial larynx although, even then, references were being made to patients who could speak 'thanks to vicarious phonatory function of the pharyngeal muscles'. In 1889 the physiologist Landois investigated oesophageal phonation following laryngectomy and Fraenkel (1893) recognized the essential mechanism. Gottstein (1900) appears to have been the first to use speech re-education with a patient following laryngectomy with development of a useful voice with a range of one octave.

An early radiological study of the mechanism of the oesophageal voice was that of Stern (1928), but he believed that the stomach formed part of the excitor and the term 'stomach speech' was frequently used to describe the oesophageal voice. Subsequent radiological studies by Beck (1931), Weiss and Grunberg (1939), Van Gilse (1950), Moolinaar-Bijl (1951), Damste (1958), and Diedrich and Youngstrom (1966) showed that the excitor lay in the oesophagus and that the downward passage of air

Reprinted by permission from *The Journal of Laryngology and Otology*, 1972, *86*, 961–990.

was accompanied by an active opening of the oesophagus and not a swallowing process. The new vibrator or pseudo-glottis was seen to be situated at the pharyngo-oesophageal junction at the approximate level of the crico-pharyngeus.

Tarnaud (1938) stressed that 'surgical technique should consider the physiology of the subsequent development of oesophageal voice'. As far as compatible with surgical care, he emphasized the importance of the preservation of certain muscles, particularly the inferior constrictor and its cricoid head and as much as possible of the recurrent laryngeal nerve which was believed to supply motor fibres to the pharyngo-oesophageal junction and upper oesophagus. Doubt has since been thrown on this point since Lund and Ardran (1964) have suggested that the recurrent nerve may play no part in the innervation of the pharyngo-oesophageal junction.

It has been generally believed, in fact, that the mode of muscle reconstruction has little or no effect on the resulting oesophageal voice.

The speech-voice muscle linkages affected by laryngectomy

In laryngectomy the basic essential is eradication of disease which must take precedence, but the post-laryngectomy reconstruction involves two additional requirements: (*a*) the purely surgical aim of achieving primary healing with the avoidance of fistulae, and (*b*) the reconstruction of the necessary voice production complex based on the new generator. (Fig. 1.)

In the normal subject, the pharyngeal resonator, controlled by the

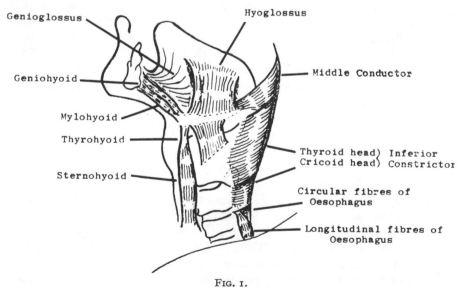

Fig. 1.

inferior constrictor, is indirectly linked to the articulators (lips, teeth, tongue and jaw), through the laryngeal generator via the thyro-hyoid muscle and membrane and the hyoid bone.

The muscle linkages divided at laryngectomy

With the removal of the larynx, the inferior constrictors lose their attachment to the generator and consequently their link with the articulators. The resection of the body of the hyoid removes the insertion of the mylo-hyoid and the genio-hyoid and still further impairs the speech voice link. At the lower end the division of the cricoid head of the inferior constrictor from its insertion destroys part of the pharyngo-oesophageal sphincter leaving only the circular fibres of the oesophagus. (Fig. 2.)

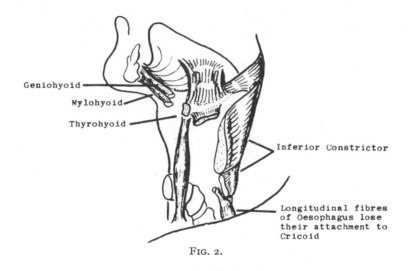

FIG. 2.

After laryngectomy the pharynx, in addition to its normal role as a resonator, is required to perform the task of driving air downwards into the oesophagus during injection. The pharynx therefore requires to be provided with full muscle control and its own muscle, the inferior constrictor, to be completely reconstructed around the pharyngeal mucosal tube. The lower end of this reconstructed inferior constrictor and merging oesophageal fibres provide the new generator in continuity with the muscle controlled pharynx above.

The upper end of the inferior constrictor must be connected to the hyoid bone and the supra-hyoid jaw and tongue muscles to produce the necessary linkages of the speech and voice complex. The cornua of the hyoid should always be maintained when compatible with surgical cure in order to preserve the hyo-glossus, sterno-hyoid and the middle constrictor. This through link retains the overall muscle influence on the pharyngo-oesophageal junction. Contraction of the supra-hyoid muscles will, as in the normal state, lift the pharyngo-oesophageal junction, aid sphincter relaxation through the 'cricopharyngeal yawn' and facilitate injection.

This paper attempts to correlate the muscle reconstruction employed, with the radiological appearances of the pharynx and the quality and efficiency of the resulting oesophageal voice.

Methods and Techniques

The investigation of the method of air intake, configuration of the pharynx and the action of the pharyngo-oesophageal junction and upper oesophagus were carried out by contrast radiography on cine film and video-tape, while an objective assessment of the quality, fluency and intelligibility of the resulting voice was obtained by asking the students of the Glasgow School of Speech Therapy to estimate the patients' voices on an assessment form compiled and subsequently analysed in the department of Speech Therapy in the Victoria Infirmary.

It was felt that this department offered a unique opportunity to compare the oesophageal voice results of a series of patients treated in the same hospital environment and by the same speech therapy rehabilitation method and in which only the surgical techniques differed.

Fifty laryngectomized patients were studied initially and thirty-eight of those were used in the final assessment.

Surgical techniques

The operations were carried out by five surgeons and the reconstructive techniques fall into four categories.

Technique A (17 cases)

This is an attempt to reconstruct a fully muscle-controlled pharynx which still maintains the through-link between the supra-hyoid tongue and jaw muscles, to reproduce the basic mechanism required for the new voice production complex. (Fig. 3.)

A mid-line incision is used and the sterno-hyoids are preserved. The thyro-hyoid and sterno-thyroid muscles are divided and the body of the hyoid is removed, preserving the cornua with the hyoglossus and middle constrictor attachments. The inferior constrictor is separated from the thyroid and cricoid cartilages and the pharynx opened from above. Care is taken to preserve as much pharyngeal mucosa as possible, particularly at the pyriform fossae, so that, when the mucosa is dissected from the cricoid and cut horizontally, the mucosal suture itself is a single, horizontal line.

The trachea is then divided and, with the larynx, stripped off the oesophagus to meet the mucosal incision above. During the removal of the larynx, care is taken to avoid tearing downwards and subsequent scarring into the post-cricoid area. The recurrent laryngeal nerves are identified and divided at their entrance into the larynx to preserve any possible cricopharyngeal branches. Single through-and-through interrupted catgut sutures are used with the knots inside the lumen for the pharyngeal closure.

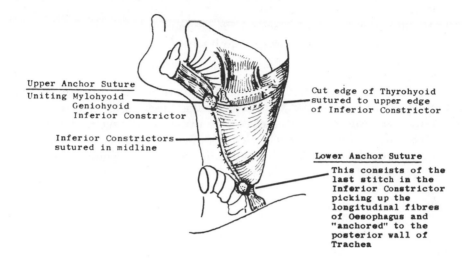

Upper Anchor Suture
Uniting Mylohyoid
Geniohyoid
Inferior Constrictor

Inferior Constrictors
sutured in midline

Cut edge of Thyrohyoid
sutured to upper edge
of Inferior Constrictor

Lower Anchor Suture
This consists of the
last stitch in the
Inferior Constrictor
picking up the
longitudinal fibres
of Oesophagus and
"anchored" to the
posterior wall of
Trachea

Sternohyoids are preserved and overlapped but have
been omitted from the diagram'for clarity.

The cut ends of the Hyoid cornua are sutured together
in front of the Upper Anchor Suture

Fig. 3.

Muscle reconstruction. The anterior edges of the two inferior constrictors are brought together throughout their length providing full muscle control for the pharynx, particular care being taken with the cricoid head (crico-pharyngeus). To reconstruct the link with the tongue and jaw muscles the upper edge of the reconstructed inferior constrictor —in the midline— is sutured to the suprahyoid muscles in the space left by the removal of the hyoid body and this has been designated the *upper anchor suture*.

The upper end of the inferior constrictor laterally is sutured to the cut upper end of the thyrohyoid and the cornua of the hyoid are then sutured firmly together in front, to buttress the weak area and to reconstitute a complete hyoid.

At the lower end, the last suture in the cricopharyngeus is brought through the longitudinal coat of the oesophagus and posterior wall of the trachea as the *lower anchor suture*. This stabilizes the pharyngo-oesophageal junction, replaces the lost insertion of the longitudinal muscle fibres of the oesophagus and re-establishes the mechanical interplay between the pharyngo-oesophageal junction and the airway as in the normal subject, thus reproducing, as far as possible, the normal muscle influences on the pharyngo-oesophageal junction.

No drainage is used apart from short 2 in. Paul's tubing wicks through separate stab wounds to the 'dead space' on either side of the trachea by the tracheostome.

These drains are removed in 24–48 hours.

Technique B. (6 cases)

The inferior constrictor including its cricoid head, is brought round the pharynx but the upper and lower anchor sutures are omitted.

This technique provides a muscle-controlled pharynx but lacks the through link of the voice production complex and leaves two areas, one above at hyoid level and one below at the lower hyopharynx, which lack muscle control. Drainage is provided to the mucosal suture line. (Fig. 4.)

Technique C (6 cases)

This method was used on certain very early cases but has not been carried out since 1962. The inferior constrictor is not brought round the pharynx as in *A* and *B*, but the mucosal suture is buttressed by stitches to the deep surface of the sterno-hyoids which are then firmly overlapped.

Some degree of anterior pharyngeal muscle buttressing is obtained

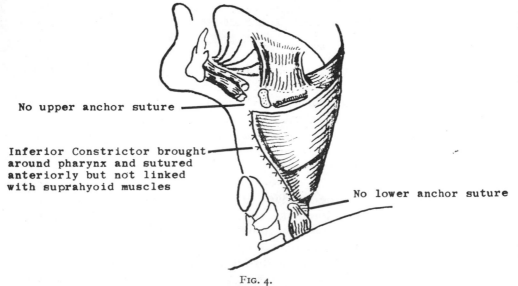

No upper anchor suture

Inferior Constrictor brought around pharynx and sutured anteriorly but not linked with suprahyoid muscles

No lower anchor suture

FIG. 4.

but no complete circular muscle control is provided for the pharyngeal mucosal tube. Through and through tube drainage was maintained for five days just below the mucosal suture line and penicillin instilled six-hourly. (Fig. 5.)

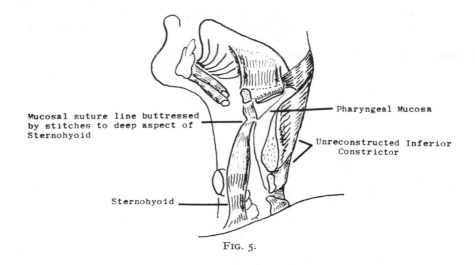

Mucosal suture line buttressed by stitches to deep aspect of Sternohyoid

Pharyngeal Mucosa

Unreconstructed Inferior Constrictor

Sternohyoid

FIG. 5.

Technique D (9 cases)

No reconstruction orientated to the oesophageal voice is carried out, the pharyngeal mucosal suture merely being buttressed by any easily available muscle tissue.

The pharyngeal tube has, therefore, no muscle control and the lack of a reconstructed inferior constrictor, and in particular its crico-pharyngeal part, breaks the muscle link with the merging fibres of the upper oesophagus thus interfering with co-ordination and control of the pharyngo-oesophageal junction. Drainage is again provided up to the mucosal suture line. (Fig. 6.)

Speech therapy techniques

Prior to 1951 all patients were under the care of one surgeon who also taught oesophageal speech, aided by those of his patients who had achieved voice. These patients were taught to introduce air into the oesophagus by swallowing but it was noted that many of them introduced air unobtrusively without swallowing, within three months of operation. Two of the patients who were taught to swallow initially are amongst the best speakers today, having themselves learned injection.

Since 1951 all patients have been given speech therapy, including any who had previously failed to develop satisfactory voice and all are taught to inject. Patients are encouraged, where possible, to imitate injection following demonstration by the speech therapist and good oesophageal speakers, as it is thought that there are different methods of initiating injection. If a patient is unable to imitate a vowel or a plosive syllable, thus showing no strongly preferred method of initiation, he is shown one of the accepted methods of injection (Gordon, 1971). Aspiration is not taught as a method of intake as in many patients it results in excessive respiratory effort with the production of marked stomal noise. It must be stressed, however, that the minor pressure changes produced in the

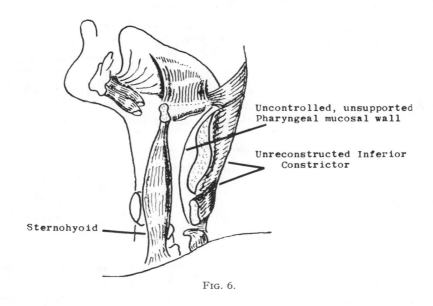

Uncontrolled, unsupported
Pharyngeal mucosal wall

Unreconstructed Inferior
Constrictor

Sternohyoid

FIG. 6.

oesophagus on inspiration are of immense value as adjuvants to injection and patients are taught to synchronize respiration and speech. Practice in synchronization of oesophageal voice with articulation and phrasing is facilitated for the patient by use of a tape repeater (Gordon, 1969).

Selection of patients for investigation. Fifty laryngectomized patients (40 male and 10 female) were assessed for suitability for inclusion in the project.

Stoll (1958), Putney (1958) and Barton and Hejna (1963) have shown psychological factors to be important in determining the success or failure of speech rehabilitation. The hospital where this series was studied provides a good environment for rehabilitation but to eliminate the possibility of adverse factors influencing the results, the criteria for inclusion were that the patient must be:

(a) Of sufficient intelligence to be employed fully under normal conditions until undergoing laryngectomy; fully employed before marrying if female, or reaching retiral age if retired prior to operation.

(b) If elderly, able to enjoy normal retirement and to maintian an interest in the environment.

(c) Free from any general condition which might affect speech ability or social integration.

(d) Well motivated towards relearning speech.

(e) Co-operative in the speech rehabilitation programme.

The selection was made from patients who had undergone operation at least eighteen months before the study and 38 patients (28 male and 10 female) who satisfied the criteria were found. Three patients were deaf and wore hearing aids but as they had all achieved satisfactory speech they were included in the survey. All three had undergone a technique *A* reconstruction. Patients who had radical dissection of lymph nodes of neck and those who had radiotherapy were also included since these factors do not affect the efficiency of speech as has been demonstrated by Hunt (1964).

Assessment of the competency of speech. Each patient was recorded under sound proof conditions on a Ferrograph tape recorder using a ribbon microphone at 7·5 i.p.s. while reading 'The Rainbow Passage' (Fairbanks, 1960) which is frequently used in speech assessment. The speech samples were assessed by final year speech therapy students from the Glasgow School of Speech Therapy, to obtain the objective opinion of a group trained to listen to the voice and its abnormalities but without specialist experience of alaryngeal dysphonia and with no knowledge of surgical techniques which might affect their judgment. The students were asked to judge as far as possible using the normal voice as a standard and their assessment was, in consequence, severe.

The group was instructed to assess each voice in accordance with the following scheme, using a four-point scale to score each heading:

1. Fluency; 2. Voice quality; 3. Volume; 4. Habitual pitch; 5. Pitch variations; 6. Intelligibility; 7. Stomal noise. Those qualities which can be measured objectively (reading rate and number of syllables per injection) or electronically (intensity, fundamental frequency and frequency range) were measured by the trained speech therapy staff as a guide to the reliability of the student assessments. The results show almost 100 per cent concordance.

A close relationship was found to exist between intelligibility and fluency in the student assessments with intelligibility consistently scoring slightly higher than fluency. For the purpose of this paper it was felt essential to simplify the assessment. Since reading rate has been reported as a reliable guide to the efficiency of oesophageal speech (Snidecor, 1962) only the scores for fluency and intelligibility were used. The assessment is thus based on the two essentials—the ability of the patient as a fluent conversationalist and the ease with which the listener can hear and comprehend without strain.

Grading the assessment. The students' assessments were divided into three speech grades according to the number of points each patient had been awarded for fluency and intelligibility.

Grade I are fluent conversationalists and superior speakers in all respects.

Grade II are also superior in intelligibility but are rated by the students as less fluent than Grade I, although many are no slower than some normal individuals using rather pedantic speech and the reading rates of two patients, who were given Grade I points by all the students are considerably slower than many in Grade II. These patients are both professional voice users.

Grade III are considered to have acquired speech that is inadequate for normal conversational needs although most of the patients in this group are capable of making themselves understood and continuing in their former employment.

Method of intake of air. This was assessed from observation of conversation and corroborated radiologically by the video-tape with sound. Thirty-five patients were classed as 'injectors' and the remaining three who are all Grade III speakers, swallowed air for speech.

Radiological techniques

The patient was seated in the left lateral position immediately in front of a 12-in. Cinelix image intensifier and a horizontal beam was centred on the patient to include lips, tongue, palate, pharynx, hypopharynx and cervical oesophagus in the field, the focal film distance being 5 ft. A microphone was placed directly in front of the patient and connected to the audio input of the video tape recorder (Fig. 7). The patient then

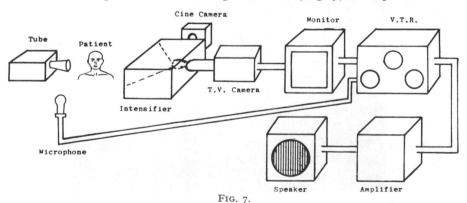

FIG. 7.
Diagram of recording system.

swallowed a mouthful of barium; injected and phonated the vowel /a/. The injection and the vowel /a/ were repeated and followed by the reading of the first two sentences of 'The Rainbow Passage' and the complete examination from before the swallow to the end of the second sentence was recorded on video-tape with synchronized sound. The procedure was then repeated, this time being recorded on 35 mm. cine film without sound at 24 frames per second. With slow speakers the duration of the examination was curtailed to reduce radiation dosage. The average dose for the examination was 3·4 rads., the dose varying slightly according to the fluency of the speakers.

At the conclusion of the examination the video-tape was immediately played back, giving an initial assessment with the advantage of synchronized sound. The processed cine film and the video-tape recordings were later examined together, the film being viewed by means of a Tage Arnø editor which allowed slow motion study and frame by frame analysis.

Radiological observations

NORMAL RADIOLOGICAL APPEARANCES. As the investigation proceeded, a pattern emerged which was accepted as 'normal'. Almost all the proficient speakers show a smooth conical hypopharynx without evidence of permanent constrictions, bulging of the wall or irregular indentations posteriorly (Fig. 8). The pharynx shows fully controlled mobility, relaxing

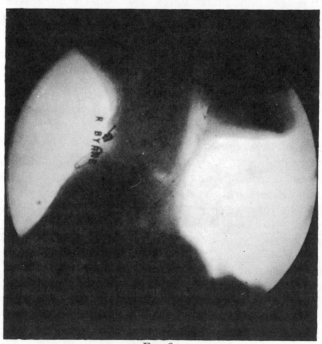

FIG. 8.
Normal picture at rest. (Technique *A*.)

to a wide space and contracting under muscle control, almost to the extent of obliterating the air space when required. The pharyngo-oesophageal junction shows free mobility in respect of relaxation and contraction but without excessive vertical movement during either injection or phonation. The vertical movement of the pharyngo-oesophageal junction in the proficient speakers is virtually the same as the movement of the crico-pharyngeus in a normal speaker using laryngeal voice to read the same passage. The length of the pharyngo-oesophageal constriction varies considerably but no definite correlation is found between the length of the generator and the quality or fluency of the resulting voice. Most of the best speakers show a long constriction, due possibly to careful reconstruction of the inferior constrictor and its cricoid head.

The normal radiological appearances of air injection for oesophageal voice
  Pre-injection phase. There is relaxation of the pharyngeal constrictors sometimes aided by a slight forward movement of the mandible to provide as much 'resident' air as possible (Fig. 9a.)
  This stage has been noticed in almost all cases reconstructed by technique *A* and has not previously been reported but may represent the initial movement of the lateral pharyngeal wall as described by Kelsey and Ewanowski (1970).
  Injection. Stage I. The pharynx is closed from the outside by air closure of the lips and soft palate, and/or active movements of the tongue against the hard palate, soft palate or posterior pharyngeal wall. (Fig. 9b.)
  The tongue may be used in any of three ways and good speakers avail themselves of one or all of the methods according to circumstances.
  (*a*) Backward movement of the tongue bringing its base against the posterior pharyngeal wall.
  (*b*) The dorsum of the tongue closes against the hard palate and the soft palate closes to complete the seal.
  (*c*) The tip of the tongue first closes behind the upper teeth then the tongue rolls back so that its dorsum contacts the hard palate (glossal press) and finally its base contacts the pharyngeal wall, thus 'milking' the air from the mouth down into the pharynx. (Fig. 9c.)
  Stage II. The inferior constrictor contracts on its contained air and the crico-pharyngeus relaxes, the air being pushed down into the oesophagus (glosso-pharyngeal press).
  Stage III. The inferior constrictor has contracted almost completely, to obliterate the pharyngeal air space, and the oesophagus is air-filled. (Fig. 9d.)
  Stage IV. The crico-pharyngeus closes, trapping the oesophageal air. The pharynx and tongue relax, the pharynx again becoming air-filled above the closed crico-pharyngeus and the patient is ready to phonate. (Fig. 9e.)
  Phonation. The pharynx and pharyngo-oesophageal junction are well controlled and the oesophagus is emptying. (Fig. 9 f.)

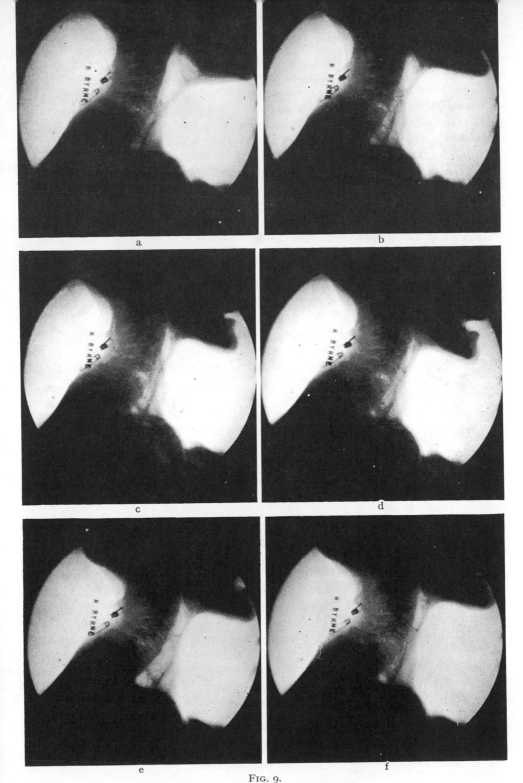

Fig. 9.
The normal injection sequence.
(a) Pre-injection phase; (b) Injection stage I; (c) Injection stage II; (d) Injection stage III; (e) Injection stage IV; (f) Phonation. (Technique A.)

Reproduced from *J. Dis. Comm.*, *1971*.

Modified injection. During fluent conversation it is essential to replenish the air reservoir without the delay of a full injection. Pharyngeal closure is made at any of the points in Stage I, according to the phonetic content of the speech and a small constrictor 'squeeze' maintains the oesophageal air reservoir. This method is intimately concerned with the plosives and allows the patient to maintain fluent conversation between natural pauses, when he has time to make a full injection.

The so-called aspiration method of air intake. No case in the series was capable of providing an oesophageal reservoir adequate for voice by aspiration alone even with a forced inspiration. This is in agreement with the observations of Isshiki and Snidecor (1965). The downward passage of air was always seen to be accompanied by active tongue and pharyngeal movement.

ABNORMAL RADIOLOGICAL APPEARANCES. These include slight variations from the accepted normal to cases showing grossly abnormal configurations and function. An attempt has been made to identify these abnormalities individually but they occur most commonly in combination.

1. *Double constriction.* This is a further area of narrowing between the oesophagus and oro-pharynx in addition to the physiological narrowing at the pharyngo-oesophageal junction, and three types may be described.

(a) *Permanent organic stricture above the pharyngo-oesophageal junction.* This is a constant area of narrowing which does not distend even during the passage of barium when swallowing. Permanent organic stricture is possibly due to (i) loss of excised mucosa, (ii) fibrosis secondary to delayed healing.

(b) *Pseudo-strictures.* These constrictions are due to bulging of the posterior pharyngeal wall into the lumen of the hypo-pharynx. These posterior bulges are variable and mobile. The barium swallow may appear normal or show only a small posterior filling defect, the bulge becoming more apparent under conditions of smaller pressure changes involved in injection and phonation. These posterior pharyngeal wall bulges or masses are believed to be due to unsutured bundles of inferior constrictor fibres which have retracted posteriorly. (Fig. 10a and 10b.)

(c) *Voluntary contraction.* Two patients in technique *A* showed a variation of their own making. Each gave a normal picture at rest, on injection and on barium swallow but on phonation the hyoid was pulled backwards to produce a second narrowing. The effect was to produce a small resonating chamber which raised the pitch of the resulting oesophageal voice. (Fig. 11a and 11b.)

2. *Pouches.* These are defined as localized forward bulging of the anterior pharyngeal wall beyond what is considered to be the normal configuration. They occur in two situations:

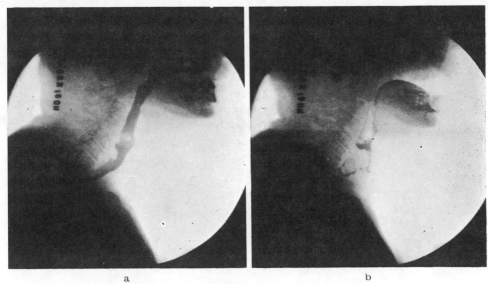

a   b

FIG. 10.

Posterior bulge.

(a) Barium swallow showing small posterior bulge above the pharyngo-oesophageal junction.
(b) The same patient showing the increased size of the posterior bulge during phonation. (Technique *B*.)

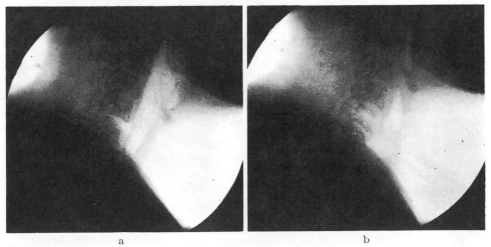

a   b

FIG. 11.

Voluntary contraction.
(a) Pharynx at rest.
(b) The same patient showing the backward movement of the hyoid bone during phonation. (Technique *A*.)

(a) *High pouches.* These are situated just below the base of tongue at hyoid level and may be due to the omission of an upper anchor suture or incomplete muscle reconstruction in this region. (Fig. 12.)

(b) *Low pouches.* These are commonly seen between the pharyngo-oesophageal junction and hyoid and may be due to incomplete reconstruction of the inferior constrictor and/or omission of the lower anchor suture leaving an unsupported area of mucosa anteriorly. (Fig. 13.)

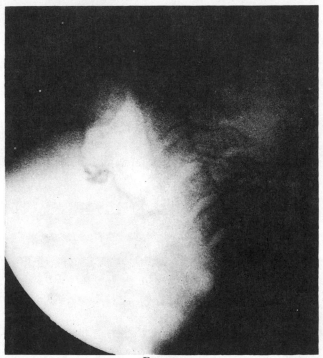

Fig. 12.
Hyoid pouch. (Technique *B*.)

In this series the pouches commonly lay between the pharyngo-oesophageal junction and a second constriction of the pseudo type (*b*), as failure to reconstruct part of the inferior constrictor leaves a weak area anteriorly with consequent retraction of the unsutured muscle fibres producing a bulge in the posterior pharyngeal wall.

3. *Inert ballooning of the hypo-pharynx.* This was found in one case only where the absence of any constrictor reconstruction left an inert pharyngeal mucosal tube (incapable of the muscle action required for injection) and separated the oesophageal fibres at the pharyngo-oesophageal junction from their link with an inferior constrictor above. The result was an uncontrolled pharynx with inco-ordination at the pharyngo-oesophageal junction incompatible with the development of adequate oesophageal speech. (Fig. 14.)

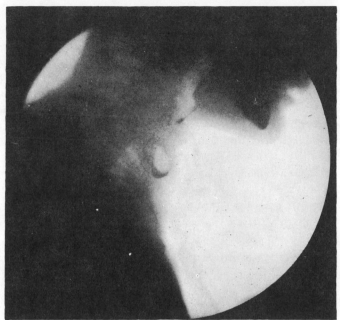

FIG. 13.
Low pouch with pseudo-stricture. (Technique *D*.)

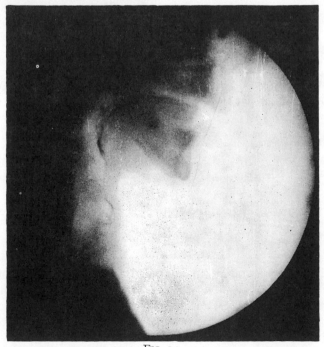

FIG. 14.
Unsupported hypopharynx. (Technique *D*.)

4. *Ballooning of the oesophagus.* This is shown as a considerable expansion of the upper oesophagus just below the pharyngo-oesophageal junction well beyond the limits of normal, with the pharyngo-oesophageal junction showing as a very thin narrow constriction between the oeso-phagus and the hypo-pharynx. The distension is most evident during phonation when there is increased pressure in the oesophagus and is associated with excessive vertical movement of the pharyngo-oesophageal junction.

The reason for this appearance is not clear but it may be due to stretching of the oesophageal wall as a result of constant increased pressure due to oesophageal speech particularly if accompanied by a poorly co-ordinated pharyngo-oesophageal junction, or it may be related to the reported atony of the upper oesophageal muscles following laryngectomy (Kirchner *et al.*, 1963). (Figs. 15*a* and 15*b*.)

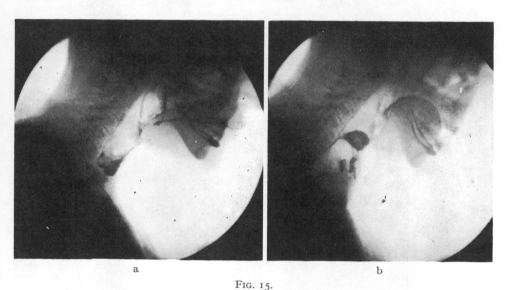

a   b

FIG. 15.
Ballooning oesophagus.
(*a*) At rest, showing lowest position of the pharyngo-oesophageal junction.
(*b*) The same patient showing excessive elevation of the pharyngo-oesophageal junction and ballooning of the upper oesophagus.
(Technique *C*.)

Radiological appearances in relation to reconstructive techniques

Technique A. All cases except three showed what has been described as the normal radiological picture. The three abnormalities were (*a*) one pseudo-stricture above the pharyngo-oesophageal junction, possibly due to a break down at the lower end of the repair. (*b*) the two subjects previously mentioned who used a voluntary muscle contraction.

Technique B. Four cases showing abnormalities were noted in this group. (*a*) One hyoid pouch. (*b*) One double constriction, posterior bulge and low pouch. (*c*) Two double constrictions.

Technique C. All showed an individual picture peculiar to this technique, namely, a very short pharynx with a long narrow pharyngo-oesophageal junction below. (Fig. 16.) Two cases showed further abnormalities. (*a*) One posterior muscle mass (pseudo-stricture). (*b*) One swallow pattern instead of injection with ballooning oesophagus.

Technique D. Eight of these nine cases showed radiological abnormalities. (*a*) One low anterior pouch. (*b*) Two posterior muscle masses. (*c*) Three cases had double constrictions with posterior bulges and anterior pouches, two of these showing a swallow pattern instead of injection. (Fig. 17.) (*d*) One had a double constriction with posterior bulge and

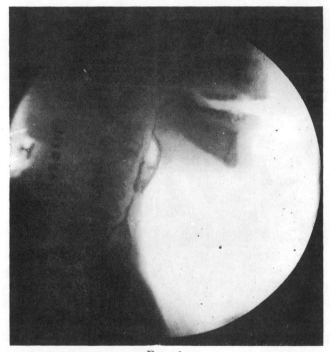

Fig. 16.
Typical picture of Type C reconstruction during phonation.

the inert ballooning anterior pharyngeal wall, previously described, and was incapable of injection and resorted to repeated swallowing efforts. (*e*) One had a posterior bulge and anterior pouch.

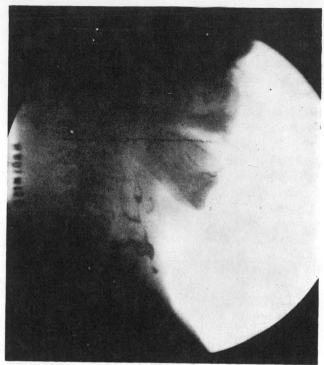

FIG. 17.

Example of posterior bulge, pseudo-stricture and distorted low pouch.

Results

Details of cases are set out in Table I. The distribution of speech grades throughout the series was:

Grade I ..	..	16
Grade II ..	..	14
Grade III ..	..	8

The results of the speech assessment are given in Table II, which shows the distribution of speech grades and surgical techniques and includes a column giving the summation of Grades I and II, to indicate the total number of adequate conversationalists. The results are expressed in number of patients under each technique. To allow a clear estimation of the standard of speech in the various grades, the mean reading rate of the grades is shown in Table III and can be compared with Snidecor's own estimates for oesophageal speakers which are shown in Table IV and with Darley's reported average reading rate for the same passage of 160 words per minute, the lowest being 129 and the highest 222 W.P.M.

Figure 18 shows a comparison of reconstruction techniques with success and failure in speech. Grades I and II (the adequate conversationalists) are accepted as successes and Grade III (the inadequate conversation-alists) as failures. This shows a 94·1 per cent success in technique A as compared with 44·4 per cent in technique D.

Figure 19 shows the distribution of speech grades through the various surgical techniques using percentages and it can be seen that there is a gradual alteration to poorer speech grades from technique A through B and C to D. The speech results of technique A when directly compared with those of the D technique appear as a mirror image. It is thought that this is due to technique A involving a fully reconstructed inferior constrictor whereas D has no wholly encircling fibres.

A statistical analysis (chi square test) of the success and failure rate (Fig. 18) of these two surgical techniques showed $\chi^2 = 8\cdot17$, $P = 0\cdot001$, which is significant.

Analysis of the results of A and B showed no significant difference as regards success or failure which is to be expected since both have an inferior constrictor repair, the only essential difference being the upper and lower anchor sutures in technique A. Technique A appears, however, consistently to produce a higher ratio of Grade I speakers, as can be seen from Fig. 19.

TABLE I.

DETAILS OF CASES.

Case No.	Sex	Age at op.	Years between op. and survey	Operation	Recon-struc-tion	Radio-therapy	Radio-logical Abnor-malities	Speech grade
1	M	58	6	Laryngectomy	A	No	No	III
2	F	64	2	Laryngectomy	A	No	No	I
3	F	33	16	Laryngectomy	A	No	No	I
4	F	45	16	Laryngectomy	A	No	No	I
5	M	74	4	Laryngectomy	B	Yes	Yes	II
6	M	70	2	Laryngectomy	A	Yes	No	I
7	M	63	3	Laryngectomy	D	Yes	Yes	III
8	M	61	2	Laryngectomy+block dissection of neck glands	B	No	No	I
9	F	51	19	Laryngectomy+ Pharyngectomy	C	No	No	II
10	M	61	3	Laryngectomy	A	No	No	II
11	M	55	25	Laryngectomy	C	No	Yes	III

TABLE I.—*continued*

Case No.	Sex	Age at op.	Years between op. and survey	Operation	Recon-struc-tion	Radio-therapy	Radio-logical Abnor-malities	Speech grade
12	F	45	1	Laryngectomy + Pharyngectomy	A	No	No	I
13	M	54	3	Laryngectomy	A	No	No	I
14	F	46	10	Laryngectomy	C	Yes	Yes	II
15	M	51	25	Laryngectomy	C	No	Yes	I
16	M	59	2	Laryngectomy	B	No	Yes	I
17	M	63	2	Laryngectomy	A	Yes	No	II
18	M	64	2	Laryngectomy + Pharyngectomy	B	Yes	Yes	III
19	M	65	1	Laryngectomy	A	No	No	I
20	M	33	14	Laryngectomy	A	No	No	I
21	M	58	13	Laryngectomy	C	Yes	No	II
22	M	59	5	Laryngectomy	A	Yes	No	I
23	M	57	8	Laryngectomy + Pharyngectomy + Anterior graft	C	Yes	Yes	II
24	M	74	2	Laryngectomy	D	No	Yes	III
25	M	64	2	Laryngectomy	D	No	Yes	II
26	F	57	5	Laryngectomy + Pharyngectomy + Block dissection	D	Yes	Yes	III
27	M	16	4	Laryngectomy	A	No	No	II
28	M	66	1	Laryngectomy	B	No	No	II
29	M	59	5	Laryngectomy	D	No	Yes	III
30	F	16	3	Laryngectomy	D	No	Yes	II
31	M	57	5	Laryngectomy	A	No	No	I
32	M	44	2	Laryngectomy	B	Yes	No	I
33	M	55	5	Laryngectomy	D	No	No	II
34	M	46	3	Laryngectomy	D	No	Yes	I
35	F	45	2	Laryngectomy	A	No	No	I
36	F	58	1	Laryngectomy	A	No	No	II
37	M	61	1	Laryngectomy	A	No	No	II
38	M	65	7	Laryngectomy	D	No	Yes	III

TABLE II.

DISTRIBUTION OF SPEECH GRADES IN THE SURGICAL TECHNIQUES

	Total	Males	Females	Grade I	Grade II	Success Grades I+II	Failure Grade III
Technique A	17	12	5	11	5	16	1
Technique B	6	6	0	3	2	5	1
Technique C	6	4	2	1	4	5	1
Technique D	9	7	2	1	3	4	5
Totals	38	29	9	16	14	30	8

TABLE III.

RANGE OF READING RATE IN THIS SERIES.

Speech grade	Words per minute		
	Average	Fastest	Slowest
Grade I	128	168	90
Grade II	121	158	101
Grade III	75	90	30

TABLE IV.

SNIDECOR'S STANDARDS FOR OESOPHAGEAL SPEAKERS.

Very superior speakers	144 words per minute
Excellent speakers ..	103–120 words per minute
Good speakers ..	60– 90 words per minute
Adequate speakers ..	60– 72 words per minute

The number of cases in B is insufficient directly to assess the functional effect of the anchor suture but a considerable difference is noticeable between the techniques when the numbers of syllables per injection are compared. (Fig. 20.)

Techniques B and C have each only six cases and show no difference as regards success or failure, i.e. five successes and one failure in each, but half of the cases in B are Grade I speakers whereas in C only one speaker is in Grade I. (Table II.) When B or C is compared statistically with D, $\chi^2 = 2\cdot26$, P = 0·20. This result does not reach significance, and it is felt that a larger number of cases would be necessary for comparison.

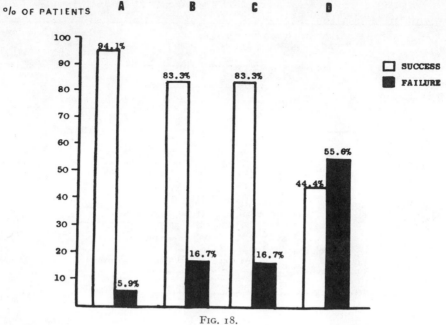

Fig. 18.

Comparison of reconstruction techniques with success and failure in speech.

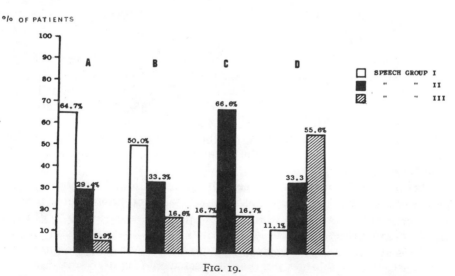

Fig. 19.

Distribution of the three speech grades through the various surgical techniques.

Comparison of syllables per injection and surgical techniques. In a further attempt to assess the mechanical efficiency of the vocal system, the patients were divided into three groups according to the number of syllables spoken on one injection. The surgical techniques were then compared on this basis and the results are shown in Fig. 20.

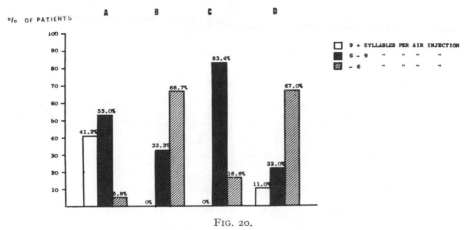

FIG. 20.

Syllables per injection throughout the techniques.

Technique *A* was the only one which showed a high percentage of patients using more than nine syllables per injection.

Although technique *D* showed 11 per cent using more than nine syllables, this represented only *one* case and the 5·8 per cent of patients in technique *A* who obtained less than six syllables per injection are also represented by only one case. *D* again showed almost as a mirror image of *A*. (Fig. 20.)

Neither *B* nor *C* included a case which achieved nine or more syllables although technique *C* showed superior results to technique *B*. A reason for this may be that the patients in technique *C* were speakers of at least nine years' experience whereas all those in technique *B* had undergone operation within the last nine years.

Inferior constrictor repair. In an attempt to assess the value of an inferior constrictor repair based on speech grade, the results of technique *A* and technique *B* (both having such repair) were added and compared with the sum of the results of technique *C* and technique *D* (neither having a constrictor reconstruction) and the results are shown in Table V.

Age distribution. As age has been cited as an important factor in the acquisition of speech after laryngectomy, the cases were divided into five age groups and the speech grades in each group were compared. (Fig. 21.)

It can be seen that the peak incidence at operation lay in the 50–59 age group (14 patients), the youngest patient being 33 years and the eldest

76 years. There appears to be a fairly even distribution of speech grades throughout the age groups.

To determine the effect of age on the speech results, expressed as success or failure, an arbitrary age of 60 was decided upon and the results above and below this age level compared. (Table VI.)

TABLE V.
COMPARISON OF SPEECH GRADES IN CASES WITH RECONSTRUCTED
AND UNRECONSTRUCTED INFERIOR CONSTRICTORS.

	Success Grades I+II	Failure Grade III	Total
A + B ..	21 (91 4%)	2 (8.6%)	23 (100%)
C + D ..	9 (60%)	6 (40%)	15 (100%)

TABLE VI.
COMPARISON OF SPEECH RESULTS ABOVE AND BELOW 60 YEARS OF
AGE.

	Success	Failure	Total
Over 60 years ..	12	4	16
Under 60 years ..	18	4	22

It would appear that in this series age at operation has little significance in the development of satisfactory oesophageal voice but may be a factor in the development of superior (Grade I) speech.

Comparison of speech grades with radiological abnormalities. Although it was not possible to state that any particular radiological abnormality was associated with poor speech, it can be seen in Fig. 22, that the incidence of such abnormalities increases from Speech Grade I to Speech Grade III.

Discussion and conclusions

Originally, Technique *A* was devised for the purpose of preventing fistula formation, and in this it has proved successful. Only one patient (a post-irradiation case) reconstructed by this method, developed a small fistula which healed spontaneously in ten days.

It was noted in the Speech Therapy Department that patients reconstructed by this method appeared to acquire oesophageal voice more quickly and easily and developed superior speech and it was this original clinical observation which instigated the present investigation. As a

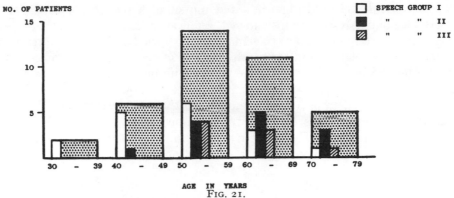

FIG. 21.
Distribution of age throughout the series.

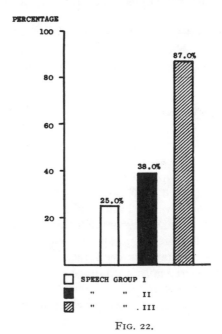

FIG. 22.
Comparison of speech groups with radiological abnormalities.

result, additions were made to the original reconstruction with the requirements of the future speech and voice mechanism in mind.

The reconstructive methods were studied from operative records and discussions with colleagues and fell within the four groups described.

The speech grades, judged by independent assessors were co-related with the reconstructions used and Technique *A* showed a significantly higher number of good speakers than the other techniques.

LARYNGECTOMY   585

Techniques B and C represented too small a number of cases for a significant analysis but B showed a lower success rate than A and qualitively higher than C. Technique D showed a high proportion of inadequate speakers and the results showed almost as a mirror image of A.

The one patient reconstructed by Technique A who was graded III by our assessors spoke with great fluency in·a pronounced Ayrshire dialect which detracted from his intelligibility to the unpractised ear.

One patient reconstructed by Technique D (according to the notes) was rated Grade I. The speech grading and radiological appearances, however, strongly suggest that a constrictor repair was, in fact, carried out.

The number of syllables spoken per injection were noted in each case and expressed in relation to the reconstructive method employed. Technique A gave significantly superior results indicating a more efficient mechanism.

Age incidence appeared to have no relevance to the speech results.

Technique A showed only one permanent radiological abnormality and this technique appears to provide a fully efficient mechanism for injection and speech and voice production.

Four cases in Technique B showed abnormalities while all cases in Technique C showed the individual picture described. Two cases showed additional radiological changes.

Of the nine cases reconstructed by Technique D, eight cases showed radiological abnormalities indicating slight to gross mechanical inefficiency.

The relationship between speech grade and radiological abnormalities was not absolute but showed a close association. Certain individuals showing X-ray changes achieved a high grade of speech indicating their capability of overcoming a basic mechanical inefficiency but, in general, the greater the radiological abnormality the poorer the resulting voice.

The radiological technique described has also proved of value in determining the mechanical cause of failure to acquire voice in some problem cases.

Healthy well-motivated patients will overcome deficiencies in their vocal mechanism and by application and effort acquire useful voice though they may never be able to acquire superior voice. Patients who are poorly motivated, elderly or in ill health may be totally unable to compensate for deficiencies in the vocal mechanism caused by a functionally poor reconstruction after laryngectomy and fail to acquire any useful speech. It is important, therefore, that every patient is given a sound reconstruction which results in an active muscular pharyngeal wall and a muscularly controlled pharyngo-oesophageal junction which will enable him to acquire speech of the highest standard possible within his physical and psychological limitations and will in no way add to his task by leaving him with an inferior mechanism which renders the production of speech difficult.

Technique A produces the highest number of Grades I and II speakers, the greatest number of syllables per injection and the smallest incidence of radiological abnormalities. The complete muscle control of the pharynx and the re-forming of the links of the speech voice complex from the articulators to the new generator of the reconstructed cricopharyngeus provides a most efficient mechanism for the production of oesophageal voice.

Summary

This paper describes in detail the four types of surgical reconstruction employed in a series of 38 patients following laryngectomy.

The type of reconstruction is correlated with the resulting radiological appearance and with the efficiency of the oesophageal voice achieved. One technique was shown to give significantly superior results.

Acknowledgements

The authors wish to thank colleagues in the Department of Otolaryngology for permission to investigate their patients; the Department of Medical Illustration for the photographic reproductions; the students of The Glasgow School of Speech Therapy for the voice assessments; the patients themselves for their co-operation, and others who have assisted in the preparation of this paper.

REFERENCES

BARTON, J., and HEJNA, R. (1963) *Journal of Speech and Hearing Association* (Virginia), **4**, 19.

BECK, J. (1931) *Zeitschrift für Laryngologie, Rhinologie, Otologie und ihre Grenzgebiete*, **21**, 506.

DAMSTE, P. H. (1958) Oesophageal speech after laryngectomy, Groningen Bolkdrukkerij. Voorheen Gebroeders, Hoitsema.

DARLEY, F. L. (1940) 'A Normative Study of Oral Reading Rate'. M.A. thesis, University of Iowa.

DIEDRICH, W. M., and YOUNGSTROM, K. A. (1966) *Alaryngeal Speech*. Thomas, Illinois.

FAIRBANKS, G. (1960) *Voice and Articulation Drillbook*, 2nd ed. Harper, New York.

FRAENKEL, B. (1893). *Berliner klinische Wochenschrift*, **30**, 758.

GORDON, M. T. (1969) *British Journal of Disorders of Communication*, **4**, 83.

—— (1971) *British Journal of Disorders of Communication*, **6**, 52.

GOTTSTEIN, G. (1900) *Archiv für klinische Chirurgie*, **62**, 126.

HUNT, R. B. (1964) *Laryngoscope*, **74**, 382.

ISSHIKI, N., and SNIDECOR, J. C. (1965) *Acta oto-laryngologica*, **59**, 559.

KELSEY, C. A., and EWANOWSKI, S. J. (1970) *Archives of Otolaryngology*, **92**, 167.

KIRCHNER, J. A., SCATLIFF, J. H., DEY, F. L., and SHEDD, D. P. (1963). *Laryngoscope*, **73**, 18.

LUND, W. S., and ARDRAN, G. M. (1964) *Annals of Otology Rhinology, and Laryngology*, 73, 599.

MOOLINAAR-BIJL, A. (1951) *Folia phoniatrica*, **3**, 20.

PUTNEY, F. J. (1958) *Annals of Otology, Rhinology and Laryngology*, **67**, 544.

REPRAND, —. (1828). First report of glottal atresia and adequate respiratory function. Academy of Science in Paris.

SIMPSON, I. C. (1971) *British Journal of Disorders of Communication*, **6**, 70.

SNIDECOR, J. C. (1962) *Speech rehabilitation of the laryngectomized*. Thomas, Springfield, Ill.

STERN, H. (1928) In *Handbuch der Hals- Nasen- Ohren- Heilkunde, mit Einschluss der Grenzgebiete*, vol. 5, p. 494. Ed. by A. Denker. and Kahler. Springer, Berlin.

STOLL, B. (1958) *Annals of Otology, Rhinology and Laryngology*, **67**, 550.

TARNAUD, J. (1938) *Les malades du larynx*. Masson, Paris.

VAN GILSE, P. H. G. (1950) Parabuccal voice with demonstration of a sound film. Int. Assoc. of Logopedics and phoniatrics. Assoc. VIII int. Speech and Voice Therapy Conference, Amsterdam.

WEISS, D., and GRUNBERG, M. (1939) *Bulletin de la Société belge d'otologie, de laryngologie et de rhinologie*, 373.

Ear, Nose and Throat Department,
The Victoria Infirmary,
Glasgow, S.2.